Children's Speech Sound Disorders

Dedication

To my dear and encouraging husband Don Bowen, whose commitment to scholarship, teaching, social justice, and keeping an open mind is my inspiration, always.

Children's Speech Sound Disorders

Caroline Bowen, PhD CPSP
Speech-Language Pathologist
New South Wales
Australia

⊛WILEY-BLACKWELL

A John Wiley & Sons, Ltd., Publication

This edition first published 2009
© John Wiley & Sons

Wiley-Blackwell is an imprint of John Wiley & Sons, formed by the merger of Wiley's global Scientific, Technical and Medical business with Blackwell Publishing.

Registered office
John Wiley & Sons Ltd, The Atrium, Southern Gate, Chichester, West Sussex, PO19 8SQ, United Kingdom

Editorial office
John Wiley & Sons Ltd, The Atrium, Southern Gate, Chichester, West Sussex, PO19 8SQ, United Kingdom

For details of our global editorial offices, for customer services and for information about how to apply for permission to reuse the copyright material in this book please see our website at www.wiley.com/wiley-blackwell.

Library of Congress Cataloging-in-Publication Data

Bowen, Caroline.
  Children's speech sound disorders / Caroline Bowen.
     p. ; cm.
  Includes bibliographical references and index.
  ISBN 978-0-470-72364-7 (pbk.)
  1. Speech disorders in children. I. Title. [DNLM: 1. Speech Disorders–therapy. 2. Child.
3. Speech-Language Pathology–methods. WL 340.2 B786c 2009]
  RJ496.S7B69 2009
  618.92'855–dc22

                                                                2008055860

A catalogue record for this book is available from the British Library.

Set in 10/12.5pt Sabon by Aptara® Inc., New Delhi, India
Printed in Singapore by Markono Print Media Pte Ltd

4 2011

Contents

Contributors

Elise Baker, PhD
Lecturer
Discipline of Speech Pathology
Faculty of Health Sciences
The University of Sydney
Sydney, NSW
Australia

B. May Bernhardt, PhD
Professor
School of Audiology and Speech Sciences
University of British Columbia
Vancouver, British Columbia
Canada

John E. Bernthal, PhD
Professor and Chair
Department of Special Education and
    Communication Disorders
University of Nebraska – Lincoln
Lincoln, Nebraska
USA

Ken M. Bleile, PhD
Professor
University of Northern Iowa
Cedar Falls, Iowa
USA

Barbara Dodd, PhD
Research Professor
Perinatal Research Centre
University of Queensland
Brisbane QLD
Australia
Department of Language and
    Communication Sciences

City University
London
UK

Lynn Flahive, MS
Instructor/Clinic Coordinator
Department of Communication Sciences
    and Disorders
Texas Christian University
Fort Worth, Texas
USA

Peter Flipsen, Jr., PhD
Associate Professor of Speech-Language
    Pathology
Department of Communication Sciences
    and Disorders and Education
    of the Deaf
Idaho State University
Pocatello, Idaho
USA

Karen Froud, PhD
Assistant Professor of Speech-Language
    Pathology
Teachers College
Columbia University
New York
USA

Hilary Gardner, DPhil
Lecturer
Department of Human Communication
    Sciences
The University of Sheffield
Sheffield
UK

Fiona E. Gibbon, PhD
Professor and Head of Department of
    Speech and Hearing Sciences
University College Cork
Ireland

Gail T. Gillon, PhD
Pro-Vice-Chancellor, College of
    Education
University of Canterbury
Christchurch
New Zealand

Karen Golding-Kushner, PhD
Speech-Language Pathologist
Executive Director
Velo-Cardio-Facial Syndrome
    Educational Foundation, Inc.
Milltown, New Jersey
USA

Sharon Gretz, MEd
Founder and Executive Director
Childhood Apraxia of Speech
    Association of North America
Pittsburgh, Pennsylvania
USA

Anne Hesketh, PhD
Senior Clinical Lecturer in Speech and
    Language Therapy
School of Psychological
    Sciences
The University of Manchester
Manchester
UK

Chantelle Highman, BSc (Hons)
PhD Candidate and Speech
    Pathologist
Curtin University of Technology
Andrea Way Child Development
    Centre
Department of Health
Perth, WA
Australia

Megan M. Hodge, PhD
Professor
Department of Speech Pathology and
    Audiology
University of Alberta
Edmonton, Alberta
Canada

Barbara W. Hodson, PhD
Professor and Doctoral Program
    Coordinator
Communication Sciences and Disorders
Wichita State University
Wichita, Kansas
USA

David Ingram, PhD
Professor in Speech and Language
Department of Speech and Hearing
    Science
Arizona State University
Tempe, Arizona
USA

Deborah G. H. James, PhD
Academic Researcher/Paediatric Speech
    Pathologist
Centre for Allied Health Evidence
University of South Australia
Adelaide, SA
Australia

Victoria Joffe, DPhil
Senior Lecturer
City University
London
UK

Gwen Lancaster, MSc
Speech and Language Therapist
Language, Learning, and Behaviour
    Support Team
London Borough of Merton
UK

Suze Leitão, PhD
Senior Lecturer
Curtin University of Technology
Perth, WA
Australia

Gregory L. Lof, PhD
Director and Associate Professor
Graduate Program in Communication
   Sciences and Disorders
MGH Institute of Health Professions
Boston, Massachusetts
USA

Brenda Louw, PhD
Professor in Speech-Language Pathology
and Head Department Communication
   Pathology
University of Pretoria
Pretoria
South Africa

Robert J. Lowe, PhD
Professor, Communication Disorders
Bloomsburg University of Pennsylvania
Bloomsburg, Pennsylvania
USA

Rebecca McCauley, PhD
Professor
Department of Communication Sciences
University of Vermont
Burlington, Vermont
USA

Karen McComas, MA
Associate Professor
Marshall University
Huntington, West Virginia
USA

Sharynne McLeod, PhD
Professor in Speech and Language
   Acquisition
Charles Sturt University
Bathurst, NSW
Australia

Adele Miccio, PhD (1951–2009)
Associate Professor of Communication
   Sciences and Disorders
Co-Director, Center for Language
   Science

Pennsylvania State University
University Park, Pennsylvania
USA

Benjamin Munson, PhD
Associate Professor in Speech Language
   Hearing Sciences
University of Minnesota
Minneapolis, Minnesota
USA

Roslyn Neilson, PhD
Lecturer
Faculty of Education
University of Wollongong
Australia

Aubrey Nunes, PhD
Director
Pigeon Post Box Ltd.
London
UK

Megan S. Overby, PhD
Assistant Professor
Department of Communication Sciences
   and Disorders
The College of St. Rose
Albany, New York
USA

Michelle Pascoe, PhD
Senior Lecturer in Speech Pathology
Division of Communication Sciences and
   Disorders
School of Health and Rehabilitation
   Sciences
University of Cape Town
South Africa

Karen E. Pollock, PhD
Professor and Chair
Department of Speech Pathology and
   Audiology
University of Alberta
Edmonton, Alberta
Canada

Thomas W. Powell, PhD
Professor
Department of Rehabilitation Sciences
Louisiana State University Health
    Sciences Center
Shreveport, Louisiana
USA

Suzanne C. Purdy, PhD
Associate Professor and Head
Discipline of Speech Science
The University of Auckland
Auckland
New Zealand

Mirla G. Raz, MEd
Communication Skills Center
GerstenWeitz Publishers
Scottsdale, Arizona
USA

Joan Rosenthal, MA
Retired
University of Sydney
Sydney, NSW
Australia

Sue Roulstone, PhD
Professor of Speech and Language
    Therapy
University of the West of England
Director of the Speech and Language
    Therapy Research Unit
Frenchay Hospital
Bristol
UK

Dennis M. Ruscello, PhD
Professor of Speech Pathology and
    Audiology
Adjunct Professor of Otolaryngology
West Virginia University
Morgantown, West Virginia
USA

Susan Rvachew, PhD
Associate Professor
School of Communication Sciences and
    Disorders
McGill University
Montreal, Quebec
Canada

Amy E. Skinder-Meredith, PhD
Assistant Professor
Washington State University
Pullman, Washington
USA

Ruth Stoeckel, PhD
Clinical Speech-Language Pathologist
Mayo Clinic
Rochester, Minnesota
USA

Carol Stoel-Gammon, PhD
Professor
Department of Speech and Hearing
    Sciences
University of Washington
Seattle, Washington
USA

Judith Stone-Goldman, PhD
Emeritus Senior Lecturer
Department of Speech and Hearing
    Sciences
University of Washington
Seattle, Washington
USA

Edythe Strand, PhD
Speech Pathologist
Department of Neurology, Mayo
    Clinic
Associate Professor, Mayo College of
    Medicine
Rochester, Minnesota
USA

Angela Ullrich, MA
Research Associate, Doctoral candidate
Department for Pedagogics and
    Therapy of Speech and Language
    Disorders
University of Cologne
Germany

Nicole Watts Pappas, PhD
Adjunct Lecturer
Charles Sturt University
Bathurst, NSW
Speech Pathologist
Mt. Gravatt Children's Developmental
    Service
Brisbane, QLD
Australia

A. Lynn Williams, PhD
Professor
Department of Communicative
    Disorders
East Tennessee State University
Johnson City, Tennessee
USA

Pam Williams, MSc
Consultant Speech and Language
    Therapist
Nuffield Hearing and Speech Centre
Royal National Throat, Nose, and EAR
Hospital
London
UK

Introduction

Children with speech sound disorders have gaps in their speech sound systems that can make what they say difficult to understand. Nevertheless, most of them persist valiantly in their struggle to communicate, despite limited speech sound repertoires, restricted use of syllable structures, and incomplete stress pattern inventories. They may fill the gaps, or constraints, with speech patterns and structures that should not really be present in the utterances of otherwise typically developing children of their ages. For instance, affected English-learning children of four or five may say *foon* for *spoon*, *bwabbit* for *rabbit*, or *dipt* for *chips*; and sometimes they simply seem to leave a gap, and the listener hears, for example, *see* for *seed*, *ine* for *mine*, or *teffone* for *telephone*. They can have poor stimulability, systemic and substitution errors, syllable structure errors, consonant distortions, vowel deviations, atypical prosody, unusual tonality, and offbeat timing. Any or all of these intriguing but bothersome speech characteristics can occur singly or in combination; and the children's speech difficulties can encompass a mixture of phonetic (articulatory), phonemic (cognitive–linguistic), structural (craniofacial), perceptual, or neuromotor bases.

Some children have minor speech production difficulties and near perfect intelligibility, likely fitting at the high end of the Percentage of Consonants Correct (PCC) scale (Shriberg 1982; Shriberg, Austin, Lewis, et al. 1997), which is displayed in Table i.1. But of those referred for screening or assessment, a large proportion of the children speech–language pathologists/speech and language therapists (SLPs/SLTs) actually see for *intervention* are at the other end of the PCC scale. They have moderate-to-severe and severe speech impairments and low intelligibility. As well as making communication arduous for the children themselves, their poor speech clarity places additional demands on their parents, siblings, and others close to them. Often, these individuals have to work overtime, listening attentively in order to decipher what the speech-impaired children are saying, regularly finding themselves in the roles of advocate, apologist, code-breaker, go-between, and personal interpreter.

Table i.1 Severity scale based on a conversational speech sample (Shriberg 1982)

Severity interval[a]	Percentage of Consonants Correct (PCC)
Mild to normal	> 85%
Mild to moderate	65–85%
Moderate to severe	50–65%
Severe	<50%

[a] The severity interval descriptors are applicable to children aged 4 and older.

Under the umbrella heading of Speech Sound Disorders (SSD), the difficulties these young clients face attract labels such as Developmental Phonological Disorder or simply Phonological Disorder, Functional Articulation Disorder or Articulation Disorder, and Childhood Apraxia of Speech (CAS). All of these diagnoses have a multiplicity of confusing synonyms and acronyms. Irrespective of diagnostic labels (Broomfield and Dodd 2004a; Shriberg, Lewis, Tomblin, et al. 2005) or psycholinguistic profiles (Baker, Croot, McLeod, et al. 2001; Stackhouse and Wells 1997) and the short-term and long-term impacts of speech impairment for the children themselves (Felsenfeld, Broen, and McGue 1992, 1994) and for their significant others, SLPs/SLTs are charged with the responsibility of dealing effectively with these gaps and are uniquely qualified to do so (Gierut 1998; Law, Garrett, and Nye 2003, 2004).

About this book

Highly unintelligible three-, four-, and five-year-old children with moderate-to-severe and severe SSD, as revealed by their PCCs in conversational speech or their performance on single-word-naming (citation naming) tasks, often have complex and difficult-to-analyse speech (Campbell, Dollaghan, Rockette, et al. 2003). Accordingly, they can pose demanding diagnostic, intervention, reporting, and information-sharing challenges for speech and language professionals. This is so whether they are seasoned therapists, experienced clinical educators, new to the workforce, or students. Addressed primarily to clinicians and clinical educators, the focus of *Children's Speech Sound Disorders* is the work clinicians do with such children and their families. It is also about the so-called 'mildly involved' children, many of whom are at school and are older than the moderately and severely affected ones (McKinnon, McLeod, and Reilly 2007; Pascoe, Stackhouse, and Wells 2006; Shriberg, Kwiatkowski, and Gruber 1994; Shriberg, Tomblin, and McSweeny 1999). These older children may have been in therapy for lengthy periods continuously or intermittently and have just one or a few persisting and seemingly intractable speech issues. Examples include a stubborn lateral or palatal /s/ or difficulty in the way they produce a long vowel, so that when they say *bird* it sounds to the listener like *bored*.

Regrettably, time constraints and conflicting priorities can make it impossible for practitioners to regularly access the literature that relates to these children; synthesise, digest, and integrate what they have read; and then apply the knowledge clinically. Consequently, potentially valuable information remains in academe, somehow refusing to cross either the theory–therapy gap (Duchan 2001) or the research–practice gap (Duchan 2001). Attempting to reduce these gaps and speaking clinician-to-clinician, clinician-to-researcher, and researcher-to-clinician, *Children's Speech Sound Disorders* sets out to make critical theory-to-evidence-to-practice connections explicit. Emphasising evidence-based practice (EBP), Part 1 concerns the theoretical and empirical developments this decade, and leading earlier work, in the classification, differential diagnosis, and management of children affected by SSD. EBP in clinical speech pathology is a dynamic three-way arrangement whose goal is to integrate three things: clinical expertise; client/patient values, interests, needs, and choices; and current best evidence (ASHA 2006a). In the EPB literature relating to our field (Dollaghan 2004, 2007; Johnson 2006;

Montgomery and Turkstra 2003; Reilly, Douglas, and Oates 2004), the important connections between the clinician's role and good science are constantly highlighted. In the words of Apel and Self (2003), 'By consciously seeking out and using scientific evidence as the foundation for their clinical services, SLPs . . . become clinical scientists. They also may become partners with researchers.' Against this scientific backcloth, the focus of Part 2 is the practicalities of day-to-day treatment of SSD and associated issues.

Expert essays

Written from the perspective of an experienced SLP involved in clinical practice, the uniqueness of this book resides in its being the work of many hands. In it, an international line-up of 51 academicians, clinicians, researchers, and thinkers representing a range of expertise, paradigms, and theoretical orientations answer questions about key theoretical, assessment, intervention, and service delivery issues. The questions, mostly multipart, are numbered consecutively Q1 through Q49 in the text, and the answers appear as sections A1 through A49. Case examples are also included throughout the book. Whereas the children—Aaron, Adam, Aidan, Andrew, Bethany, Bobby, Brett, Brian, Bruno, Ceri, Christopher, Daniel, David, Dorothy, Emeline, Emma, Fiona, Gerri, Greg, Huia, Iain, Joanna, Jessica, Josie, Kenny, Luke, Madison, Max, Nadif, Nina, Olaf, Owen, Peter, Precious, Quentin, Ricky, Robert, Sebastian, Shaun, Sigrid, Simon, Sophie, Tessa, Tumi, Uzzia, Vaughan, William, Xing-Fu, Yoshi, and Zach—are real, their names and family members' names are pseudonyms. And although many of them *are*, not all questions are necessarily the author's. Most are based on frequently asked questions from students, clinical educators, and clinicians in continuing professional development (CPD) or continuing education unit (CEU) events, private correspondence, and postings to the phonological therapy list (Bowen 2001). It is hoped that the essays will provide a unique resource for SLPs/SLTs, wherever they work.

World Health Organization

In an individual child, intelligibility concerns may come bundled co-morbidly with other communication impairments, for example, voice or fluency disorders, semantic and pragmatic difficulties, and language-processing and production issues. Some children have other issues of health, development, and well-being, such as physical or sensory challenges, chemical allergies and food intolerances, intellectual impairment, learning difficulties, and auditory processing and attention deficits. In culturally and linguistically diverse clinical settings, numbers of them face the added complication of attempting to acquire more than one language and hence more than one speech sound system (Yavas 2007). Whether they are monolingual or multilingual, have an isolated SSD, or have an SSD as one of several issues, their lives will be affected in the areas of Body Function, Body Structure, Activity and Participation, Environmental Factors, and Personal Factors. These are the headings itemised in the World Health Organization's ICF-CY: the children and youth version of the *International Classification of Functioning, Disability and Health* (World Health Organization 2001). The first question is about the ICF-CY, and it goes to speech-language pathologist, Sharynne McLeod.

A tireless worker in speech research and pedagogy, Dr. McLeod is Professor of Speech and Language Acquisition at Charles Sturt University, Australia. She is vice president of the International Clinical Linguistics and Phonetics Association (ICPLA), editor of the *International Journal of Speech-Language Pathology*, a Fellow of Speech Pathology Australia, and a Fellow of ASHA. Her research has focused on the production of speech sounds in children and adults, and a specific area of inquiry she pursues is the application of the ICF-CY to children with speech impairment.

Q1. Sharynne McLeod: The ICF-CY and children with speech impairment

In at least two respects, the ICF-CY (WHO 2007) is more than a general way of viewing behaviour, ability, and health status in children. First, when applied to individual children with SSD, it affords an orderly, holistic framework within which to perform an evaluation, select an appropriate therapy, deliver it, and measure and analyse its effects and outcomes, in the process of evidence-based management. Second, it is a vehicle for involving close people in a child's life—family, friends, teachers, and others—in intervention and a means of connecting with the more distant people concerned for the child's well-being in agencies, funding bodies, and policy-making teams: the ultimate providers and determiners of services. How do these elements fit together, and what are the interrelationships between the ICF-CY components and clinical practice? As a vibrant work-in-progress, responsive to a changing world, the ICF-CY will probably never be quite finished! What would you like to see added to or taken from the current schema, and how can clinicians working with children and youth with unintelligible speech apply the principles of the ICF-CY and keep abreast of any changes?

A1. Sharynne McLeod: The contribution of the ICF-CY to working with children with speech impairment

Children with speech impairment bring more than their mouths to the clinic. Each of the children on our caseloads brings a unique combination of factors, such as relationships with family, friends, teachers, and acquaintances; aspects of their lives that are important to them; their personalities, learning styles, and so forth. As SLPs we often take these factors into consideration, but rarely do so in an explicit fashion (McLeod 2004). Instead, our reports and clinic files predominantly contain information about children's speech output, such as their abilities to produce consonants and vowels correctly.

For over two decades, the World Health Organization has been developing an extensive classification system to be used throughout the world to support the health and wellness of all people. This started with the *International Classification of Impairment, Disabilities and Handicaps* (ICIDH; World Health Organization 1980) and the most recent version of this is the *International Classification of Functioning, Disability and Health – Children and Youth* (ICF-CY; World Health Organization 2007). A description of the history and application of the ICF-CY to children with communication impairments is contained in McLeod and Threats (2008). The five components of the ICF-CY (listed below) have direct relevance to children with speech impairment (McLeod and McCormack 2007; also see McLeod 2006 for a case study).

1. Body Structure

Structures of the ear, nose, mouth, larynx, pharynx, and respiration are routinely screened by SLPs to determine their potential contribution to speech impairment. For the majority of children with speech impairment, Body Structure is not considered to be a causal factor (Shriberg, Kwiatkowski, Best, et al. 1986). In some cases, such as when a child has a craniofacial anomaly (e.g., cleft lip and palate), an impairment in Body Structure can impact his/her ability to speak intelligibly and may also have an impact on activity and participation in society.

2. Body Function

Articulation, voice, fluency, hearing, respiration, and intellectual and specific mental functions, such as temperament and personality functions, are classified among Body Functions in the ICF-CY. SLPs working with children with speech impairment routinely consider these aspects in their assessment and intervention practices. The majority of SLP assessment, analysis, and intervention tools for children with speech impairment fall under the category of Body Function. Thus, although not specifically stated in the ICF-CY, Body Function can include measures such as the PCC, the occurrence of cluster reduction, and the inventory of consonant phones (McLeod and Bleile 2004).

3. Activities and Participation

Learning and applying knowledge; general tasks and demands; communication; interpersonal interactions and relationships; major life areas such as education; and community, social, and civic life are all included in the ICF-CY as categories of Activities and Participation. Due to the paucity of available tools to consider this component, the *Speech Participation and Activity Assessment of Children* (SPAA-C) (McLeod 2004) was developed by SLPs to facilitate conversations with children, their siblings, parents, friends, teachers, and significant others. When we as SLPs set goals for children with speech impairment, it is important that we acknowledge and include these broader aspects of the lives of children with speech impairment. Thus, communicating intelligibly on the sporting field and during the school play are relevant goals for SLPs working in this framework. It is also helpful if we consider the possible mismatch between capacity and performance in these life areas. As children grow older, the impact of speech impairment on individuals' Activities and Participation may include an impact on social, educational, occupational, and behavioural outcomes as well as on quality of life for these individuals and their families (McLeod 2007b).

4. Environmental Factors

Products and technology; support and relationships; attitudes; and services, systems, and policies are all included as Environmental Factors in ICF-CY. Each of these areas can act as a facilitator and/or barrier to children with speech impairment. In most children's lives, perhaps the most prominent Environmental Factor is their family. As SLPs we need to be aware of facilitating involvement of parents and siblings in assessment and intervention (Watts Pappas, McLeod, McAllister, et al. 2008). We also need to be aware of the impact a child with a speech impairment can have on families, particularly mothers (Rudolph, Kummer, Eysholdt, et al. 2005) and siblings (Barr, McLeod, and Daniel 2008). Another relevant Environmental Factor is the attitudes of family, friends, acquaintances, and people in authority (such as teachers), health professionals, and society. The attitudes people hold towards children with speech impairment can either be facilitative or act as a barrier in these children's lives. Consequently, there may be times when our intervention goals need to be directed towards others, rather than the children with speech impairment. Finally, Environmental Factors include the policies and services that are available for children with speech impairment. In some nations, such as the USA and UK, legislation ensures that children with speech impairment are provided with relevant services, and these act as an environmental facilitator. In other nations, such as Australia, SLP services are not legislated, and access to services may be difficult, particularly for those living in rural areas (Wilson, Lincoln, and Onslow 2002), acting as an environmental barrier.

5. Personal Factors

Age, gender, race, other health conditions, coping styles, overall behaviour pattern, and character style are all included in the ICF-CY as relevant Personal Factors. Unlike the other components of the ICF-CY, detailed descriptions of Personal Factors are not included in the manual. However, it is helpful if SLPs explore relevant Personal Factors for each child they engage with.

Finally, the ICF-CY is far more than these five discrete components. The interaction between each of these components is essential for visualising the goal of health and wellness. In my view, the advantage of engaging with this comprehensive classification system is that it enables holistic consideration of children with speech impairment in order to envisage and facilitate fuller participation in society.

Evidence, belief, and practice

EBP is a process and a responsibility. It is located at the juncture between clinicians' engagement with scientific theory and research, and their engagement with clients and their worlds. The onus for *adopting* EBP rests with individual clinicians and cannot be imposed by professional associations, workplaces, educators, legislators, or policymakers. But most clinicians probably only have a small part to play in *constructing* the evidence side of the EBP equilateral triangle.

Academic SLPs/SLTs and Linguists are largely responsible for developing, evaluating, adapting, synthesising, reporting, and teaching about new research, theory, therapy, and best practice. They usually do so in laboratory, classroom, and CPD/CEU circumstances. Meanwhile, clinicians apply the outcomes of this research endeavour (in anything but laboratory conditions) wherever and with whomever their clients happen to be. So doesn't it seem unreasonable that the burden of converting speech-language pathology into an evidence-based discipline is frequently allocated to practitioners? And that it is done so without providing them with necessary skills, time, and resources to keep up with the available evidence and integrate it into practice? Might it not be fairer if the lion's share of the responsibility for the *evidence* aspect of EBP rested with the individuals who educate SLPs/SLTs, that is, the researchers whose job it is to address and answer clinical and educational questions and the policy-makers who channel reform?

As well as being unreasonable, it provides an environment in which gaps in communication between researchers, academics, policy-makers, and practitioners are perpetuated and exacerbated, oftentimes manifesting as uncertainty, antagonism, and uncomfortable relationships. Where co-operation and sharing would be highly desirable, instead we hear the doubtful voices of academic researchers who are uncertain whether the produce of their hard work is valued or used by clinicians. Then we find conscientious academic teachers whose students complain that they do not teach enough—or indeed *anything*—about the nitty-gritty of practice, as well as exasperated clinicians and CPD/CEU participants criticising messages from the laboratory and the lecture hall as out-of-touch, unrealistic, impractical, and impossible to implement. Such criticisms point to the importance of *modelling* and *teaching* principles of EBP in the academic preparation of new SLPs/SLTs by delivering higher education that is *itself* rooted in and guided by EBP.

Having put their student days behind them, CPD/CEU participants often clamour for content that is useful and not too theoretical or research-focused. Perhaps it was in the context of unrelenting requests for practical professional development subject matter, almost stripped of theory, that Vicki Lord Larson and the late Nancy McKinley (Larson and McKinley 2003, p. 26) invoked the famous maxim of gestalt psychologist Kurt Lewin. Lewin (1951, p.169) asserted that, 'there is nothing more practical than a good theory to enable you to make choices confidently and consistently, and to explain or defend why you are making the choices you make'. Alternatively, their use of the quotation may have been prompted by conversations with students fresh from clinical placements who had been told by experienced SLP/SLTs that what they had learned in lectures and from textbooks 'was great in theory' but that in the real world we do it *this* way!

When 'doing it this way' means implementing atheoretical, untested assessment protocols, goal-setting strategies, target-selection approaches, or treatment methodologies that have remained essentially unmodified for decades, there may be any number of explanations. It may not be due to a reluctance to move out of a comfort zone and try something new. Rather, it may relate to a need to rationalise the purchase of particular materials and equipment, or to individual clinicians' gaps in knowledge of alternatives. For example, applications of optimality theory in nonlinear phonology (Bernhardt and Stemberger 1998, 2000), the psycholinguistic framework (Stackhouse and Wells 1997), *Metaphon* (Dean, Howell, Waters, et al. 1995), Core Vocabulary Therapy (Dodd, Holm, Crosbie, et al. 2006), and Patterns (Cycles) Therapy (Hodson 2007; A5) are not taught in some undergraduate and graduate programs, and clinicians may never encounter them in workshops or readings. Furthermore, management pathways within some agencies dictate that the nature of any therapy delivered is determined by personnel concentrations and waiting list management strategies, as opposed to clinical reasoning around the best possible fit between client (and that includes family), therapist, and therapy. Or it may be because most of what a particular professional or agency 'does' in SSD management is consultative: working through aides, assistants, and teachers (McCartney, Boyle, Bannatyne, et al. 2005), rarely seeing clients one-on-one. Or it may even have to do with a mindset that equates 'research findings' with 'impossible to operationalise'.

Controversial practices

Our field has an assortment of commonly practised, heavily promoted, and unbelievably popular controversial practices (Duchan, Calculator, Sonnenmeier, et al. 2001) that are currently unsupported by empirical evidence or theory. They include oral motor treatments (OMT) with their non-speech oral motor exercises (NS-OME), tools, and toys (Beckman 1986; Boshart 1998; Chapman Bahr 2001; Marshalla 2001; Rosenfeld-Johnson 1999; Strode and Chamberlain 1997) and auditory integration therapies or 'sound therapies' (ASHA 2004d). Then there are exclusive therapies that may have some theoretical support, but which, on the evidence side, only enjoy limited testimonial support, such as PROMPT: Prompts for Restructuring Oral Muscular Phonetic Targets (Chumpelik 1984; Hayden 2006). They are exclusive in that qualified, certified speech and language professionals must pay to gain additional basic and advanced training and accreditation in order to own 'the knowledge' in the form of special techniques (the prompts), therapy administration manuals, and materials.

When clinicians elect to 'do it this way' with therapies that await scientific evaluation, they may justify their choices in terms of confidence, faith, or resolute *belief* that the treatment in question works. Questioned on their use of a favoured but hotly debated methodology many 'believers' (Gruber, Lowery, Seung, et al. 2003) will respond that, in their estimation, the intervention approach does not *require* theoretical justification or scientific evaluation because they 'know' it is effective! Examples of woolly, occasionally evangelistic, 'it works for me' or 'we don't know how it works but it does' reasoning abound in mailing lists and are inevitably commented on in clinical forums relating to NS-OMT (Lass and Pannbacker 2008; Lof and Watson 2008; Powell 2008a, b; Ruscello 2008a).

As well as expressing confidence in NS-OMT, proponents also proffer arguments in favour of their continued use that emphasise their discernment of a weak or absent 'no' case. Moderate thinkers like Kerridge, Lowe, and Henry (1998) have cautioned that we must not confuse the fact of 'currently without substantial evidence' with the idea of 'without substantial value'. Nonetheless, we need to think seriously and critically about the theoretical bases and proposed therapeutic mechanisms (Clark 2003) of techniques that lack (and in the NS-OMT and PROMPT instances mentioned above, for a *long* time have lacked) empirical support.

Defending the NS-OMT component in the *Nuffield Centre Dyspraxia Programme* (Williams and Stephens 2004), Williams, Stephens, and Connery (2006) advise: 'We should not stop using treatments that we have seen to be effective through years of clinical practice just because there is as of yet no peer-reviewed published evidence to support their use. Of course, we need to be mindful of what the evidence base is saying, but we cannot wait for absolute proof that something works - we have to continue clinical work, alongside informing the research process. It is likely to be many years before we know exactly what works and for which groups of children.' These words are in keeping with Van Weel and Knottnerus (1999) who said: 'In EBP, there will always be interventions for which no evidence is (yet) available, but that is no reason to withhold the intervention' going on to note that, 'where research provides unequivocal evidence of the absence of effects, the situation is much clearer'.

Theory–therapy and research–practice gaps

Although there is unequivocal evidence (Gierut 1998) at a range of levels (ASHA 2004c; Reilly, Douglas, and Oates 2004) supporting many intervention approaches for SSD, there is scant research that provides practitioners with *explicit* clinical guidance. To date there is one randomised control trial study of treatment efficacy (Almost and Rosenbaum 1998); few studies have examined rate of change relative to duration and frequency of therapy, and most studies have measured accuracy of word production rather than the intelligibility of communicative discourse. Accordingly, it would be difficult—if not impossible—to institute best clinical practice guidelines in SSD based on research findings. And perhaps that is one of the reasons why many practitioners appear to marginalise (Baker and McLeod 2004) and possibly trivialise the relevance of published research as a guide to practice.

Regardless of the reasons some clinicians have for their reluctance to implement new research or to relinquish theoretically unsupported interventions, the outcome is that the principles of practice are frequently incongruent with the research findings (Duchan 2001; Ingram 1998). Musing on Lewin's famous assertion, and conceding that he may have been right about there being nothing more practical than a good theory, Rothman (2004, p. 6) maintains that Lewin's dictum relied on an assumption that 'good' (accurate and applicable) theories are *available* to address practical problems. Arguing the need for a stronger sense of interdependence and collaboration between those engaged in research and those occupied with professional activities, Rothman writes: 'If critical advances in health behavior theory depend on an iterative process by which theoreticians and interventionists cooperate in the testing and evaluation of theoretical principles, individuals in both camps need to not only recognize the goals and values of each group, but also trust each other's ability to advance our understanding of both theory and practice.'

Positive collaborations

Standing back from accounts of partition between theorists, researchers, and practitioners in medicine, education, and health sciences for a moment, and looking closely at our own SLP/SLT profession, committed as it is to issues of communicative competence and communicative effectiveness, we see encouraging signs of bridge-building. This is particularly noticeable within the doctoral degree process (Bernthal and Overby, A46). Conference presentations and proceedings provide heartening examples of clinicians who have completed or are pursuing clinically oriented research or coursework doctorates while continuing to work as clinicians during their studies and beyond. Examples of people who have done so include Highman (A36), Leitão (A48), Neilson (A17), Stoeckel (A35), and Watts Pappas (A25). Relationships forged between doctoral candidates, supervisors, and advisors, around scholarship and the publication process, can help cement strong collaborative connections between laboratory and clinic or classroom.

Two important questions

What can a child speech interventionist do when faced with inescapable gaps in the evidence base? Clinical science research and clinical reasoning (Kamhi and Pollock 2005) are not all about incontrovertible evidence and elegant theories. But they do have a lot to do with plausibility, healthy scepticism, the questions we ask, and how we ask them. According to a highly recommended article by Clark (2003), there are at least two lines of enquiry we can adopt in setting about choosing an intervention methodology for one of our clients. First we can ask, 'Is this treatment beneficial?' or, '*Does* it work?' To answer this, the therapist examines the evidence base, looking for adequately documented evidence of the effects, effectiveness, and efficacy (Olswang 1998) of the treatment under consideration. If that evidence is unavailable, Clark advises posing a second question: 'Is the treatment approach theoretically sound?' or, '*Should* it work?' This second line of investigation can be successful, according to Clark, only if the practitioner clearly understands (a) the nature of the targeted impairment, and (b) the therapeutic mechanism of the proposed treatment—or how it is *supposed* to work. In this regard, intervention approaches should be based on a theory of the particular speech behaviour in question and should be what Rosen and Davidson (2003) called 'dismantle-able', or able to be broken down into components for the purpose of examining them for rationale and effects, or (their term) 'empirically supported principles of change' or 'explicitly principled therapy' (Crystal 1972).

Keeping up with the literature

Key peer-reviewed publications hold a wealth of clinically relevant reports on SSD, but some clinicians do not have easy access to libraries, journals, and proceedings. The accessibility of research findings is also sometimes reduced because vast numbers of the reports are expressed in densely technical and statistical language that is unfathomable for readers who are not researchers. In fact, at times it seems that researchers, revelling in their intellectualism, write their reports *only* for their co-authors and a handful of other researchers to read!

Despite bridge-building that occurs in doctoral research and discipline-specific electronic mailing lists, phenomena of information sharing, new research-to-practice links, and harmonious collegial communication between academe and therapy room are barely perceptible in many clinics. For there, busy therapists hardly ever have the time to integrate new research into day-to-day practice. Neither do they have the time to *discuss* what they do manage to read or *modify* for their own cultural settings enticing new techniques that worked well in one country but which need help to travel to another part of the world, or to a different 'world' that may be culturally remote but geographically quite close by. How, for instance, can clinicians working with indigenous populations in remote Australia, or clinical consultants in the UK advising families from the former Soviet Union with English as their second or third language, adapt and apply a powerful clinical insight from a research laboratory in Madison, Wisconsin and make it work for their clients?

Impediments to implementing research findings clinically are not all about time constraints and the propensity for complex literature reviews, research methods, experimental results, statistical data, and discussions to be expressed in impenetrable scientific prose, or unfamiliar language, in much of our literature. There is also therapists' inclination to stay with what they know. In terms of treatment approaches, for instance, information has been available for a long time about the advantages for the client, by way of clinical efficiency, of working on error *patterns* (Grunwell 1983, 1992; Hodson 1982, 1994; Ingram 1974, 1986, 1989) rather than laboriously targeting individual phonemes one-by-one. Similarly, nonlinear phonology, so relevant to theory and therapy for phonological disorders, has been around for at least three decades, but it is still generally seen as something new, difficult, and 'out there' by many practitioners and not to be incorporated into practice. As well as being conservative in the choice of treatment approach, clinicians have been slow to move on some of the more up-to-date target selection criteria (displayed in Table 8.1, p. 282) that are now supported by research evidence. Tending to follow traditional guidelines by targeting sounds that are *early developing*, *less complex*, and *stimulable in isolation*, many therapists remain cautious when it comes to embracing new guidelines that would have them work on sounds that are *later developing*, *more complex*, and *non-stimulable* (Baker, A11; Williams 2003a).

Ingram (1998) struck a cautious note when he wisely advised against rushing new theory and research into practice as soon as it hits the journals. But the probability of a *widespread* rush to apply new research actually happening is remarkably low. Indeed, according to a survey of 270 Australian speech-language pathologists (McLeod and Baker 2004), for almost all clinicians, it may be that little is adopted from the current literature, in that just 1.1% of those surveyed reported that research influenced their choice of intervention approach. And what an astonishing choice of evidence-based interventions there is!

Cultural and linguistic parochialism

Or is there? Do therapists around the world *know* about the available options? Pascoe (2006), for example, says: 'While there are undoubtedly some issues specific to phonology therapists on different sides of the Atlantic, in general the clients we serve are similar and the theoretical and clinical issues the same', but that, 'it sometimes feels as if there are fewer links between British/European speech and language therapy, and American/Canadian speech and language pathology than there should be.' This redirects attention to another gap: the tendency for British and European books and key journals in our field to focus on British and European research and North American publications tending to focus on US and Canadian research. Admittedly there has been more international representation within individual works in recent years, but take for example the predominantly UK 'feel' of the books by Dodd (2005) and Pascoe, Stackhouse, and Wells (2006), and the journals *Child Language Teaching and Therapy*, *Clinical Linguistics and Phonetics*, and *The International Journal of Language and Communication Disorders*, compared with the North American 'feel' of the books by Bauman-Waengler (2004), Bernthal, Bankson, and Flipsen, Jr. (2009), Kamhi and Pollock (2005), and Pena-Brooks and Hegde (2000), and the *Journal of Speech, Language, and Hearing Research; Language, Speech and Hearing Services in Schools; Seminars in Speech and Language;* and *Topics in Language Disorders*. Michelle Pascoe reflects on these issues in her response to Q2.

Dr. Michelle Pascoe qualified as a speech and language therapist/audiologist at the University of Cape Town, South Africa in 1995. She has worked as a speech and language therapist with children with speech, language, and literacy difficulties in South Africa and the UK. Michelle's PhD focused on intervention for school-age children with speech difficulties and was supervised by Professors Joy Stackhouse and Bill Wells at the University of Sheffield. She subsequently co-authored books on children's speech and literacy difficulties (Pascoe, Stackhouse, and Wells 2006; Stackhouse, Vance, Pascoe, et al. 2007). Michelle is now a Senior Lecturer at the University of Cape Town, where she continues to develop her research into intervention for children with speech and literacy difficulties.

Q2. Michelle Pascoe: Child speech practice: an international view

As a South African Speech Language Therapist who has worked in clinical and academic settings in both the UK and South Africa and who has co-authored a book (Pascoe, Stackhouse, and Wells 2006) on child speech that reflects an appreciation of theory, research, and practice, you have a unique international perspective. What is your take on there being 'fewer links between British/European speech and language therapy and American/Canadian speech and language pathology than there should be'? And how does child speech practice in your country resemble or differ from what happens—according to both the literature and you own observations—in the UK, Europe, and North America?

A2. Michelle Pascoe: Going between: intervention for children's speech sound difficulties from an international perspective

British author L. P. Hartley began his brilliant novel with the line: _'The past is a foreign country: they do things differently there'_ (Hartley 1953). This quotation—now almost proverbial—reminds me of how our practice as speech and language therapists has changed since the early origins of the profession in the 1950s and 1960s.

In our book _Persisting Speech Difficulties in Children_ (Pascoe, Stackhouse, and Wells 2006, Chapter 1), we review historical shifts in intervention for children with speech sound difficulties and consider how, in some cases, the shift from articulation to phonological approaches has resulted in the (again, proverbial) 'baby being thrown out with the bathwater'. But, there are other ways in which we can reflect on differences and similarities in practice: by looking at intervention for children with speech sound difficulties in countries around the globe, both foreign and more familiar.

There are many differences in how practitioners around the world assess and manage children's speech difficulties. For a start, the terminology used gives an obvious clue as to how differently practitioners within the English-speaking world approach speech difficulties. In the US, practitioners talk about 'speech pathology'; in the UK, reference is made to 'speech and language therapy'; and in South Africa . . . well, sometimes we talk about 'speech-language pathology', sometimes 'speech and language therapy', and sometimes 'speech and hearing therapy'. The latter reflects the way in which South African speech therapists have, up until recently, received a dual training comprising both speech and language therapy and audiology. There are parts of the world where 'apraxia of speech (AoS)' is preferred over 'developmental verbal dyspraxia (DVD)' and other places where the term 'childhood apraxia of speech (CAS) prevails'. To a large extent, these differences reflect the different contexts in which we work. Practitioners funded by and working within health care may naturally align themselves with medical models of working, more than those working in educational contexts. The former may talk more easily of 'speech pathologies' and 'speech disorders' than the latter, who may feel more comfortable with the notions of 'delays' and 'difficulties.' The contexts in which we work differ widely, and it is inevitable that these will shape our terminology and how we approach our work with children with speech difficulties.

The context in which I carried out my undergraduate training was in South Africa in the first part of the 1990s. On the brink of a new democracy, at the end of the apartheid years, the country was not only geographically isolated from the world's leading countries but also politically isolated. The effect of this isolation was for those working in the field to look outwards: my training in speech and language therapy seemed to involve a carefully integrated perspective on approaches to speech difficulties in the UK at that time (e.g., PACS, Metaphon, Nuffield, Psycholinguistic Approaches) and approaches in the USA and Canada (e.g., Cycles Therapy, Multiple Exemplars, Distinctive Feature approaches). My perspective as a new clinician working with children's speech sound difficulties was thus informed by an amalgamation of some of the most exciting developments happening around the globe, making up in breadth what it lacked in depth. My own sense, years later, working in the UK as a clinician and a clinical educator, was that it was easier to be 'spoiled for choice' in a country home to several of the key proponents of particular approaches to children's speech difficulties. The need to look outwards may be less urgent when you have a wealth of knowledge, research, and the associated infrastructure right on your doorstep.

Back in South Africa, things have changed and, although still aware of the bigger picture, the profession is more inward-looking as we seek to address the enormous challenges in addressing children's speech and associated literacy difficulties in our own unique context. The country has 11 official languages, yet few resources for the assessment of languages other than English and Afrikaans. Furthermore, our knowledge about phonological development in languages other than English and Afrikaans is limited, and clinicians who can speak the indigenous languages of the country are few, although this imbalance is slowly changing. The challenges extend beyond those posed by the rich language diversity of the country: HIV/AIDS and poverty affect a large proportion of the population, for whom speech difficulties are necessarily a low priority. Nevertheless, our work in promoting emergent literacy and the links between phonological awareness and speech processing is vital and should be seen as more than just a luxury. There is research taking place into emergent literacy, speech development, and the role of speech and language therapy in linguistically diverse classrooms. Some of this research demonstrates the important role of our work in a primary health care context, but further studies are needed to demonstrate the pressing importance of these issues. In a recent issue of the *South African Journal of Communication Disorders*, Kathard, Naude, Pillay, and Ross (2007) urged practitioners to carry out relevant research for relevant practice, urging that 'the kind of engagement required involves more than relocating services to community clinics or re-focusing an empirical research lens to, for example, Black African languages. All this may serve to do is re-produce the same kind of restrictive ways of knowing'.

Although the contexts in which we practice differ, there are surely more similarities than differences when working with children's speech difficulties around the world. South African therapists—and other therapists working in developing countries—need to be careful about chucking out the baby with the bathwater yet again. Instead we should be forging links wherever we can. There is a core of knowledge about linguistics, phonetic transcription, anatomy, target selection, reinforcement, and relevance that seems common no matter where we work or in what language. For SLPs in South Africa to ignore this core knowledge would be foolish, but as Kathard et al. (2007) urge, we need to adapt ways in which we research and practice so that they are relevant and useful for the population we serve. The psycholinguistic approach to children's speech and literacy difficulties (Stackhouse and Wells 1997, 2001) is an approach that exemplifies much of this core knowledge and has been shown to bring about positive changes in children with persisting speech difficulties under ideal (or relatively ideal) circumstances. However, the approach is a flexible one, and an important next step, for example, in the South African context, is to demonstrate the effectiveness of the approach in different contexts which may include in group settings working through untrained assistants using a variety of languages and with minimal resources.

Communication between practitioners through resources such as Caroline Bowen's Web site (http://www.speech-language-therapy.com) and through books such as Sharynne McLeod's *International Guide to Speech Acquisition* (McLeod 2007a) helps develop this global perspective. The application of these concepts in a particular service delivery context will differ. How much therapy can you offer? Do you do it yourself or through co-workers? How involved are the parents? How long to see the child for? On their own or with others? At home, in the classroom, or clinic? It is the different ways we approach these service delivery issues that make the links with others so interesting.

My view is that we should all consider ourselves as 'go betweens' building bridges between countries. There will always be countries where things are done differently, but that it what makes our field exciting. We should embrace that foreignness, and dialogue with the differences.

A plethora of gaps and questions

Finally, public and private Internet discussions between speech and language professionals have stories to tell. They are noteworthy for demonstrating a plethora of gaps in international communication about SSD. We find experienced therapists in the UK hearing, for the first time, about Patterns or Cycles Therapy (Hodson 2006), Phonotactic Therapy (Velleman 2002), or Multiple Oppositions Therapy (Williams 2000a, b), and US therapists discovering the Psycholinguistic Framework (Stackhouse and Wells 1997) or *Metaphon* (Dean, Howell, Waters, et al. 1995) also for first time, many years after they first appeared in the international literature. But how 'international' is the literature and who reads it anyway?

So we have it. Questions galore! There are burning questions about clinicians and the evidence-base. Where empirically supported intervention guidance exists, will clinicians have time to find it and read it? Will they be able to evaluate it and see it as a professional obligation to do so? Gaps galore! Children with gaps in their speech sound systems and clinicians working to fill those gaps, surrounded by disparities in communication be-tween academe and therapy room; gaps in knowledge, service delivery, and evidence; theory–therapy and research–practice gaps; and gaps in international communication. Undoubtedly the list goes on and should include the gaps that can exist between the needs, goals, expectations, roles, and responsibilities of therapists and the needs, goals, expectations, roles, and responsibilities of individual children, their families, and com-munities. There are even gaps in the way our profession's histories have been recorded (Duchan 2001), as Chapter 1 reveals.

Part I

A practical update

Chapter 1

The evolution of current practices

Conceptual frameworks are easy to ignore. Like the air we breathe, their presence is everywhere, once they are looked for. Yet, they are often taken for granted, under-estimated and under-examined. One way to reveal the influence of frameworks today is to study their use in the unfamiliar contexts. For example, an examination of past practices of speech therapists raises questions about what practitioners did then as well as how and why they did it. Such an investigation creates the distance needed for clinicians to apprehend aspects of their own practice that are ordinarily taken for granted.

Duchan 2006

One of our profession's few historians, Duchan (2001) believes there has been too little work on the evolution of current practices. She observes that most histories of the origins of speech pathology in the US focus on organisational matters and place the genesis of the profession in about 1925, when workers in the field of speech disorders and speech correction established their own organisation. This same institutional focus is found in chronologies by Margaret Eldridge, recording the development of speech therapy in Australia (Eldridge 1965) and the Commonwealth of Nations (Eldridge 1968a, b). Beginning in the 19th century, Duchan has produced a fascinating history that is broader in scope than its predecessors and different because it includes a systematic record of the science and ideas underlying practice. All of this and more is freely available on the Internet (Duchan 2001).

Aubrey Nunes, who has a PhD in Linguistics from the University of Durham, shares Duchan's interest in our history. But as a Speech and Language Therapist (SLT), Linguist, perennial student, and thinker, he prefers to take an even longer view. Graduating as an SLT from the National Hospital College of Speech Sciences in 1979, Aubrey worked for 10 years in the 1980s as a National Health Service SLT with children and youth, and he has been engaged in child speech-related research since 1976. In A3, Dr. Nunes explains why he believes 'modern' speech therapy had its genesis in 17th century England.

Q3.   Aubrey Nunes: The British origins of child speech practice

An aim of this book is to provide a practical update for clinicians working with children with speech sound disorders (SSDs), with reference to about 70 or 80 years of the history that underpins what we do as speech-language clinicians in assessment and therapy. You have said (Nunes 2006) that speech-language pathology (SLP)/SLT can be seen to originate in the 17th century, and not the 20th. Can you expand on that theme, and comment on what you have called 'the very practical, anti-theoretical, and subjectivist stance of SLT in Britain'?

A3.   Aubrey Nunes: A legacy lost

Eldridge (1968a, b) traces a century of the treatment of speech disorders, starting over 200 years after its genesis in England in 1667, when William Holder proposed the theory of distinctive features and described its application to work with the deaf. Scarcely remembered or acknowledged as pioneers of speech intervention, William Holder (1616–1698), John Thelwall (1764–1834), and Alexander Melville Bell (1819–1905) took a 'top-down' approach to speech impairment, highlighting the need to understand what constitutes 'normal speech'. But in relation to the academic preparation of SLTs, the British professional association, the Royal College of Speech and Language Therapists (RCSLT), and the Health Professions Council (HPC) have a quite different perspective.

In 2005, the University of Essex had just obtained the funding for an SLT course. Martin Atkinson (personal communication 2007) tells how the University pitched one aspect of the proposed curriculum to an Accreditation Panel from the HPC and an observer from the RCSLT. Students would be taught linguistics by world-class researchers in speech and language development and pathology. The unanimous reaction was that these proposals were unacceptable. 'The problem,' the Panel said, 'is that there's too much linguistics.' This unanimity reflects a paradigm that is bottom-up and anti-theoretical; starts from pathology, not normality; disdaining categories not detectable at the beginning of normal speech development, such as the prosody.

Linguistics is the science of speech and language. The RCSLT mentions speech, language, and communication as aspects of SLT (RCSLT 2006, p. 2), but the responsibility for SLT training now lies with the HPC. The HPC (2007, p.13) specifies linguistics as one of 10 bodies of knowledge relevant to 'profession-specific practice' that also includes anatomy and psychology. But this says nothing about what SLTs should know about linguistics and the scientific basis of that discipline from the invention of the alphabet 3,000 years ago to works such as Chomsky (1965), Chomsky and Halle (1968), Smith (1973), and their academic progeny. The most serious likely shortfall in course content is key information around the discovery, by Chomsky in particular, that there is interest in *how* most children learn to talk during what Lenneberg (1967) calls 'the critical period'—from infancy to puberty. In remedying the superficiality and apparent 'dumbing down' of the SLT linguistics curriculum, any addition to it could be reconciled with all the other competing pressures by defining more precisely the irreducible core of SLT through a process of discussion between practitioners, academics, and researchers of the appropriate balance between the 10 topics.

Generative linguistics and an acquisition module

For Chomsky, Halle, and Smith (see above), there are not just words like *browning* and *brownish*, but possible words like *unbrown* and *brownable*. This is why typically developing children as young as two or three find it fun to hear parents calling themselves, for example, *Mumanimumpy* and *Dadamadandy*, since *Mummy* and *Daddy* are recoverable by what is known as a 'grammar', and such a grammar is 'generative', hence 'generative linguistics'. Chomsky (1965, pp. 3–62) stresses the need to explain the acquisition of a grammar from an initial state to an end-state of 'competence'. At 2;6 the child's errors, which are not always consistent, can involve phonotactics (e.g., cluster reduction), phonemics, (e.g., fronting), phonetics, (e.g., production errors with /s/), prosody, (e.g., unstressed syllable deletion), and rules (e.g., *a elephant*). The notion of an error presupposes a standard of comparison, called 'competence' in generative linguistics. Linguistic competence is different from other proficiencies. For instance, in singing, there is a continuum with Amy Winehouse near one end, this contributor near the other, but insoluble arguments about the ranking in between. There is a distinction between the capacity, that competence represents, and the use of that capacity in speech. Competent speakers of a language generally have no difficulty distinguishing between normal and impaired speech, and their language spoken in a variety of dialects and accents, and their expectation is that other competent speakers can do the same.

No matter how the grammar is expressed, it must be finite—like a book with so many pages and words—and acquired within the critical period. And there is an expectation that this is possible. The expectation is only surrendered under diagnoses such as Down syndrome, where competence is rarely found. This expectation, obvious to all parents, is defined by 'learnability'. There are theories about how such an acquisition module might work, with Nunes (2002) arguing that, because all languages have *featural*, *segmental*, and *prosodic* structure, it may use nothing more than these three components. But because the grammar is finite, if acquisition works separately for each aspect (phonotactics, prosody, phonemics, and rules), the finiteness has to be separately defined for each one. It is simpler to assume just one acquisition module: simple, abstract, powerful, but developmentally vulnerable.

By deduction from generative linguistics, learnability theory, and biology, the acquisition module is the most likely focus of disorder. But this is at odds with the informal RCSLT paradigm, which happens to converge with the radical liberal sociolinguistics of Labov (1966). Following such radical liberalism, defining all linguistic variables sociologically, Law (1992) emphasises developmental variation (rather than universal capacity and an end state of competence). By this disavowal of both competence and the notion of a critical period, a therapy outcome of 'improvement', rather than normal speech, becomes a legitimate, ethical, and expeditious goal, and terminating therapy at 5;0 or 6;0, long before speech acquisition is typically complete (possibly at around 9;0 according to Nunes 2002), becomes acceptable practice. This handicaps the description of developing speech and denies crucial insights that offer potential to assist and expedite intervention. One solution is to embrace and update the work of our three forgotten pioneers. Nunes (2002, 2006) describes how this can be done, not by abandoning accumulated practical wisdom or by adopting a fashionable terminology, but by invoking Chomsky's subtle insight: that the normality of acquisition is itself remarkable.

The three pioneers

Holder (1669) defined phonemes in terms of features that combined to create a 'derivation', rendering any independent existence for phonemes impossible. The features Holder identified were place, voice, nasality, continuance, sonorance in consonants, and tongue position, 'tension' and the use of the lips in vowels. He described his intervention for one boy's speech as progressing from consonant–vowel combinations repeated in sequences, such as BAH-BAY-BEE-BAW-BOO and DAH-DAY-DEE-DAW-DOO, to words. He used *theory* to justify treatment. Also theoretically driven, and several lifetimes later, Thelwall (1812) developed a theory of prosody. He treated children with various speech disorders, who would come to stay with him and his wife for months at a time, with his wife responsible for education and pastoral care.

Like Holder, Alexander Melville Bell was familiar with the speech difficulties of hearing-impaired speakers because his wife was deaf. In Bell (1849), he advanced Holder's work with fuller schedules of nonsense words for therapy and a more complete theory of distinctive features. Both Holder (1669) and Bell (1886) recognised that features had to be universal. Bell charted vowel height and 'backness' as positions on a V-shaped diagram with EE, AH, and OO at the extreme points. At the same time, he started developing 'Visible Speech', expressing features systematically, for clinical use.

The three British SLT pioneers all reasoned from theory and stressed the importance of fun and empathy with children. Their notion of featural and prosodic elements, combining in language-specific ways, provides the basis for extended series of nonsense words in therapy, foreshadowing 'possible words' in generative phonology.

Enter Henry Sweet (1845–1912). A phonetician and scholar of English, Sweet (1908) refers to the 'inestimable privilege' of having being taught by Bell, but omits him from the bibliography. Intrigued, the Irish playwright, critic, political activist, and spelling reformer George Bernard Shaw immortalized the story in the Higgins, Pickering, and Eliza trio in his 1913 *Pygmalion*. Bell's wife was Eliza, and there is Bell in Higgins and Pickering. Sweet was a Henry, and the gracelessness of Higgins is clearly his.

At the zenith of the British Empire, Sweet and Daniel Jones (1881–1967) were preoccupied with the teaching of English as a foreign language, taking no interest in impairment. Jones (1967, first published in 1918) used Bell's notion of the V to define his own idealisation of 'cardinal vowels'. His narrow elitism sacrificed the insight from Bell and Holder that features define phonemes, not vice versa. Bell and Holder were interested in universality. Jones was interested in 'educated' speech or that of 'persons educated in one of the great English public schools' (Jones 1967, p. 4). Jones artfully obliterated Bell's legacy, putting in its place a covertly prescriptive system of phonetic transcription that is unhelpful to clinical practice in a sociolinguistically complex world (Munson, A45, p. 342), where subtle judgments are needed about transcription (Müller 2006) and where the standard is neither given nor obvious.

The balance sheet

In the UK in child-speech pedagogy and clinical practice, linguistics is now replaced by a clinical linguistics that can only describe the most typical delays and disorders. It exaggerates the dichotomy between the cognitive and sensori-motor aspects of speech, and is incapable of defining the possible limits of disorder (its most severe forms). In my view, it thereby diminishes the potency and probability of success in the treatment of the very disorders that are most likely to cause lifelong communicative frustration, educational and vocational limitations, and social penalties (Van Riper 1939; Gierut 1998). Suspiciousness of theory opens the door to subjectivism, easily mistaken for the right to believe what one wants. This can allow false claims, such as those put forward by the proponents of non-speech oral motor therapies (NS-OMT), to become the cornerstones of therapy modalities (Lof, A30). A prominent British example of this is in Williams and Stephens (2004), who implausibly hold that the most problematic aspect of speech acquisition is that which is least variable, namely movement, and that the least problematic is that which is most variable, like the phonological detail of /t/ and /d/ before sonorants in unstressed syllables.

Clinical practice driven by learnability is a way of thinking and more. In the treatment of speech sound disorders (SSD), it looks for the totality of what is missing, not by counting phonemes or processes, but by clinical description of the smallest possible number of words, maybe just 10 or 20. Given an acquisition module that normally and finitely extracts a target grammar from the random accidents of the input, this should be the main initial focus of SLT/SLP clinical enquiry if there is no clear medical diagnosis or social catastrophe. Intervention can take many traditional SLT forms. But the essence is to mimic nature, subtly enhancing normal child-experience, aiming for normal speech, not as particular outputs, but as empowerment.

Suppose a child says *potato* as '*popoTAYto*' with two adjacent unstressed syllables on the left. In such speech, the acquisition module misconstrues how stress in English is mostly on *alternating* syllables. It might take a treatment session to show that non-continuance, labiality, voice, place, and schwa-features, can all go once, contrastively into one initial, unstressed syllable, followed by a particular sort of foot. So *potato* can facilitate *tomato*. The outcome is greater, faster, and more complete because the decisive events are in the child's mind. In a way consistent with current developmental psychology, the process is advanced positively by revelation, not negatively by correction. This cannot be emulated in computer software; no two children are the same; the grammar can develop in the child's mind in minutes of therapy. This cannot be devolved to parents, volunteers, classroom assistants, by worksheets, handouts, or home programs; it can only be done by skilled clinicians. It is efficient; it makes optimal use of precious time; and it leads to the most nearly complete possible outcomes.

The modern roots of therapy for children's speech

As Nunes (A3) proposes, by rights our history begins with William Holder, John Thelwall, and Alexander Melville Bell, but our swift trip will not be as rich in detail as the Duchan (2001) account. Rather, it will resemble a 'sampler tour', summarised as a timeline in Table 1.1 It provides a glimpse of the notable SLP/SLT and Linguistics influences on contemporary child speech practice, in a breakneck dash from the 1930s to the millennium and beyond. Connections are made between our history of practice and practice today.

Our timeline jumps from Holder, Thelwall, and Bell to the 1930s and Lee Edward Travis (1896–1987), whose *Speech Pathology: A Dynamic Neurological Treatment of*

Table 1.1 Timeline: Milestones in the history of children's SSD

Pioneers	William Holder (1616–1698) John Thelwall (1764–1834) Alexander Melville Bell (1819–1905)	
1931	Lee Edward Travis	'The Travis Handbook' contained one paragraph on articulation and a word list
1934	Irene Poole	Produced a developmental schedule for 'normal' articulatory proficiency
1937	Robert West	Published *The Rehabilitation of Speech*
1937	Samuel T. Orton	Published *Reading, Writing and Speech Problems in Children*
1938	Sara Stinchfield & Edna Hill-Young	Treated delayed/defective speech with a motor-kinaesthetic therapy
1939	Charles Van Riper	Developed a social theory of speech acquisition coupled with an auditory–phonetic therapy
1940	Grant Fairbanks	Published a voice/articulation drill book with listening lists and minimal pairs
1940	Theory–Therapy Gap—Research–Practice Gap	The principles of practice were often at odds with theory and research
1941	Roman Jakobson	Developed a linguistics theory of phonological universals
1943	Mildred Berry & Jon Eisenson	Linked a linguistic–mentalist acquisition theory with articulatory–motor therapy
1945	World War II ended	SLP/SLT was informed by physiology, psychology, and psychiatry (not linguistics)
1948	Kurt Goldstein	Discussed symbol formation, and this sort of thinking lead to the novel idea of 'underlying representation' and 'psycholinguistic processing' in phonology
1952	Helmur Myklebust	Used the same term: symbol formation
1957	Charles Osgood	Talked about mediation/psycho-linguistic processing
1957	Mildred Templin	Published *Certain Language Skills in Children*
1959	College of Speech Therapists	Formulated a definition of dyslalia
1959	Margaret Hall Powers	Defined functional articulation disorder
1968	Noam Chomsky & Morris Halle	Wrote SPE presenting distinctive features theory and generative phonology
1968	Jon Eisenson	Presented the notion of symbol formation
1968	Charles Ferguson	Developed contrastive analysis
1970s	American Behaviourism	3-position testing and Traditional Articulation Therapy dominated assessment and intervention
1972	Muriel Morley	Implied that 'functional articulation disorder' did not have a neuromotor basis
1973	David Stampe	Explicated natural phonology and phonological processes
1975	Pamela Grunwell	Showed the relevance to SLP/SLT of Clinical Linguistics
1976	David Ingram	Changed the SLT/SLP view of SSD with his book *Phonological Disability in Children*
1979	Frederick Weiner	Published *Phonological Process Analysis* (Test)
1980	Lawrence Shriberg and Joan Kwaitkowski	Published *Natural Process Analysis* (Test)

Table 1.1 (*Continued*)

1980	Barbara Hodson	Published *Assessment of Phonological Processes* AAP (Test)
1981	Frederick Weiner	Presented an account of conventional minimal pairs therapy
1982	Stephen E. Blache	Applied distinctive features theory to phonological assessment and therapy
1983	Barbara Hodson and Elaine Paden	Published *Targeting Intelligible Speech*: Patterns therapy/Cycles approach
1984	Dana Monahan	Published (perhaps the first) phenological Assessment and Therapy Package
1985	Pamela Grunwell	Published *Phonological Assessment of Child Speech*: PACS
1985	Marc Fey	Published the 'Inextricable constructs' article, making everybody think!
1985	Carol Stoel-Gammon and Carla Dunn	Published the groundbreaking *Normal and Disordered Phonology in Children*
1986	Elizabeth Dean and Janet Howell	Published the Developing linguistic awareness article, heralding *Metaphon*
1986	Mary Elbert and Judith Gierut	Published the *Handbook of Clinical Phonology*
1989	Gwen Lancaster and Lesley Pope	Described auditory input therapy for under 3s, and 'difficult' young clients
1990	Elizabeth Dean, Janet Howell, Anne Hill and Daphne Waters	Published *Metaphon* as an assessment and therapy resource pack
1992	Marc Fey	Headed up a challenging LSHSS clinical forum
1993	Lawrence Shriberg	Looked at development differently with the early, middle and late 8
1997	Martin Ball and Raymond Kent	Published The *New Phonologies: A Book for Clinicians and Linguists*
1997	Joy Stackhouse and Bill Wells	Published the first volume of a book series on the psycholinguistic framework
1998–1999	B. May Bernhardt and Joseph Stemberger	Developed clinical applications of non-linear phonology
2001	World Health Organization	Introduced the *International Classification of Functioning, Disability and Health* (ICF-CY)

Normal Speech and Speech Deviations (Travis 1931) contained just one paragraph on articulation therapy and a list of initial–medial–final-sound production practice words in an appendix. Although 'the Travis handbook', as it was affectionately or even reverently called, offered a minuscule contribution as far as articulation therapy was concerned, it was highly regarded as a standard text, providing outlines of the neurophysiological bases for and clinical subtypes of fluency, articulation and voice problems, and aphasia. Uninfluenced by linguistics theory, Travis presented a view of disorders that had the speech sound (or segment) as the basic unit of speech. There was a hopeful sign in the same year that more was to come with the appearance of and article by Wellman, Case, Mengert, and Bradbury (1931), reporting on the development of 'speech sounds' in young children. Publications by other American SLPs soon followed with such revealing titles as: *The Rehabilitation of Speech* (West, Kennedy, and Carr 1937), *Reading, Writing and Speech Problems in Children* (Orton 1937), and *Children with Delayed or Defective Speech: Motor-Kinesthetic Factors in Their Training* (Stinchfield and Young 1938). Robert West (1892–1968) wrote the first section of West, Kennedy, and Carr (1937) and introduced information about articulation difficulties due to oral deformities and hearing impairment. Speech remediation suggestions in the second half of the book included muscle relaxation, non-speech oral motor exercises (NS-OME), phonetic placement strategies, and drill.

There was another flurry of influential 'child speech' speech pathology publishing activity between 1939 and 1943. It started with the first of nine editions of *Speech Correction: Principles and Methods* (Van Riper 1939). Ahead of his time in many ways, Charles Van Riper (1905–1994) emphasised the significance of social context on the day-to-day experience of speech-impaired individuals, with portents of the ICF-CY (McLeod, A1). His social perspective is revealed in his famous definition: 'Speech is defective when it deviates so far from the speech of other people in the group that it calls attention to itself, interferes with communication, or causes its possessor to be maladjusted to his environment' (Van Riper 1939, p. 51). Van Riper's cultural sensitivity and inimitable insight into what he called the 'penalties' of communication impairment may have stemmed in part from his intrapersonal and interpersonal experiences of stuttering. Discussing what people with communication 'differences' might make of their social situations, and what they might perceive others to read into their symptoms, he wrote, 'The difference in itself was not so important as its interpretation by the speech defective's associates' (p. 66). Reflecting sourly on the likely reactions of the said associates, he wrote, 'Personality is not merely individuality but evaluated individuality' (p. 67). So intensely important was the social level for Van Riper that he recommend trainee speech correctionists undertake assignments, such as lisping for a day, to develop empathy for individuals with speech difficulties and appreciation of their emotional landscapes. The social aspect was present in his intervention advice, too, when he suggested that correctionists should work with *teachers and parents* in pursuing therapy goals.

Paradoxically, although Van Riper espoused and sustained a sincerely held social view of speech impairment and of disability when it came to presenting his treatment approach—classically referred to as 'Traditional Articulation Therapy' or 'Van Riper Therapy'—it could never have been regarded as communication-focused. He incorporated many disparate elements in an atomistic array of peripheral procedures that included stimulus–response routines; sensory training that he called auditory stimulation, comprising auditory discrimination, 'ear training', and auditory sequencing; and production drill. These all became part of an auditory–phonetic (or sensory–motor) therapy that is still practised today (Hegde and Pena-Brooks 2007; Raz, A4). In the same highly productive period, practical manuals, books of exercises, source books, and workbooks for the speech correctionist began to appear, replete with practise word and sentence lists, listening lists, rhymes, stories, therapy tips, advice and ideas, and techniques and activities to be used in speech lessons (Fairbanks 1940; Nemoy and Davis 1937; Robbins and Robbins 1937; Twitmeyer and Nathanson 1932).

In work whose impact was far-reaching, Irene Poole, a school speech teacher at the University Elementary School in Ann Arbor, Michigan, produced, for her doctoral research, a developmental schedule for phonetic development (Poole 1934). This was consistent with the prevailing, and persisting, view that therapy for child speech should be based on normative expectations. Other accounts of normative phonetic proficiency

Table 1.2 Developmental schedules for phonetic development

Age of acquisition[a] (Kilminster and Laird 1978)	Order of acquisition[b] (Shriberg 1993)
3;0 p b t d k g n m ŋ w j ʒ h	Early-8
3;6 f	m n j b w d p h
4;0 l ʃ tʃ	
4;6 z s dʒ	Middle-8
5;0 r	t ŋ k g f v tʃ dʒ
6;0 v	
8;0 ð	Late-8
8;6 θ	ʃ ʒ l r s z ð θ

[a] Data source: single-word citation-naming.
[b] Data source: conversational speech samples.

criteria have followed, up to the present day (McLeod 2009), including Arlt and Goodban (1976); Kilminster and Laird (1978); Prather, Hedrick, and Kern (1975); Sander (1972); Smit, Hand, Freilinger, et al. (1990), and Templin (1957). Following Poole's pioneering lead, one study of phonetic mastery (Kilminster and Laird 1978) involved single-word citation-naming by children age three to eight and a half in Queensland, Australia and determined the typical ages, in years and months, by which 75% of children had mastered 24 English phones. Most of the available developmental profiles for speech sound acquisition are similarly structured, but Shriberg (1993) took a novel approach when he produced a clinically useful breakdown of the 'early-8', 'middle-8', and 'late-8' acquired sounds, based on conversational speech samples, with 8 phones in each category. The norms provided by Kilminster and Laird, and Shriberg's early-, middle-, and late-8 are contrasted in Table 1.2.

Inconsistencies between theory, therapy, and practice

The release in 1943 of *The Defective in Speech* (Berry and Eisenson 1942) provided an alternative view, with a swing away from Van Riperian auditory perceptual and ear training, refocusing on auditory memory span, and the motor execution component of speech output, in treatment that saw the therapist administering general bodily relaxation procedures and speech musculature exercises, which today are generally referred to synonymously as non-speech oral motor exercises, oral motor therapy, oral motor treatment, or oro-motor exercises (the preferred UK term). Apparently ignoring the social context of and consequences for the client of his/her communication impairment, Berry and Eisenson wrote about the mechanism of first-language learning for the first time in the speech pathology literature. They embraced the associative–imitative model (Allport 1924) from psychology theory, conceptualising speech in linguistic–mentalist terms. But again, these insights were not reflected in their intervention suggestions. Like Van Riper's, their therapy belied any appreciation of language, and they proceeded from bottom up, starting with tongue, lip, and jaw exercises, with stimulation of individual phones, and using phonetic placement techniques and repetitive motor drill. In her analysis of these disparities, Duchan (2001) highlights the genesis of 'a familiar trait in our professional development, the theory-therapy gap' and also comments that 'a second identifiable gap was between research findings and therapy practices', pointing to a sort of interdisciplinary gap that saw speech pathologists failing to take much advantage of the developmental psychology research that flourished from the 1920s to the 1950s.

Throughout the 1940s and beyond, linguistics theory blossomed in the hands of individuals like Jakobson (1941), who studied child language, aphasia, and phonological universals; Velten (1943), who investigated in the growth of phonemic and lexical patterns in infants; and Leopold (1947), who explored sound learning in the first two years of life. These developments in linguistics later proved highly relevant to practice, but, during and immediately following World War II, the profession tended towards physiology, psychology, and psychiatry for elucidation, and not linguistics or education. By the 1950s, however, the literature revealed that thinkers knew something more was going on in speech besides auditory, visual, and tactile perception and motor execution of sounds. The idea of an inner process or underlying representation as a clinical construct was imminent. Eisenson (1968) talked about symbol formation, Goldstein (1948) and Myklebust (1952) alluded to inner language, and Osgood (1957) used two terms: mediation and psycholinguistic processing.

Dyslalia or functional speech disorder

SLP/SLT was a young profession when SSD were called 'dyslalia' or 'functional articulation disorders'. In its *Terminology for Speech Pathology*, the College of Speech Therapists (1959) defined dyslalia as: 'Defects of articulation, or slow development of articulatory *patterns*, including: substitutions, distortions, omissions and transpositions of the sounds of speech.' Almost simultaneously in the US, Powers (1959, p. 711) defined it, with a different name, using the word 'functional' in its medical pathology connotation 'of currently unknown origin' or 'involving functions rather than a physiological or structural cause'. Powers said: 'The term functional articulation disorder encompasses a wide variety of deviate speech *patterns*. These can be described in terms of four possible types of acoustic deviations in the individual speech sounds: omissions, substitutions, distortions, and additions. An individual may show one or any combination of these deviations.' How interesting it is to find that as early as 1959 SLPs in Britain and the US had an agreed definition and terminology and included the notion of speech *patterns* when they described speech development and disorders. Nonetheless, it must be remembered that they did so without taking into account speech sounds' organisation and representation, cognitively. The 'phoneme' and constructs like it were the domain of clinical linguistics, and it would not be until twenty years or more after the formulation of the British and American definitions that the beginnings of a practical assessment and 'therapy connection' (Grunwell 1975; Ingram 1976) would be forged between phonological theory and SLP practice.

In Britain and Australia, the designation dyslalia remained in vogue until the 1960s, when the preferred American term, functional articulation disorder, gained currency. The ongoing preoccupation of therapists, in the 1960s through to the mid-1970s, with individual sounds in the so-called 'three positions' (initial, medial, and final) still constituted a strictly phonetic approach to the problem and somehow isolated the linguistic function of speech from the mechanics or motoric aspects of speech. It is enlightening to return to Grunwell's 1975 critique of contemporary practice and her proposal for a more linguistically principled approach to assessment and remediation than the ones that had evolved from practice in the 1930s.

Functional articulation disorders were graded in severity as mild, moderate, or severe. In the severe category were the children with 'multiple dyslalia' or 'multiple misarticulations' whose speech was generally unintelligible to people outside of their immediate families. It was readily acknowledged that children with severe functional articulation disorders could usually imitate or quickly be taught how to produce most speech sounds (Morley 1972). In other words, the supposed motor execution problem or 'articulation' disorder appeared to reside in the children's difficulty in employing speech sounds for word production, which they could produce in isolation. Intervention concentrated on the mechanical aspects of establishing the production of individual phonemes, one at a time, context by context. By defining the problem in articulatory terms, and focussing in therapy on speech and accuracy of production, SLPs/SLTs failed to take into account something that they already knew: that speech serves as the spoken medium of language in a system of contrasts and combinations that signal meaning-differences. That is, when children are acquiring the agreed pronunciation patterns of a language and learning the correspondences between articulatory *movements* and sounds, they also discover relationships between *meanings* and sounds.

Linguistic theory and sound patterns

The linguistic linkage that enticed speech-language clinicians to consider speech disorders in terms of sound systems or patterns came about when researchers in the area of generative linguistics, Chomsky and Halle (1968), expounded distinctive features theory in *The Sound Patterns of English*, a book so famous and influential in linguistics circles that it is commonly referred to simply as SPE. Contemporaneously, Ferguson (1968) looked at contrastive speech analysis and phonological development (see also Ferguson 1978; Ferguson and Farwell 1975; Ferguson, Peizer, and Weeks 1973). Then, Stampe (1973, 1979) forged another link, but this time in the area of natural phonology; leading most saliently for us to Ingram and his innovative work (Ingram 1974, 1976) uniquely dedicated to the understanding of disordered speech. Finally, what had been interpreted by SLPs/SLTs as multiple individual errors came to be seen as sound class problems, involving multiple members of those classes. From this solid beginning, grounded in scholarship, stemmed the development of clinical applications of phonology—linear and, in due course, non-linear (Bernhardt and Stemberger 1998, 2000) quickly acquiring in the process both an international and a cross-disciplinary flavour.

But, we have to remind ourselves that all of this clinically relevant information emerged in the 1970s environment in which practice was still heavily influenced by the medical model and American Behaviorism; 'SODA' articulation analysis of errors of (S) substitution, (O) omission, (D) distortion, and (A) addition; and 'Traditional Articulation Therapy'. This therapy, or at least close variations of it, is still widely implemented today. For example, Mirla Raz, an experienced licensed speech pathologist certified by the American Speech-Language-Hearing Association, regularly uses the approach in her practice. Furthermore, she has written three workbooks, intended for clinicians, aides, and parents working with children with SSD and marketed on the Internet.

Q4.   Mirla G. Raz: A clinician's interpretation of 'Van Riper therapy'

Your *Help Me Talk Right* workbooks (Raz 1993, 1996, 1999) have their roots in the so-called 'traditional approach' to articulation assessment and intervention. These sound-by-sound hierarchical therapies still have a place in the speech and language clinician's repertoire, but perhaps not always in a form that would be instantly recognisable to Van Riper (1978). Can you provide an account of the way you implement traditional assessment and therapy for the later developing sounds (/s/, /l/, and /r/), explaining what attracts you, as an experienced SLP, to use this methodology. What have you retained from the original Van Riper methodology. What, if anything, have you discarded or added? Are there ethical concerns associated with selling 'self-help' articulation workbooks directly to consumers whose children may or may not have received diagnosis by a certified SLP/SLT?

A4.   Mirla G. Raz: One clinician's streamlining of traditional articulation therapy

In my first job as a SLP in the US in the mid-1970s, I serviced three schools in a public school district, where the majority of my clients could not say /r/, /l/, and/or /s/. Suddenly everything I learned, as a Master's level speech pathology student, had to be put into practice. But which approach was best? Stumped, I turned to my supervisor. She suggested an adaptation of the 'traditional' approach to articulation therapy described by Charles Van Riper in *Speech Correction: Principles and Methods* (Van Riper 1939) and subsequently with John V. Irwin in *Voice and Articulation* (Van Riper and Irwin 1958). The 1958 book informs my implementation of traditional therapy.

In the Van Riper and Irwin approach, a sound is targeted sequentially: in isolation, syllables, words, and, finally, in 'normal speech'. The authors emphasise the 'corrector function', with the first therapy task being '. . . to make our case interested in the articulation of others, to make him learn to listen to the exact sound sequences of words spoken by his therapist and friends.' They also stress 'searching for the target', with the tongue exploring the mouth, in 'tongue training exercises', 'babbling' or 'random, relaxed, free vocalizations', 'modification of other sounds', and phonetic placement through 'hunting.' When 'hunting', clients experiment with tongue placement until they hit on the target. They explain, 'Like the hunter who targets his rifle, the articulation case must learn to get the range, then shoot a series of shots to the right and left and up and down, until he knows exactly where to adjust the sights' (p.138). Once 'found', the target is 'fixated' in key words through drill.

> The teacher writes the word on one of several cards (or pictures representing it). Then she asks the student to go through the series one at a time, saying the word on each card ten times. Finally, the special word to be used is repeated a hundred times, accenting, and prolonging, if possible, the sound which in other words is made incorrectly. (p. 148)

Finally, the client enters the 'terminal therapy' phase, during which stabilisation of the sound is emphasised under conditions of speed (increased tempo) and various emotions.

Although the traditional hierarchy was appealing, there were several niggling questions. Can anyone 'make' a child interested in the speech of others, and is it necessary? If it is necessary, I speculated, might it not be more effective to *demonstrate* how the child's production of a sound differed from standard production? Why require children to search for phonetic placement when it can be easily taught? Why administer tongue exercises when they are valueless (Lof 2003)? What is the point of boring, unchallenging drill? Might it be more time-efficient to move to the next level once a child showed proficiency at the level just mastered (let us say 80% proficiency with 20 different words, where 'proficiency' implies accurate production of the target at a specified level: single sound, syllable, word, phrase, or sentence)? Further, might therapy sessions be used more efficiently if sounds were stabilised over time, with increasing *contextual* challenges, up to and including the conversational level rather than with different speech-rates and emotions?

With the benefit of clinical experience, I found satisfactory answers, for me as a therapist, to these questions and in the process developed a system of sound correction that I felt was more streamlined than the original. My hierarchy moves from the target sound in: (1) isolation, (2) CVs and VCs, (3) word pairs, (4) simple sentences, (5) the within word position, (6) clusters, (7) random sentences, (8) elicited conversations, and (9) conversational speech. Here follow examples of stimuli for my additional steps.

- Target /s/ in word pairs and simple sentences: 'see seven', 'pass dress', and 'I see a seven'
- Target /r/ within words and in clusters: 'carrot', 'turtle', 'green', and 'scrub'
- Target /l/ randomly in sentences: 'The pilot flew the plane.'
- Target /l/ in elicited conversation: The therapist manipulates input to encourage the child to use the target conversationally. For instance, playing an airport game, I might ask, 'Who flies the plane?' to elicit 'pilot'.

Case example

On initial assessment in July 2007, 'Aaron', 6;3 achieved receptive and expressive standard scores of 81 and 76 on the PLS-3 (Zimmerman, Steiner, and Pond 1991). His expressive vocabulary (Williams 1997) was poor. His literacy skills, according to his parents and teacher, were well-below grade level, although his score on the Lindamood Auditory Conceptualization Test (Lindamood and Lindamood 1979) was grade-appropriate. Aaron's speech was characterised by /w/ for /r/ and /f/ for /θ/ replacements, and interdental production of the alveolars /s/, /z/, /l/, /n/, /t/, and /d/, which I felt could be corrected as a sound class.

Therapy began in August 2007. Aaron was seen individually for 45-minute sessions, which were increased to 60-minute sessions. Receptive and expressive language (including vocabulary), reading, and the alveolars were targeted in each session with approximately 10-15 minutes devoted to his speech for the first six sessions, and 20 minutes in sessions 7–9. Thereafter, errors were corrected incidentally while we worked on other areas of deficit during the 60-minute sessions. In all, approximately 5 face-to-face hours over 27 sessions were devoted to correcting his alveolars, plus time spent on homework. By session 27, his sound targets were used conversationally in all obligatory contexts.

In therapy session 1, I explained to Aaron what his error was and, using imagery, what he needed to do to correct it. He had to 'keep the tiger (his tongue) in the cage (his teeth closed)'. Aaron practised saying the six targets in isolation, remembering to 'keep the tiger in the cage'. As this was easy, I immediately introduced production of CVs and VCs. As the session progressed, I increased the challenge to producing the targets SIWI (e.g., 'took', 'dip', sick'), avoiding words with the targets word-finally (e.g., 'lot'). In session 2, I noted that he had maintained the ability to produce the targets SIWI, so words with the targets SFWF (e.g., 'kiss' and 'ball') were introduced. Before long, he could produce the targets initially *and* finally in the same word (e.g., 'lace' and 'date'). By session 3, Aaron easily produced word pairs (e.g., 'see soup' and 'pass bell'), so we advanced to simple sentences with targets SIWI and SFWF, continuing this in session 4. By session 5, at single word level, he was producing the targets within words and in initial consonant clusters. Progress was steady, so in sessions 5 and 6, we worked on the sounds in random sentences. Elicited conversation in play began in session 7, using airport and space centre games and characters and 'setting him up' to produce utterances containing all targets. Elicited conversation continued in sessions 8–10. With targets produced with 30% accuracy by session 11, Aaron was ready for a motivational program to encourage generalisation to conversation. His mother was provided with typewritten instructions on modelling and a photocopy of the motivational home program from Raz (1993), encouraging revisions and repairs and instating a simple reinforcement schedule, using pennies as rewards. All targets were in 100% use conversationally by session 13. Correct alveolar production continued in sessions 14 and 15, so Aaron was allowed to select a toy from the toy chest. His father had already purchased a longed-for DVD as Aaron's reward for completing this aspect of therapy, and when I said the word, he presented it to him!

Homework was complicated because Aaron's parents are divorced and share custody. In all sessions, I wrote the homework in his speech notebook. He attended once weekly with his mother, with whom he lives most of the time, and once weekly with his father or one of his paternal grandparents. His mother observed three sessions, but this was avoided because Aaron became demanding and clingy with her. His grandmother did not observe, but his father and grandfather sat in when they attended. When his mother came, a few minutes at the ends of sessions were devoted to explaining the homework. Homework was designed to take 10 minutes daily, increasing to 20-minute elicited conversation sessions with his mom. Prior to each therapy session, Aaron's mom reported on homework, always commenting that he had co-operated and performed well.

Discussion

Motivational program

When introducing a motivational program, I talk to children about using their sound(s) *all* the time. I tell them it is really their responsibility to remember to use their sound at home, at school, and when talking to friends. If they forget, I or their parents (if that can be arranged) will remind them. To further motivate them, I tell them that whenever they use their sound in the therapy room, they will earn a chip (to put in a cup decorated with a happy face) and the number of chips they need to earn in that session. For instance, in motivational session 1, children must use the target three times in order to earn three chips. This increases to five chips in the next session. I continue to adjust the reinforcement, increasing the challenge in each consecutive session, to a maximum of 15 chips. Earning the minimum number of chips or better for that session earns them a candy or small toy. Once successfully using the target conversationally, a child selects a toy from my treasure chest, as Aaron did.

Parent involvement

Motivational programs work best, I believe, with parental involvement. I discuss, by phone or in person, what motivates their child: pennies, stars, happy faces, a favourite toy, or treat? We also explore what *they* can do to help the child focus on using the target habitually. Once the child is successful in integrating the target into conversational speech, I encourage parents to provide a special reward, such as a restaurant meal or a toy that the child wants.

Homework

As with Aaron, the goal of speech homework is to reinforce and carry-over what a child accomplishes in therapy sessions. For example, if a child produced a target SIWI, the picture sheet used is sent home with written instructions in his/her homework notebook. This is done for every session, whether parents work with the child or not.

Parent-administered therapy

In a tightly regulated and 'ethics driven' profession like SLP/SLT, the question arises of whether there are ethical concerns associated with selling 'self-help' articulation workbooks (e.g., Raz 1993, 1996, 1999) directly to consumers to use with their own children, whose speech may or may not have been assessed by a SLP/SLT. The overriding issue, I believe, is what happens to children for whom there are no viable alternatives. Ultimately, it is important that the child benefits, even if it is the parents who do the therapy. Unfortunately, for many children, therapy administered by a speech and language professional is not an option. Many school districts in the US offer therapy only for problems that negatively impact *educational* outcomes. A misarticulated sound or two does not necessarily qualify a child for speech services (ASHA 2004a). Some home-schooling parents elect not to access school-based services. Furthermore, there are families who cannot afford, cannot travel to, or do not wish to avail themselves of private practitioner services. The goal of the *Help Me Talk Right* books (Raz 1993, 1996, 1999) is to provide such parents with a structured approach to the remediation of their children's /l/, /r/, /s/, and /z/ difficulties.

There are four final points I would like to highlight. First, feedback from parents (which can be viewed at the Web site http://www.speechbooks.com) about the books has been uniformly positive. Second, had they been available, the books would have been of great help to *me* when I first started out as a clinician. Third, the books can be used by para-professionals (speech assistants). And fourth, most of the *Help Me Talk Right* books have been purchased by speech pathologists and school districts, so for me there is tremendous satisfaction in knowing that the books are accepted by colleagues in our profession and are used in their work.

Clinical phonology

In the 1970s, linguists and academic and clinical SLPs/SLTs were talking to each other about language in general and clinical phonology in particular. For phonologists Pamela Grunwell and David Ingram, there was a clear mission to help the SLP/SLT profession in the practical application of phonological principles to the treatment of children with 'phonological disability': and many clinicians, the author included, devoured every word they wrote! Clinical phonology, according to Grunwell (1987), a British linguist working in the UK, was the clinical application of linguistics at the phonological level. Ingram (1989a), an American located in Canada at the time, considered that phonology embraced the study of: (1) the nature of the underlying representations of speech sounds (how they are stored in the mind); (2) the nature of the phonetic representations (how the sounds are articulated); and (3) phonological rules or processes (the mapping rules that connect the two). To complete the international (but English language) flavour of all of this, in the US, Stoel-Gammon and Dunn (1985) provided further theoretically principled guidance in a book about assessment and therapy, as did Elbert and Gierut (1986).

From a therapy point of view, the most radical aspect of the new principles was their focus on changing phonological patterns by stimulating children's underlying systems for phoneme use. There was an apprehensive feeling abroad in the clinical community that, because of the theoretical paradigm shift, therapeutic approaches, intervention goals, and therapy procedures and activities should now be different, or at least revamped. Fey (1985, p. 255) answered these concerns and uncertainties in a reassuring article, in which he wrote:

> . . . adopting a phonological approach to dealing with speech sound disorders does not necessitate the rejection of the well-established principles underlying traditional approaches to articulation disorders. To the contrary, articulation must be recognized as a critical aspect of speech sound development under any theory. Consequently phonological principles should be viewed as adding new dimensions and new perspectives to an old problem, not simply as refuting established principles. These new principles have resulted in the development of several procedures that differ in many respects from old procedures, yet are highly similar in others.

What revolution?

Did the hackneyed term 'paradigm shift' (Kuhn 1962) overstate what actually happened? *Was* there a phonological revolution? *Did* the new principles change practice? Certainly there were changes in the way assessments were being conducted (Grunwell 1975, 1985a; Hodson 1980; Ingram 1981; Shriberg and Kwiatkowski 1980; Weiner 1979), but did the *intervention* work of Elbert, Dunn, Gierut, Grunwell, Hodson, Ingram, Paden, Stoel-Gammon, and others alter what happened in therapy? The answer probably has to be, 'not much'. As recently as December 2004, when Barbara Williams Hodson, co-developer in the mid-1980s of patterns or cycles therapy (Hodson and Paden 1983, 1991), was asked in an online interview for *Thinking Big News* (Thinking Publications 2004): 'If you could change one thing in how SLPs work with clients what would it be?' Her response was: 'The one thing I wish most is that SLPs would work on patterns when serving an unintelligible child, rather than to focus on teaching isolated sounds to a criterion.' This resonated with something she wrote some 12 years before (Hodson 1992, p. 247) about the relative lack of application of phonological principles, by North American SLPs to either assessment or intervention:

My own observation, based on interactions with practising clinicians while giving clinical phonology presentations in some 40 states and 5 Canadian provinces, is that even now in the early 90s, only about 10% of the practising clinicians across the United States and Canada seem to be incorporating any phonological principles in their assessment and/or remediation.

Dr. Barbara Hodson is a Professor and Doctoral Program Coordinator at Wichita State University. A Fellow of ASHA, in 2004, she received the ASHF Frank Kleffner Lifetime Clinical Achievement Award. In A5 she discusses the continuing adherence by many therapists to sound-by-sound therapy.

Q5. Barbara Hodson: A therapy that focuses on phonological patterns

In the preface of *Evaluating and Enhancing Children's Phonological Systems: Research and Theory to Practice* (Hodson 2007, p. 177), there are echoes of the statements you made in 1992 and 2004, warning colleagues of the pitfalls for severely and profoundly involved clients, of focusing on individual phonemes (e.g., /f/ as a singleton) until mastery as opposed to cycling patterns. You go on to write:

> *Most treatment programs are phoneme-oriented. The majority of these focus on mastering each phoneme before progressing to the next target. Some use contrastive techniques (e.g., minimal pairs, maximal oppositions, multiple oppositions). A few target word structures, referred to as 'phonotactic' by Velleman (2002). Our preference for children with severe/profound disordered expressive phonological systems is to target patterns that are deficient, including word structures related to omissions (e.g., /s/ clusters, final consonants) as well as phoneme categories (e.g., velars, stridents). Phonemes are considered to be a means to an end rather than the true targets.*

Given the empirical evidence for Cycles (for a review, see Baker, Carrigg, and Linich 2007), it really is unfathomable that this still needs to be said. How do you account for the apparent reluctance of so many clinicians to abandon hierarchical therapies based around phonetic execution, and how would you convince them of the advantages, for the client, of doing so?

A5. Barbara W. Hodson: Enhancing phonological *patterns* to expedite intelligibility gains

Most likely, it is not as much that SLPs/SLTs have a reluctance to abandon phoneme-oriented traditional therapy, as Q5 suggests, as it is that a good many apparently do not really know how or exactly what to do differently to facilitate the development of phonological patterns in children with highly unintelligible speech. Recent graduates, as well as veteran practitioners, have informed me during numerous national and international presentations over the past three decades that the common practice in their college SSD/phonology classes has been for professors to discuss a number of treatment approaches briefly, but not to really help students learn how to implement phonological approaches. This information was the impetus for Hodson (2007).

SLPs/SLTs also report that many professionals who supervise university clinical and school practicum experiences remain focused on having all children with speech sound errors, including those with highly unintelligible speech, master each phoneme one at a time (e.g., to 90% criterion). We do know that virtually every treatment approach helps children improve their speech (Ingram 1983). The issue remains, however, that we need to expedite intelligibility gains so that children have adequate phonological/metaphonological skills necessary for success in literacy (Larrivee and Catts 1999). Literacy difficulties have been found to correlate strongly with phonological deficiencies (Gillon 2004). Children with severely disordered phonological systems have repeatedly experienced difficulties in the area of phonological awareness (Gillon 2004), phonological representation (Nathan, Stackhouse, Goulandris, et al. 2004; Stackhouse 1997), reading (Bird, Bishop, and Freeman 1995), and spelling (Clarke-Klein and Hodson 1995).

Time considerations

If a child has only a few sounds in error, targeting one phoneme at a time to mastery seems to suffice. Children with numerous phonological deviations and unintelligible speech, however, typically require years of treatment when targeting phoneme by phoneme to mastery (personal communications). Time is critical for children with disordered phonological systems. According to the Critical Age Hypothesis (Bishop and Adams 1990), children need to be intelligible by age 5;6 or literacy acquisition most certainly will be hindered. It must be noted, however, that simply being intelligible does not guarantee literacy acquisition, because other factors (e.g., dyslexia, hearing loss) may also be involved.

Assessment considerations

Another concern pertains to clinicians and researchers still relying mostly on phoneme-oriented assessment measures (e.g., Goldman and Fristoe 2000) that do not differentiate between omissions, substitutions, and distortions in the scores (Prezas and Hodson 2007). A common practice is to note the number of phonemes in error in the final tally, with all types of errors receiving equal weighting. Thus, a child with distortions often appears to be as severe as a child with the same number of omissions, even though omissions have a much more deleterious effect on intelligibility and underlying phonological representations. Moreover, children's improvement over time is often 'clouded' by phoneme-oriented tools (Velleman 2005). It is imperative that assessment measures differentiate types of errors and also document improvement over time (Hodson 2003, 2004).

Evidence considerations

Evidence for the effectiveness of a modified Cycles Phonological Remediation Approach (with minimal pairs) has been provided by group studies (Almost and Rosenbaum 1998), and the effectiveness of the Cycles approach (unmodified) has also been reported in a number of case studies (Hodson 1997). Moreover, videos are available demonstrating dramatic changes in intelligibility of children after approximately 40-50 contact hours in less than 2 years (Hodson 2005). Kamhi (2006b) stated that the Cycles Approach combines an 'efficient goal attack strategy with traditional speech therapy and metaphonological activities' (p. 275) and appears to be 'effective', but he noted that more research is needed to investigate efficiency aspects. Clearly, a large, randomised, well-designed, controlled study comparing results of approaches (e.g., oral motor, contrasts, patterns, phoneme mastery) for highly unintelligible children is needed—with the proponents of the respective methods being involved for fidelity, but with independent investigators conducting the study.

Summary comments

Even though phonological analyses and phonological intervention approaches often require greater knowledge, skills, and effort, we must provide the most efficacious services possible for all clients. Moreover, helping a young child with highly unintelligible speech to develop the phonological/metaphonological abilities necessary for success in school is one of the most rewarding experiences an SLP/SLT can have.

> *. . . it is notable that the development and acceptance of new revelations within our profession is a surprisingly slow process. Many individuals are just now encountering the concept of the Cycles Approach for the first time almost 30 years after it was introduced. In a broader sense, that ours is a healthy profession is revealed in that the search for knowledge and improvement in service delivery is never-ending. May this ever continue to be the case for our healthy, inquisitive profession.*

(Paden 2007)

Models of phonological acquisition

It has become axiomatic in the literature to say that, because so little is known about normal phonological development, a cohesive and convincing linguistic theory of phonological disorders has yet to be formulated. Ingram (1989a) surveyed various attempts in the field of linguistics to construct a phonological theory that covered both normal and disordered phonological acquisition, indicating that the most likely sources of elucidation of *normal* acquisition might be universalist/structuralist theory (Jakobson 1941/1968), natural phonology theory (Stampe 1969), or the Stanford cognitive model (Macken and Ferguson 1983). Of the three, only Stampe's was directly tied to a phonological theory.

The behaviourist model

The behaviourist model dominated linguistics from the 1950s to the early 1970s. It applied a psychological theory of learning to explain how children came to distinguish and produce the sound system of the ambient language. Its adherents, like Mowrer (1952, 1960), Murai (1963), and Olmstead (1971), identified the role of contingent reinforcement in gradually 'shaping' a child's babbling to meaningful adult forms through classical conditioning. An important aspect of the model was the emphasis on *continuity* between babbling and early speech. The behaviourists believed that the infant came to associate the vocalisations of the mother (usually) with primary reinforcements, such as food and nurture, with adults' vocalisations assuming secondary reinforcement status. Eventually, the infant's vocalisations would become secondary reinforcers (providing self-reinforcement) due to their similarity to adult models. From this point, the caregiver could refine the sound repertoire of the infant through selective reinforcement. The behaviourist framework did not presuppose, or indeed show any interest in, an innate order of speech sound acquisition. The sounds acquired depended on the reinforcement obtained from the linguistic environment.

The structuralist model

The structuralist model (Jakobson 1941/1968), which stemmed from structuralist linguistic theory, proposed *discontinuity* between babbling and speech. In addition, the structuralists postulated an innate, universal order of acquisition, with distinctive features emerging hierarchically and predictably. Jakobson regarded babbling as a random activity virtually unrelated to the development of the sound system. Research evidence of regularities in prelinguistic vocal patterns (Ferguson and Macken 1980; Oller, Wieman, Doyle, et al. 1976) has, however, weakened this position. As well, mid-1970s research challenged Jakobson's hypothesis of a sequence of phonemic oppositions as the basis for the earliest stages of phonological development. Kiparsky and Menn (1977) demonstrated that the child's word count is too small to provide objective evidence of the distinctive features 'unfolding' in the way proposed by Jakobson. Really, the developmental order of phonemic oppositions has proved difficult to ascertain, because analysis has to take into account the adult targets attempted as well as the child's phonetic repertoire. To complicate matters, children seem to selectively *avoid* saying words containing certain consonants that are difficult for them to produce (Ferguson and Farwell 1975; Schwartz and Leonard 1982). Studies of evidence of lexical avoidance (or 'lexical selection') lent weight to the theory that, in the first-50-words-stage, children target whole words (Ingram 1989a, pp. 17-22). The phonetic variability readily observed in children in the 9- to 18-month age range may also provide evidence against a universal order of phoneme acquisition. Irrespective of such shortcomings, Jakobson's views exerted a tremendous, enduring influence on linguist thought. Ingram (1989a) for one, counted the structuralist model as one of the 'most likely candidates' (p. 162) for a theory of normal phonological acquisition. He talks about this in A6.

Dr. David Ingram received his PhD from Stanford University in 1970, where he studied language universals under Professor Joseph Greenberg and phonological acquisition in children under Professor Charles Ferguson. His interest in language disorders was developed during two subsequent years as a Research Associate at the Scottish Rite Institute for Childhood Aphasia. He was a professor at the University of British Columbia from 1972 to 1998 and has been a professor at Arizona State University since 1998. His research is on language acquisition in typically developing children and children with language and phonological disorders. The focus is on both English-speaking children and children acquiring other languages. The language areas of primary interest to him are phonological, morphological, and syntactic acquisition. He has published over 100 articles and is particularly known for his seminal work, *Phonological Disability in Children* (1976), and his comprehensive textbook, *First Language Acquisition* (1989).

Q6.   David Ingram: Theory and SSD

Can you comment on this quotation from Powell, Elbert, Miccio, et al. (1998) who said, 'Perhaps we err in our attempt to find a single theory to support all of our work with children with phonological disorders. When we acknowledge the heterogeneity of this target population, we are logically moving towards acknowledging that different theoretical approaches may have to guide our work with different subgroups. We seem to have moved past the more simplistic "one theory fits all" view.' It is a moot point in SLP/SLT circles whether clinicians spend much time thinking about theories, but most clinicians probably incorporate into their 'theory of intervention' (Fey 1992b) the idea that you cannot work effectively with children with SSD unless you have a good grasp of normal development. In this context, the notion of 'typical acquisition' is usually around age-of-acquisition and order-of-acquisition schedules that focus on surface forms and not much to do with theories of development and models of phonology. Do you continue to regard the structuralist model as a frontrunner in the formulation of a theory of normal phonological acquisition (Ingram 1989a), and what are the other contenders? How do you see a theory of acquisition informing the development of theories of disorder and intervention, and how can clinicians use this information?

A6. David Ingram: The role of theory in SSD

This quotation by Powell, Elbert, Miccio, et al. (1998) is a well-intended comment on the complexity of determining a theoretical account of children's SSD. The effort to do so has a long history of moving from simpler to more complex explanations. Originally, SLP began with little if any theory, treating speech sound errors as errors with individual sounds, and subsequent treatments based on the intuitively reasonable assumption that improvement would result from drill and repetition. These early efforts were supported by subsequent acceptance in many circles of behaviourism, a movement clearly described in the present book.

With the demise of behaviourism (Chomsky 1959), a new era of linguistic explanations emerged, with the result over time being a daunting range of possible theoretical accounts (c.f. summaries in Ball and Kent 1997). In the 1970s, the field of SLP was sympathetic to these efforts, and the proposals have constituted major sections of most textbooks since (Stoel-Gammon and Dunn 1985; Bauman-Waengler 2004). At least two potential problems arose with these efforts at theoretical explanation. For one, phonological theories became more and more complex and abstract, and de facto harder to assimilate and make clinically relevant. Second, no clear theoretical approach has won out, in the sense of demonstrating it is, without argument, the best and clinically most relevant account. The positive from all this is the impression that a range of approaches 'work' (with some debate whether one or another might be even more effective). The Powell et al. suggestion captures this state of the art. That is, they reflect the impression: (1) that many theories have shown success, and (2) that children with a range of speech sound problems respond to different approaches. This leads the authors to the intuitively reasonable conclusion that specific theories, and their subsequent treatment approaches, may work better for some disorders than others.

Like behaviourism, however, this intuitively reasonable assumption is wrong. It errs on both the side of treatment and the side of theory. Concerning treatment, it is certainly good news that a range of treatment approaches work and also good news that SLPs/SLTs know them. There is the implication, however, that a reasonable arsenal of treatment approaches is sufficient to treat SSD. Unfortunately, a range of available treatment approaches is no guarantee of future success without some theoretical grounding. There is no foundation to the prediction that what worked with one child will work with another child, just because the two children appear to be similar based on some assessment. Nor does it make sense simply to run a child through the approaches until one clicks. We need to understand the disorders better than that, and a better understanding can only come from a sound theoretical approach.

Let me try to make this more concrete. Let's say I am a practicing SLP with excellent skills at two quite different treatment approaches. On the one hand, I am very experienced in using a cycles approach (in a group setting) with target selection based on using developmentally appropriate sounds. At the same time, I am also well trained at using a maximal contrast approach, involving intense one-on-one intervention with target sounds well beyond the child's current developmental level. On Tuesday, I evaluate two children, Barbara and Judy. I conclude from my clinical intuitions that Barbara will benefit from a cycles model, whereas Judy will be best served with the maximal contrast therapy.

At one level, this is evidence-based practice. When I meet with Barbara's parents, I will discuss the cycles approach and refer to Hodson (2004) and other references as needed. When meeting with Judy's parents, however, my justification will be through discussing work by Gierut (2001) and the references therein. I will also be doing exactly what Powell et al. suggest, that is, moving past the simplistic 'one theory fits all' view. I will rely on my clinical experience over many years of practice, an invaluable part of my decision-making process. Given the latitude afforded to me by Powell et al., I also have one additional option. If one or both children don't meet my treatment goals, I can just switch them to the other approach. Or, if I get to attend a national convention in the interim, I can bring home a new approach I might learn at a workshop there. I have also satisfied Powell et al. by not thinking too much about theories throughout the whole process.

Is what I have just described 'best' practice? I don't think so. The bottom line is that knowing a range of treatment approaches and selecting from them as needed for specific subgroups is not sufficient. There needs to be a single theoretical basis for these decisions. In Ingram and Ingram (2001), we discuss a situation similar to the one above. We offer the hypothesis that there may be two subgroups of children with SSD: one with poor whole-word skills and one with good whole-word skills. The former group will be children with poor intelligibility, who are having difficulties matching their speech sounds to the target models. The latter group, on the other hand, are matching the target words relatively well (over 50% of the segments) but are possibly delayed in terms of their speech. We go on to suggest that the former children are candidates for a developmental approach, such as the one described for Barbara. The latter children, however, with good matching skills, may respond well to the maximal contrast approach as mentioned for Judy. Importantly, these decisions follow a single theory, a theory that incorporates whole-word abilities into our account of how children acquire their phonological systems. Within this theory, it makes sense to select the treatments as mentioned, and no sense to do it the opposite way.

Turning to the implications about theories by Powell et al., they make a false assumption about what theories are about. While referring to the 'one approach fits all' view as simplistic, they replace it with a Rodney King 'why can't we all get along' view. Rodney King was an American whose arrest was videotaped and found to include an excessive use of force by the police. This quote was his response to the arrest. He later went on to make significant contributions to the American civil rights movement. Oops, that was Martin Luther King.

Here's an example of how this point of view could be applied. In Ingram (1989a), I contrast two theories of language acquisition: a maturational approach and a constructionist (Piagetian) approach. These theories make very different claims about how language is acquired. For example, it is known that certain syntactic constructions are acquired late, for example, more complex forms of passive sentences. A maturational account would say that this is because the grammatical principles needed to form passive sentences do not mature until later, say age 6. A constructionist approach would predict that these sentences could be acquired earlier through the right combination of exposure to them and internal developments of the child's language acquisition.

Can these theories co-exist? They can, according to Powell et al. Let's again turn to a concrete example from speech sounds disorders. We know that children acquire certain English sounds late, such as the dental fricatives. On Wednesday, I assess two four-year-olds, both referred with problems with these fricatives and a concern that intervention may be appropriate. I reach the following conclusions. One child, Dan, strikes me as very constructionist in his learning, whereas the other child, Tom, appears maturational. My recommendations are as follows. Dan will start an intervention program where we will use auditory bombardment to stimulate his acquisition of the dental fricatives. We will work on a selective vocabulary with these sounds, which in turn will lead to internal gains in his language knowledge. Poor Tom, however, cannot learn these sounds because his speech development needs to mature. No amount of intervention will help Tom, who will be left alone to acquire these sounds at age six when his maturation is complete. If this makes sense to you, there's some land in Florida I'd like to talk to you about.

The Rodney King approach underlies a basic misunderstanding that somehow theories can co-exist. Here's one further demonstration of this misconception. Let's consider a theory of phonological acquisition that proposes children use phonological processes to simplify speech. This theory has many processes, including Fronting (which changes k to t, e.g., 'key' is [ti]), and Backing (which changes t to k, e.g., 'tea' is [ki]). Another theory, NeoJakobson Theory, says that children's productions reflect their underlying distinctive features. This theory allows Fronting, but not Backing, as a natural process. On Thursday, I assess two children: one who shows Fronting (David) and one who is doing Backing (Caroline). My conclusions are that David is using the phonological process theory to acquire his speech sounds, whereas Caroline is using the NeoJakobson theory. Again, this is nonsense. The problem with the phonological process theory (as stated) is that it makes up any process it needs, and is therefore too powerful. By explaining everything, it explains nothing. The more restricted theory is to be preferred. How then, can the NeoJakobson Theory account for our data? The theory states that children's first feature distinction is between a labial consonant and a non-labial consonant. The first non-labial consonant can either be a [t] or a [k]. Most children will opt for the [t], a more common sound in early productions, and this choice is the predicted, or unmarked, sound. Some children, however, may select to produce [k] instead, since it still has the same underlying value of the [t], that is, both being non-labial. This becomes, therefore, the less common, or more marked, choice. It is not always easy to evaluate theories and decide that one is more explanatory than the other, but the bottom line is that such evaluations are the way theories are assessed, not by saying they all happily coexist.

If I am to stand by and defend the simplistic (sic) view that one theory fits all, then I should provide some suggestions on what this theory might look like. In Ingram (1997), I outline the basic properties of such a theory. The first point to make is that our theory for SSD has, in the short term, different goals than phonological theory. The latter has as its goal the characterization of the phonological systems of the thousands of languages that exist in the world. Our goal, by no means trivial, is to have a theoretical account of the phonological systems of children's first words, often less than a thousand in number. This goal does not require the extent of theorisation or formalism needed in linguistic theory. As suggested in Ingram (1997), it is possible to isolate the shared assumptions of phonological theory in general to form the basis of our theory of SSD. Here are some of those shared characteristics: the acquisition of an early lexicon involves the acquisition of phonological representations; these early representations, like adult representations, consist of phonological features; the early representations of children are underspecified, that is, they do not contain the full range of features of those for adult speakers; children first acquire a subset of the features underlying all languages; my research leads me to suggest these early features are consonantal, sonorant, labial, dorsal, continuant; voice; the child's productions are speech sounds that have one or more of these features; the first syllables are constructed from a small set, that is, CV, CVC, VC, CVCV, CVCVC; children's productions attempt to match the adult models, in typical development around 70%.

I'll finish with one of my favourite quotes: 'Theory without practice is speculation, practice without theory is dangerous.'[1]

The biological model

Like Jakobson, Locke (1983) stressed universality in his proposal of a biological model of phonological development. However, Locke emphasised *biological* constraints rather than linguistic ones. Rejecting Jakobson's idea of discontinuity between babbling and speech, Locke postulated relatively rigid maturational control over the capabilities of the speech production mechanism. For Locke, phonology began before 12 months of age with the pragmatic stage when certain babbled utterances gained communicative intent. At the same time, the phonetic repertoire was essentially 'universal', constrained by the anatomical characteristics of the vocal tract. During the 'cognitive stage' that followed, the biological constraints persisted while the child learned to store and retrieve relatively stable forms of phonemes learned from adult language models. At 18 months, in the 'systemic stage', biologically determined babbling production patterns gave way to more adult-like speech. These speech attempts reflected phonologically the target language. Patterns found *only* in adult speech were acquired and patterns not contained in it were 'lost'.

The natural phonology model

Meanwhile, Stampe (1969) had proposed his natural phonology model of phonological acquisition. He posited that children come innately equipped with a universal repertoire of phonological processes: Stopping, Fronting, Cluster Reduction, and so on. These

---

[1] Source lost in time.

processes were 'mental operations' that change or delete phonological units, reflecting the natural limitations and capacities of speech production and perception. In Stampe's view, natural processes amounted to articulatory restrictions, which came into play like reflexes. The effect of these 'reflexes' (which were not reflexes in the physiological sense) was one of preventing accurate production of sound differences. This occurred despite the sounds being perceived correctly auditorily and stored as 'correct' adult phonemic contrasts in the linguistic mechanism in the brain. The processes operated to constrain and restrict the speech mechanism per se. Stampe held that these universal, innate simplifications of speech output involved children's cognitive, perceptual, and production domains. In essence, he believed that the processes simplified speaking in three possible ways. Given a potential phonological contrast, a process favoured the member of the opposition that was the:

1. least complex to produce;
2. least complex to perceive; or,
3. least complex to produce and perceive.

For instance, given the choice of saying /d/ or /ð/, the assumption was that /d/ was easier, because, in typical development, it was acquired earlier; for example, 'this' (/ðɪs/) is often realised by young children as /dɪs/ (an example of Stopping).

The child's developmental task was to suppress the natural phonological processes to achieve full productive control of the phonemes of the ambient language. He also believed that, from the time they began using speech meaningfully, children possessed a fully developed, adult-like, phonological perceptual system. Thus, while they exhibited natural processes in output, they already had an underlying representation (a mental image or internal knowledge of the lexical items) of the appropriate adult target form (so 'this' would be /ðɪs/ underlyingly and /dɪs/ on the surface). Stampe relied heavily on a deterministic explanation of phonological change. He maintained that children 'used' processes for the phonological act of simplifying pronunciation.

The progression to adult-like productions (for instance, the use of consonant clusters) represented mastery of increased constraints (upon output phonology). This development occurred through the suppression of natural processes and consequent revision of the universal system. Change occurred through a passive mechanism of suppression as part of maturation. Stampe did not consider cognitive constraints related to the pragmatics of communication, or of the active learning of a language-specific phonology through problem-solving, as in the Cognitive Model. Possibly the most contentious aspect of Stampe's interpretation of Natural Phonology was his claim that the processes were psychologically real, with Smith (1973, 1978) concluding that there was no psychological reality to the child's system because there was no evidence for the 'reflex mechanism' proposed by Stampe in applying, or rather 'using', phonological processes.

The prosodic model

The prosodic model of Waterson (1971, 1981) introduced another novel theoretical construct. It involved a perceptual schema in which 'a child perceives only certain of the features of the adult utterance and reproduces only those he is able to cope with' (Waterson 1971, p.181) in the early stages of word production. Waterson (1971),

Braine (1974), Macken (1980), and Maxwell (1984) asserted that, in infants, perception and production are both incomplete at first. Both developed and changed before they could become adult-like. Unlike the more generally applied phonological process-based (segmental) description, Waterson's schema provided a gestalt of child production rather than a segment-by-segment comparison with the adult target. Waterson's approach is particularly useful in describing the word productions of toddlers and may explain those that do not readily appear to be reductions of adult forms.

The cognitive/Stanford model

The Stanford or cognitive model of phonological development (Ferguson 1968; Kiparsky and Menn 1977; Macken and Ferguson 1983), and also Menn's (1976) 'interactionist discovery model', construed the child as *Little Linguist*, a captivating idea that dates back at least as far as Comenius (1659). Comenius insisted that, for a child, language-learning was never an end in itself but rather a means of finding out about the world and forming new concepts and associations. In problem-solving mode, the child met a series of challenges and mastered them, thereby gradually acquiring the adult sound system.

Because the child was considered to be involved actively and 'cognitively' in the construction of his/her phonology, the term cognitive model was used. Phonological development was an individual, gradual, and creative process (Ferguson 1978). The Stanford team proposed that the strategies engaged in the active construction of phonology were individual for each child and influenced by internal factors: the characteristics and predispositions of the child; and external factors: the characteristics of the environment. The external factors might include the child's ordinal position in the family, family size, child-rearing practices, and interactional style of the adults close to the child.

Levels of representation

Both Stampe and Smith recognised only two levels of representation. Stampe saw phonological processes as mapping from the underlying representation to the surface phonetic representation, whereas Smith (1973) saw realisation rules assuming this function. Stampe *and* Smith insisted that the child's phonological rules or processes were innate or learned extremely early. Then, Ingram (1974) coined the term 'organisational level' to connote a third, intervening component, related to, but distinct from, the perceptual representation of the adult word. A similar three-level arrangement, implicit in Jakobson's distinctive features theory, was central to cognitive or Stanford theory.

Smith rejected the hypothesis that each child has a unique system, and assumed full, accurate perception and storage of adult speech targets. He proposed a set of ordered and universal phonological tendencies and realisation rules. Realisation rules were physical expressions of abstract linguistic units. Any underlying form had a corresponding realisation in substance. In this instance, phonemes were 'realised' or manifested in 'phonic substance' as phones (whereby meanings were transmitted). Smith's view was that the processes acted as a filter between the correctly stored adult word and the set of sounds produced by the child. Again, the problem arose of the child being perceived as passively allowing the realisation rules to 'apply' in reflecting the adult word.

Theories of development, theories of disorder, and theories of intervention

The theoretical assumptions upon which any speech-intervention approach is based derive first from a theory or theories of normal phonological development, or how children normally learn the speech sound system through a combination of maturation and learning. Exploring this idea, Stoel-Gammon and Dunn (1985) posited four basic interacting components necessary for the formulation of a model of phonological development.

1. An auditory–perceptual component, encompassing the ability to attend to and perceive linguistic input.
2. A cognitive component, encompassing the ability to recognise, store, and retrieve input and to compare input with output.
3. A phonological component, encompassing the ability to use sounds contrastively and to match the phonological distinctions of the adult language.
4. A neuromotor component, encompassing the ability to plan and execute the articulatory movements underlying speech.

From the practitioner's beliefs and assumptions about *normal* development comes a theory of *abnormal* phonological development: that is, a theory of disorders that explains why some children do not acquire their phonology along typical lines. Then, from the theories of normal and abnormal acquisition, and their formalisms, a theory of *intervention* can evolve. The nature of a theory of intervention (or theory of therapy) depends on how the individual clinician understands, interprets, incorporates, adapts, and modifies knowledge of normal and abnormal acquisition, and what theoretical assumptions are made in the process. Michie and Abraham (2004) suggested that intervening without a theory of therapy can lead to 'reinventing the wheel rather than re-applying it'. Expanding on this point, they explained that, if we can isolate which parts of a treatment are doing the work of facilitating desired goals, it is possible to 'fine-tune' therapy to maximise those effective components while reducing components that do not seem to exert much effect on the outcome.

A theory of therapy, that is, how best to improve the speech of a child with SSD beyond the progress expected with age, must logically rely on *assessment procedures* that are congruent with the interventionist's theories of development, disorders, and intervention (Fey, 1992a, b; Ingram, A6). In this regard, our timeline should record the development, mainly in the 1980s, of new speech assessments based around Natural Phonology theory and emphasising phonological process analysis. These included, in order of publication: Weiner (1979), Shriberg and Kwiatkowski (1980), Hodson (1980), Ingram (1981), Grunwell (1985b), and Dean, Howell, Hill, et al. (1990). Phonological process analysis introduced the concept of an abstract level of knowledge. This was revolutionary in its time, and was the phonological version of syntactic deep structure.

The first minimal pair therapy, inspired by Natural Phonology, appeared in the literature when Frederick Weiner had a dazzling idea! Calling it 'the method of meaningful contrast' (Weiner 1981a), he described what we now know as conventional minimal pairs therapy (Barlow and Gierut 2002). More therapy ideas based on linguistic principles followed rapidly. For example, a year later, Blache (1982) presented a systematic approach to minimal pairs and distinctive feature training in a book chapter; Hodson and Paden (1983) produced the first edition of *Targeting Intelligible Speech*, which described their 'patterns' approach, popularly called 'cycles therapy' (Hodson, A5); Monahan (1984, 1986) devised a minimal pairs therapy kit called *Remediation of Common Phonological Processes*; and Elbert and Gierut (1986) wrote the *Handbook of Clinical Phonology*. In the same period that all this activity was going on in the US, in the UK, Grunwell (1983, 1985b) provided intervention guidance in peer-reviewed journal articles; Dean and Howell (1986) wrote an inspiring article about the metalinguistic aspect of therapy for child speech that heralded the development of the *Metaphon Resource Pack* (Dean, Howell, Hill, et al. 1990); and Lancaster and Pope (1989) developed a therapy manual, *Working with Children's Phonology*, that focused on an auditory input therapy (thematic play) approach suitable for very young children and older children with cognitive and attention-span challenges (Lancaster, A20). Still in the UK, the first of a series of books (Stackhouse and Wells 1997) devoted to an influential psycholinguistic framework appeared (Gardner, A21).

A clinical forum on phonological assessment and treatment, edited by Marc Fey, was published in 1992 in one of the ASHA journals, *Language, Speech, and Hearing Services in Schools* (LSHSS). Other such forums followed in 2001, 2002, 2004, and 2006, but this particular one, with articles by Edwards (1992), Elbert (1992), Fey (1985, 1992a, b), Hodson (1992), Hoffman (1992), Kamhi (1992), and Schwartz (1992), is still extraordinarily helpful as a comprehensive introduction. In one of the articles, Fey (1992b) captured the clear distinction between intervention approaches, intervention procedures, and intervention activities when he described and applied a structural plan for analysing the form of language interventions, such as phonological therapies. This hierarchical plan (displayed in Table 1.3) was adapted by Bowen (1996a) and discussed in Bowen and Cupples (1999a).

For clinicians, one good reason for knowing the theoretical underpinnings of the 'therapies' in his/her repertoire is that it enables them to pick and choose among them, or even to combine aspects of them, based on client need. In suggesting that we should be more aware of theories, it should not be assumed that theories are only incorporated into intervention if we, as clinicians, are conscious of them. As Duchan (personal correspondence 2008) points out, 'I feel that we can look at any intervention and deduce its theoretical underpinnings or at least the assumptions it is based on, even if the clinician cannot articulate them. For example, drill is based on an assumption or theory that learning is like exercise, the more you practice saying a sound or word, the better you "know" or can say it next time.'

Fey's useful hierarchy covered the steps involved in modifying and adapting theoretical principles into a practicable intervention approach. It shows the progression from (1) a given phonological theory (e.g., Natural Phonology) to (2) a phonological analysis that is congruent with that theory of phonological development (e.g., Independent and Relational Analysis) to (3) the phonological therapy approach under consideration (e.g., Conventional Minimal Pairs Therapy), informed by (1) and (2). It then allows description of three levels of intervention goal—basic goals, intermediate goals, and specific goals—with goal-selection and goal-attack as critical components. From these arise (4) the intervention procedures of choice within the selected therapy model or a coherent combination of models and (5) workable intervention activities that are both consistent with the preceding four levels and suitable for a particular client.

The 'other' clinical forums, so useful to clinicians, referred to above include one in LSHSS edited by Barlow (2001, 2002); one in the *American Journal of Speech-Language*

Table 1.3 Theory to intervention hierarchy

---

1. PHONOLOGICAL THEORY

Clinician's <u>own</u> Theory of Development ~ Theory of Disorders ~ Theory of Intervention

CONGRUENT WITH

↓

2. PHONOLOGICAL ASSESSMENT APPROACHES

↓↑

CONGRUENT WITH

↓↑

3. PHONOLOGICAL THERAPY APPROACHES

Incorporating goal selection and goal attack via 3 levels of intervention goals:

<u>LEVEL 1</u>

Basic Intervention Goals

(1) To facilitate cognitive reorganisation of the child's phonological system and phonologically oriented processing strategies; (2) to improve the child's intelligibility.

<u>LEVEL 2</u>

Intermediate Intervention Goals

To target *groups* of sounds related by an organising principle (e.g., Phonological Processes or Phonological Rules)

<u>LEVEL 3</u>

Specific Intervention Goals

To target a sound or sounds or structure, using <u>vertical strategies</u> , working on a goal until a criterion is reached, then treating a new goal; or <u>horizontal strategies</u> , e.g., targeting several sounds within a process, and/or targeting more than one process simultaneously, and/or targeting syllable structures, metrical stress, etc. simultaneously with a process or processes.

↓

4. INTERVENTION PROCEDURES

e.g., stimulability training, or phonetic production

↓

5. INTERVENTION ACTIVITIES

Contexts and events, such as games and tasks

Pathology edited by Williams (2002a, b); another in *Child Language Teaching and Therapy*, guest edited by Bernhardt (2004); and, one in *Advances in Speech-Language Pathology* (now renamed the *International Journal of Speech-Language Pathology*) edited by McLeod (2006). More specific clinical forums dealing with particular therapy approaches are also available to guide the clinician. For example, there is one on *Metaphon* (Dean, Howell, Waters, et al. 1995) in *Clinical Linguistics and Phonetics*, and one on Parents and Children Together: PACT (Bowen and Cupples 1999a, b) in the *International Journal of Language and Communication Disorders*.

Looking at Table 1.1 and the seventy years from the Travis articulation paragraph in 1931 to the impact of phonology in the 1970s, via the information explosion of the Internet era, to the ICF-CY view of speech impairment post 2001, we see the dominant influence of linguistics on child speech practice. Interestingly, Bleile (personal correspondence 2005) sees the effects of linguistics, and particularly the impact of phonology, on our practice as being less than we thought it would be. He uses the analogy of waves crashing onto a beach, and a 'wave height' metaphor from surfing. The first wave, distinctive features theory, was 'over head' and went way, way up the beach; then came natural phonology theory and phonological processes, 'head high' and not so far up the beach; following that, nothing was quite 'shoulder high' or even 'waist high', with metrical phonology, auto-segmental phonology, and other nonlinear approaches creating small ripples that barely dampened the sand. Can it be that linguistic theory is now exhausted as a source of ideas and insights about phonological disorders, like behavioural psychology that ran out of puff in the 1970s? Perhaps information processing models like the psycholinguistic model of speech processing and production (Stackhouse and Wells 1997, 2001) hold promise of enticing waves on the intervention side in the future. Maybe it is time for big new insights to come from biology, particularly developmental neurology, and genetics. This notwithstanding, there are aspects of linguistic and psycholinguistic theory that we clinicians should be well acquainted with, because certain linguistic principles can help in devising evidence-based therapies that are conducive to treatment efficacy.

Communication and advocacy

Our recent history has unfolded alongside the creation and expansion of the Internet, comprising the World Wide Web (Berners-Lee 2002) and e-mail, and the growing use of information and communication technology (ICT) by academics in general (Hallett 2002), speech and language professionals in particular (Bowen 2003), and consumers of SLP/SLT services. E-mail, electronic mailing lists, message boards, and other Web-based discussion have facilitated quick, easy, and enjoyable international sharing and collaboration among academics and specialist clinicians who have the time to devote to it, and have provided novel opportunities for professionals and consumers to engage with each other. Part of this Internet expansion has included the growth of child speech-related advocacy Web sites, the most prominent of which is the Apraxia-KIDS Web site (Gretz 1997). Frustrated in 1997 by the lack of information on childhood apraxia of speech (CAS), consumer advocate Sharon Gretz worked with local SLP academics and clinicians to develop training programs for SLPs and accessible Web-based information for families new to diagnosis, those seeking ongoing support, and individuals interested in the research side. She talks about this in A7.

Q7. Sharon Gretz: Consumer advocacy and CAS

As the parent of a teenager who had severe CAS at the age of three, founder and Executive Director of Apraxia-KIDS and the Childhood Apraxia of Speech Association of North America (CASANA), and a doctoral student in communication sciences and disorders, you have made an extraordinary contribution to our field and have a unique perspective on SLP/SLT child speech practice. Impressively, CASANA has become the only national non-profit organization in the US and internationally with the sole focus of CAS. Can you provide a little of the history of what inspired you to follow this path and share your thoughts on the mutual needs, goals, expectations, roles, responsibilities, and costs for the child (or adolescent or young adult), family, and therapist in the assessment, therapy, and management of CAS? Where do consumer advocacy and Web-based communication fit, and what is your vision for the future of organisations like CASANA and smaller, more local 'CAS associations' that currently need to raise funds in order to operate?

A7. Sharon Gretz: Apraxia-KIDS[SM] and the Childhood Apraxia of Speech Association of North America (CASANA)

Beginning in 1994 and for a span of several years, from my seat behind a one-way mirror, I witnessed my child's emergence as a speaker and communicator. I witnessed his incredible struggle, effort, resolve, and, ultimately, success. Eventually, after over 200 individual speech therapy sessions, my son (who had been diagnosed with severe CAS and dysarthria) was a 'talker', his speech intelligible. To say that observing the painstaking, persistent work of both clinician and child was inspiring is an understatement. Fuelled by an appreciation for the good outcomes possible with proper diagnosis, treatment, and clinician–parent partnerships, I turned my thoughts to what I could do to help others in similar circumstance. At the time, little information on CAS existed that could be interpreted by families. The Apraxia-KIDS listserv, followed by the Web site, were created to address gaps in information and to create an international community of concern regarding children affected by this disorder.

Clearly, in the mid to late 1990s, CAS did not appear to be a speech disorder receiving adequate time or attention in the professional literature. Additionally, training opportunities on the topic for practicing professionals were infrequent. These professional circumstances existed alongside several critical needs of parents and caregivers, including the need to:

- gain support for the emotional and practical aspects of raising children with CAS;
- develop advocacy skills to benefit children with CAS; and,
- learn how to help their children with speech and communication practice at home.

CASANA was founded in 2000 to address the above areas of need. Perhaps more importantly, the association has served as a catalyst and a galvanising force for heightened professional interest, education, research, and support worldwide for children with CAS and their families. High-quality Web sites and online communities, such as the Apraxia-KIDS Web site and its companion e-mail listserv, appear to play a vital role in providing reliable information and support. For example, in a survey, Boh, Csiacsek, Duginske, et al. (2006) found that 93% of parents of children diagnosed with CAS used Internet sites as information sources regarding their child's disability. Overwhelmingly, parents report that the *most* helpful information they receive is not obtained from treating SLPs/SLTs, but rather from the Apraxia-KIDS listserv (Lohman 2000). Furthermore, SLPs/SLTs report that they routinely visit specific consumer group Web sites, such as Apraxia-KIDS.org, to gain information relative to clinical cases (Nail-Chiwetalu and Bernstein Ratner 2007).

Apraxia-KIDS and CASANA at work

To illustrate the impact that Apraxia-KIDS and CASANA resources have on families and children, consider the story of a mother named 'Jenna' and her five-year-old son 'Greg'.

Jenna subscribed to the Apraxia-KIDS listserv in a panic. Greg had been receiving both private and school-based speech therapy for nearly three years. He was identified through public early intervention as having CAS near his third birthday, and yet, in the several years that he had seen three different SLPs, he continued to have just a handful of single-syllable words that were intelligible enough for unfamiliar listeners to understand. Through both reading of listserv e-mail, Apraxia-KIDS website articles, and her active questions to the listserv regarding her son's situation, Jenna learned that several key issues might be influencing her son's poor progress. First of all, she learned that his school speech therapy group, comprised of her son and five other children, was not the recommended service delivery model for a child with severe CAS. She also learned that by law (Individuals with Disabilities Education Improvement Act [IDEA] 2004) she was considered a team member in her son's individual education planning (IEP) and that there were rules governing the process that might help her advocate for improved services for Greg, including individual speech therapy. Jenna also learned that the bubbles and horn-blowing activities that occupied most of her son's private speech therapy time were not likely to make a significant difference in his speech production skills (Lof, A30). Additionally, Jenna came to realise that she should be working at home with her son in specific ways that would benefit carry-over of skills learned in treatment. Through local parents involved with CASANA's groups, Jenna located a different, private SLP. She now felt prepared to interview the new SLP to assure herself that the professional understood both the nature of CAS and its treatment and the need to actively involve Jenna in helping her son at home. Jenna was also able to attend a national conference on CAS held in a city in a nearby state. At the conference, Jenna attended sessions where she learned more about CAS, but also about other associated problems that Greg was facing and could possibly face in the future. Ecstatically, Jenna reported to her online community (the Apraxia-KIDS listserv) that, for the first time, Greg was making significant progress in his speech and communication skills. He also had several friends at school, his handwriting was improving, and his reading difficulties were being addressed. Jenna now had hope for Greg's future and also felt more competent and confident as his chief advocate. She also reported with delight that Greg's new school SLP was attending a CASANA workshop to learn more about appropriate assessment and treatment of children with CAS. After several years of involvement and with increased frequency, Jenna now often *answered* questions posed by new parents to the listserv, sharing the information she had learned with others in similar circumstances.

Because of life situations like that of Jenna and Greg, CASANA's board of directors believes that its work is of an urgent nature. The presence of severe speech disorder, and thus communication impairment, has serious ramifications on the quality of life for youth growing up with this disorder. Above and beyond the complicated and challenging speech disorder and its frequent co-morbidities, issues regarding the children's inclusion, relationships, education, emotional functioning, and social well being and independence are also likely to be at stake (Markham and Dean 2006).

Roles and challenges for the future

As more research is produced and knowledge is gained about best assessment and treatment practices and the long-term ramifications of CAS, undoubtedly consumer groups will have a role in the widespread dissemination of information regarding toddlers, children, and youth of all ages with this disorder. One challenge will be to educate professionals and parents to evaluate readily available Internet information and to critically judge its authority, reliability, and credibility. An additional challenge is likely to be ongoing funding for consumer non-profit groups like CASANA. In some ways, the organization is a victim of its own success. Through the work of CASANA, there is increased interest in and attention to CAS. This interest and attention leads to increased demand for assistance and education, which in turn requires more funding. Financial resources to support ongoing operations or new programs, such as research, will need to develop for long-term sustainability of these efforts.

Barriers made of words

Gretz (A7) includes, among the motivational factors driving the development of CASANA, the paucity of information on CAS that could be interpreted by families. Her observation accords with the view of McNeilly, Fotheringham, and Walsh (2007) that terminology in comunication sciences and disorders 'presents a significant barrier to the profession's advancement in research, clinical effectiveness, public image and political profile'. Insisting that change is imperative, McNeilly et al. are clear that, 'influencing attitudes and understanding about something as fundamental and closely tied to one's professional identity as terminology is no small task'. They also underscore the need for sufficient will, resources, and cooperation, as well as a realistic timeframe within which to effect such change. Against the historical backdrop provided here in Chapter 1, the following chapter covers a range of currently applied systems of terminology and the issues that surround them, as well as accounts of the classification, description, and assessment of children's speech.

Chapter 2
Terminology, classification, description, and assessment

In the area of child speech, the barriers engendered by difficult nomenclature are considerable. Picture new students, individuals re-entering the profession, and practitioners switching from adult to child caseloads facing the task of reading the SSD literature from the 1970s onwards and encountering an agglomeration of conceptual, classificatory, and descriptive terms. These terms come primarily from medicine, linguistics, and psychology, only to be enveloped in a mystifying array of like-sounding terms, drawn from the study of literacy in the fields of education and psychology. Within and across disciplines, the same words are sometimes used to denote different concepts and phenomena: 'phonological processes' being a case in point (Scarborough and Brady 2002). One of the first things to strike the reader will be the influence of the medical model and symptomatological and aetiological frameworks, adopted singly or in tandem. Quickly realising the need for a medical or nursing dictionary and a glossary of key genetics terms (as in Table 2.1), he or she will discover broad, trichotomous *symptomatic distinctions* between *articulation disorder*, *phonological disorder*, and *childhood apraxia of speech* (CAS). Historically, this was not the case. For example, Grunwell (1975), who really understood the difference, wrote an article with the paradoxical title: 'The phonological analysis of articulation disorders' that reflected the jumbled state of the terminology at the dawn of the phonological revolution.

The most commonly used classification system in clinical settings is based around three *aetiological* distinctions: *unknown* cause, *putative* or supposed cause, and *known* cause. SSD is usually considered to have 'no identifiable causal factor' and is often given the designation 'functional speech disorder'. Here, 'functional' implies 'unknown cause'. Children with functional SSD comprise the largest sub-group within child speech impairment, whereas children who have SSD of *known* (or 'organic') aetiology fall into several, much smaller sub-groupings. In a survey, Broomfield and Dodd (2004a) established that functional SSD affects 6.4% of *all* children in the UK; an interesting finding in relation to Shriberg and Kwaitkowski (1994) in the US, who proposed that 7.5% of *all* children age 3–11 experienced SSD (of known and unknown aetiology).

Table 2.1 Glossary of genetic terms

AETIOLOGY	*The study of causes or origins.*
ALLELES	*Humans carry two sets of chromosomes, one from each parent. Equivalent genes in the two sets might be different, for example, because of single-nucleotide polymorphisms. An allele is one of the two (or more) forms of a particular gene.*
DNA Deoxyribonucleic acid	*The molecule that encodes genetic information and is capable of self-replication and synthesis of **RNA**. DNA consists of two long chains of nucleotides twisted into a double helix and joined by hydrogen bonds between the complementary bases adenine and thymine or cytosine and guanine. The sequence of nucleotides determines individual **HEREDITARY** characteristics.*
ENVIRONMENT	*All circumstances surrounding an organism or group of organisms, especially: (a) The combination of external physical conditions that affect and influence the growth, development and survival of organisms. (b) The complex of social and cultural conditions affecting the nature of an individual or community.*
GENE	*A **HEREDITARY** unit consisting of a sequence of **DNA** that occupies a specific location on a chromosome and determines a particular characteristic in an organism.*
GENE EXPRESSION	*The process by which a gene's coded information is converted into the structures present and operating in the cell.*
GENOME	*The complete DNA sequence of an organism.*
GENOTYPE	*The genotype is the genetic makeup, rather than the physical appearance (**PHENOTYPE**), of an organism or group of organisms. It involves the combination of **ALLELES** located on **HOMOLOGOUS CHROMOSOMES** determining a specific characteristic or trait.*
HEREDITARY	*(a) Transmitted or capable of being transmitted genetically from parent to offspring. (b) Appearing in or characteristic of successive generations. (c) Of or relating to heredity or inheritance.*
HOMOLOGOUS CHROMOSOMES	*A pair of chromosomes containing the same linear gene sequences each derived from one parent.*
INCIDENCE	*The number of new cases of a disorder or disease during a given time interval, usually per annum, expressed as **INCIDENCE PROPORTION** (**RISK**) or as **INCIDENCE RATE**.*
INCIDENCE PROPORTION	*The number of new cases divided by the size of the population at risk. For example, if a stable population contains 1,000 preschoolers and 2 develop a condition over 2 years of observation, the incidence proportion is 2 cases per 1,000 preschoolers.*
INCIDENCE RATE	*The number of new cases per unit of person-time at risk. Using the previous example, the incidence rate is 1 case per 1,000 person-years, because the incidence proportion (2 per 1,000) is divided by the number of years (2). Using person-time rather than just time covers circumstances in which participants exit studies before they are completed.*
INHERITANCE	*(a) The process of genetic transmission of characteristics from parents to offspring. (b) A characteristic so inherited. (c) The sum of characteristics genetically transmitted from parents to offspring.*
LOCUS	*Locus (pl. loci): The position on a chromosome of a gene or other chromosome marker; also, the DNA at that position. The use of locus is sometimes restricted to mean regions of DNA that are expressed. See **GENE EXPRESSION**.*
MONOGENIC DISORDER	*A disorder caused by a mutant allele of a single gene.*
OLIGOGENIC DISORDER	*A phenotypic trait produced by two or more genes working together.*

Table 2.1 (*Continued*)

PHENOTYPE	*The phenotype comprises the observable physical or biochemical characteristics (**PHENOTYPIC TRAITS**) of an organism, as determined by both genetic makeup (**GENOTYPE**) and environmental influences. It is the expression of a specific trait, such as stature or blood type, based on genetic and environmental influences.*
POLYGENIC DISORDER	*Genetic disorder resulting from the combined action of alleles of more than one gene (e.g., heart disease, diabetes, and some cancers). Although such disorders are inherited, they depend on the simultaneous presence of several alleles; thus, the hereditary patterns usually are more complex than those of single-gene disorders.*
PREVALENCE	*The total number of cases of a disease or condition in a given population at one time.*
RNA Ribonucleic acid	*A polymeric constituent of all living cells and many viruses, comprising a long, usually single-stranded chain of alternating phosphate and ribose units with the bases adenine, guanine, cytosine, and uracil bonded to the ribose. The structure and base sequence of RNA are determinants of protein synthesis and **TRANSMISSION** of genetic information.*
SINGLE-NUCLEOTIDE POLYMORPHISM	*Single nucleotide polymorphisms or SNPs (pronounced 'snips'), are DNA sequence variations that occur when a single nucleotide (A.T.C. or G) in the genome sequence is altered.*
SYMPTOM	*A symptom is a sign or an indication of disorder or disease, especially when experienced by an individual as a change from normal function, sensation, or appearance. Symptomatic classifications of SSDs are based on speech characteristics or 'symptoms' such as limited phonetic repertoire, or persistence of normal phonological patterns.*
TRANSMISSION	*Genetic transmission is the transfer of genetic information from genes to another generation or from one location in a cell to another location in a cell.*

Where does 'functional' fit?

For some researchers (e.g., Gierut 1998 in an important 'state of the art' article), the large 'functional' component includes children with CAS, children with articulation disorders, and children with phonological disorders, all included in the same category. Other scholars (Ruscello 2008a), who also make the known-versus-unknown aetiological distinction, place children with phonetic (articulatory) and phonemic (phonological) difficulties in the populous 'unknown origin' grouping, followed by small, separate subgroupings of children who have at least one observable explanation for their speech difficulties. From Ruscello's perspective, children in these special categories may exhibit a range of organic issues: *craniofacial anomalies*, such as cleft lip and palate or dental malocclusion; *sensory impairments*, such as hearing loss (Purdy, A47); and *motor speech disorders*, such as one of the dysarthrias, apraxia due to a known neurological cause, or CAS, affecting speech–motor planning and/or speech–motor execution, in varying combinations. Ruscello uses the overarching term 'sound system disorder(s)' (abbreviated SSD) to embrace all possibilities as opposed to this author's preferred term, 'speech sound disorder(s)' (*also* abbreviated SSD). An interesting aspect of the so-called 'functional' speech disorders is that we now have suggested subgroups that are linked to *causes* (Flipsen 2002). Drawing on data from several hundred case studies, Shriberg (2006) summarised seven putative subtypes of SSD (listed below) based on genetic (inherited) and environmental risk factors. Furthermore, he suggested clinical prevalence percentages for the first four of these seven, coding them with 'working terms' and abbreviations as subtypes of *speech delay*.

Prevalence was not estimated for a fifth speech delay subtype, Speech Delay-Dysarthria (SD-DYS), but potentially it would amount to less than 2% of the SSD Speech Delay population. In a separate SSD category of *speech errors*, Shriberg (2006) included Speech Errors-Sibilants (SE-/s/) and Speech Errors-Rhotics (SE-/r/). To complete the picture, he added two additional (unnumbered) categories of SSD, also based on genetic and environmental risk factors whose working terms and abbreviations were Undifferentiated Speech Delay (USD) and Undifferentiated Speech Sound Disorder (USSD).

1. Speech Delay-Genetic (SD-GEN), 56%
2. Speech Delay-Otitis media with Effusion (SD-OME), 30%
3. Speech Delay-Developmental Psychosocial Involvement (SD-DPI), 12%
4. Speech Delay-Apraxia of Speech (SD-AOS), <1%
5. Speech Delay-Dysarthria (SD-DYS)
6. Speech Errors-Sibilants (SE-/s/)
7. Speech Errors-Rhotics (SE-/r/)
   Undifferentiated Speech Delay (USD)
   Undifferentiated Speech Sound Disorder (USSD)

Shriberg classified the *primary origin* or probable aetiology of the putative subtypes as:

1. SD-GEN: Polygenic/Environmental
2. SD-OME: Polygenic/Environmental
3. SD-DPI: Polygenic/Environmental
4. SD-AOS: Monogenic? Oligogenic?
5. SD-DYS: Monogenic? Oligogenic?
6. SE-/s/: Environmental
7. SE-/r/: Environmental
   USD: Any of 1–5
   USSD: Any of 1–7

With regard to the *processes affected*, Shriberg's breakdown was:

1. SD-GEN: Cognitive-Linguistic
2. SD-OME: Auditory-Perceptual
3. SD-DPI: Affective-Temperamental
4. SD-AOS: Speech-Motor Control
5. SD-DYS: Speech-Motor Control
6. SE-/s/: Phonological Attunement
7. SE-/r/: Phonological Attunement
   USD Processes Affected: Any of 1–5
   USSD Processes Affected: Any of 1–7

When classification systems based around aetiological distinctions with causal subgroups are applied, clinicians attempting differential diagnosis discover that the speech of some children is impossible to pigeonhole because it seems to 'belong' in more than one category. Broomfield and Dodd (2004b) discuss the unsurprising elusiveness of neat clinical categorisation, pointing out that it has caused several authors (Fox, Dodd, and Howard 2002; Stackhouse and Wells 1997) to question the clinical utility of the aetiological approach. Commenting on Shriberg's (1997) aetiological system, Broomfield and Dodd note three difficulties: (1) children do not fall easily into one subgroup or another;

it bears doubtful universality since it has not been trialled with non-English-speaking
children; and (3) it provides no mechanism to account for developmental change. They
go on to suggest that one alternative to the medical model approach is the theoretically
strong psycholinguistic profiling approach proposed by Stackhouse and Wells (1997).
But again, Broomfield and Dodd (2004b) are unconvinced, querying its utility on three
points: one, its having little regard to surface phonology; two the lengthy diagnostic
process involved in applying the framework; and three, the uncertainty of its universal
applicability.

By contrast, Dodd (1995, 2005) proposed a model with psycholinguistic underpinnings that is based primarily on linguistic profiling and speech subtypes. In it, specific
speech subtypes are matched to discrete areas of psycholinguistic difficulty or breakdown that are 'testable' or 'differentially diagnosable'. Dodd's model enjoys growing
support for its universal applicability (Goldstein 1996; So and Dodd 1994). It embraces
four subtypes that can occur at any age or stage of speech development, plus CAS. They
are:

- **Phonological delay:** in which all phonological rules or processes evident in a child's
  speech output are attested in typical development, but are characteristic of children
  chronologically younger than the child in question;
- **Consistent deviant phonological disorder:** in which children have co-occurring non-
  developmental or unusual errors *and* developmental rules or processes, with the presence of unusual processes signalling that the child has impaired understanding of the
  target phonological system;
- **Inconsistent deviant phonological disorder:** in which children exhibit delayed *and*
  non-developmental error types *and* variability of production of single word tokens
  equal to or greater than 40%; and,
- **Articulation disorder:** in which children are unable to produce particular perceptually
  acceptable phones.
- **Childhood Apraxia of Speech:** Broomfield and Dodd stress that children with CAS, as
  described by Ozanne (1995, 2005), have 'deviant' surface speech production patterns
  that may sound *similar* to those of children with inconsistent deviant phonological
  disorder. They point to key differences between the two, in terms of *proposed level
  of breakdown* and in terms of *symptomatology*. These differences are summarised in
  Table 2.2 and the reader is referred to Dodd (2005) for interesting discussion.

The use by clinicians of classificatory cover terms

Faced with a range of approaches to classification, clinicians and researchers tend to use
cover terms differently from each other, and there is variation from clinician to clinician
and from researcher to researcher, sometimes relative to 'what they grew up with'.

'Articulation disorder' as a cover term

Clarity is achieved in recent literature where 'articulation disorder' implies phonetic-
level difficulties and 'phonological disorder' implies phonemic or cognitive–linguistic

Table 2.2 A comparison of CAS and Inconsistent Deviant Phonological Disorder

Childhood Apraxia of Speech (CAS) (Ozanne 1995, 2005)	Inconsistent Deviant Phonological Disorder (Dodd1995, 2005)
Level of breakdown Children's speech processing breaks down at the phonetic program assembly level, with associated phonological planning and motor speech program implementation difficulties	Children's speech processing difficulties are primarily at the phonological planning level.
Spontaneous vs. imitated speech Spontaneous speech is closer to their intended target than imitated speech.	Imitated speech is closer to their intended target than spontaneous speech.
Phonological awareness skills Children tend to have intact phonological awareness skills.	Children are likely to have an associated deficit in PA.
Oromotor or feeding difficulties Children often have oromotor or feeding difficulties.	Children do not often have oromotor or feeding difficulties.
Clarity and precision Children have an overall lack of clarity and precision.	Children are likely to be more precise.
Suprasegmental characteristics Children's voice, prosody, and fluency may be affected.	Children's voice, prosody, and fluency are usually intact.

difficulties with organisation of the speech sound system. Nevertheless, in clinical settings, some speech and language therapists and speech-language pathologists (SLTs/SLPs) use the term 'articulation disorder' loosely and inaccurately. This is noticeable, and understandable, when they opt for 'articulation disorder' to refer to *any* SSD, in explaining a child's speech difficulties in what they perceive to be simple language, to people who do not have a background SSD. Less understandably, they also do it when they use professional patois to communicate with SLP/SLT colleagues, referring to *all* speech disorders as 'articulation disorders' (or 'artic' disorders).

'Phonological disorder' as a cover term

Confusingly, some authorities use 'phonological disorder' as an overarching heading that embraces phonological disorder, articulation disorder, and other SSDs. For example, Gierut (1998) uses 'functional phonological disorder' synonymously with 'phonological disorder' and under that heading includes five groupings. The first two are *phonetic disorders* and *phonemic disorders*, and she is careful to note that these two are not mutually exclusive. The third is *motor speech disorders*, including 'childhood apraxia'. Gierut's fourth category encompasses *'functional phonological disorders associated with more global involvement of multiple aspects of the linguistic system'*, for example, in children with specific language impairment (p. S86). The fifth is *phonological disorders with organic bases*, such as hearing impairment, craniofacial anomalies, 'mental retardation' (intellectual disability), and 'childhood apraxia' (again). She also mentions a sixth group of children: those with 'phonological differences' or 'phonological difficulties' who are culturally and linguistically diverse, pointing out that these children with 'dialect differences, or native language differences' may not have a phonological disorder as such (Munson, A45).

'Sound system disorder' as a cover term

Ruscello (2008a) accomplishes simplicity and clarity with Shelton's (1993) inclusive classificatory term 'sound system disorders'. It denotes children with clinically significant sound production errors of unknown aetiology who have either phonetic (articulatory) production errors, or phonemic (phonological) production errors, or both, and children with craniofacial anomalies, sensory impairments and, motor speech disorders who have sound system disorders of known aetiology.

'Speech sound disorder' as a cover term

In its policy and clinical guideline documents, ASHA uses the rather consumer-friendly cover term 'speech sound disorder', with the articulation/phonology dichotomy, noting that, 'Intervention in speech sound disorders addresses articulatory and phonological impairments, associated activity and participation limitations, and context barriers and facilitators by optimizing speech discrimination, speech sound production, and intelligibility in multiple communication contexts' (ASHA 2004b). Speech sound disorder is also the preferred term of Bernthal, Bankson, and Flipsen (2009) and within the influential Phonology Project, at the Waisman Center at the University of Wisconsin-Madison. An interpretation of Shriberg's (2006) conceptualisation of how 'speech sound disorder' evolved from 'articulation disorder' is displayed in Table 2.3.

Terms related to intervention

The inevitable confusion engendered by having several approaches to the classification and description of SSD spills over into intervention-related terminology and nomenclature. Gierut (1998), for example, talks about four 'phonological treatments': traditional sensory-motor articulation therapy, Cycles Therapy, the *Metaphon* approach, and conventional minimal pair therapy. Describing the traditional sensory-motor articulation approach, Gierut cites Van Riper and Emerick (1984) and Winitz (1969, 1975), whose work in speech intervention well and truly predated any explicitly motivated *phonological* intervention, and possibly even predated the term 'phonological therapy'. She then provides an account of the Cycles approach (Hodson and Paden 1991), with its traditional *and* metaphonological flavour (Kamhi 2006b, p. 275), about which Fey (1992b) famously remarked, 'there is nothing inherently phonological about the use of cycles' (p. 279). At the same time, he added that because the approach aims to encourage gradual system-wide change, it is highly consistent with the goal common to all phonological approaches of facilitating reorganisation of the child's system. The third account Gierut provides is of conventional minimal pair therapy (Weiner 1981a), the only one on her list

Table 2.3 From articulation disorder to childhood SSD: 1920–2005

Articulation			→			Speech
One Cover Term	**Two Cover Terms**	**No Preferred Cover Term**	**Overlapping Cover Terms**	**One Cover Term**	**One Cover Term**	**One Cover Term**
'Articulation disorder' covered the UK term 'dyslalia' and later 'functional articulation/speech disorder' in the US.	Children had an articulation OR a phonological difficulty. Phonology impacted error description and assessment, but intervention was 'articulatory'.	Articulation disorder and phonological disorder were used confusingly and almost synonymously in the literature and by clinicians.	Children had a phonological difficulty OR an articulation difficulty, with the emphasis on phonology, and frequently observed overlap between the two.	'Phonological Disorder' incorporated delayed or disordered phonology, with phonetic and phonemic levels, and mapping rules.	'Phonological Disorder' now incorporated Phonological Awareness and Phonological Memory acknowledging the speech–literacy link.	SSDs was preferred in the literature, but clinicians still referred to children's articulation or phonology difficulties.
ARTICULATION	ARTICULATION & PHONOLOGY	ARTICULATION or PHONOLOGY	ARTICULATION-PHONOLOGY	PHONOLOGY	PHONOLOGY	SPEECH SOUND DISORDERS
1920–1970	**1971–1980**		**1981–1990**		**1991–2004**	**2005···**

of four that meets all of Fey's (1985, reprinted 1992) strict criteria for a 'phonological' therapy following 'phonological principles' (see below). In Weiner's approach, the therapist works at word (meaning) level, confronting children with their own homonymy, and providing a semantic motivation to change production, thereby facilitating phonological reorganisation. The fourth 'phonological treatment' Gierut outlines is *Metaphon* (Dean, Howell, Waters, et al. 1995), an approach that sets out to eliminate persisting phonological processes via metalinguistic awareness tasks (Howell and Dean 1994) involving imagery, minimal contrast activities, feigned listener confusion, and guided discussion to promote self-monitoring of output.

Phonological principles

Like Grunwell (1975) and Ingram (1976), Fey (1992b) observed three basic principles underlying what he called phonology-based approaches to treatment such as conventional minimal pairs therapy (Weiner 1981a).

1. Modifying groups of sounds or particular syllable structures

The first principle concerned the modification of *groups* of sounds attacked according to an organising feature or systematic rule (of the child's), rather than the correction of individual phonemes. Targeting groups of sounds acknowledges the systematic nature of phonology and aims to promote generalisation of new learning across the child's speech sound system. The speech production errors that the systemic rules represented fell into two main categories: *substitution errors*, where one sound or sound class is substituted for another (as in stopping, fronting, gliding, backing, and assimilation); and *structural errors*, where the structure of the syllable or word changes (as in cluster reduction, diminutisation, schwa insertion or epenthesis, final consonant deletion, and weak syllable deletion). For example, if a child who was 'stopping' treated all fricatives as stops, producing, systematically, *fun* as /pʌn/, *sum* as /dʌm/, and *shoe* as /du/, and so on, the therapist would target fricatives as a sound class, or frication as a feature, rather than treating, say, /f/ then /s/, then /ʃ/, and so on, position-by-position in word-initial, within-word, and word-final contexts. Similarly, if a child's speech was characterised by prevalent final consonant deletion, with many open syllables and productions like /kɒ/ for *cough*, /bʌ/ for *bus*, /pɛ/ for *pet*, and /ɛ/ for *edge*, the therapist would tackle final consonant inclusion across his/her system, in preference to treating /t/, /f/, /s/, and /dʒ/ individually and serially as word-final singleton omissions.

2. Establishing feature contrasts

The second principle was around establishing feature contrasts as opposed to perfecting articulatory execution sound-by-sound and word position-by-word position. Phonetic placement techniques, such as *hunting* (Van Riper and Irwin 1958), the 'trail blazing' (*sic*) *progressive approximations* method (Van Riper 1963), the *successive approximation* procedure (Kaufman 2005; McCurry and Irwin 1953), and *shaping* (Bernthal and Bankson 2004; Shriberg 1975), are all goal attack strategies used as intermediary steps towards adult-like phonetic execution of a therapy target. In the process of fostering such articulatory precision, clinicians may encourage children to produce 'a good crisp /s/', 'a clear /tʃ/', 'a perfect /k/', 'a sharp /t/', 'a beautiful /ŋ/', or 'a lovely /l/'. But in phonological therapy, the child is rewarded for creating *contrast* by using a sound in the target sound class, or a reasonable approximation of the target. For instance, with a child working at the systemic level to eliminate stopping of fricatives, a production like /ʃʌn/ for *sun* rather than /dʌn/ for *sun* would be rewarded, because /ʃ/ and /s/ are in the same (fricative) sound class. With the same child, or another child, working at the structural, syllable shape level, trying to learn final consonant inclusion, a production such as /bim/ for *bean* rather than /bi/ for *bean* would be rewarded. This acceptance of phonemic contrast and the lack of emphasis on fine-tuning of phonetic form, particularly in the early stages of therapy, can be difficult to explain to parents and caregivers, especially if they are anxious and keen to see progress. Their expectation of a clinicians' role may be that we are 'supposed to be' encouraging perfection, and they can find it hard to understand that, if a goal in therapy is to eliminate stopping of fricatives, then /fɪp/ for *ship* is 'more correct' than /dɪp/ for *ship*, and /sɪp/ for *ship* is even more of an improvement!

3. Working at word level and making meaning

The third principle had to do with the goal of making *meaning*, with the implication that the therapy itself must perforce be constructed around listening to, discriminating between, decoding, and saying 'real' words. In fact, it is a truism that phonological therapy *must* be at word level or above (i.e., word, phrase, sentence, or conversational level) in order to signal to the child that the purpose of having a system of sound contrasts, or a phonological system, is to communicate (or to make meaning). The child discovers that homophony must be avoided and appropriate contrast established. If *come*, *crumb*, *drum*, *gum*, *plum*, *some*, and *thumb* are all collapsed and realised homonymously as [dʌm], they come to appreciate that something (phonological) has to change!

Characteristics of phonological disorder

Stoel-Gammon and Dunn (1985) reviewed the small (at the time) literature on the relationship between normal and disordered child phonology, finding a general view that, as well as many similarities between normal phonology and disordered phonology, there were also substantial differences between the two. Their useful list of the most frequently described characteristics of developmental phonological disorders (as opposed to 'phonetic' or 'articulation' disorders) included the presence of:

1. Static speech sound systems that had plateaued at an early level of development.
2. Extreme variability in production, without gradual improvement.
3. Persistence of phonological processes beyond typically expected ages.
4. 'Chronological Mismatch' (Grunwell 1981) with mastery of 'later', 'difficult' sounds and structures, and errors with sounds usually acquired early in development.
5. Idiosyncratic rules or processes that rarely occur in normal phonology.
6. Restricted use of contrast.

Misuse of terms

There is an unfortunate tendency among SLPs/SLTs to 'improve on' the term phonological disorder, replacing it with: *'phonological processing disorder'*, *'phonological process disorder'*, or *'phonological processes disorder'*. Although they have crept into the vernacular, achieving prominence in the workplace, on the Web, in e-mail discussion, and on professional association Web sites, none of these three inappropriate terms is an acceptable synonym for 'phonological disorder'.

Four 'phonological terms' that are easily confused

Phonological disorder in the area of speech (Grunwell 1987; Ingram 1989a), phonological processes in the area of speech (Stampe 1969), phonological processes in the area of literacy (Scarborough and Brady 2002), and phonological processing in the area of literacy (Snowling, Bishop, and Stothard 2000) are four different things.

1. Phonological disorder (speech)

Phonological disorder, also known as developmental phonological disorder (DPD), is an SSD at the cognitive–linguistic level, manifested in (surface) speech error patterns. In clinical settings, it is unusual to hear phonological disorder called 'phonological speech disorder' (Gillon 1998) or 'expressive phonology disorder' (Bird, Bishop, and Freeman 1995). We obviously do not need *more* terms, but if we *did*, these would be good, explanatory ones to use because they help to distinguish (a) phonological impairment in terms of speech error patterns, from (b) phonological impairment in terms of literacy, specifically in relation to phonological awareness (PA) and phonological processing (Gillon 2004, pp. 89–90).

2. Phonological processes (speech)

As recounted in Chapter 1, Stampe's (1969) natural phonology theory introduced the concept of phonological processes. A phonological process was a *descriptive rule or statement* that accounted for structural or segmental speech errors of substitution, omission, or addition. Natural phonology theory stressed the importance of natural phonological processes as a set of universal, obligatory rules governing a particular phonology. These innate processes represented the *constraints* a child modifies or suppresses in order to learn more *advanced forms* in the process of mastering spoken language. The constraints, according to Stampe, disallowed the production of all but the simplest pronunciation patterns in the early stages of phonological development. 'Advanced forms' really implied the correct 'adult' realisation of the sound. Recall from Chapter 1 that Stampe saw the processes as being universal, innate, and psychologically real, operating to constrain and restrict the speech mechanism, and that he believed children actively 'used' processes for the phonological act of simplifying pronunciation via a 'reflex mechanism'. In this sense, because he thought the processes were real 'mental operations', Stampe believed that the processes provided an *explanation* of children's speech sound errors.

Stampe's legacy includes a range of useful descriptors for the speech characteristics of typically developing children and children with SSD, such as 'stopping of fricatives', 'velar fronting', 'deaffrication', and 'cluster reduction', that are widely utilised by SLPs/SLTs. But descriptions they *are*, and explanations they are *not*. Table 2.4 displays a selection of the common phonological processes (or phonological deviations or phonological rules in some literature) that can be used to describe error patterns in phonologies that are developing *normally*, phonologies that are *delayed*, and phonologies that are *disordered*. The cut-off ages for the elimination of the deviations displayed in the table in simplified form to share with families are those suggested by Grunwell (1987), for whom the term 'deviation' implied that the child's production deviated from the adult target.

3. Phonological processing and phonological processes (literacy)

Scarborough and Brady (2002) provide a must-read glossary (for the literacy enthusiast or phonology tragic) of what they call the 'phon words', carefully distinguishing between

Table 2.4 Common phonological processes and their *approximate* ages of elimination in typical (Grunwell 1987)

Phonological Process (Phonological Deviation)	Adult Target vs. Child's Realisation		Description	Eliminated by ≈ Age
	Adult	**Child**		
Context sensitive voicing	PIG: pɪg KISS: kɪs	bɪg gɪs	A voiceless sound is replaced by a voiced sound. In these examples, /p/ is replaced by /b/, and /k/ is replaced by /g/. Other examples might include /t/ being replaced by /d/, or /f/ being replaced by /v/.	3;0
Word-final devoicing	RED: rɛd BAG: bæg	rɛt bæk	A final voiced consonant in a word is replaced by a voiceless consonant. Here, /d/ has been replaced by /t/, and /g/ has been replaced by /k/.	3;0
Final consonant deletion	HOME: houm ROUGH: rʌf	hou rʌ	The final consonant in the word is omitted. In these examples, /m/ is omitted (or deleted) from 'home' and /f/ is omitted from 'rough'.	3;3
Velar fronting	KISS: kɪs GIVE: gɪv WING: wɪŋ	tɪs dɪv wɪn	A velar stop or nasal is replaced by an alveolar stop or nasal respectively. Here, /k/ in 'kiss' is replaced by /t/, /g/ in 'give' is replaced by /d/, and /ŋ/ in 'wing' is replaced by /n/.	3;6
Palatal fronting	SHIP: ʃɪp TAJ: taʒ	sɪp taz	The palato-alveolar fricatives /ʃ/ and /ʒ/ are replaced by alveolar fricatives /s/ and /z/.	3;9
Consonant harmony	CUPBOARD: kʌbəd DOG: dɒg	pʌbəd gɒg	The pronunciation of the whole word is influenced by the presence of a particular sound in the word. Here, /b/ in 'cupboard' causes the /k/ to be replaced /p/, which is the voiceless cognate of /b/, and /g/ in 'dog' causes /d/ to be replaced by /g/.	4;0
Weak syllable deletion	AGAIN: əgɛn TIDYING: taɪdiɪŋ	gɛn taiɪŋ	Syllables are either stressed or unstressed. Here the weak syllables in 'again' and 'tidying' are omitted.	4;0
Cluster reduction	SPIN: spɪn ANT: ænt	pɪn æt	Consonant clusters occur when two or three consonants occur in a sequence in a word. In cluster reduction part of the cluster is omitted. Here, /s/ has been deleted from 'spin' and /n/ from 'ant'.	4;0

Table 2.4 (*Continued*)

Phonological Process (Phonological Deviation)	Adult Target vs. Child's Realisation		Description	Eliminated by ≈ Age
	Adult	**Child**		
Gliding of liquids	REAL: ril LEG: lɛg	wil jɛg	The liquid consonants /l/ and /r/ are replaced by the glides /w/ or /j/. In these examples, /r/ in 'real' is replaced by /w/, and /l/ in 'leg' is replaced by /j/.	5;0
Stopping	FUNNY: fʌni JUMP: dʒʌmp	pʌni dʌmp	A fricative consonant or an affricate consonant is replaced by a stop. Here, /f/ in 'funny' is replaced by /p/, and /dʒ/ in 'jump' is replaced by /d/.	See below

Approximate ages of elimination for stopping of fricatives and affricates

/f/, /s/	FUNNY: fʌni ← pʌni SIP: sɪp →tɪp	3;0
/v/, /z/	VAN: væn → bæn ZOO: → du	3;6
/ʃ/, /dʒ/, /tʃ/	SHIP: ʃɪp → dɪp JUMP: dʒʌmp → dʌmp CHIP: tʃɪp → tɪp	4;6
/θ/, /ð/	THING: θɪŋ → tɪŋ THEM: ðɛm → dɛm	5;0

the many phonological concepts and terms that are found in contemporary literacy theory, research, practice, and pedagogy. In such contexts, 'phonological processing' is a collective term that refers to the phonological information-using abilities and codes (or phonological processes) that are fundamental to learning to read and write. These are 'abilities', or 'mental operations', that cannot be directly measured. They include phonological *representations*, phonological *memory*, phonological *knowledge*, phonological *awareness*, and phonological *naming*. Scarborough and Brady define phonological processing as: 'The formation, retention, and/or use of phonological codes or speech while performing some cognitive or linguistic task or operation such as speaking, listening, remembering, learning, naming, thinking, reading, or writing' (p. 318). They note that these phonological processes do *not* require conscious awareness, asserting that PA is sometimes treated as a separate category because it deals with tasks and constructs that *do* require conscious reflection on the phonological structure of words (Neilson, A17; Hesketh, A22). Scarborough and Brady believe the term 'phonological processing' obscures important distinctions between *constructs* (underlying mental operations that cannot be directly observed or measured) and *tasks* (that can be), and between 'the various tasks themselves with regard to their requirements for other sorts of processing'.

Web questions

In light of the confusion surrounding child speech terminology, it is interesting to find that, in the decade 1998–2008, several hundred questions asked by consumers (mainly parents) and SLP/SLT professionals and students visiting the author's Web site (http://www.speech-language-therapy.com) have concerned this very topic. For example, the parent of an unintelligible four-year-old asked, 'Can you please tell me the difference between an articulation disorder and a phonological disorder; how can you tell them apart; and are they treated differently?' Another parent wrote, 'My five year-old was diagnosed by one therapist who said he had a phonological disorder, but the therapist who is actually treating him says he has "a phonological processing disorder" and that we need to work on "his artic". I am so, so confused by this: help!' And this came from a colleague: 'Although I have been an ASHA-certified school-based SLP for over 20 years, and most of my caseload is "artic", I have to say I am confused about the difference between phonetic speech sound disorders, and phonemic speech sound disorders. In simple terms, what exactly is the difference, and can they exist concurrently in the same child?' Such questions prompted the development of a plain English response on the Web site, a variation of which is displayed in Box 2.1. Predictably, it is one of the most-retrieved pages there and much used by students, clinical educators, and practitioners, including those preparing talks for consumer groups. Why 'predictably'? Just over 67% of site visitors and 50% of e-mail correspondence generated by the site come from the US, where children with SSD comprise the largest proportion of the caseloads of school-based speech-language professionals (ASHA 2004a). Indeed, almost 91% of SLPs in US schools serve children with SSD (ASHA 2006b).

Two major sub-groups

Within the SSD client population, there are two major sub-groups of children: (1) poorly unintelligible preschoolers with low percentages of consonants correct (PCCs) and multiple errors; and (2) acceptably intelligible school-aged students with high PCCs and 'residual errors' (Pascoe, Stackhouse, and Wells 2006; Shriberg, Tomblin, and McSweeny 1999; Smit 2004a, b). In practice, clinicians often reserve the terms 'articulation disorder' and 'functional articulation disorder' for the reasonably intelligible children of all ages—preschoolers and school students—with one or just a few speech production difficulties, characteristically involving /s/, /z/, /l/, and /r/ and, in some settings, /θ/ and /ð/ also. A high proportion, but we don't know precisely *how* high, of the unintelligible preschoolers have a phonological impairment ('phonological disorder') entailing linguistic difficulties with organising speech sounds into patterns of sound contrasts. A small proportion (<1% of the paediatric SLP/SLT SSD caseload) have CAS thought to be due to a deficit in speech motor control (ASHA 2007a, b; Shriberg 2004, 2006; Shriberg, Campbell, Karlsson, et al. 2003). Each and every SSD can co-occur (e.g., phonetic and phonemic issues in the same child), and each can occur with other communication disorders (e.g., CAS and stuttering in the same child) or with other conditions (e.g., phonological disorder and ADHD in the same child).

Speech assessment: screening

Speech assessment involves careful, informed observations and hypothesis testing. The process typically begins with the referral followed by a preliminary, informal *screening*

Box 2.1 How do articulation disorder and phonological disorder differ?

A PLAIN-ENGLISH EXPLANATION FOR CONSUMERS

How do articulation disorder and phonological disorder differ?

To answer this question accurately, it is important to know that SLPs/SLTs make a distinction between speech and language. Human language is partly innate and partly learned from our interactions with the people in our world. The 'learned' part is like a code, or systematic rules that enable us to communicate ideas and express wants and needs. Reading, writing, gesturing, and speaking are all forms of language. For convenience, we can think of language as having two main divisions: first, receptive language, or understanding what is said, read, or signed; and second, expressive language: speaking, writing, or signing. Our overall grasp of what Linguistics, Neurology, Psychology, and related disciplines reveal about the nature of typical speech and language development, and what can go wrong with them, is critical to our understanding of a particular child's speech and or language difficulty.

When we think about speech as the spoken medium of language, we find, among other things, that it has a phonetic level and a phonemic level. The phonetic level takes care of articulation: the motor act of producing the vowels and consonants, so that we have a repertoire of all the sounds we need in order to speak our language or languages. The phonemic level is in charge of phonology: the 'brainwork', if you like, that goes into organising the speech sounds from the phonetic level into patterns of sound contrasts that enable us to make sense when we talk.

In essence, an articulation disorder is a *speech* disorder that adversely affects the phonetic level so that the child has difficulty saying particular consonants and vowels. The reason for this may be *unknown* or poorly understood as is the case for children who do *not* have serious problems with muscle function; or the reason may be *known* and well-understood as is the case for children with dysarthria who do have serious problems with nerve and muscle function (like children with cerebral palsy), or children with anatomical (craniofacial) differences, such as some children with cleft lip and palate. By contrast, in essence, a phonological disorder is a *language* disorder that affects the phonemic organisation level. The child has difficulty organising his/her speech sounds into a system of sound contrasts, often referred to as phonemic contrasts. One way of understanding this is to think of the phonetic or articulation level as happening 'in the mouth' or even 'on the lips' and the phonemic or phonological level as happening 'in the mind' (Grunwell 1989). The phonemic level is sometimes referred to as the linguistic level or the cognitive level.

Can phonetic and phonemic difficulties co-occur?

Yes, they can: the same child can have both at the same time. Some of their intelligibility challenges can have a phonetic or articulatory basis and others of their challenges can have phonological bases.

Can they occur with other speech or language disorders?

Again, the answer is 'yes'. For example, the same child may have co-occurring difficulties at the phonetic level, the phonemic level, the motor planning level, and perceptual level.

Can individuals with CAS have some combination of all these other issues too?

Yes, they can. In addition to having difficulties with planning the movements required for speech, children with CAS can have phonetic and/or phonemic issues. Because of their knowledge-base, SLPs/SLTs are able to distinguish between the many speech and language disorders they have to assess (or 'differentially diagnose') in the course of their work, and they can also recognise these co-occurrences.

Where can I find out more?

There is further information, written for a general readership, about children's SSDs at this Web page: http://www.speech-language-therapy.com/phonol-and-artic.htm.

procedure in which the SLT/SLP listens to and watches the child speak. Usually without discussion or collaboration, the SLP/SLT develops a tentative explanation, or hypothesis, about the nature of any apparent difficulties with a view to conducting further investigations if needed. This initial screening may be as simple as making observations of the child in conversation, either with the therapist or with a parent, sibling, or peer, or it may involve a short screening test. Appropriate screening reflects sensitivity to cultural and linguistic diversity. In family-centred practice (Watts Pappas, A25), which is by no means universal, there is collaboration around the nature and conduct of further assessment. The SLP/SLT provides pertinent information, but it is a family's decision whether to proceed, who should be present in assessment sessions, and so on.

Initial screening may be conducted by a person who is not an SLP/SLT and may involve the use of computer software. For example, the 66-picture computerised *Phoneme Factory Phonology Screener* developed in the UK is designed for teachers to administer to children whom they suspect have speech sound difficulties, before referring them to SLP/SLT services for assessment. The teacher listens as the student names the pictures, writing down alphabetically or phonetically the child's production of one particular sound per word. The software has the capability of generating a report, based on what the teacher records, specifying the errors and patterns revealed, with normative comparisons and an indication of whether the child's speech difficulties are 'developmental' or 'disordered'. Any recommendation to refer to speech therapy is based on this report. The report also guides the teacher to appropriate activities to use in an associated software title in the series, the *Phoneme Factory Sound Sorter* program. In testing the software, 408 children were assessed on the screener by a teacher–researcher and by an SLT using the phonology subtest of the DEAP (Dodd, Hua, Crosbie, et al. 2003). These two measures of the children's speech were used to determine the screener's sensitivity (71%), specificity (99%), and positive predictive values (81%). The order of testing was randomised (i.e., sometimes the children were assessed first by the teacher and sometimes first by the SLT) so as to control for order effects.

The first author of the *Phoneme Factory* software packages, Dr. Sue Roulstone, was Chair of the Royal College of Speech and Language Therapists (RCSLT) from 2004 to 2006. She has worked as a clinician, an educator, a manager, and a researcher, mainly with children and always with an interest in the interface between therapy and education. Her research interests include evaluation of SLT service delivery, children and family perspectives on speech and language impairment, epidemiology of speech and language impairment and professional judgement and decision making, and her response to Q8 reflects these interrelated topics.

Q8.   Sue Roulstone: Child speech screening and *Phoneme Factory*

Screening and assessment practices vary widely. In its preamble to *Preferred Practice Patterns*, ASHA (2004b) states that the document provides 'an informational base to promote delivery of quality patient/client care. They are sufficiently flexible to permit both innovation and acceptable practice variation, yet sufficiently definitive to guide practitioners in decision making for appropriate client outcomes'. The document goes on to say, 'Pediatric speech-language screening is conducted by appropriately credentialed and trained speech-language pathologists, possibly supported by speech-language pathology assistants under appropriate supervision.' How do screening practices in the UK differ from those specified in the ASHA guidelines? Has the *Phoneme Factory* been a successful innovation as a referral tool, and can you clarify teachers' use of the screener in relation to the *Phoneme Factory Sound Sorter* intervention component? Is this work children do while waiting for SLT intervention?

A8.   Sue Roulstone: Screening for speech impairments

I'd first like to draw attention to the different uses of the word 'screening' that are in common usage within the profession and more widely in health and education services. Generally, screening is used to suggest a level of assessment that provides a pass/fail outcome, which indicates whether or not a child has a speech and language difficulty that requires more in-depth, confirmatory assessment. However, there are several stages along the diagnostic pathway at which 'screening' might be used, and for the purposes of this discussion, I'd like to identify three.

1. Early identification screening of at-risk populations

Firstly, screening is used to describe a public health process in which children within a defined population are tested in order to identify those who are at risk of speech and language problems so that they might be referred for further diagnostic testing; the aim of such screening is to provide early identification, preferably in a pre-symptomatic stage, in order to provide treatment at the earliest appropriate opportunity (Hall and Eliman 2003, p. 135).

2. Informal SLP/SLT triage screening

A second use of screening describes part of the initial assessment process carried out by an SLT/SLP. In Q8, Caroline has described an 'informal screening procedure' carried out by SLPs/SLTs at the first assessment of a child following referral. Pickstone (2007) has referred to this as a 'triage' process whereby the experienced SLP/SLT makes judgements about the priority status of the newly referred child in order to make the best use of resources and monitor the urgency and needs of those being referred.

3. Formal screening assessment

Thirdly, screening assessments might be used to decide whether an aspect of speech and language requires further investigation. The screening assessment components of the DEAP (Dodd, Hua, Crosbie, et al. 2003) and HAPP-3 (Hodson 2004) probably fall into this category; by using them, the therapist gains a quick overview of the child's articulation and phonology in order to establish whether or not to carry out full diagnostic testing of the child's speech output.

These different stages of screening represent a gradual focusing of the identification and diagnostic process, and in order to decide who could or should carry out screening, it can be helpful to determine which stage in the diagnostic process is being described and the purpose of screening at that point. Within the UK, the first type of screening would be regarded as a public health role, to be carried out by health and education professionals. This might include health visitors; teachers and nursery (daycare and preschool) staff, who work in primary care; and paraprofessionals in some community settings, who have been trained for a particular procedure (Pickstone, Hannon, and Fox 2002). In the UK, a health visitor is a qualified and registered nurse or midwife who has undertaken further (post registration) training in order to be able to work as a member of the primary health care team. The role of the health visitor is about the promotion of health and the prevention of illness in all age groups.

The RCSLT (Gascoigne 2006) would see the role of SLTs in the public health arena to be strategic in nature—advising on the type of procedures to be used and training the other professionals involved. Indeed, it would be rare for SLTs in the UK to carry out this kind of screening directly themselves. Occasionally, where SLTs are establishing the needs in a particular population (e.g., setting up a new service in a school or a preschool setting), SLTs might be directly involved in population screening. However, following this, the screening and referral process would be handed back to the people in regular contact with the child; the SLT would see it as his/her role to support the process by providing materials and training. On the other hand, the second and third types of screening for speech and language impairment would be regarded as the role of the state-registered SLT, perhaps supported by a SLT assistant within some constrained contexts. Furthermore, Pickstone (2007) reports the use of more experienced therapists in the triage process in order to utilise their expertise in decision making.

Population screening

In the rest of the discussion, screening is used in the first sense, where the testing is part of a public health process aiming to identify which children should be referred for further confirmatory or diagnostic assessment. Screening is defined by the UK National Screening Committee (n.d.) as follows:

> *Screening is a public health service in which members of a defined population, who do not necessarily perceive they are at risk of, or are already affected by a disease or its complications, are asked a question or offered a test, to identify those individuals who are more likely to be helped than harmed by further tests or treatment to reduce the risk of a disease or its complications.*

In a systematic review of screening programs, Law, Boyle, Harris, et al. (1998) concluded that, although there were a number of screening assessments which had adequate sensitivity and specificity (i.e., they were able to identify a reasonable proportion of cases [sensitivity] and a reasonable proportion of children who were not cases [specificity]), no comparisons had been made between the different procedures. The impact of these assessments on actual referral and identification practices is rarely evaluated. Furthermore, they noted the lack of consensus regarding which children *should* be identified for treatment and the uncertainty that the ones identified by screening procedures would be the ones who would most benefit from intervention. Currently, although there are preferred assessments for screening for early language impairment, the emphasis is on primary prevention and providing universal access to advice for parents (Hall and Eliman 2003, p. 262; Pickstone, Hannon, and Fox 2002). As a result, there is no nationally recommended process for screening for speech and language impairment in the UK, and most SLT departments, in collaboration with local primary care and education settings, will have developed and publicised referral criteria to guide referrals; in some cases, particular screening assessments will be recommended.

Phoneme Factory

Given this UK policy context, it was not our original intention to develop a screening assessment when we started the development of *Phoneme Factory* [a software suite comprising the *Phoneme Factory Sound Sorter* (Wren and Roulstone 2006) and the *Phoneme Factory Phonology Screener* (Wren, Hughes, and Roulstone 2006)]. In the UK, where therapists are working with children of school age (i.e., children from the age of four), therapy is typically school-based and curriculum-focused (Gascoigne 2006, p.224). The original aim of the *Phoneme Factory* project, therefore, was to develop a therapy tool that could be set up by therapists for use by teachers in class and that had credence for teachers as useful to the speaking and listening and pre-literacy curriculum. Our view was that therapists frequently left picture- and paper-based activities for teachers that were of poor quality (e.g., photocopied sheets), that got lost and crumpled and separated from instructions and therefore either were not carried out at all, or were carried out in ways that might deviate from the SLTs' original intentions. We felt that computer software had much to offer in providing materials that were fun, interactive, and maintained their quality. Furthermore, because the activities need little adult input, they are less likely to be unintentionally and unhelpfully modified by the teacher or assistant working with the child. Conscious that the software, once left in the classroom, would inevitably be used more widely by education staff, we developed seven software games that were primarily PA activities and were therefore unlikely to cause children harm, even if the games were used indiscriminately for children other than those under the care of the SLT. The games could be configured to fit with the individual child's targets and error patterns. As we predicted, once we had piloted the software games in classroom, teachers were keen to have greater access to them. Our advisory therapist group, too, felt that they could be of general applicability to a greater number of children, who perhaps had minimal speech output immaturities or who had literacy problems. Our position has been that engagement of teachers with the work of SLTs is crucial to the success of intervention for children of school age, and therefore, if we are to introduce the use of software as one of our tools, then we should make this accessible to teachers, too. So our challenge became how to make *Phoneme Factory* therapy software [i.e., the Sound Sorter component (Wren and Roulstone 2006)] more accessible without the risk of teachers perceiving that they now had a tool that would replace the need for therapy referral. It was this dilemma that led to the development of the screener (Wren, Hughes, and Roulstone 2006).

The aim was to produce a screener that could be used reliably by teachers to identify children whose expressive phonological systems were not age-appropriate in order to refer for further investigation by a SLT. Further, we aimed to produce a screener that would provide teachers with feedback about the child's phonology and with suggestions for activities that could be carried out by the teacher using the therapy software. The original therapy software was designed to allow therapists to configure the games to suit an individual child's phonological system, target sounds, and contrasts. So the first stage was to further develop the therapy software to include some teacher settings that did not require detailed analysis of a child's system, but that would nonetheless provide appropriate activities (or games). The software now includes these teacher settings, which include a random selection of PA games as well as pre-set games for developing PA related to developmental substitutions and simplifications, on a phonological process basis. This component of the *Phoneme Factory Sound Sorter* includes games for stopping, fronting, final consonant deletion, context-sensitive voicing, gliding, and deaffrication. The games aim to fulfil four purposes:

- Provide interim activities whilst a child is awaiting an SLT appointment;
- Provide relevant activities should the therapist not be able to visit the school to program the software him/herself or to provide a teacher with support activities;
- Provide activities for children whose articulation or phonology is perhaps a little immature but does not warrant further referral; and,
- Provide general phonological awareness activities that might be of use to any child as pre-reading activities.

Having developed the screener, the next stage of the research program is to assess the impact of the use of both the screener and the sound sorter software on referral processes and on the development of children's phonology, using a wider sample of SLT and teacher views of the software. So there is still research to be done on how the software works in practice. However, here is an illustrative example of how things might work out.

Case illustration

'Christopher' is a new student in his Year 1 class at primary school. Aged 5;3, he has moved home during the summer. No information is available to the class teacher at the start of term, and she immediately notices that Christopher is very difficult to understand. The teacher allows Christopher a couple of weeks to settle into class and then completes the *Phoneme Factory* screener with him. The screener report indicates that Christopher is using developmental and non-developmental errors and should be referred for assessment by an SLT. The teacher prints out a copy of the report to discuss with Christopher's parents and then, with their permission, refers him to the SLT service. The screener report has also suggested some activities on the sound sorter; the report recommended that Christopher uses the pre-set teacher settings for 'fronting', 'final consonant deletion', and also for 'general phonological awareness'. The SLT has a waiting list of about 2 months, so when she sees Christopher, the information from the screener report provides a baseline against which Christopher's progress over the last 2 months can be measured. The therapist's in-depth assessment of Christopher's phonology showed that he is consistently using alveolar voiced plosives for all velar plosives and consistently using /h/ for all word initial fricatives; all word final consonants are omitted. On her next visit to the school, the therapist configures the *Phoneme Factory* sound sorter to target Christopher's systematic sound preference for /h/ SIWI. Having played the games already in class, Christopher is able to use the software independently, and his teacher allows him some time each day to work on the PA activities. Therapy continues, using a combination of the individually configured software games and individual sessions with the therapist, Christopher and his mother working on a combination of phonological awareness/input tasks using the sound sorter, and activities to remediate the child's errors in production.

Speech assessment: diagnostic evaluation

Child speech assessments are prompted by: (1) referral, including referral by a child's family; (2) a child's medical, sensory, or developmental status, for example, the speech of children with cleft palate is routinely assessed in most of the industrialised world (Golding-Kushner, A13); or (3) failing a speech-language screening (see ASHA 2004, for further information). They are conducted by appropriately credentialed SLPs/SLTs, working individually or as members of collaborative teams that may include the child, family members/caregivers, and others (Louw, A28; Watts Pappas, A25). Speech assessments are administered to children as needed, requested, or mandated or where there are indications that individuals have articulation and/or phonology impairments associated with their body structure/function and/or communication activities/participation (McLeod, A1). Depending on the presenting picture, the SLP/SLT examines, among other aspects, the phonetic, phonological, perceptual, phonotactic, prosodic, speech motor, and intelligibility aspects of the child's speech. In Evidence-based Practice, the particular tests chosen depend on the child's presentation, the educated preferences and theoretical orientation of the clinician, and client/patient values and wishes.

The case history interview and/or questionnaire

The case history interview and/or a history questionnaire provide helpful information about the child and the family that may help the therapist manage assessment and intervention sensitively and appropriately. Ideally, information gathering is conducted with an eye to the potential 'red flags' for speech impairment (summarised in Box 2.2) that alert the clinician to a range of important risk factors.

Independent and relational analysis

Stoel-Gammon (1988) considered that an analysis of a child's phonology should involve an independent analysis and a relational analysis. The analyses are based on data from a single word (SW) and conversational speech (CS) sample, of around 200 words if possible. In recording results, it is important to differentiate between what was found in the SW sample, as opposed to the CS sample. For Stoel-Gammon, a completed independent and relational analysis includes:

1. What the child attempted to produce (an independent analysis of adult forms);
2. What the child actually produced (an independent analysis of child's corpus);
3. What was produced correctly by the child (a relational analysis);
4. What was produced incorrectly by the child (a relational analysis);
5. The nature of the child's incorrect productions (a phonological process analysis and other errors); and
6. The extent (percentage of occurrence) of phonological processes and other errors.

Box 2.2 Red flags for speech impairment

Red Flags	Information
Failure to babble or late onset of canonical babbling	Infants start to produce canonical (speech-like) CV and VC strings of babble at around 7 months, and all infants should be producing canonical babble, at least some of the time, before their first birthday. Canonical babbling may go hand-in-hand with all sorts of other perfectly normal baby noises, including strange vocalisations, squeals, and gurgles. Babble and real speech overlap for months, with the baby producing both. Failing to babble or late-onset of canonical babble are associated with hearing impairment and motor speech disorders; and late onset of canonical babbling is predictive of delayed language development. Normative guidelines are available at http://www.vocaldevelopment.com.
Middle ear disease (OME) 12–18 months of age	Otitis Media with Effusion (OME) between 12 and 18 months is associated with speech delay.
Glottal replacement	Glottal replacement, when it is not dialectal, should alert the clinician to the possibility of speech delay or disorder.
Initial consonant deletion (ICD)	ICD is only attested in first language learners of Finnish, French and possibly Hebrew and alerts the clinician to the possibility of moderate and severe phonological disorder and/or CAS.
Small phonetic inventory	A small repertoire of consonants, and/or vowels may signal moderate and severe phonological disorder and/or CAS.
Backing	Backing may indicate an early history of OME (Shriberg, Kent, Karlsson, et al. 2003).
Widespread or inconsistent vowel errors	Prevalent or inconsistent vowel errors are a diagnostic marker for CAS. Children with CAS and children with moderate and severe DPD frequently experience difficulties producing vowels. Studies show that at least some vowel errors may occur in as many as 50% of children with these diagnoses (Eisenson and Ogilvie 1963; Pollock and Berni 2003). In typically developing children under 35 months, 24–65% have a high incidence of vowel errors. By 35 months, errors are far less prevalent (0–4%) (Pollock and Berni 2003).
Persistent final consonant deletion (FCD) (beyond about 2;10)	FCD coming up to the third birthday should alert the clinician to the possibility of speech delay or disorder.
PCC <50 in beginning readers	A PCC below 50% when formal reading instruction starts is associated with literacy acquisition difficulties (reading, reading comprehension, and spelling).
Speech difficulties >6;9	Persistent, mild speech production difficulties beyond age 6;9 are associated with literacy acquisition difficulties.

We can think of the *independent analysis* as a handful of inventories and the *relational analysis* as a handful of percentages. The independent analysis is a view of the child's unique system without reference to the target (adult) phonology. It consists of a consonant inventory, a vowel inventory, a syllable–word shapes inventory, and a syllable–stress patterns inventory. By ascertaining what is *not* present in the sample, the examiner develops an account of inventory constraints (absent phones and phonemes), positional constraints (e.g., a sound such as /k/ might not occur word initially in CVC words like *cap*, although it occurs word finally in CVC words like *pack*), and sequential or phonotactic constraints (the C and V combinations that the child does not use). The relational analysis is a normative comparison that looks at the child's system relative to an idealised version of the target (adult) phonology, as it would be with each sound said 'perfectly', and comprises:

- PCC in SW and CS;
- Percentage of Vowels Correct (PVC) in SW and CS; and,
- Phonological Processes in SW and CS expressed as percentages of occurrence.

Combining elements of SODA analysis (described in Chapter 1) and place-voice-manner (PVM) analysis (Hanson 1983; see Table 2.5), production errors, or mismatches between the child's realisations and the adult target (or 'standard sound'), are identified by sound class and position within words.

Errors are described in terms of patterns (e.g., using the HAPP-3), phonological processes (e.g., via the ALPHA-R, DEAP, KLPA-2, GFTA-2, or PACS), or phoneme collapses (via the SPACS), depending on the clinicians' theoretical orientation and the assessment needs of the child, and, in the clinical reality, depending on the test instruments available. Citations for the tests mentioned here are included in Table 2.6.

Table 2.5 Place-Voice-Manner (PVM) chart for PVM analysis

Manner Voiceless-voiced cognates (pairs): voiceless on the left		Place							
		Labial			Coronal			Dorsal	
		Bilabial	Labiodental	Interdental	Alveolar	Palato-alveolar	Palatal	Velar	Glottal
Obstruent	Stop	p b			t d			k g	
Obstruent	Fricative		f v	θ ð	s z	ʃ ʒ			h
Obstruent	Affricate					tʃ dʒ			
Sonorant	Nasal	m			n			ŋ	
Sonorant	Liquid				l		r		
Sonorant	Glide	w					j	w	

Obstruent: A consonant formed by obstructing outward airflow, causing increased air pressure in the vocal tract.
Sonorant: A vowel or a consonant produced without turbulent airflow in the vocal tract. A sound is sonorant if it can be voiced continuously at the same pitch.

Table 2.6 Commonly cited child speech assessments

Test	Citation	Scope
ALPHA-R	Lowe, R. (2000). *Assessment Link between Phonology and Articulation - Revised*. Mifflinville, PA: ALPHA Speech & Language Resources.	ARTICULATION PHONOLOGY
AP	Hickman, L. (1997). *Apraxia Profile*. San Antonio, TX: The Psychological Corporation.	APRAXIA (CAS)
BBTOP	Bankson, N. W., & Bernthal, J. E. (1990). *Bankson-Bernthal Test of Phonology*. Austin, TX: Pro-Ed.	PHONOLOGY
CAAP	Secord, W. A., & Donohue, J. S. (2002). *Clinical Assessment of Articulation and Phonology*. Greenville, SC: Super Duper.	ARTICULATION PHONOLOGY
CAPES	Masterson, J., & Bernhardt, B. *Computerized Articulation and Phonological Evaluation*. San Antonio, TX: Psychological Corporation.	ARTICULATION PHONOLOGY
DEAP	Dodd, B., Crosbie, S., Zhu, H., Holm, A., & Ozanne, A. (2002). *Diagnostic Evaluation of Articulation and Phonology (DEAP)*. London: The Psychological Corporation.	ARTICULATION PHONOLOGY
GFTA - 2	Goldman, F., & Fristoe, M. (2000). *Goldman-Fristoe Test of Articulation-2*. Circle Pines, MN: American Guidance Service.	ARTICULATION
HAPP - 3	Hodson, B. (2004). *Hodson Assessment of Phonological Patterns* (3rd Edition). Austin, TX: Pro-Ed.	PHONOLOGY
	Khan, L. M. L., & Lewis, N. P. (2002). *Khan–Lewis. Phonological Analysis* (2nd ed.). Circle Pines, MN: American Guidance Service.	PHONOLOGY
KSPT	Kaufman, N. (1995). *Kaufman Speech Praxis Test for Children*. Detroit, MI: Wayne State University Press.	APRAXIA (CAS)
	Dean, E., Howell, J., Hill, A., & Waters, D. (1990). *Metaphon Resource Pack*. Windsor, Berks: NFER Nelson.	PHONOLOGY
NDP - 3	Williams, P., & Stephens, H. (Editors) (2004). *Nuffield Centre Dyspraxia Programme Third Edition*. Windsor, UK: Miracle Factory.	APRAXIA (CAS)
PACS	Grunwell, P. (1985a). *Phonological Assessment of Child Speech* (PACS). Windsor: NFER-Nelson.	PHONOLOGY
PAT - 3	Pendergast, K., Dickey, S. E., Selmar, J. W., & Soder, A. L. (1997). *Photo Articulation Test* (3rd Edition). San Antonio, TX: The Psychological Corporation.	ARTICULATION
QS	Bowen, C. (1996). The Quick Screener. Available from http://www.speech-language-therapy.com/tx-a-quickscreener.html.	ARTICULATION PHONOLOGY
SPACS	Williams, A. L. (2003b). *Speech Disorders: Resource Guide for Preschool Children*. Clifton Park, NY: Thomson Delmar Learning.	PHONOLOGY
STAP - 2	Armstrong, S., & Ainley, M. (1992). *The South Tyneside Assessment of Phonology* (2nd Edition). Northumberland: Stass Publications.	ARTICULATION
TSSS	Kirkpatrick, J., Stohr, P., & Kimbrough, D. (1990). *Test of Syllable Sequencing Skills (TSSS)*. Tucson, AZ: Communication Skill Builders.	SYLLABLE SEQUENCING
Blakeley	Blakeley, R.W. (2001). *Screening Test for Developmental Apraxia of Speech* (2nd Edition). Austin, TX: Pro-Ed.	APRAXIA (CAS)
VMPAC	Hayden, D., & Square, P. (1999). *Verbal Motor Production Assessment for Children*. San Antonio, TX: The Psychological Corporation.	APRAXIA (CAS)

Dr. Carol Stoel-Gammon joined the Speech and Hearing Sciences faculty at the University of Washington in 1984 and has a PhD in Linguistics from Stanford University. Her many research interests include linguistic and early linguistic development; cross-linguistic studies of phonological acquisition; early identification of speech and language disorders; phonological acquisition in children with speech and language disorders; relationships between phonological and lexical acquisition; effects of hearing loss on phonological development; and phonological development of children with Down syndrome. She teaches graduate and undergraduate classes, including Language Science, Phonetics, and Phonological and Articulation Disorders. In her reply to Q9, she considers the practical realities for the SLT/SLP in administering an appropriate, effective, and efficient speech assessment when time is limited.

Q9.   Carol Stoel-Gammon: Speech data collection and analysis

As Masterson, Bernhardt, and Hofheinz (2005) wrote, 'efficient treatment depends on many factors, one being a valid and reliable assessment from which to derive a treatment plan. Conversational data are potentially representative of a client's everyday speech and in that regard are an ecologically-valid basis for planning effective and efficient treatment. A clinician-controlled single-word sample, in comparison, may not elicit a client's typical speech production patterns.' Taking into account the unavoidable trade-off between the available time and choosing an appropriate sampling and analysis methodology, how would you guide a clinician with just 1 hour in which to administer a speech assessment for an unintelligible preschooler and 1 more hour to complete the analysis? How can the 2 hours be best spent?

A9.   Carol Stoel-Gammon: Assessment of the speech of an unintelligible preschool child

Meet 'Brett', 4;9, referred by his preschool teacher, who is concerned because she has rated his intelligibility at just 50%. His parents, 'John' and 'Vicki', have little difficulty understanding his speech, but are anxious to act on the teacher's concerns because even close relatives often need them, or Brett's sister 'Dorothy', 3;6, to interpret for them. Brett has received no previous SLP/SLT assessment or intervention when he becomes acquainted with 'Eric', the new graduate SLP/SLT who has just 1 hour to gather speech assessment data and related information. Sensibly, Eric has assigned Brett an early morning appointment, hoping that he will be fresh enough to perform well. Dorothy is at preschool and Brett is reassured to have both parents in the unfamiliar clinic room during the assessment, observing, participating, and responding to Eric's questions and clarification requests when Brett is difficult for *him* to understand.

Eric has already viewed Brett's normal audiogram and tympanogram, read the teacher's brief report, and reviewed the family's responses to a case history questionnaire mailed to them 3 weeks previously and returned a few days ago. He knows that Brett: (a) is reserved at preschool, seldom talking with peers; (b) shows frustration on the rare occasions that family members ask him to repeat himself, usually responding crossly with 'never mind'; (c) is sometimes teased by older neighbourhood children because he says *bwett* for *Brett*; (d) relies on Dorothy to interpret his wishes at times; (e) is a happy, confident boy in general, with good athletic skills, and is eager to speak more clearly.

The first 30 minutes of the consultation has comprised the case history interview, an unremarkable (but nonetheless essential) oral muscular examination, and conversing with Brett to establish rapport and gain an initial impression of his communication skills. The history uncovers nothing of note. Language development is age-appropriate and there are no indications of CAS or dysarthria. Rather, everything points to phonological impairment with the possibility of both phonemic and phonetic issues.

Like many SLPs/SLTs, Eric is equipped with a good-quality audio recorder, but does not have video. He has assembled a suitable standardised articulation and phonology assessment (such as the HAPP-3, the GFTA-2, or DEAP) and books, games, and toys to tempt Brett to talk, so that Eric can gather SW and spontaneous CS samples, imitated utterances, and intelligibility and stimulability data. It is important to note that a CS sample is essential in speech assessment, providing information that is unavailable from a SW articulation test. Analyses of aspects of these data will occur within the assessment hour, and, if required, Eric will do additional analyses later.

In my view, the most important parts of the assessment are twofold: first, the data collected should reveal the general nature of Brett's speech production patterns; second, the analyses should provide a basis for a treatment plan. Although the clinician may not be able to determine the precise substitution and deletion patterns for each phoneme of English, the data should show Brett's phonetic inventory in terms of sounds and syllable/word structures; voice quality; prosodic features; consistency of productions at the segmental and word levels; and his stimulability for absent sounds and syllable and word structures.

CS sample

Potentially, the spontaneous speech sample, gathered and recorded over 10-15 minutes, will bring to light Brett's: (1) 'everyday' language abilities in terms of mean length of utterance (MLU) and vocabulary; (2) production patterns in terms of speech rate, phrasal intonation, and fluency; (3) ability to perform revisions and repairs; and (4) overuse, if any, of a particular phoneme in running speech, a phenomenon referred to 'systematic sound preference' (Grunwell 1985a). Eric will obtain a sample of Brett's conversation with his parents and with Eric himself. John and Vicki will be asked to repeat any words Eric does not understand, to facilitate later analysis. Using the clinician as a conversational partner in sampling should demonstrate how Brett responds when his (relatively unfamiliar) conversational partner does not understand him. Does he simply repeat the utterance, modify it, refuse to respond, or pretend not to hear?

SW sample

In SLP/SLT contexts, the SW sample is typically drawn from a phonology or articulation test, such as the three mentioned above. The SW information it provides complements that gained from the CS sample. Because Eric knows what the intended targets are in his chosen test, he will be able to perform a relational analysis that displays which aspects of word productions do and do not match the target. Relational analysis is impossible with poorly intelligible CS samples with a high proportion of unknown target words.

Stimulability assessment

The term stimulability assessment refers to a dynamic evaluation (Edythe Strand, A40) wherein a clinician provides verbal, visual, tactile, or auditory cues to determine whether the child is able to adequately produce a sound or syllable structure with clinician support and scaffolding (Miccio, A15; Glaspey and Stoel-Gammon 2007). Having first ascertained from his SW and CS data Brett's sound and syllable structure constraints (absent phonemes and phonotactic combinations), Eric will determine whether Brett can produce, with support, his missing consonants and vowels in isolation, and consonant phonemes in at least two syllable positions (e.g., initially and finally).

Consistency assessment

Consistency of production refers to the degree to which the pronunciation of a word (or sometimes a phoneme) remains the same across various productions (Stoel-Gammon 2007). To assess variability, Eric will have Brett repeat five or six words, produced in error in the SW sample, several times. Then, to determine any effects of utterance length on consistency of production, he will elicit words (both those in error and those produced accurately) in increasingly complex environments. (e.g., by having Brett imitate *ball*, *basketball*, *basketball player*, and *big basketball player*).

Analysing the data

The time needed for analysis rests on several factors, including Eric's transcription skills, his familiarity with the analysis measures, and the intelligibility of the sample, but it should be 'doable' within an hour if the SLP/SLT is experienced. The procedure can be streamlined by following steps 1 to 5 below.

1. SW relational analysis

Let's assume that Eric has gathered and transcribed, online, using broad transcription and a few helpful diacritics, 45 known words. He will check his online transcriptions against his audiotape and make necessary corrections and additions, and then compare Brett's productions with idealised adult targets, in *relational* analyses that will provide numerical measures of accuracy. The quantitative measures of Brett's productions thus gained will be: (a) PCC, (b) PVC, and (c) percentage CV structure correct. The latter measure allows Eric to quantify the degree to which segment and syllable deletions occur in Brett's speech. In addition, Eric examines the *nature* of Brett's errors in terms of error patterns (often referred to as phonological processes). The error analysis allows Eric to see whether Brett's errors resemble those of younger, typically developing children or are disordered or idiosyncratic. Taken together, these relational measures will give Eric an idea of Brett's accuracy levels in elicited SW productions and of his error-types. He will also examine the accuracy of polysyllabic words, including stress placement, using the words and phrases from the consistency assessment.

2. SW independent analysis

Now Eric will focus exclusively on Brett's productions without reference to the adult target. Using a checklist, he simply notes the presence or absence of certain sound classes and syllable structures. The checklist is based on responses to the following seven questions, and they relate to Brett's word productions regardless of accuracy of pronunciation. Does the single-word sample include: (1) Stops at three places of articulation? Voiced and voiceless stops? (2) Nasals at three places of articulation? (3) Voiceless and voiceless fricatives and/or affricates, and how many of each? (4) Liquids? (5) Closed syllables? (6) Consonant clusters? (7) Three-syllable words? From this analysis, Eric will be able to determine the number and diversity of consonants and word structures Brett produces in SW productions.

3. CS analysis

Now Eric listens to the CS sample, glossing (i.e., writing down the words) 50–70 fully or partially intelligible utterances, half from the Brett–parent conversation and half from the Brett–Eric one. He will also record the number of unintelligible (to him) utterances. By dividing the intelligible utterances by the total utterances, and multiplying by 100, Eric gains an idea of Brett's percentage of intelligible utterances in CS. If Brett produces full sentences, yielding a relatively high MLU, a sample of 50 partially or fully intelligible utterances will suffice. One word responses such as '*yes*' and '*no*' should not be included in the utterance count, as they provide little information about Brett's phonological system.

After glossing, Eric listens once again to portions of the CS (about 100–120 utterances in all) and uses the checklist above to determine presence/absence of the sound classes and word structure forms in Brett's spontaneous speech. This independent analysis will be based on both intelligible and unintelligible utterances, and accuracy of production is not considered. In addition, Eric rates the 'normalcy' of Brett's voice quality, speech rate, lexical stress patterns, sentence rhythm, and prosody (Skinder-Meredith, A37), noting any systematic sound preferences.

4. Comparing the SW and CS analyses

The final step in Eric's analysis (and this should be considered a 'first pass' or 'overview') is to determine how Brett's SW and CS production patterns compare. In many cases, particularly for children who have received SLP/SLT intervention for their speech, SW phonetic inventories are relatively large, word structures are fairly complex, and accuracy of pronunciation may be quite good. In contrast, CS may be characterised by simple CV syllable structures and limited consonant and vowel inventories.

5. Looking further

The procedures outlined above can provide a broad, rather than deep, understanding of Brett's speech. If, for example, the assessment indicated that Brett had particular problems with vowels and multisyllabic words, Eric would later use relevant, more in-depth instruments to gain a more fine-grained analysis. It must be acknowledged that many published SW articulation tests do not assess all the vowels of English (see discussion in Stoel-Gammon and Pollock 2008) and even fewer assess words of more than two syllables; therefore, a full understanding of difficulties in these areas is only possible via additional assessments.

Interpreting the analyses

Now Eric must interpret his findings carefully in order to plan an effective and efficacious program of treatment. Speculatively, possible outcomes of the analysis and potential treatment approaches are summarised in the following three scenarios.

Scenario 1

Brett exhibits small SW and CS consonant and syllable structure inventories, and consequently a low PCC, low percentage of word structures correct, and of course, limited intelligibility. Accordingly, Eric thinks fast and considers treatment that focuses on phonetic inventory expansion, across place and manner classes and across syllable structures.

Scenario 2

SW and CS comparisons indicate high PCC scores for Brett's SW productions but a low PCC for spontaneous speech. Eric decides that the focus of intervention must be on transferring Brett's abilities in single words to running speech, and he talks to John and Vicky about how they can help with this generalisation.

Scenario 3

Brett's SW and CS phonetic inventories are large, and he has a good range of word structures, but he has low accuracy in terms of segments and word structures, and is highly inconsistent. So Eric sets about developing an intervention program to stabilise Brett's productions and encourage segmental and structural accuracy.

Summary

The key points of this assessment are as follows:

1. Assessment data gathering should be broad-based, examining productions in a variety of imitated, elicited, and spontaneous contexts: single words; spontaneous speech; word repetitions; and words/phrases produced with and without clinician support.
2. The analysis should involve both relational and independent approaches and focus on a variety of parameters: segmental accuracy; nature and consistency of segmental errors and word structure errors; vowel inventory and vowel accuracy; presence/absence of sound classes and word structures; stress at the word and sentence levels; and rate, rhythm, and intonation patterns of spontaneous sentence productions.
3. The assessment procedures identified will provide a broad overview of Brett's speech. The time needed for analysis is reduced by the use of a checklist approach. Once preliminary analyses are completed and areas of concern are identified, additional assessments should be performed, as needed.

Summarising assessment data

The sheer volume of analysed data collected from more talkative children can be overwhelming, but there is a range of ways to organise them to provide a quick but detailed overview of a child's speech. For example, Baker (2004) provides a practical 4-page phonological analysis summary and management plan, and, in the same volume there is a user friendly assessment of vowels summary (Watts, 2004).

Severity measures

Having analysed and organised a child's speech data, the clinician may want to quantify severity for his/her own information; to inform parents, as part of the process of ensuring appropriate services for the child; or for insurance purposes. The issue of determining and reporting severity of involvement has exercised the research skills of Dr. Peter Flipsen, Jr., a Professor of Speech Pathology in the department of Communication Sciences and Disorders, and Education of the Deaf at Idaho State University, Pocatello. So, he seemed the ideal person to answer the question posed in Q10. Widely published, he has the distinction of being third author of the sixth edition of the highly respected classic text *Articulation and Phonological Disorders* (Bernthal, Bankson, and Flipsen 2009). A proportion of Dr. Flipsen's current research program is devoted to examining atypical acquisition of speech sound production skills in children.

Q10.   Peter Flipsen, Jr.: Assessing and measuring severity of SSD

There appears to be considerable uncertainty about the best way to rate severity of involvement in child speech disorders, and it is also difficult to get a sense of how it is attempted in current clinical practice, and why clinicians want or even need these ratings. The findings of Flipsen, Hammer, and Yost (2005) indicate that the use of impressionistic rating scales for determining severity of involvement in children with speech delay is problematic. What alternative procedures and measures have better clinical utility, and what do you see as the best 'next step' in further investigation of severity measures?

A10.   Peter Flipsen, Jr.: Severity and speech sound disorders: a continuing puzzle

When we begin discussing severity of involvement, one question my students often ask is 'why do we even need to assess severity? Isn't it enough to just say that the child qualifies for services?' In some instances, it isn't necessary, but sometimes it is. In an era of personnel shortages and expanding demands for SLP services, we often need to prioritise our time. Where the law permits (not in the United States), children with milder problems may be placed on waiting lists, whereas those with greater degrees of involvement are given higher priority for services. Severity ratings may also be of value for clinicians who try to improve their efficiency by working with children in groups, with the groups often being defined by level of severity (I've not seen much evidence for the effectiveness of group interventions, however). Finally, I have even heard that some insurance companies determine the amount of service they will pay for based on severity ratings (i.e., children with milder problems would be entitled to fewer treatment sessions).

When the situation demands it, my sense is that most clinicians typically rely on impressionistic severity rating scales. But as indicated in the question, such scales are problematic. In our study (Flipsen, Hammer, and Yost 2005), we looked at ratings from a group of 10 very experienced clinicians (with at least 10 years of clinical experience working with children), and even they did not agree very well on their ratings of severity for a group of 17 children with speech delay of unknown origin. Admittedly, the scale we gave the clinicians was just a set of numbers on a line, with 1 being 'normal' and 7 being 'severe'. And we didn't tell them what to think about; we just said, 'tell us how severe you think their problem is'. Some clinicians and some of my students have since suggested that we should tell clinicians what specifically to focus on when they make their ratings. Some existing rating scales do that, and I can't honestly say I know whether clinicians agree any more than usual with such scales. In any event, ratings from rating scales may not be reliable because clinicians may simply be considering different things in their ratings. But then we have to decide what the most important things are that clinicians should focus on. As it turned out, in our study, we did try to figure that out by identifying the clinicians who agreed the most with each other (we found six who did), and we looked at what they were considering. We looked at how their ratings correlated with a long list of possible severity measures. It appeared that they were considering number, type, and consistency of errors at both the single-sound and whole-word levels. But we based our analysis on the ratings of only six clinicians, so we really can't generalise these findings to all clinicians. Perhaps more importantly, we didn't have enough data in our study to allow us to figure out whether any of the things they considered were more important than any of the others. Clearly, a much larger study is needed.

So what's a clinician to do? There is not yet a definitive answer, but one measure that continues to show up in the research literature is PCC (displayed in Table i.1, p. xii). Back in 1982, Shriberg and Kwiatkowski developed this measure and showed that it correlated very nicely with severity ratings of conversational speech samples obtained from a much larger group of clinicians (who used the same scale as in Flipsen et al. 2005). Shriberg and Kwiatkowski showed that, if PCC was less than 50%, then clinicians rated the sample as severe; if PCC was 50–65%, they rated the sample as moderate to severe; if PCC was 65–85%, they rated it as mild to moderate; and if PCC was greater than 85%, they rated the sample as mild. It should be noted that the samples used for the ratings were obtained from children age 4;1 to 8;6 (mean 5;9), so it isn't clear whether these severity categories are valid for children outside of this age range.

The calculation of PCC requires recording a conversational speech sample that includes at least 200 intelligible words. It should be a conversation; it is not clear whether similar severity ratings would be obtained with narrative samples. The sample should then be transcribed using narrow phonetic transcription. It is important to use narrow transcription because the severity categories determined by Shriberg and Kwiatkowski (1982c) were based on a definition of PCC which assumes that omissions, substitutions, and distortions (indicated by the presence of diacritics) are all errors. If broad transcription were to be used, distortions are being ignored, and the resulting measure is actually called PCC-R (Percentage Consonants Correct-Revised). See Shriberg, Austin, Lewis, et al. (1997) for a discussion of different variations on PCC, including measures that consider vowels. In any event, once the narrow transcription of the sample is completed, all of the consonants that were attempted should be examined and a tally made of those which are correct and those which are not (any omissions, substitutions, or distortions). Here is the formula for calculating PCC:

PCC = (# of correct consonants/total # of consonants attempted) × 100.

PCC is not perfect, however. One practical problem with using it clinically is that age differences are not accounted for. If two children both have a PCC score of 75%, would it really mean the same thing if one child was three years old and the other was eight years old? Probably not. In addition, error types may not be the same at different ages. That three-year-old may be producing mostly omission and substitution errors, whereas the eight-year-old may be producing mostly residual distortion errors (Gruber 1999). One way to get around the age question (though it doesn't directly address the error type issue) would be to know how PCC normally changes with age. Normative studies don't yet exist and clearly need to be developed, but Austin and Shriberg (1996) have developed 'reference data' based on several hundred children with normal or normalised speech (who happened to have been part of various research projects). That report provides means and standard deviations for PCC over a wide range of ages. These PCC data can be freely downloaded from http://www.waisman.wisc.edu/phonology/BIB/Bib.htm and could be used by American clinicians (since the children all spoke dialects of American English) to estimate how many standard deviations the child is from his/her age peers. For clinicians in other countries, such reference data could be developed.

A related 'concern' with PCC is the fact that it only is valid to translate the scores into severity categories if your PCC values come from conversational speech. I refer to this as a concern (and not a problem) only because many clinicians still fail to assess conversational speech. Several studies over the years (e.g., Andrews and Fey 1986; DuBois and Bernthal 1978; Healy and Madison 1987; Morrison and Shriberg 1992; Wolk and Meisler 1998) have shown that performance in SW is usually different from performance in conversation, and thus conversational speech should probably be evaluated directly. On the other hand, Masterson, Bernhardt, and Hofheinz (2005) showed that PCC values derived from one particular single word task were not significantly different from PCC values derived from conversational samples. Arguments from clinicians against evaluating conversational speech are twofold. They say they don't have the time, and they say they aren't sure they will get a good sample of all the speech sounds. In response to these concerns, Johnson, Weston, and Bain (2004) developed a sentence repetition task that includes a representative sample of the consonants of English, and they showed that PCC scores on their task are not significantly different from PCC scores obtained from conversational speech samples. Administering and scoring the sentence-repetition task is much faster than recording and transcribing conversational speech. The task itself is shown in an appendix of their publication and includes a phonetic transcription and a formula for calculating PCC. Each sentence is read aloud to the child, and, as the child repeats it, the clinician simply crosses out any consonant phoneme that was not produced correctly (again any omission, substation, or distortion). Johnson and colleagues did not, however, directly examine whether severity ratings would be the same on the two tasks. This probably does need to be done, as the link from PCC scores on their task to PCC scores from conversation to severity rating from conversation is an indirect one at best. But if you really can't do conversational speech analysis, it may be a place to start.

Parents' concerns and questions

> *If parental involvement in SLT is a requirement, there should be a greater focus on their perceptions, needs and concerns, particularly during the early phase of their involvement... Where recognition of the parental perspective could influence future decision making and negotiation of treatment... it emerged from the parents' accounts that even where they became involved in their child's therapy, this did not lessen, in their eyes, the need for the therapist to be involved. The therapist was perceived by parents as the provider of the direction and means for therapy.*
>
> Glogowska and Campbell 2000

The questions parents ask

Once their child's speech has been assessed, parents or caregivers are provided with a report. This may be a verbal report in some instances, but often it is a written report; and, in some settings, reports in writing are mandatory. The initial questions parents ask their SLP/SLT, and often *keep* asking, arising from such reports, are usually related to *severity* ('How serious is my child's problem?'), *prevalence* ('Do many children have this problem?'), *aetiology* ('What caused this problem?'), *prognosis* ('Can the problem be corrected?'), *therapy* ('What are you, or we, going to do about the problem?'), and *target selection* and *goal setting* ('Where do we start working on the problem?'). Severity, prevalence, and aetiology are discussed above, and will be addressed briefly again here, relative to the kinds of answers clinicians can provide to families.

The questions families ask: severity

Other than presenting them with impressionistic estimates based on experience with similar children, there are three simple-to-use aids available to help in answering parent's questions about severity, each of which is based on objective measures. The three: PCC, percentage of occurrence of processes or patterns, and normative data, can be used in combination with each other, alongside informal intelligibility ratings.

PCC

Although it has its limitations (Flipsen, A10), PCC can be useful in providing an impression of 'severity of involvement' to parents. It is important to explain to them that not everything to do with speech impairment can be neatly classified in terms of mild, moderate, and severe, and that the severity increments suggested by Shriberg (1982; displayed in Table i.1 p. xii) cannot be applied with children below 4;1 or older than 8.6.

An advantage of using this simple scale is that it can become the basis for demonstrating progress (or lack of progress) over time, to families. Some children, from the age of about 4;0 (particularly those who are entranced by numbers or who like to see progress represented graphically), enjoy seeing their PCCs rise and find it encouraging. Simple imagery using a drawing of a ladder, mountain, flight path, or train journey (with a PCC of 50% shown at the half-way mark and 100% at the summit or destination and gradations between) can provide pleasure and motivation.

Percentage of occurrence of processes/patterns

Similarly, when the presence of phonological patterns or phonological processes is expressed in percentage terms (e.g., Cluster Reduction 100%) in initial reporting to parents, it provides a straightforward way for them to appreciate their child's therapy gains as the percentage drops. Again, this can be conveyed to those children who are spurred on by performance feedback and extrinsic reinforcers (Lowe, A16).

Normative data

Age norms for the typical ages of elimination of processes (see Table 2.4) may be helpful for parents and can allay anxiety in those who are inclined to expect too-much–too-soon, like the many parents the many parents who worry unnecessarily about gliding of liquids and interdental /s/ and /z/ in three year olds!

Intelligibility ratings

Intelligibility ratings are notoriously unreliable, but they have considerable clinical utility. As well as being informative for parents, it can be quite a useful exercise for clinicians to ask for impressionistic ratings of intelligibility on a five-point scale from parent(s) or a significant other, such as a grandparent or preschool teacher, and compare these with the therapist's own rating. Those doing the rating are asked, 'How intelligible is ___ in day-to-day conversation. How much of what s/he says do *you* understand?' They then select a point on the following scale. Sometimes they will qualify their ratings, for example, by observing that the child is less intelligible when tired, unwell, or rushed, or that intelligibility often seems better when the child speaks on the telephone, and this is useful information for the clinician to have.

1. Completely Intelligible
2. Mostly Intelligible
3. Somewhat Intelligible
4. Mostly Unintelligible
5. Completely Unintelligible

Reviewing the original ratings and comparing them with current ratings once intervention is underway and progress is evident can provide encouragement to parents, which they may convey to their child receiving therapy. Occasionally, it is enlightening to ask children how intelligible they believe they are by getting them to rate a familiar adult as a listener ('How well does Dad understand your words?' and 'How well does he understand ___'s [naming another child or adult] words?').

The questions families ask: prevalence

Work cited by the Waisman Phonology Project indicates that around 15% of three-year-olds have difficulties with speech intelligibility that are not associated with currently known causes. When they enter Grade 1, their second year of school, about 25% of these children (some 3.5% of all children) retain a significant, diagnosable speech disorder of currently unknown origin. The National Institute on Deafness and Other Communication Disorders (NIDCD) and ASHA, drawing on the work of Gierut (1998), have reported that 10% of children entering Grade 1 have a moderate-to-severe speech disorder, and that 16 in every 1000 children under age 18 have a chronic speech disorder.

The questions families ask: aetiology

As discussed above, we still do not know in *precise* terms the causes of the so-called SSDs of unknown origin, but their aetiology is no longer such a mystery (Flipsen 2002; Shriberg 2006). In view of this, perhaps we could relinquish the use of 'functional' in clinical settings, as it has become something of a misnomer. We can now provide parents with suggestions as to *likely* causes relative to three putative aetiological subtypes. This is surely preferable to unsatisfactory (to parents) responses like 'We don't really know'. Current research suggests that 'functional' SSD may be due to genetic transmission of a linguistic processing deficit, middle ear disease, or genetic transmission of a speech motor control deficit. Each can occur co-morbidly, in varying degrees, in the same child.

Genetic transmission of a linguistic processing deficit (60%)

The first putative cause, accounting for about 60% of referrals, is the genetic transmission of a linguistic processing deficit, expressed as a problem with speech production. There are findings to support the theory of aetiology for this group in the form of large family studies, particularly the K.E. family study of a rare genetic disorder in the UK (Vargha-Khadem, Watkins, Alcock, et al. 1995). Exploration of the risk factors for childhood speech disorder by Fox, Dodd, and Howard (2002) led to a finding that between 28% and 60% of children with a speech and language deficit have a similarly affected sibling or parent, or both. Family history is also commonly revealed in the day-to-day experience and informal 'genotype research' (see Table 2.1) of clinicians, not only in case history taking, but also in the frequent appearance on our speech caseloads of siblings, cousins, or otherwise closely related children.

Middle ear disease (30%)

In the second group, covering about 30% of referrals, are the children who have experienced or who are experiencing fluctuating ('fluctuant') conductive hearing loss, typically associated with episodic otitis media with effusion (OME), or middle ear disease (Casby 2001). Otitis media is the most frequently diagnosed disease in infants and young children (Dhooge 2003). Findings that have arisen from structural equation modelling techniques (Shriberg, Flipsen, Kwiatkowski, et al. 2003) suggest that speech effects are most closely tied to hearing loss associated with frequent OME occurring in the 12–18 months age range (for further discussion, see Purdy, A47).

Genetic transmission of a speech motor control deficit (10%)

The remaining 10% are understood to have a genetically transmitted deficit in speech motor control, and in this grouping are the children with CAS. There are several ongoing collaborative genetic projects around CAS aimed at developing the phenotype for this disorder. Perceptual and acoustic techniques are being used to gather, analyse, and quantify affected children's and family members' speech, speech motor control, and prosody.

In fact, all three putative subtypes are the subject of active investigation by teams of researchers. The goals of this research are to understand the origins of the disorders and to support the development of assessment and treatment methods that enable consumers and SLPs/SLTs to make optimal clinical decisions for affected children. Data collection and data analysis are centered around epidemiologic, molecular genetic, and speech-language data on each of the three, in the contexts of both genotype and phenotype research.

The questions families ask: prognosis

Questions about prognosis and anticipated duration of therapy may be posed in a variety of ways, from 'How much treatment does my child need?' (which may sound like an enquiry about the probable cost in money and time) to a more direct, 'Will my child's speech be normal by the time he/she starts school?' and even 'Will my child's speech improve to the point that no one would know there was ever a speech difficulty?' Such questions are commonly asked early in the therapeutic engagement, often before any assessment or therapy has taken place. For most children with SSD, the outlook is optimistic (Gierut 1998; Kamhi 2006b; Shriberg 1997). Shriberg reported that approximately 75% of children with speech delay had normal range speech performance by the age of six (with or without therapy), and that the balance (25%) normalised by nine, with just a few exhibiting residual errors, typically /s/, /r/, and /l/ distortions. Because we do not have robust outcome figures for the small CAS subgroup, statements to parents must be more guarded, but we can say that therapy for CAS has been shown to be effective even in severe cases (Jakielski, Kostner, and Webb 2006; Strand, Stoeckel, and Baas 2006).

The questions families ask: therapy approaches, target selection, and goal setting

It is quite usual for parents to ask their new therapist, 'Which method do you use?' especially if they have been advised that a particular method is preferable. There is a range of evidence-based treatment approaches to phonetic and phonemic issues (Baker and McLeod 2004; Joffe and Serry 2004) and CAS (Strand, Stoeckel, and Baas 2006) as well as many commercially available materials and programs, with varying levels of empirical support, for SSD, and particularly for CAS. These materials and programs are available on the open market, and some parents purchase them with a view to 'going it alone' with therapy or augmenting what the SLP/SLT puts in place. Without patronising, it may be important to counsel some parents that not all treatments suit every child and that all treatments have to be individually and expertly tailored in response to the child's needs, strengths, challenges, co-morbidities, assessment outcomes, and response to intervention. In that sense, they must appreciate that there is no one 'preferred method', and that a 'good method' is one that is adaptable to changes in the child (in terms of attention, interest, motivation, and well-being) and flexible over time (as the child develops) and across settings (clinic, home, preschool, and 'out') and conditions (one-to-one in a dyad, and in a group). Whereas it is common for parents to ask about the overall therapy approach, or combination of approaches, a clinician uses, it is quite rare for them to ask about target selection and goal setting, except perhaps to suggest working on a particular sound that worries them. For example, some parents are keen to work on interdental substitutions for /s/ and /z/, or difficulties with /r/ and /l/ because of issues of stereotyping and social indexing (Munson, A45).

Question families seldom ask: phonological generalisation

Parents rarely ask about phonological generalisation, but it is something that we as clinicians think about all the time—carefully choosing targets with an eye to maximal impact. If parents do ask, they may be reassured if we convey, in accessible terms, that we:

- exercise clinical judgement in selecting targets (breaking 'the rules' advisedly at times);
- select targets using linguistic criteria while taking into account motivational factors;
- take into consideration attributes of the child and the parents;
- are flexible in choosing targets and feature contrasts;
- are mindful of, and refer periodically to, the growing evidence-base for explicitly principled target selection criteria (listed in Table 8.1, p. 282).

One person who is vitally interested in the impact of target selection upon phonological generalisation is Dr. Elise Baker, an SLP and lecturer with The University of Sydney. Elise has almost two decades of clinical and research experience in the area of speech impairment in children. She has a particular interest in treatment efficacy research, exploring how theory informs practice, and how intervention research informs theory. Elise is also interested in how SLPs/SLTs across different workplaces put research into practice.

Q11.   Elise Baker: Prioritising complex treatment targets

The term 'phonological generalisation' refers to a change in a child's phonological system that goes beyond the treatment words or treatment (sound or structure) targets used during therapy. How can a clinician set about using theoretical concepts in phonology, such as markedness, implicational relationships, sonority, and complexity to prioritise intervention targets in order to facilitate widespread change in children's phonological systems for less SLP/SLT time?

A11.   Elise Baker: The why and how of prioritising complex targets for intervention

SLPs/SLTs have a tradition of prioritising early developing and stimulable speech sound intervention targets. Such targets are reasoned to be easier and less frustrating for children to learn. Other time-honoured criteria influencing target selection are sounds that are in the child's name, important to the child or family, or prominent in the ambient language; and production patterns that attract teasing, are unusual, highly variable, or greatly affecting intelligibility. Such factors may be relevant, but the logic and principles they reflect are rarely grounded in phonological theory.

Theories guide clinicians' actions, potentially explaining and predicting their consequences (Apel 1999). The likely consequence of targeting a sound deemed 'easier' for an unintelligible preschooler to learn is that it will be learned. Will there be an overall effect on other gaps in the child's speech output? That we cannot predict. But target selection guided by theoretical principles helps SLPs/SLTs predict likely systemic changes to a child's speech production, when intervention addresses a particular target. This handy crystal ball tells the SLP/SLT, 'If I select sound X then I might not only get X, but also Y and Z.'

Children need to be intelligible by the critical age of 5;6 (Nathan, Stackhouse, Goulandris, et al. 2004), so improvements must be timely. For over 20 years, research has accrued favouring treatment of complex targets that induce system-wide phonological change (Gierut 2007). What are *complex* targets? To answer this question, several theoretical phonological principles need cumulative definition. Understanding a definition in the following list requires understanding of prior definitions.

Linguistic universals

phonological characteristics or traits across (nearly) all languages. Universals may be *absolute* in nature, such as all languages have stops; or universals may be *tendencies* across many languages, such as most languages have at least one nasal phoneme (O'Grady, Archibald, Aronoff, et al. 2005).

Markedness

phonological characteristics that are uncommon across languages such as /θ/ are termed marked (Velleman 1998). Universal characteristics such as stops are unmarked. Marked traits are usually more complex and later developing, like /θ/ in English. Ordinarily, a marked trait occurs in a language if its unmarked (implied) counterpart also occurs (O'Grady et al. 2005).

Implicational relationships/universals

the existence of a marked trait in a language implies the existence of the unmarked counterpart. For instance, stops and fricatives are related by implication because fricatives' existence in a language implies the existence of stops. This next point is highly relevant to target selection. If a child has stops, they will not, by implication, have fricatives. If a child has fricatives, however, by implication they will have stops. How can this impact target selection? If an unintelligible four-year-old has few stops (e.g., only /t, d, b/) and is taught the more marked trait of fricatives, then by implication this child might acquire the targeted fricatives *and* the previously absent stops. A comparable situation exists with clusters implying affricates. Clinical illustrations provided by Gierut (2007) tell of child '154' (3;2) and child '147' (3;1). Pre-treatment neither used affricates phonemically nor produced clusters. Child 154's treatment target was /tw-/. Post-treatment, this child learned /tw/, both affricates /tʃ, dʒ/, and other clusters. Child 147's treatment target was /tʃ/, and only /tʃ/ was learned. Post-treatment child 147 'showed little or no further generalisation, either to other affricates or clusters' (Gierut 2007, p. 10), indicating that clusters may be the targets of choice.

Sonority

the amount of stricture or 'sound' in a consonant or vowel (Roca and Johnson 1999). This concept has proved interesting in clinical phonology application recently and is germane to target selection. Steriade (1990) proposed a numerical sonority hierarchy: a list of phones, ordered according to degree of oral stricture and sound. Most sonorous are vowels (0), then glides (1), liquids (2), nasals (3), voiced fricatives (4), voiceless fricatives (5), voiced stops (6), and finally, voiceless stops (7). If you say [i] versus [p], the vowel is obviously the more sonorous. We like to articulate words with a rise and fall in sonority. For instance, in a word like *print*, we start with the least sonorous segment (voiceless plosive) followed by liquid with the vowel at the peak, then the less sonorous nasal, finally falling to the least sonorous voiceless stop. It would be unnatural to say [rpɪtn]. This rise-then-fall tendency is called the sonority sequencing principle. How does this principle relate to markedness, implicational relationships, and target selection? Consonant clusters are more marked than singletons, but are some clusters *more* marked than others? One approach to classifying two-element consonant clusters according to markedness is to rank them according to their sonority difference score, using their respective numerical values from a sonority hierarchy (Ohala 1999). For example, /kw/ (7 minus 1) has a sonority difference score of 6, whereas /fl/ (5 minus 2) scores 3. Classifying clusters according to sonority difference, Gierut (1999) reported that those with small sonority difference scores (e.g., /fl/, scoring 3) are more marked than consonant clusters with larger sonority difference scores (e.g., /tw/ scoring 6). For example, Child 6 (3;8), detailed in Gierut (2007), produced no clusters prior to intervention for /bl/. Following intervention, the child acquired /tw, kw, pl, bl, sw, fl, sm, sn, sp, st/ in addition to varying but improved production of: /f, v, θ, ð, s, z, t, ʃ, h, l, r/. Child 2 (4;2) in the same study was taught the relatively less marked /kw/ with its larger sonority difference score. This child did not acquire clusters in response to intervention, but showed generalisation to two untreated singletons, /ʃ, dʒ/. In a similar study of 12 children with phonological impairment, Baker (2007) reported that targeting /s/+C, specifically, /sn, st, sp/, saw some children learning /s/ clusters *and* other untreated clusters (e.g., pre-treatment David used /kw/ only, whereas post-treatment he acquired /sp, st, sk, sm, sn, pr, br, kr, bl, str/). Not all of Baker's participants had such far-reaching changes, with some only learning initial /s/ clusters. Further, it was noted that the participants' pre-treatment productive phonological knowledge influenced what they learned about the phonological system. Morrisette, Farris, and Gierut (2006) postulate that initial /s/+ stop 'clusters' are adjuncts, not true clusters, and therefore are not subject to the implicational relationships amongst clusters with respect to sonority. It seems that clusters with a small sonority difference of 3, like /sl, fl/, or 4, like /bl/, may better promote generalised change to singletons and clusters. Gierut (1999), Gierut and Champion (2001), and Morrisette et al. (2006) provide compelling evidence and consonant cluster target selection guidelines.

Complexity

a useful abstract concept for studying systems, the constituents of systems, and how they inter-relate in organised hierarchies. The interested reader is referred to Rescher (1998), who provides a philosophical overview of complexity. Consider a speech sound. It is part of a child's phonological system, abiding by laws or rules determining its relationship to the other sounds and structures (e.g., syllables, word shapes, and stress patterns). It has a relative complexity status being either more or less complex than other system constituents. Furthermore, the phonological system interacts with other linguistic and cognitive systems. A metaphor illustrates what this means for selecting intervention targets. Elbert (1989) suggested that the phonological system is a puzzle children solve as they learn to talk. Imagine a jigsaw puzzle depicting an elephant on bare, dry ground. Some puzzle-pieces are 'complex', containing more information about the bigger picture. These have more spaces where other pieces can attach. A child with a severe phonological impairment characterised by a limited phonetic inventory may have a few puzzle pieces depicting dry ground, but they are unhelpful in informing the bigger picture. Upon receiving a 'complex' puzzle piece, like the elephant's head and trunk, the child possesses important bigger picture information, enabling quicker, more efficient completion of more parts of the puzzle than would be possible had they received another less informative puzzle piece depicting dry ground. This idea has research support: selecting complex targets for intervention helps children learn *efficiently* about the phonological system. The complexity of a phonological constituent triggers the aspects of the system learned. Using the basic tenets of learnability theory, Gierut (2007) argues that, to learn efficiently, children with phonological impairment must be taught complex parts of the system, beyond what they have already learned. This idea is not limited to child phonology. The benefit of preferring complex over simpler targets manifests excitingly in other language domains, including syntax (Thompson and Shapiro 2007) and semantics (Kiran, 2007). In a clinical forum on the complexity account of treatment efficacy (CATE), Thompson (2007, p. 3) noted that 'while challenging the long standing clinical notion that treatment should begin with simple structures, mounting evidence points towards the facilitative effects of using more complex structures as a starting point for treatment.' In a discussion on complex targets within the context of phonological intervention, Gierut (2001) proposed four general, evidence-based categories. A brief summary with examples follows.

1. Complex linguistic structures

Marked properties or structures of the phonological system are complex and have been shown to imply unmarked properties. For example, consonants imply vowels (Robb, Bleile, and Yee 1999); fricatives imply stops (Elbert, Dinnsen, and Powell 1984); affricates imply fricatives (Schmidt and Meyers 1995); clusters (except for /sp, st, sk/) imply affricates (Gierut and O'Connor 2002); and true clusters with small sonority differences imply true clusters with larger sonority differences (Gierut 1999). See Gierut (2001, 2007) for helpful reviews.

2. Complex psycholinguistic structures

Psycholinguistics explores children's speech and language processing (Baker, Croot, McLeod, et al. 2001). The study of complexity and treatment target selection attests interactions between the phonological system and the lexicon. Morrisette and Gierut (2002) reported that words occurring frequently in a language facilitated more system-wide improvements in children's phonological systems compared with low-frequency words, indicating that sounds in high-frequency words are more complex.

3. Complex articulatory phonetic factors

Stimulability reflects an individual's capacity for articulatory complexity. According to Powell (2003), as non-stimulable sounds are more complex, they should take priority over stimulable sounds to facilitate generalisation to both stimulable and non-stimulable sounds. Powell, Elbert, and Dinnsen (1991) provide supporting evidence. Rvachew's (2005b) research supports an alternative view: selection of stimulable sounds. Rvachew also notes the importance of phonemic perception training alongside phonetic place procedures for improving stimulability.

4. Conventional clinical factors

Developmentally later acquired sounds are more complex, facilitating greater system-wide changes than earlier acquired sounds (Gierut, Morrisette, Hughes, et al. 1996). Sounds consistently in error, underpinned by least productive phonological knowledge, are considered more complex (Gierut, Elbert, and Dinnsen 1987). Simultaneous selection and pairing of two or more sounds that differ by major class and have maximal feature differences is more complex, facilitating greater system-wide changes compared with targeting one sound (Gierut 1992). Indeed, Williams' (2005) systemic approach to target selection requires targeting up to four sounds (including clusters) within one session, with target selection based on phoneme collapses, irrespective of markedness, stimulability status, or age norms.

The steps a clinician can take in applying the principles of complexity are as follows. Firstly, discover what the child knows about the phonological system they are learning through an independent and relational analysis. List any singleton consonants and clusters not used by the child. Discard stimulable, early-developing, relatively less marked targets. This will probably leave just late-developing sounds and clusters. Recalling that targeting clusters is demonstrably efficient in achieving much progress in exchange for relatively little SLP/SLT time, scrutinise all two- and three-element clusters. Identify clusters with small sonority differences, excepting /sp, sk, st/. Consider prioritising three-element clusters (e.g., /spl, str/) or those with small sonority difference scores, such as /fl, sl, ʃr/ in light of your analysis of the child's phonological knowledge of the cluster constituents; this step is important. See Gierut (2004a) and Morrisette et al. (2006) for clear guidelines and case studies. With complex targets identified, intervene using high-frequency words. Finally and crucially, although target selection guided by theory and evidence offers predictive insight into possible system-wide changes, the predictions do not *guarantee* a child's response to intervention. Phonological generalisation data *must* be collected regularly throughout intervention to monitor progress, guiding ongoing clinical decisions (Baker and McLeod 2004). Watch for changes to the singletons and clusters originally listed. Treatment target(s) may change sluggishly, but subtle, easily missed changes may occur unnoticed, unless phonological generalisation is closely monitored. This is a brief, prescriptive account of the complexity approach to theoretically principled target selection, a deeper understanding of which can be gained by reading the fascinating references suggested here. The complexity approach is one of a few recent approaches for selecting targets. For example, see Williams' (2005) systemic approach and Bernhardt and Stemberger's (2000) constraint-based nonlinear approach for alternative perspectives on treatment target selection.

Communicating with clients

In a much thumbed chapter on terminology and nomenclature, Kenneth Scott Wood wrote:

> *All areas of scientific study are afflicted with a certain amount of ambiguity, duplication, inappropriateness, and disagreement in the use of terms. Like other sciences, speech pathology, audiology, and the entire cluster of studies associated with the production and perception of speech have been developing over the years a terminology and nomenclature that leave much to be desired in logic and stability. Many terms and their meanings are not well crystallized because the subject matter is always changing; concepts themselves are often tentative and fluid, and many writers have liberally coined new terms whenever they felt a need to do so. This growth of speech pathology and audiology, stimulated as it has been by so many workers, has generated hundreds of terms, some of which are interchangeable, some of which have different meanings to different people, some of which are now rare or obsolete, and some of which for various reasons have had only a short literary life.* Wood, 1971, p. 3

What might Wood have made of 'prioritising complex targets', 'linguistic universals', 'markedness theory', 'the sonority sequencing principle', 'implicational relationships', 'psycholinguistic structures', 'most' and 'least' productive phonological knowledge, 'phoneme collapse', and 'constraint-based nonlinear phonology'? Onerous and confusing though it may be, however, technical language is essential to professions like ours. It enables us to define precisely what we are talking about, so facilitating unambiguous communication within our profession, with other professions, and, when appropriate, with consumers of our services. Meanwhile, a crucial role for SLPs/SLTs is that of clarifying jargon for consumers of our services, if and when they want such explanations. Conveying such information can be difficult. The information itself may be distressing; it is not an easy thing, for instance, to explain the prognostic implications of CAS or dysarthria to a troubled parent. The recipient of the information may be distressed, unprepared for answers, or have difficulty understanding or accepting them. The situation in which the information is being transmitted may be unfavourable and the available time inadequate. And the manner in which the information is conveyed may be problematic: detailed written reports, for example, with no face-to-face verbal explanation, may be alienating and too confronting for many clients.

Many of us have had the unfortunate experience of trying unsuccessfully to explain complex concepts and issues, for clients or caregivers, without misinforming them by oversimplifying the message. At the same time, we know that, for some consumers, the use of correct terminology is a sign (to them) that professionals are prepared to share information openly and respectfully without making condescending value judgements about their capacity to understand, accommodate, and 'use' such information appropriately. Indeed, numerous families (and clients, if they are old enough) prefer to be told the correct name of a disorder, symptom, anatomical feature, assessment procedure, or therapy technique.

On the other hand, the last thing many families of children with communication difficulties want to hear when they are attempting to understand and help their child's speech development is a torrent of incomprehensible jargon. For a lot of families, this is particularly true in the early stages of diagnosis and at times when they are anxious and upset. They do want facts, but until they are confidently engaged in a constructive program for their child, most can do without the complications of having to understand the differences between, for example, the astonishing number of 'speech pathology words' that seem to start with 'phon' or 'dys'! We also have to bear in mind that people deal with the information we present in different ways and at different rates. In situations where just one parent brings a child to therapy, so that the other parent gets all the information by proxy, it is not uncommon for the accompanying parent to reach a degree of acceptance and insight into the child's difficulties in advance of their partner. In such a situation, the parent who actually meets with the clinician may be more prepared to 'trust' the information being conveyed. These and other issues around terminology, classification, description, assessment, and 'breaking the news' are often highlighted in our engagement with the various 'special populations' described in Chapter 3.

Chapter 3
Special populations

All children with speech sound disorders (SSD) require 'special consideration', but there are certain individual clients and client-groups that seem to warrant *extra* special consideration. In this chapter, issues that manifest clinically for these individuals and groups and their families are examined. The topics are: parents' perceptions of their child's SSD at the point of initial referral; children with co-occurring speech *and* language disorders (McCauley, A12); children with cleft palate, craniofacial anomalies, and velopharyngeal dysfunction (Golding-Kushner, A13); children who have been internationally adopted (Pollock, A14); children with limited stimulability (Miccio, A15); children with SSD and issues of self-efficacy (Lowe, A16); children with speech *and* literacy difficulties (Neilson, A17); and children with speech impairments in culturally and linguistically diverse settings (Bleile, A18).

Parents' initial perceptions of their child's SSD

In general SLT/SLP paediatric practice, some of the children whose parents bring them for initial screening and assessment have problems with speech as their *only* voice, speech, language, or fluency issue, and others have a SSD as their obvious and *primary* communication disorder perhaps in conjunction with minor language delays. For the majority of them, SLP/SLT management is straightforward from the therapist's perspective. In these cases, parents will have identified their child's speech issue and arranged for an assessment, whereupon the clinician assessed the child's speech and initiated an appropriate intervention regimen, suggested a 'watchful waiting' approach, or informed the parent that the child's speech was within normal limits in the context of discussion of normal expectations (see Tables 1.3, p. x and 2.4, p. x). Some parents contact the SLP/SLT indicating descriptively that their child has severe, moderate, or mild speech issues. Within the 'mild' group, parents may report difficulties with one or two sounds: /k/ and /g/; /s/ and /z/; /r/, /l/, or /θ/ and /ð/. When some of these children with supposedly minor difficulties actually attend for assessment, it transpires that the parents' observations were accurate and sufficient, but often this turns out *not* to be the case. In fact, most clinicians can probably produce examples of times when, given a parent's description during the intake process, they were expecting to evaluate a child with little amiss with their speech, only to find a complex speech picture, on occasion with additional issues.

Similarly, parents may come to the SLP/SLT because, or partly because, they have been encouraged to do so by a nursery or daycare worker ('carer') or preschool teacher or school teacher ('teacher'), all of whom regularly assume an important role as referrers to SLP/SLT services. Sometimes parents, suspecting a problem, will have approached the carer or teacher for referral advice ('I think my son needs to see a speech therapist; do you agree?'; 'Is my daughter's speech development on-track for a child of her age?'). On the other hand, sometimes the carer or teacher makes the first move, with the parents apparently unaware of any difficulty ('Your son's speech is difficult to understand; have you considered an assessment by a speech professional?'). Other parents notice a speech problem but actually *wait* for carers or teachers to prompt them into action. In these situations, carers and teachers can be understandably tentative and overly reassuring, not wanting to alarm parents or appear to be critical of their child-rearing prowess. So, when the parent contacts the SLP/SLT, they may quote the referring person as saying that the child's pronunciation errors are quite minor and that the referral is precautionary. They may even report to the SLP/SLT that the referrer mentioned that 'just a few sessions' of therapy or home management advice would quickly rectify the problem. Again, this sort of low-key initial presentation can be the opening gambit with children who prove to have complex intervention needs. Meanwhile, the reverse happens, too, with parents reporting severe difficulties that turn out to be mild (though perhaps not 'mild' from the parents' perspective). Further, they may express concerns about *speech* when issues with *language* or *fluency* appear, to the therapist, to be more in need of attention. Such situations may require a perceptual shift by parents, and necessary support while this is happening should be in place. It may not be a big step for a parent to accept that he or she has been worrying unnecessarily, but it can be a painful adjustment for those who unexpectedly discover that a so-called mild problem is serious, especially when the advice of a trusted carer or teacher conflicts with the therapist's expert advice. No matter how serious or mild the child's difficulty appears to be, it is the clinician's responsibility to determine the presence or absence of speech impairment, to diagnose the nature of it if there is one, and to determine if any *other* types of communication disorder, or 'special considerations' are present.

Three special populations

Referral of children with co-occurring speech *and* language difficulties is a frequent occurrence and, according to reviews by Tyler (2002) and Tyler and Tolbert (2002), language-based approaches appear to be the best possible intervention choice for them. Even with timely, appropriate intervention, these children may be in therapy for lengthy periods (Ruscello, St. Louis, and Mason 1991; Tyler and Watterson 1991), so there is often a strong desire on everyone's part for intervention to start without delay. But there is a period for some children with speech impairment when the treatment of their poor intelligibility is a low intervention priority. For example, there are the children with such severe language delays or disorders, including pragmatic language limitations with accompanying behaviour difficulties, that it is extremely problematic to know how to tame and engage with them, what to treat first, or what combination of issues to address.

Then there are the sickest children with cleft palate and craniofacial anomalies, many of whom run a physical and emotional marathon—with their families—of heroic medical management, surgical intervention, degrees of recovery, and hard-won survival before they ever reach us (Kummer 2008). And third, there are the internationally adopted infants, toddlers, and children who may have travelled to foreign countries from places where SLP/SLT services are unavailable and for whom initial consultation may be late by the usual standards of the industrialised world.

All three of these groups *may* contain *some* children who are behaviourally challenging: actively acting out, depressed, or unduly passive, possibly as a consequence of their life experiences, in terms of health and wellbeing, surgery, trauma, malnutrition, dislocation, and separation. Their communication issues may have been exacerbated by insufficient stimulation in orphanages or hospitals, late identification, communicative frustration, or shifting linguistic influences. There may be powerful co-morbidities, such as medical fragility and the complex of psychosocial disturbances, sensory issues, and seizures, that appear to go hand-in-hand with some craniofacial anomalies and certain syndromes. The following three questions to our experts are about these particularly special groups of children and their families.

Children with co-occurring speech and language disorders

In a thoughtful piece about spoken language, Kent (2004, p. 1) may have summed up the view of many parents about the elite status of speech, when he made the arresting statement that:

> *Speech is but one modality for the expression of language; however, speech has special importance because it is the primary, first-learned modality for hearing language users. Speech is a system in the sense that it consistently and usefully relates the meanings of a language with the sounds by which a language is communicated.*

Many parents will wistfully tell clinicians early in an initial meeting something along the lines of, 'If he could talk clearly, it would solve a lot of problems.' These same parents may be surprised or worried if a clinician appears not to be focused on the child's speech but more interested in evaluating a range of *other* aspects of the child's presentation, such as levels of comprehension in differing conditions. Then, when it comes to therapy, parents of children who are speech- *and* language-impaired may feel that their genuine concerns about speech intelligibility are being sidelined, as they see it, while language objectives are given undue precedence.

In A12, Rebecca McCauley talks about the issues involved in assessment, treatment planning, and intervention for severely involved children with co-occurring speech and language issues, including those with complex presentations and worrying behaviour, where families in particular, but also at times, trans-disciplinary team members, find it difficult to come to grips with customary, evidence-based SLP/SLT intervention priorities and hierarchies. For related discussion, see Watts Pappas, A25; Louw, A28; and Stoeckel, A35.

Dr. Rebecca McCauley began teaching at the University of Vermont in 1986 in the Department of Communication Sciences. In 2008, she became a professor at Ohio State University in the Department of Speech and Hearing Science. She has authored or co-edited three books: *Language, Speech, and Reading Disorders in Children: Neuropsychological Studies* (1988), *Assessment of Language Disorders in Children* (2001), and *Treatment of Language Disorders in Children* (2006). She has published several articles and book chapters on SSD and participated in preparation of the ASHA documents related to childhood apraxia of speech (CAS). With Lynn Williams (A19) and Sharynne McLeod (A1, p xiv), she is working on a fourth book, *Interventions for Speech Sound Disorders in Children*.

Q12.   Rebecca McCauley: Children with co-occurring speech and language issues

How would you set about prioritising and implementing speech and language treatment; in what ways would you involve parents in the intervention team? When parents' or team members' perception of the SLP/SLT needs of the child, and their expectations of the focus therapy will have, are at odds with the speech-language clinician's findings and recommendations, how would you approach the task of information sharing and reaching consensus treatment priorities and goals?

A12.   Rebecca McCauley: Prioritising goals for children with speech and language disorders

Children with severe language delays and disorders who also show evidence of SSDs represent a large heterogeneous group with diagnoses such as specific language impairment, one of the autism spectrum disorders, or developmental delay. Almost invariably, these children find it difficult to make themselves understood in everyday communication; in fact, usually that is the reason they have been found eligible for intervention. In addition, such children may exhibit co-occurring or core challenges in attention or behaviour (e.g., tantrums or withdrawal) that sorely affect their lives at home and at school. Prioritising intervention goals for children whose needs span speech, language, communication, and sometimes management of problem behaviours, represents a delicate balancing act.

That balancing act is both facilitated, in the long run, and complicated, in the short run, by the involvement of teams of educators, health professionals, SLPs/SLTs, and families. Parents or other primary caregivers play a central role in the teams constituted to address the child's communication needs. Within a philosophy of family-centred practice (Crais 1992), parents' expertise about, investment in, and access to the child are seen as potentially invaluable resources. In order to realise that potential and establish a strong alliance across all members of the team, I find it helpful to introduce at least three concepts: *speech production* (what sounds were used and whether they were used for communicative purposes), *language* (words and larger units of meaning that were understood or attempted in production), and *communication* (verbal and nonverbal means of sharing and receiving information). Ideally, I incorporate examples from our shared observations of the child to illustrate these concepts and their interrelationships. For children exhibiting problem behaviours, I would also point out that such behaviours are increasingly seen as efforts to communicate, which can be replaced when more conventional communications are identified, learned, and rewarded (Halle, Ostrosky, and Hemmeter 2006).

To the extent that all members of the child's team share a common understanding of *speech, language,* and *communication*, they are in a better position to react to any plan that I might propose based on evaluation results and my knowledge of what research exists to support a given set of intervention goals and strategies. Team collaboration on such a plan facilitates changes ranging from subtle refinements to major modifications that more effectively incorporate knowledge of the child, his or her surroundings (including his or her family's needs and values), and team members' abilities to contribute.

Plans for children with significant speech and language needs usually incorporate augmentative alternative communication (AAC) strategies that can help optimise the child's current communicative effectiveness as well as specific strategies aimed at improving the child's more specific speech and language skills. Although parents are sometimes reticent about the inclusion of AAC strategies (e.g., a communication board or signing) because of fears that it represents a lowering of expectations and may hamper speech and language development, reassurance on two fronts usually allays those fears. First, available evidence suggests that the use of AAC is more likely to facilitate than retard advances in other forms of communication (Mirenda 2003; National Research Council 2001). Second, helping the child become a more effective communicator can be expected to have immediate effects on the quality of his/her life and the lives of those around him/her, thus producing a highly valuable outcome independent of future effects.

Intervention methods used for speech and language facilitation vary depending on the child's level of development in each area, but often include those described by several other contributors to this volume as well as a variety of methods described in McCauley and Fey (2006). How I involve parents in implementing an intervention plan depends on their interest and resources. Often, at the outset of therapy, I will suggest that we start small and consider greater involvement as we go. At the most basic level, I ask that parents keep me abreast of times when they see advancement, or suspect special unanticipated challenges that might affect the course of our work. Most parents will also be happy and able to reward spontaneous use in the home setting of target behaviours that I can let them know are emerging in treatment sessions.

For parents with the time and interest who have children whose communication is in its earliest stages of development, parent-implemented programs are especially appropriate and well supported by evidence. In such intervention programs, parents are taught several facilitating strategies to use in play and/or book reading with their child (Cole, Maddox, and Lim 2006; Girolametto and Weitzman 2006). For parents with similar children, but less time or interest, I might teach them a single specific strategy, such as focused stimulation (frequent modelling of a target structure without a request for imitation) (Ellis Weismer and Robertson 2006). Yet another area in which parents and I have had success is in approximating stimulability activities, such as those described by Miccio (A15), or phonological awareness activities, such as those described by Gillon (2006).

To illustrate how these various components may work together, let me describe a hypothetical child who shares many features with a number of children we have seen at our university clinic. 'Zach', 3;8, presents with apparently age-appropriate receptive language and nonverbal cognitive ability. However, he uses fewer than 50 single words—all with limited intelligibility in part due to a moderate SSD. His parents are busy professionals who have two other children, one younger and one older than Zach. Although Zach effectively uses elaborate gestures with family members, and during circle time at his preschool, he shows considerable frustration when other children fail to understand him, resulting in his refusing to participate or acting out against particular children.

In an initial plan for Zach, I would propose elements designed to address his communication, language, and speech needs, then work with his parents and other team members to decide how best to finalise and implement it. With that group, I would initially identify 10 target words that could form a core vocabulary to increase his expressive language, increase his mastery of missing sound patterns (e.g., final consonants, clusters), or both. In clinic sessions, I would target these words through the use of Hodson's cycles approach as well as focused stimulation in play. In order to examine progress in both speech and language domains, I would examine his acquisition of intelligible productions (those that were understandable even if misarticulated) as well as accurate ones (those in which the target structure was used correctly). As we moved through the list of words, I would enlist Zach's parents, older sibling, and team members from his preschool in using focused stimulation for these same words. Given his frustration in the preschool setting, I would also discuss what AAC strategy or strategies, such as the classroom's use of some sign language or shared use of a topic board, might work best to increase Zach's communicative effectiveness and possibly help settle his behaviour as well. I would work with the school personnel to see if sounds or sound structures targeted in Zach's treatment might also be highlighted in phonological awareness activities occurring as part of the preschool curriculum. Although in this case, combined treatment of expressive language and speech are facilitated because Zach is at the single-word level of development, for any child with a similar range of needs, team planning can ensure that goals for speech, language, and communication co-exist and often overlap at various times in the child's day.

Working with parents and other professionals in a team context can be an immensely satisfying process, even as it is a challenging one. That satisfaction comes because the diverse perspectives presented in a team not only produce a plan that better fits the child and his/her needs, but also because they help me do my very specific job better. When children have many missing speech and language skills, it is easy to get lost in the 'trees' of their many potential goals. Other team members, especially parents, can help us all keep track of the 'forest', that is, the child's overall communicative effectiveness.

Children with cleft palate, craniofacial anomalies, and velopharyngeal dysfunction

Whereas children with co-occurring speech and language difficulties form a typical component of the generalist child SLP/SLP caseload, children with cleft lip and palate, craniofacial anomalies, and velopharyngeal dysfunction (or velopharyngeal insufficiency, VPI) may or may not be frequent referrals. In Australia, Canada, and the US, and in most other parts of the industrialised world, the majority of children with cleft palate and craniofacial disorders receive speech and/or language therapy at school or in the community, and not from cleft palate 'specialists'. The flow of referrals to generalist settings is likely to increase as the sickest babies increasingly survive infancy. In the US, there are public laws (e.g., Public Law 107-110, *No child left behind*, of 2001) *requiring* school personnel to meet the needs of children with all types of impairments and legislation (Individuals with Disabilities Education Improvement Act [IDEA], 2004) that ensures that, if they desire it, parents are full participants in the process (Gretz, A7; Watts Pappas, A25).

Fortunately located generalist SLPs/SLTs have opportunities to refer to, or consult with by phone, teleconference, e-mail or in person, more experienced colleagues; collaborate with a craniofacial team; or seek the opinion of a specialist in velopharyngeal dysfunction. But many do not have such resources to call upon and are left to handle the task of reading up on and then managing a wide range of difficulties related to cleft lip, cleft palate, submucous cleft, maxillary retrusion, malocclusion, and nasal and nasal cavity abnormalities.

It is generally advised that a child who has had early palate surgery should be reviewed at least annually by an SLP/SLT to monitor speech development. The majority of these children will require 'some' through to 'intense' SLP/SLT intervention, and about one in five requires additional (secondary) palate surgery to optimise their potential for typical voice quality, resonance (eliminating hypernasality), and speech production. In terms of speech output, the therapy itself may target articulation, phonology, and voice quality and aim to expand restricted sound repertoires and eliminate or reduce abnormal compensatory articulation patterns. Children with craniofacial anomalies often have concomitant difficulties with hearing, including chronic otitis media and all that it implies (Purdy, A47), and additional health and medical issues.

Dr. Karen Golding-Kushner tackles Q13, lending her extraordinary expertise to the important questions that immediately arise for clinicians who see youngsters with craniofacial anomalies infrequently. Well known for her role as the Executive Director of the Velo-Cardio-Facial Syndrome Educational Foundation, Inc., Dr. Golding-Kushner is the former Clinical Director of the Center for Craniofacial Disorders at the Montefiore Medical Center, Bronx, NY, and is currently in private practice in central New Jersey. An ASHA Fellow, she has specialised in craniofacial disorders, cleft palate, and velopharyngeal function for the best part of 30 years.

Q13.   Karen Golding-Kushner: Children with craniofacial anomalies

For the generalist SLP/SLT and others who are inexperienced with craniofacial disorders, cleft palate, and velopharyngeal function, what are the important issues in speech development, assessment, and intervention? Are there circumstances in which the generalist is best advised to step back and recommend to families that they seek experienced, expert guidance? Some children with craniofacial anomalies have been adopted nationally or internationally, often by parents who have already raised a family and feel they have something to offer a child with special challenges, and in so doing they can face unexpected complications. How would you guide these parents?

A13.   Karen Golding-Kushner: Issues in speech development, assessment, and intervention for children with craniofacial disorders, cleft palate, and velopharyngeal dysfunction

Soon after a new baby with a cleft is born, and prior to any surgery, the SLP/SLT should meet baby and parents, providing information on normal communication development and guidelines for stimulating oral sound development and feeding. Every child with a cleft palate or craniofacial disorder should have a complete speech and language evaluation by the age of one year. In the industrialised world, cleft palate is usually repaired at around 12 months, and because of the high risk in this population for otitis media, pressure-equalising tubes (ventilation tubes or 'grommets') are frequently surgically inserted at the same time. It is important that both middle-ear health and hearing be closely monitored. Provided these things happen in a timely manner, for the majority of children with cleft lip only, or non-syndromic cleft palate, speech and language development proceeds along typical lines. For about 20% of children with cleft palate, however, and for children with craniofacial disorders associated with syndromes, development of language and speech and the quality of voice and resonance may be compromised by risks related to associated anomalies potentially affecting hearing, cognition, morphological (anatomic) structure, and dentition (Hall and Golding-Kushner 1989; Golding-Kushner 2001). Some studies have suggested the number of children with speech disorders is as high as 75%, and that those disorders may even persist into adolescence (Peterson-Falzone, Hardin-Jones, and Karnell 2001; Peterson-Falzone, Trost-Cardamone, Hardin-Jones, et al. 2006). Further, some syndromes are associated with *specific* patterns of articulation, voice, resonance, and language disorders.

Hearing

The association between palatal clefts, even submucous clefts, and middle ear disease is strong because the *levator veli palatini* and *tensor palatini* and other palatal muscles are abnormally positioned and oriented. The eustachian tube, designed to ventilate the middle ear, leads from each middle ear to the back of the throat. The *tensor palatini* is responsible for opening the eustachian tube orifice, and its abnormal placement and function limits or prevents ventilation. In some cases, the eustachian tube itself may be angled or positioned abnormally. To make matters worse, the belly of the *levator veli palatini* often elevates to fill the opening to the eustachian tube, occluding it during speech and swallowing, preventing it from fulfilling its proper function of ventilating and equalising pressure on either side of the middle ear cavity (Shprintzen and Croft 1981; Gereau, Steven, Bassila, et al. 1988; Shprintzen and Golding-Kushner 2008). Some syndromes, such as Treacher Collins syndrome, are associated with severe conductive hearing loss. Others, such as Stickler syndrome, are associated with sensorineural hearing impairment. For affected infants and toddlers, early detection, medical or surgical treatment, and, if appropriate, amplification, are essential (Purdy, A47).

Associated syndromes

Over 400 syndromes are associated with cleft palate, and some, including velo-cardio-facial syndrome (VCFS) and foetal alcohol syndrome, are known to be associated with cognitive impairment, language delays or disorders, and/or significant hearing loss. These risks, caused by the same genetic defect responsible for the cleft, are inherent to the particular syndrome under consideration. Further, some syndromes, such as VCFS, which is caused by a microdeletion on chromosome 22 in the 22q11.2 region, are associated with syndrome-specific patterns of speech and language disorders (Golding-Kushner 2005, 2007a, 2007b).

Voice

Vocal quality, pitch, and volume each reflect activity at the level of the larynx. Although cleft palate is not a direct risk factor for any of these features, it appears that individuals with borderline velopharyngeal competence may exhibit degrees of hyperfunctional voice use, vocal fold changes, and dysphonia (hoarseness), due to attempts to compensate for loss of intraoral air pressure (D'Antonio, Muntz, Marsh, et al. 1988; Lewis, Andreassen, Leeper, et al. 1993). Some syndromes are associated with laryngeal anomalies that result in voice disorders. For example, among the characteristics of VCFS are unilateral vocal fold paralysis and laryngeal asymmetry, both of which may cause hoarseness; and laryngeal web, which may cause elevated vocal pitch and loss of volume (loudness) (Chegar, Tatum, Marrinan, et al. 2006; Miyamoto, Cotton, Rope, et al. 2004; Shprintzen 1999). Vocal loudness also may be reduced in speakers with conductive hearing loss and increased in speakers with sensorineural hearing loss, both of which might be associated with specific syndromes.

Oral resonance

Severe oral crowding or hypertrophy (enlargement) of the gingival tissue, or, more commonly, tonsillar hypertrophy, can cause oral damping of the acoustic signal and muffled resonance. Enlarged tonsils may or may not appear to be infected, but in most cases, removal and pathology analysis reveals they are bacteria-laden. Infection aside, their presence can cause a 'potato-in-the-mouth' tone or cul-de-sac resonance. Extremely hypertrophied tonsils in toddlers acquiring speech are also associated with habitual forward tongue carriage as the child works to open the airway by maintaining the tongue in an anterior position. Oral resonance abnormalities typically require physical management (e.g., tonsillectomy) and are not amenable to speech therapy.

Hyponasality

Too little nasal resonance may result from adenoid hypertrophy, deviated septum, other nasal anomalies, or obstruction of the nasopharynx following pharyngoplasty (secondary surgery to eliminate VPI). Because hyponasality can co-occur with hypernasality, both should be rated separately during evaluation (see Table A37.1, p. x). While the treatment of hyponasality is usually medical or surgical, increasing the duration of nasal consonants during connected speech may effectively reduce the perception of hyponasality (Golding-Kushner, 2001).

Hypernasality

Excessive nasal resonance during vowel production, due to communication between the oral and nasal cavities, is one of the greatest risks associated with cleft palate. Hypernasality, the consequence of VPI, discussed below, is best diagnosed by a trained listener, not instrumentally, because it is *only* of significance if it can be perceived. On the other hand, VPI can *only* be diagnosed using instrumentation to visualise the region, as discussed later. Hypernasality permeates connected speech and occurs when the speaker is unable to fully separate the oral and nasal cavities at the right time during connected speech due to a physical inability to effect velopharyngeal closure, timing errors, or both. Hypernasality is a vowel phenomenon but commonly co-occurs with a consonant event. Nasal emission is nasal air escape through the nose during speech, especially during production of pressure consonants. Nasal air escape is an obligatory articulation error that occurs in the presence of VPI.

VPI, velopharyngeal incompetence, velopharyngeal dysfunction

VPI (or VPD), which primarily requires physical management, has several causes including deficient velar tissue, abnormal or asymmetric movement of the velum, lateral pharyngeal walls, or posterior pharyngeal wall, tonsillar hypertrophy (Shprintzen, Sher, and Croft 1987), and errors in learning. If present, an oronasal fistula may exacerbate the effects of VPI (Isberg and Henningsson 1987). The presence of compensatory articulation errors may also exacerbate VPI (Hoch, Golding-Kushner, Sadewitz, et al. 1986; Henningsson and Isberg 1986). Neuromotor problems may also cause VPI, but cleft palate is not a risk factor for neuromotor problems and they occur rarely in children with cleft palate.

Treatment efficacy always rests on accurate diagnosis, and diagnosis of VPI requires direct visualisation of velopharyngeal function during unimpeded connected speech. The gold standard for assessing velopharyngeal closure is direct visualisation using both flexible fibreoptic nasopharyngoscopy to analyse anatomy and airway patency (openness) and multiview videofluoroscopy to view pharyngeal wall motion and tongue activity during speech. Unfortunately, my experience has been that many clinicians continue to rely on indirect measures like pressure-flow techniques or nasometry to diagnose disorders of resonance and velopharyngeal function. They confuse data that appear 'objective' with an assessment that is valid (relevant). Indirect assessment techniques such as these provide no information about the location, configuration, consistency, or cause of VPI, and so their value in treatment planning is controversial (Peterson-Falzone, Hardin-Jones, and Karnell 2001).

People often ask, 'Why not do trial therapy to see if hypernasality can be reduced without surgery?' There is no therapy technique to eliminate velopharyngeal closure when VPI is consistently present. Other than for errors of learning (see below), speech therapy is ineffective in eliminating VPI. Nevertheless, despite an absence of evidence in their favour (Lof, A30), clinicians persist with non-speech oral motor exercises (horn-tooting, whistle-blowing, pushing manoeuvres), electrical stimulation, palatal massage, and other nonsense, wasteful of time and resources. Regrettably, I have seen more than a few patients in whom these procedures caused additional, *avoidable* problems, including habituated abnormal tongue position, substitution of /m/ for /n/ because of the focus on lip closure around chewy tubes and wind instruments, and vocal fold nodules. A few reports (Kuehn 1991, 1997) indicate that, under specific conditions involving inconsistent closure, *improvement* has occurred with continuous positive airway pressure (CPAP) or nasopharyngoscopic biofeedback. However, results were inconsistent across subjects, and it was not clear that velopharyngeal closure could be completely established or maintained long-term. If closure is short-term, or 'improved' but not eliminated, hypernasality will persist, so the use of CPAP at this time must be considered experimental (Kummer 2001b).

Errors in learning

Some speech learners, with or without clefts, exhibit adequate velopharyngeal closure on all but one phoneme or sound class, typically involving a nasal snort or nasal fricative substitution for /s/, /z/, /f/, /v/, /ʃ/, /ʒ/, /tʃ/, and /dʒ/. Occluding the nares during stimulability testing results in production of /k/ or nothing at all, and the speaker may exhibit discomfort at not being able to emit air. Such errors in learning are easily treatable with speech therapy, and physical management is inappropriate and unwarranted. In contrast, a speaker with nasal emission, that is, passive loss of air through the nose, sounds better with the nares occluded because he or she was directing air orally, and closing the nose eliminated the passive 'leak'.

Articulation

Articulation errors in children with cleft palate, VPI, and craniofacial syndromes may be obligatory, maladaptive, developmental, or compensatory (Golding-Kushner 1995, 2004). Of these, all but developmental errors may be related to malocclusion, palatal fistulae, VPI, severe oral crowding, or hearing loss. It is important to note that children with cleft palate do *not* typically have CAS, oral–motor weakness, dysarthria, or other speech problems of neuromuscular origin. Extensive clinical experience shows that, unfortunately, they are frequently misdiagnosed with these disorders, leading to the application of inappropriate therapy procedures (Golding-Kushner 2002). Even when correctly diagnosed, many SLPs persist in the inappropriate use of non-speech oral motor exercise, despite a complete lack of evidence of any benefit (Powers and Starr 1974; Ruscello 1982; Starr 1990; Van Demark and Hardin 1990; Lof 2002, 2003; and see Ruscello, A42).

Expert guidance

Before starting treatment, it is incumbent on the speech pathologist to sort out which part of the speech disorder can be treated therapeutically and which part cannot. Unfortunately, most SLPs lack specific training in cleft palate and VPI. If the child presenting to them is followed by a cleft palate team, the therapist can consult with the SLP/SLT who is part of the team for guidance.

But what about children who are not known to have a cleft or VPI? A decision tree can be helpful. If you hear hypernasality and all speech errors are obligatory, refer for velopharyngeal imaging. If you hear nasal airflow on only one sound, one cognate pair, or one sound class, but nasal airflow is appropriate on other sounds, the problem is likely nasal snorting (also called nasal fricative or phone-specific VPI), treatable with speech therapy. Nasal airflow can be detected easily by holding a sensitive mirror beneath the nares while the child produces words that exclude nasal phonemes, or by holding one end of a drinking straw at the edge of a nostril and holding the other end of the straw to your ear (Skinder-Meredith, A37). If you are not sure, pinch the nose and see if speech seems better. If it is better, the airflow was likely obligatory. If it sounds the same or even worse, the error was likely phone-specific, requiring speech therapy. If one is unsure, a referral to an SLP/SLT with expertise in this area, a craniofacial team, or both should be made. Similarly, an SLP/SLT treating a child with a compensatory articulation disorder may lack training in this area. Although the basic procedures are those used in 'traditional' articulation therapy, an SLP/SLT with expertise in this area will be able to offer special techniques and 'tricks' to the treating clinician. I have also had excellent results working with children (and their parents) who live long distances from my office using videoconferencing (Golding-Kushner 2007b). Teletherapy, which is gaining in application and popularity in many aspects of medicine, habilitation, and rehabilitation, is an exciting new frontier.

International adoption

I have worked with many families who adopted a child they were told had a repaired cleft palate, only to discover at the time of, or even after, the adoption that the palate had not been repaired, that it was poorly repaired, or that the repair had dehisced (ruptured or broken open). This might have been due to poor surgical technique or inadequate post-operative care. These adoptive families are faced with making a decision about surgery while, at the same time, helping their child adjust to their home-family, culture, and life (Pollock, A14). In many instances, these children were three years old or even older when the palate repair was finally done, invariably leading to the development of a severe compensatory articulation disorder. With the support of their home-family, the ultimate speech outcome for these children has a good prognosis.

Most of the time, children waiting for adoption have not had the benefit of examination by a clinical geneticist, and biological family history may be unknown. This means that, at times, a cleft palate is 'just' a cleft palate, but at others, the cleft may be only one feature of a syndrome. This may or may not be apparent until after the child has been placed, and those considering adoption should be prepared for that possibility.

Summary

The prognosis for normal speech in children with cleft palate is excellent but is often dependent on a combination of surgery and speech therapy. There are many different surgical procedures, and the one that will work best for an individual patient should be determined by the configuration of the velopharyngeal gap as visualised according to the procedures described above.

Children who have been internationally adopted

International, 'inter-country', or 'overseas' adoption is a prevalent practice throughout the industrialised world. According to the U.S. Department of State, 22,728 visas were issued to orphans entering the United States in 2004 and 22,884 in 2005, but see Pollock (2007) for a more comprehensive view. Anecdotally, most of these children acquire their new home language with relative ease, even though they may have been quickly transported from orphanage to family home, and from one language to another. A contrary view, well supported by evidence, comes from research effort by Karen Pollock and others into language acquisition of adopted children from non-English-speaking environments, showing that they can have significant difficulties, necessitating SLP/SLT assistance. Dr. Pollock emphasises the need for more research into why, when, and how to intervene with these children, stressing the urgent need for normative data on early language development in internationally adopted children, especially during the first year or two post-adoption.

Head of the Child Phonology Laboratory at the University of Alberta, Dr. Karen Pollock is a professor and chair of the Department of Speech Pathology and Audiology with a background in both linguistics and SLP, and is co-editor of one of *this* author's favourite child speech references (Kamhi and Pollock 2005). Her recent research has been concerned with vowel errors in children with phonological disorders, speech-language acquisition in internationally adopted children, and the phonological characteristics of African American Vernacular English. Suppressing, with some difficulty, the urge to ask about her important vowel research as well, the author asked her to cover some of the international adoption issues that are important for SLPs/SLTs to understand.

Q14.   Karen E. Pollock: Language acquisition of international adoptees

What do we now know about the about the nature and course of speech-language acquisition in typically developing internationally adopted children? When should we encourage parents to seek professional services, such as speech-language therapy or early intervention, and how can they be supported in the process? And what preparation, in terms of professional consultation, might parents undertake if they are planning to adopt a child from overseas with a known cognitive or communication disability?

A14.   Karen E. Pollock: Internationally adopted children learning English as a second first language

Children adopted internationally experience a unique pattern of linguistic exposure. They typically hear only the language of their birth country prior to adoption, and then, because most English-speaking adoptive parents do not speak the child's birth language, they hear only English after adoption. Consequently, children lose their birth language abilities rapidly, within weeks according to some estimates. In essence, they become monolingual English speakers shortly after adoption, but have not yet had sufficient time to acquire age-appropriate English skills. Obviously, the older the child at adoption, the more linguistic catching up is required to match monolingual non-adopted peers, and the more likely their overall language proficiency and academic success will be affected. Because language acquisition in children adopted internationally differs from that of other bilingual or second language learners, the term 'second first language' learners has been proposed (Glennen 2002; Roberts, Pollock, Krakow, et al. 2005). Lacking ongoing first language capabilities as a scaffold, the reality for these children is that they have to 'start over' with learning the new language (Geren, Snedeker, and Ax 2005).

Early empirical investigators of second first language acquisition anticipated various delays based on two assumptions. First, they believed the second first language learning situation was bound to impact development detrimentally. Second, they expected early environmental deprivation related to orphanage care to evoke significant delays in cognition and language. Indeed, studies of children adopted from Romania during the early 1990s supported these hypotheses, with the prevalence of language delays extending from 60% to 94% (Johnson 2000; Rutter and The English and Romanian Adoptees Study Team 1998).

Optimistic findings from subsequent studies of children adopted from Russia, China, and elsewhere suggest that the Romanian situation was extraordinary. The extreme neglect/deprivation suffered by Romanian orphans and their struggles post-adoption appear to be atypical of internationally adopted children generally. In fact, many internationally adopted children have been found to demonstrate average or better English language skills within a year or two post-adoption (see summary of studies reviewed below), demonstrating that, for many children, second first language learning proceeds relatively smoothly and the effects of early institutionalisation may be counteracted by placement in an enriched environment (Glennen 2007b; Windsor, Glaze, Koga, et al. 2007).

Language acquisition in internationally adopted children

Most communication research with this population deals with lexical and syntactic development. Results show that, for children adopted under 2;0, vocabulary and morphosyntax increase rapidly during the first year home, continuing to improve during the preschool years. For example, Glennen (2007a) found that children adopted from Eastern Europe had language abilities that were comfortably within normal limits (WNL), using standard monolingual English norms, by one year post-adoption. Roberts et al. (2005) found that 95% of the adopted Chinese preschoolers they studied scored within or above the normal range on standardised speech and language measures, and 27% demonstrated exceptional language skills. Less research has been completed on children adopted at older ages (2–5 years), but preliminary studies (Glennen 2007c) indicate equally impressive progress, with most children scoring WNL on standardised test measures from one to two years post-adoption.

Results of recent investigations of longer-term outcomes (early elementary school) for language and literacy skills in children adopted under 2;0 are mixed. For example, Scott, Roberts, and Krakow (2008) found that children adopted from China who had completed Grade 1 or 2 performed at or above average on measures of oral and written language. By contrast, Glennen and Bright (2005) found a higher incidence of pragmatic and higher-level language skills difficulties in school-age children adopted from Eastern Europe. Approximately 11% of them received diagnoses of either a speech-language impairment or learning disability, and 25% had attention deficits and/or were considered hyperactive. These discrepant results may relate to the different birth countries, gender (all girls in the group adopted from China), age at testing, or methodology (hands-on assessments vs. parent/teacher surveys).

Speech acquisition in internationally adopted children

There is little research on speech (i.e., phonetic or phonological) development in these children, with Pollock (2007) and Pollock and Price (2005) providing detailed summaries of the available studies. Two longitudinal small-N group studies (Pollock, Price, and Fulmer

2003; Price, Pollock, and Oller 2006) of children adopted from China as infants/toddlers found considerable individual variation in early phonological measures, such as canonical babbling ratio, phonetic inventory size and diversity, and proportion of monosyllables. However, the majority (7 out of 8) of participants performed WNL on the *Goldman Fristoe Test of Articulation – 2nd Edition* (GFTA-2) at 3;0 and/or had normal range PCCs. Errors were primarily familiar developmental ones seen in monolingual English-speaking children, like cluster reduction, gliding, stopping, and derhotacisation. The one child whose GFTA-2 score was below average also had a low PCC, explained by prevalent cluster reduction and stopping, and an idiosyncratic pattern of consonant addition. Interestingly, none of the early speech measures taken at 6 months post-adoption appeared to predict performance at 3;0.

Two larger group studies of toddlers/preschoolers included a standardised measure of articulation proficiency, the GFTA-2, in their assessment battery. Glennen (2007) found that 3 (or 11%) of 27 two-year-olds adopted from Eastern Europe scored below average on the GFTA-2 at one or more years post-adoption. Similarly, in their study of 55 three- to six-year-olds adopted from China under 2;0, Roberts et al. (2005) found that only 4 of the 55 (or 7%) had below average standard scores. Although studies of school-age internationally adopted children have not included expressive phonology measures, Scott et al. (2008) reported that 3 of the 24 first and second grade children studied were receiving services for mild articulation disorders.

Aiming to explore phonological abilities in more detail, Pollock, Chow, and Tamura (2004) phonetically transcribed spontaneous language samples from a subset (25) of the preschoolers in the Roberts et al. (2005) study. Analyses included PCC-Revised (PCC-R), phonological mean length of utterance (PMLU), and phonological process usage. Three children (12%) had low scores on one or more measures, but no common trends emerged. Mostly, they produced developmental errors commonly seen in non-adopted monolingual English-speaking peers, and evidence of cross-linguistic interference from Chinese was absent. In summary, the bulk of children studied demonstrated age-appropriate phonology following one or two years of English exposure. The error types of those with delays were comparable to those often seen in their monolingual English-speaking peers with phonological delay.

Implications for assessment

Parents considering adoption or waiting for a child's arrival need to gather all available information about the child's communication status in their birth language. Such information is not routinely provided, but can be critical in diagnosing true disorders and determining eligibility for services. Glennen (2002) provided a comprehensive list of suggested questions about language development and abilities to ask caregivers during pre-adoption interchanges or at the time of adoption and communication skills to observe during initial meetings.

Communication assessment of internationally adopted children presents challenges for SLPs/SLTs, particularly during the first year post-adoption. While the birth language is undergoing rapid attrition and the transition to the emerging adopted language is proceeding, it is difficult (if not impossible) to determine whether apparent delays relate to this natural transition or are evidence of developmental communication delays that predated adoption.

Glennen (2005, 2007a) proposed guidelines for the assessment of speech-language skills in newly adopted children, combining prelinguistic (foundational) measures like joint attention, gestures, and symbolic play [using the Communication and Symbolic Behaviour Skills-Developmental Profile (Weatherby and Prizant 2002)] and linguistic measures like vocabulary comprehension [using the MacArthur Communicative Development Inventories (Fenson, Dale, Reznick, et al. 1993)]. Applied to a group of 27 toddlers (aged 11–23 months) adopted from Eastern Europe, these guidelines accurately predicted those with persistent language delays at 2;0. Glennen stressed the benefit of including prelinguistic measures in early assessments, noting that they are not language-specific and remain unchanged post-adoption. When using language-specific measures with newly adopted children, comprehension measures are more likely to accurately reflect abilities, as comprehension typically precedes production. Pollock and Price (2005) offered similar suggestions for phonetic/phonological assessment, emphasising that, during the first weeks or months post-adoption, observations of the quality and quantity of vocalisations (whether actual words or not) and size and diversity of the phonetic inventory could yield important diagnostic information. For example, typically developing children, regardless of adoption status or language environment, are expected to produce canonical syllables by 10 months of age.

Over the first year or two post-adoption, preliminary normative data are available for vocabulary size and utterance length from two longitudinal studies. Glennen and Masters (2002) followed 130 children adopted from Eastern Europe, and Pollock (2005) provided similar data for 141 children adopted from China. These data, organised by chronological age or months post-adoption, can be used to compare a child's scores to those of other children adopted at similar ages. In terms of phonetic/phonological development, Pollock and Price (2005) suggest periodic reassessments to monitor the size, diversity, and distribution of sounds in the phonetic repertoire to monitor the rate and amount of change over time. These measures may also be compared to normative data for monolingual children but interpreted according to length of exposure to English rather than chronological age.

Finally, based on the results of numerous studies of preschool and school-aged children adopted from China and Eastern Europe as infants/toddlers (e.g., Glennen and Bright 2005; Pollock et al. 2004; Roberts et al. 2005; Scott et al., in press), it appears that standard English tests can be used (although cautiously) one or more years post-adoption. Children adopted as preschoolers may be assessed with such instruments two or more years post-adoption (Glennen 2007c).

Intervention considerations

Any child adopted internationally is potentially 'at risk' for speech-language delays, by virtue of the abrupt language switch and inadequate stimulation in orphanages. This necessitates parents being watchful regarding development during the first year home, and, if concerns emerge, seeking an SLP/SLT opinion. As a rule of thumb for families, if vocabulary, utterance length, and intelligibility gains are sluggish, a comprehensive speech-language evaluation is indicated, and intervention may be necessary.

Well-established guidelines for determining eligibility for speech-language intervention services for children adopted internationally are currently unavailable, with intervention decisions often made randomly (Glennen 2007b). Glennen found that about half of the newly adopted toddlers she followed were assessed by early intervention teams and provided speech-language intervention, even though many were *already* functioning at the top of their peer group. At the other extreme, stories of older internationally adopted children being denied services are even more concerning. For example, Glennen (2007b) shared an example of a girl aged 8;0, floundering academically four years post-adoption, who was denied assessment and treatment services in English because she was classified as an English as a Second Language (ESL) student. Incredibly, even though she had not been exposed to her birth language for four years, the school insisted on testing her in that language. I also have personal knowledge of a child for whom a school postponed speech-language assessment until the child had 'graduated' from their ESL program: a glaring catch-22! The ESL program was not designed to meet the needs of second first language learners or children with language delays/impairments. It is unclear whether such stories are common, but there is a clear need for the development and implementation of evidence-based guidelines for assessment and intervention. Meanwhile, when such situations arise, parents and SLPs/SLTs should advocate for appropriate services and educate other professionals about the unique circumstances of children adopted internationally and the nature of second first language acquisition. Just as it is inappropriate to hold newly adopted children to unreasonable expectations based on non-adopted monolingual speech-language norms, service eligibility guidelines developed for bilingual and ESL children cannot simply be generalised to children adopted internationally.

To date, there have been no investigations of treatment efficacy for internationally adopted children with speech-language delays/disorders, but we do have descriptions of such children with true speech-language disorders (Pollock, 2007). They include little evidence of either cross-linguistic (birth language) interference or communication patterns unique to this population. Apparently the children mimic the same process of development as monolingual English-speaking children, but at later ages. Thus, when intervention is warranted, it is appropriate to employ the procedures and materials commonly used with monolingual clients. As Glennen (2007b, p. 6) notes, intervention should 'target each child's diagnosis and symptoms, not the adoption status.'

Children with limited stimulability

The aim of stimulability assessment is to discover whether the production of an error-sound or missing sound is enhanced or made possible when elicitation conditions are modified or simplified. Traditionally, in child speech *assessment*, a child was said to be stimulable for a sound if he/she could produce it correctly in isolation when given auditory and visual models, encouragement, and support while ensuring that distractions and linguistic demands on the child were minimal. Also traditionally, the developers of *treatment* approaches for child speech disorders have had no difficulty in persuading clinicians to focus on early developing and stimulable (in isolation) sounds first on the basis that these sounds are easier for children to learn. As this made logical good sense, these rationales for treatment target selection remained unchallenged for decades; but eventually, challenges did come (Miccio, Elbert, and Forrest 1999; Powell and Miccio 1996; Rvachew, Rafaat, and Martin 1999). The profession is now in a position to appreciate that stimulability data are of most interest in young children with severely restricted phonetic inventories, and of most use when they are collected for sounds absent from a child's inventory. But what is the current understanding of the term 'stimulable'?

In the more recent speech *assessment* literature, the term 'stimulability', and even 'true stimulability', has been used to mean that a child is stimulable for a consonant phoneme in at least two syllable positions, rather than simply being able to produce it imitatively in isolation. Schmidt and Lee (2000) define motor learning as 'a set of processes associated with practice or experience leading to relatively permanent changes in the capability for movement.' The three precursors to motor learning are: (a) motivation, (b) focused attention, and (c) pre-practice. Pre-practice involves phonetic placement training prior to entering the practice phase; so, for many clients, it is inextricably bound up with stimulability training. Irrespective of speech diagnosis, for those clinicians who see their clients infrequently, such as those working consultatively, and for those who have virtually unlimited access to their clients, the modern notion of true stimulability for consonants has major ramifications.

In many clinical settings worldwide, SLTs/SLPs see their clients with speech disorders infrequently. There are at least three common service delivery scenarios. First, some SLPs/SLTs working in consultative models may only see a given client once or twice a school term, and then only briefly. Second, other SLPs/SLTs see children for between six and ten assessment/treatment sessions and then hand over the entire business of intervention to a parent in the form of a home program, or to a teacher, aide, assistant, or other non-SLP/SLT as a school program, perhaps reviewing the child's progress at intervals, but possibly not. And third, and literally quite close to home for the author, children attending publicly funded agencies are allocated, by legislation, a maximum of ten SLP/SLT appointments. Not ten per school term or ten per year: ten full stop! Against this background, we know that SLPs/SLTs are uniquely qualified to make non-stimulable sounds stimulable, whereas most non-SLPs/SLTs probably have to rely on luck to achieve success in this area!

Dr. Adele Miccio (1952–2009) explored the role of stimulability in the treatment of children with SSD in A15. At the time of writing Dr. Miccio was Associate Professor of Communication Sciences and Disorders and Applied Linguistics and Co-Director of the Center for Language Science at Pennsylvania State University, where she taught courses in phonetics and phonology and conducted research on typical and atypical phonological acquisition, the relationship between bilingual phonological development and later literacy abilities, bilingual phonological assessment, and treatment efficacy. Formerly a clinical SLP in Colorado, she received her PhD in Speech and Hearing Sciences from Indiana University–Bloomington. She was an Associate Editor of the *American Journal of Speech-Language Pathology* and on the editorial board of *Clinical Linguistics & Phonetics*. Her contribution to scholarship in our field was immeasurable and she is sorely missed.

Q15.   Adele Miccio: Stimulability and phonetic inventory expansion

Should clinicians focus on stimulability training with infrequently seen 'home/school program' clients, and what should the parents' or other helpers' role be in this situation? In other situations, where the clinician has reasonably unfettered access to a client, how would you prioritise and implement work on stimulability?

A15.   Adele Miccio: First things first: stimulability therapy for childre. with small phonetic repertoires

Stimulability has been defined a number of ways since the term first appeared in the speech pathology literature in the 1950s (Carter and Buck 1958; Milisen 1954), although the concept was described even earlier by Travis (1931). Simply put, stimulability is a client's ability to immediately modify a speech production error when presented with an auditory and visual model (Lof 1996; Powell and Miccio 1996).

Bain (1994) noted that stimulability testing determines the difference between a child's abilities during a highly supportive imitative condition and a typical spontaneous condition where the phonetic environment as well as lexical and syntactic issues may restrict articulatory abilities. To determine stimulability, target sounds are elicited in isolation, syllables, and/or words (Carter and Buck 1958). Earlier studies (Sommers, Leiss, Delp, et al. 1967) referred to a child's general stimulability or overall likelihood to self-correct. In other words, if a child's performance improves from that in spontaneous speech, a child is judged to have good stimulability skills—a positive prognosticator for future success in treatment. Thus, treatment is most important for children with poor stimulability skills.

Although more sophisticated phonological assessments that identify patterns of errors and illuminate a child's knowledge of the phonological system have been developed (Bernhardt and Stemberger 2000; Elbert and Gierut 1986; Ingram 1981; Shriberg and Kwiatkowski 1980; and see Stoel-Gammon, A9; Bernhardt and Ullrich, A32) and have increased our understanding of generalisation patterns, researchers have also documented a relationship between sound-specific stimulability and generalisation (Miccio, Elbert, and Forrest 1999; Powell, Elbert, and Dinnsen 1991). Consequently, stimulability continues to be used to prioritise caseloads. Children who are stimulable for consonants absent from their phonetic inventories will most likely acquire these sounds without treatment. Sounds absent from the inventory that are not stimulable, however, are unlikely to be acquired without direct treatment.

Stimulability is also a consideration in treatment target selection. Treating non-stimulable sounds is most likely to result in the acquisition of both treated and non-treated sounds. Non-stimulable sounds tend to be more complex. Targeting more complex sounds promotes system-wide generalisation and increases the learnability of less complex sounds (Tyler and Figurski 1994; Gierut 2007; and see Baker, A11). Targeting both stimulable and non-stimulable sounds promotes early success (Edwards 1983; Rvachew and Nowak 2001).

Furthermore, stimulability testing may also be used to probe for learning during the course of treatment. Adaptations of Carter and Buck's (1958) protocols are still widely used today for this purpose (Miccio 2002; Powell and Miccio 1996). Recently, Glaspey and Stoel-Gammon (2005, 2007) developed the Scaffolding Scale of Stimulability, a hierarchical scale of cues and linguistic environments, to monitor discrete changes in production in response to treatment. This scale also quantifies improved responses to cues as well as the change in the number of cues needed over time.

Despite the positive aspects of using stimulability for assessment purposes, it has met with resistance, by clinicians, with regard to treatment target selection (Fey and Stalker 1986; Hodson and Paden 1991; Rvachew 2005b). This generally relates to the difficulty of teaching non-stimulable sounds, the time involved in instruction, or the increased frustration of children who have difficulty imitating sounds absent from their phonetic inventories.

...rns have motivated the development of treatment programs for young children ...onetic inventories who are not stimulable for production of sounds missing ...ntories (Miccio and Elbert 1996; Miccio 2005; Powell and Miccio 1996).

...target non-stimulable sounds and still achieve early success, Miccio and ...rt (1996) proposed teaching all consonants at once during every session (both stimulable and non-stimulable). The important components of this treatment strategy include directly targeting non-stimulable speech sounds, making targets the focus of joint attention, associating speech sounds with hand/body motions, associating the sounds with alliterative characters of interest to the child, encouraging vocal practice, and ensuring successful communicative attempts.

Because the primary goal is to enhance stimulability, speech sounds are taught in isolation (e.g., [s::::::::::]) or in a CV context (e.g. [kʌ]). Each consonant is associated with a character and a hand or body motion. Details regarding the characters and their associated movements are shown in Table A15.1. Information on how stimulability probes are conducted and generalisation data are gathered across sessions may be found in Miccio (2005). A typical treatment is described below for 'Fiona', age 4;3. Pre-treatment, Fiona's phonetic inventory consisted of [m n p b t d w j h]. None of the English consonants absent from her phonetic inventory were stimulable.

Table A15.1 Stimulus characters and associated motions.[a]

Manner	Consonant	Character	Associated Motion
Stop	/p/	Putt-Putt Pig	Glide hands in a skating motion.
	/b/	Baby Bear	Pantomime rocking a baby.
	/t/	Talkie Turkey	Raise a pretend phone receiver to ear.
	/d/	Dirty Dog	Make digging motion with hands.
	/k/	Coughing Cow	Place hand near top of throat.
	/g/	Goofy Goat	Roll eyes toward ceiling.
Fricative	/f/	Fussy Fish	Fussily push hands away from body.
	/v/	Viney Violet	Move arms up as a winding vine.
	/θ/	Thinking Thumb	Move thumb in a circle.
	/s/	Silly Snake	Move finger up arm.
	/z/	Zippy Zebra	Zip coat.
	/ʃ/	Shy Sheepy	Clutch hands together and push down.
Affricate	/tʃ/	Cheeky Chick	Move hand sassily toward cheek.
	/dʒ/	Giant Giraffe	Move hand upward in stair steps.
Nasal	/m/	Munchie Mouse	Push lips together and rub tummy.
	/n/	Naughty Newt	Shake finger in a scolding motion.
Liquid	/l/	Lazy Lion	Stretch arms in "L" shape.
	/r/	Rowdy Rooster	Rev motorcycle gears.
Glide	/w/	Wiggly Worm	Shiver.
	/j/	Yawning Yo-Yo	Yawn and move hand to suppress it.
	/h/[b]	Happy Hippo	Laugh and shake shoulders.

[a]Adapted from Table 3 in Miccio, A. W., & Elbert, M. (1996). Enhancing stimulability: a treatment program. _Journal of Communication Disorders_, 29, 335–352. Used with permission from Elsevier.
[b]From a phonological perspective, /h/ is considered a glide in English. It has no cognate and patterns as a glide (e.g., is not phonemic in coda position). Thus, all the sounds are listed from the front to the back and by sound class with stops, fricatives, and affricates first, then the nasals, and finally, the liquids and glides. Because /h/ cannot be strictly continuous like the other fricatives, it has a CV motion, [ha].

At the beginning of the session, following the administration of a brief stimulability probe, large 5 × 7-inch (13 × 18 cm) character cards were reviewed with the associated speech sound and motion. To focus Fiona's attention on each character, the cards were shown one at a time. Doing so ensured that Fiona understood the target sounds and their associated motions. Research on semantic development shows that children are more likely to spontaneously repeat the names of objects that are the focus of joint attention and that were previously labelled for them (Baldwin and Markham 1989). For this reason, speech sounds are associated with characters of interest to children. The character for /z/, for example, is Zippy Zebra. Alliterative characters also provide an immediate opportunity to generalise new information to larger linguistic units and to facilitate phonological awareness and the alphabetic principle that are important for emerging literacy skills (Adams, Treiman, and Pressley 1998; Hesketh, A22). Each consonant is also associated with a motion. The motion for [z] is zipping up a coat. All fricatives are associated with continuous motions. All stop consonants, on the other hand, are associated with ballistic motions to draw a child's attention to these features of speech sounds. All consonants, including those that are present in the phonetic inventory, are reviewed, and associated body movements are always used concurrently with speech production. Fazio (1997) found that children with specific language impairment remembered poems after a 2-day delay when the poem was learned with accompanying hand motions. The hand motions appeared to serve as retrieval cues. To learn new speech sounds, children must be able to retrieve the new articulatory information at a later date and to use the new sounds in words. Multimodal input increases the ability to remember new sounds (Rauscher, Krauss, and Chen 1996).

To facilitate speech sound production, treatment was embedded in play-like activities that provided Fiona with multiple opportunities to imitate consonants. Although direct imitation of the correct production of sounds in error is not required in this program, vocal practice is encouraged and children make verbal requests. For example, Fiona's favourite character was Happy Hippo. She would say, 'I'm happy like Happy Hippo. Ha Ha Ha! Are you happy, too?' Doing so is an important element for acquisition and generalisation to larger linguistic units (Powell, Elbert, Miccio, et al. 1998; Saben and Ingham 1991). In this program, children are encouraged to speak through turn-taking activities. A typical session utilises a maximum of three turn-taking activities that are designed specifically around the target speech sound characters. Both Fiona and the clinician were fully involved in turn-taking activities so that the clinician was constantly modelling the target sounds and Fiona had multiple opportunities to imitate them. Sometimes Fiona's parents participated in treatment activities. They also took turns and modelled the target sounds. Characters were printed on playing cards to easily facilitate sound production. Fiona's favourite activity was Go Fish. In this familiar game, everyone had a set of cards and took turns asking for a desired card. Because both stimulable and non-stimulable sounds were included, Fiona often failed to produce the intended sound when requesting a card. The associated movement, however, provided the clinician with the information needed to identify the intended sound. When Fiona produced [d] but mimed zipping up her coat, for example, the clinician knew the intended sound was [z]. Because the clinician handed Fiona a Zippy Zebra card, Fiona's communication attempt was successful. At the same time, the clinician provided feedback about how to produce [z] while miming zipping her coat: 'Let me see, do I have Zippy Zebra? Zippy Zebra says [z::::::::::].' When Fiona requested Putt Putt Pig, a sound she knew, she said [pʌ pʌ] while making a skating motion with her hands (Putt Putt Pig is wearing roller skates). The clinician provided positive feedback, 'Great! You made the Putt

Putt Pig sound, [pʌ pʌ]' while making the skating motion. Every time Fiona took a turn, she was free to request any character she wished. Giving Fiona the freedom to choose any sound enabled immediate success. Successful communication, in turn, encouraged more verbalisation (Rescorla and Bernstein Ratner 1996). Whenever the clinician took a turn, she requested a non-stimulable sound. In this way, Fiona was always assured of successful production attempts with stimulable sounds and had multiple opportunities to attempt non-stimulable sounds. In addition, the clinician had many opportunities to provide instruction without resorting to drill-like activities. Fiona was given an assertive role involving requesting and directing attention to sounds of interest. Because all characters are alliterative, multiple opportunities arose to indirectly target generalisation of newly learned sounds to lexical items and to use them spontaneously. Baby Bear, for example, has a bib and a bottle. Putt Putt Pig is pink and wears a purple dress. Fiona commented on these characteristics when she requested these characters and again received feedback about the sounds she made with accompanying motions. Fiona, as well as other young children, preferred simple games. Simple games also provide the most opportunities to attempt speech sounds. After playing Go Fish, Fiona played a game where she took turns requesting character cards to place in a space ship. At the end of the session, the space ship took off and a door opened with a sticker inside for Fiona to wear home. It is important to remember that Fiona was never required to imitate correct production after the clinician. The clinician identified the intended target by the associated motion even when it was produced incorrectly. The clinician drew attention to the correct production through modelling and phonetic placement cues. As Fiona became more comfortable with the clinician and had more successful communicative attempts, she also began to imitate the clinician more frequently and to attempt to correct herself. The treatment activities provided a supportive framework that encouraged speech production and enhanced Fiona's awareness of the properties of speech sounds. At the end of the session, a short probe of palindromes (dad, mom, pop, bob, etc.) was administered to assess generalisation to the coda position. Fiona's parents had a set of character cards at home. At the end of the session, we suggested a few sounds to work on at home. These are always stimulable sounds, for example, [n] and [d], and the parents were advised to always use the corresponding motions. Thus, the parents assisted with generalisation but did not force production of sounds that were difficult. At the end of the session, Fiona said, 'Mommy starts with the Munchy Mouse sound.' Fiona participated in this program twice weekly for 12 weeks. Sessions were 50 minutes in length. Post-treatment, she had added all fricatives, affricates, and [r] to her phonetic inventory and was stimulable for the production of [k, g, l]. Pre-treatment, Fiona produced complete sentences, but with only stops, nasals, and glides in her consonant inventory, and she was unintelligible to all but her immediate family. When she began treatment, she substituted [d] for velars, affricates, and voiced fricatives, [h] for voiceless fricatives, and [w] for liquids. Following 12 weeks of treatment to enhance stimulability, she was stimulable for all targeted sounds and produced many of them in simple words or used typical developmental substitutions in more difficult contexts. When Fiona returned to the clinic after a winter break of 4 weeks, she began a minimal pair treatment approach using *maximal* oppositions to directly target the contrastive nature of speech sounds and to continue to encourage generalisation across the phonological system.

This program to enhance stimulability for speech sound production is based on findings from treatment research. As noted above, non-stimulable sounds are least likely to change without treatment, and targeting non-stimulable sounds results in acquisition of the treated non-stimulable sounds as well as untreated stimulable sounds (Miccio, Elbert, and Forrest 1999; Powell, Elbert, and Dinnsen 1991). For children with small inventories, it is important to rapidly increase the size of the phonetic inventory for intelligibility reasons. This program is designed especially for young children with small phonetic inventories who are not stimulable for production of the speech sounds absent from their phonetic repertoires. Once children are stimulable for the majority of consonants, they move on to treatment using a contrastive approach or a combination of stimulability and phonological contrasts. In addition, children are ready for direct phonetic placement training if needed.

Roles and responsibilities: Child, family, and therapist

For therapy to work, child, family, and therapist all need to share the inherent responsibilities of the therapeutic encounter. There is a mutual obligation for families and clinicians to work with each other to facilitate progress, and for children to be as cooperative in the process as they can be. Simply put, we are unable to work effectively with children who cannot attend—even if only for brief flashes—to the business of therapy. At a minimum, they must possess some level of competence, focus and intrinsic motivation.

Intrinsic motivation: Self-efficacy, valence, and attributions

Intrinsic motivation as it relates to children's contributions to progress in therapy has been a strong interest of Dr. Robert J. Lowe. A graduate of Ohio University, Dr. Lowe received his doctorate in speech pathology in 1986. His work experience includes several years as a school clinician in Iowa before beginning university teaching at the University of South Dakota. Since 1985, he has been a professor at Bloomsburg University of Pennsylvania, where he teaches courses in phonetics, diagnostics, fluency, and phonology. Dr. Lowe is author of the *ALPHA-R Phonology Test* (Lowe 2000), a textbook on phonology (Lowe 1994), a workbook on phonological processes (Lowe 2002), co-author of two workbooks for articulation and phonology intervention (Lowe and Weitz 1992a, b), and author of a text on speech-language pathology and related professions in the public schools (Lowe 1993).

Q16. Robert J. Lowe: Motivation and generalisation of treatment targets

There is a certain pre-occupation in our work with speech-impaired children with the tasks of choosing the right therapy approach, treatment objectives, reinforcement schedules, and initial target words. These are important priorities that tend to focus practitioners on assessment data analysis and matching those data with suitable interventions and therapy materials that will trigger new learning, new patterns of generalisation, new levels of intelligibility, and hopefully a new and improved PCC. Amid this busy process, we probably sometimes do not look closely at the characteristics of the child, the family, and ourselves, and how these qualities might impinge upon speech progress. Can you explore for us the place in the therapy equation of levels of self-efficacy, valence (the degree of attraction or aversion that an individual feels towards a specific object or event), and attribution of behaviour, on the part of the child?

A16.   Robert J. Lowe: The role of intrinsic motivation in learning of new speech behaviours

In 1993, Kwiatkowski and Shriberg proposed a framework for intervention in which the two parameters of capability and focus were viewed as an interactive system impacting the learning and generalisation of speech sounds. They called this two-factor approach the 'capability-focus treatment framework'. Capability included linguistic variables, such as productive phonology and risk factors (e.g., mechanism constraints, cognitive-linguistic constraints). Kwiatkowski and Shriberg (1998) elaborate on capability and ascribe to it both the ability to produce sound targets and the ability to use self-monitoring processes in the learning of new targets. Focus included attention, motivation, and effort that basically would reflect the child's interest or disposition towards change. In Shriberg's (1997) review of the model, he points out clinician comments suggesting that lack of focus is associated with minimal treatment progress. Clinicians made comments such as: 'lack of motivation for speech change', 'fear of failure', 'unwilling to risk being incorrect', and 'easily frustrated'. He suggests that, for some children, this lack of focus will interfere with learning and generalisation, even when they have strong capabilities.

Weiss (2004) expanded this view of focus as she explored the research literature outside of the speech-language field. Her paper looked at the role the client plays in the intervention process, and she notes that this role is largely ignored in the treatment of children with speech and language disorders. The exception appears to be the area of stuttering, which has looked at the roles of motivation, temperament, the client's belief in the clinician, and belief in the potential success of treatment.

Weiss tells of an unintelligible five-year old client (Sid) who made remarkable progress over a 4-week period during which he was not seen for therapy. The progress followed a conversation in which Sid asked if Weiss could understand his younger sister's speech better than his own. The answer was 'yes', to which Sid replied, 'But she's a baby.' Four weeks later, they met again for a therapy session and his speech had improved remarkably. Weiss suggests that the dramatic improvement was in part due to a change in the child's motivation or perhaps to a realisation that his speech was something that he must take responsibility for and work to correct. In other words, the child had chosen to change his speech system, believed he could, and did. In terms of the Kwiatkowski and Shriberg model, the child's disposition had changed, and he was now willing to apply his production skills and make use of self monitoring and regulation to learn the new sound targets.

This choosing to change and believing that it can be done are associated with the constructs of intrinsic motivation, self-efficacy, and valence. Speech-language clinicians are familiar with the construct of motivation. We typically motivate our clients by offering rewards for their good work. Sometimes it is verbal praise or a pat on the back, and often we use prizes (e.g., stickers, toys, and special privileges). These are *extrinsic* motivators in that they come from outside of the client. Intrinsic motivation comes from within the individual. It is all about doing something because you want to do it and is considered to be more powerful than extrinsic motivation. In the Weiss example, her client displayed intrinsic motivation by showing that he wanted to change his speech.

Intrinsic motivation can be developed by the use of extrinsic reinforcers. Henderlong and Lepper (2002), in their review of the literature on praise, note several studies that have shown verbal praise to increase a child's desire to engage in tasks or spend more time at a task. However, in some cases, reinforcers have also been shown to actually inhibit the development of intrinsic motivation. This phenomenon is sometimes referred to as the 'over justification effect'. The child may initially engage in an activity because it has some intrinsic value, but as the adult continues to reinforce or reward the behaviour, there is a shift so that the activity is done to gain adult approval or the prize. In other words, the adult's judgment or approval of the performance becomes the child's goal. As a result, when there is not the likelihood of a reward, the child will not voluntarily engage in the behaviour. This effect has been documented in children as young as four years of age.

Henderlong and Lepper (2002) and Malone and Lepper (1987) note several factors that can promote intrinsic motivation. Several of the factors are described below.

Praise

Verbal praise is a common component of the speech therapy session. Praise is more effective when it is perceived by the client to be sincere and if it is associated with a specific aspect of the client's performance rather than just a general 'Good job!' Sincerity is more important for older children than it is for preschoolers, who are not as discerning. Older children have a good sense of how well they should perform, thus praising a child's effort for work on a task that should be easy may not be well received and could actually lead to discouragement. On the other hand, praise for effort on a difficult task would be appreciated and promote intrinsic motivation.

Praise can function to recognise a client's work, and recognition in itself can be a strong motivator. Who doesn't feel some satisfaction when others recognise our efforts and results? One cautionary note: when giving praise, be sure to centre that praise on the client's efforts and successes towards reaching his/her goals. If the child begins working to please the clinician and meet the clinician's goals, then intrinsic motivation suffers.

Cameron, Banko, and Pierce (2001) reviewed more than 100 experimental studies on the impact of praise and rewards on intrinsic motivation. They conclude that rewards given for low-interest tasks increase intrinsic motivation. For high-interest tasks, rewards have a negative effect if they are tangible, offered beforehand, and if loosely tied to performance level. If the rewards are clearly linked to performance, the measures of intrinsic motivation increase or are equivalent to non-rewarded controls.

Attributions

What the child attributes success or failure to can also influence the effects of praise. Performance attributions refer to the inferences children make about the causes of their successes or failures. Healthy attributions are those that the child can control. For example, a child believing he was successful because he kept trying shows a healthy attribution because the child has control of how hard he/she tries. But, if the child attributes his success to luck or to the task being easy, then that is not a healthy attribution as the child does not have control of how lucky they are or the difficulty of the task. The clinician can encourage healthy attributions through his/her comments and use of praise. Pointing out that their continued efforts resulted in success reinforces a healthy attribution ('If I keep at it, I can succeed.').

Meaningful goals

Setting goals that are meaningful to the client can promote motivation. In the Weiss article, Sid recognised that his younger sister, 'a baby', was a better talker. After that realisation, his goal was to improve speech production. That, of course, was the clinician's goal from day one. The difference was that now it was also *Sid's* goal. Choosing goals that are meaningful to the client and that are seen as obtainable work to promote intrinsic motivation. Valence is the perceived strength or value of the reward that will result from the performance. In the case of Sid, the value of talking better than his baby sister was very motivating. Whenever the clinician can 'sell' the value of change, motivation will result.

Fantasy

Children love to play games. Placing speech activities within game or fantasy contexts will tap into a natural play mode of young children. It is okay to practice production of the /s/ sound in different word contexts, but it is much more motivating to practice those words if they are the key to finding clues to a hidden treasure. Once children understand the concept that speech is a tool to help them acquire their needs, then activities can be designed to use this tool in fantasy games, which are highly motivating. An example would be a game where the child is searching for clues that would help locate a hidden treasure. The clinician would serve as the 'clue master', and in order to reveal a clue to the child, a secret code would have to be uttered. It might simply be the saying of three target words in a particular order with correct articulation. The clinician would be aware of the order (it could be written down), and the child would try the different sequences until he/she hit on the correct one. The target words could be pictured so that the child could change the order as each attempt is made. This activity points out the value of correct articulation in accomplishing a desired end (finding the treasure), while at the same time being fun!

Self-efficacy

Self-efficacy is an individual's belief in their ability to perform a particular task. More formally, Bandura (1994) described it as a person's beliefs in their capabilities to produce designated levels of performance. Self-efficacy beliefs can determine how you feel, think, and behave.

They can also influence motivation. Individuals with good self-efficacy for a particular task are more likely to engage in the task, show more perseverance in completing the task, and are more likely to use self regulation in learning.

It should be emphasised that efficacy appears to be task- or behaviour-specific. For example, you may have good self-efficacy for successfully reading a romance novel, but poor self-efficacy for reading a textbook on organic chemistry. Bandura (1994) notes several influences on the development of self-efficacy. Past experiences, for example, can promote good self-efficacy. In relation to speech and language, a client is much more likely to approach learning a new speech sound if they have already had success in learning other speech sounds. Successful past experiences build a child's confidence or belief that they can succeed in the future. On the other hand, a series of past failures would increase the child's belief that they will fail at future attempts. It is here that I would suggest that some of the recent literature on choosing sound targets may be misleading. Some of the work summarised by Gierut (2001) suggests that treatment of more complex properties of the phonological system appears to result in the greatest generalisation. I'd argue that it may depend on the child's temperament. For a child who is a risk taker, this may be the approach to take; but for a shy child who is reluctant to try new sound targets, I would suggest starting with easier, less phonologically complex sound targets. Once the child has a history of success, then I would move to more complex sound targets.

Another factor that promotes self-efficacy is vicarious learning. If a client sees a peer successfully learning a new sound target, it may increase his/her confidence and encourage him/her to keep trying. Again, it would be important for the client to hear praise for efforts so that the idea of perseverance is being promoted. Along with that, the clinician can also express his/her confidence in the client's abilities, which also promotes self-efficacy.

The last influence on the development of strong self-efficacy is the reduction of stress reactions. The client must recognise that it is okay to fail. Failing is part of the process of learning the new skill. Any emotional distress associated with failing will only interfere with learning the new behaviour. In the clinical situation, the client should be experiencing success more than failure. An occasional failure is needed to develop perseverance, but those failures need to be surrounded by successes. The speech-language clinician can be pro-active in this area by developing an atmosphere where failure is recognised as part of the learning process but not penalised. We all fail, and often it is by failing that we learn how to succeed.

Summary

Intrinsic motivation represents an intangible that can be tapped by the speech-language clinician and used to promote the learning of new speech targets. It is influenced by a number of factors, including praise, attributions, goals, and self-efficacy. Its value is that it can take the speech and language goals of the clinician and make them into what the client wants to accomplish. Once that occurs, our job becomes a whole lot easier!

Children with speech and literacy difficulties

Output phonological representations play an important role in learning to read (Snowling, Goulandris, and Stackhouse 1994), and children with impaired phonological output are at greater risk for impaired phonological awareness skills. Within the SSD population, many children diagnosed with CAS also exhibit phonological awareness (PA) difficulties, if we take PA to mean the ability to reflect on and manipulate the structure of an utterance as distinct from its meaning (Stackhouse 1997, p. 157). PA is an essential skill in literacy acquisition and a necessary aspect of making sense of an alphabetic script. Having said that, it is important to mention Larrivee and Catts (1999), who cautioned that phonological disorder *alone* is not closely related to problems with early reading skills, but that when phonological disorder is accompanied by another speech or language impairment, such as CAS, reading and writing disabilities may emerge. This takes us to school and to the interface between teachers, mentioned previously in this chapter for their frequent role in making referrals, and clinicians.

Dr. Roslyn Neilson is a Private Speech Pathologist who has, over many years, completed a PhD in Psychology in the area of phonological awareness and reading difficulties, taught in the Faculty of Education at the University of Wollongong in Australia, published two innovative tests of phonological awareness, and presented numerous in-services to working teachers. Her clinical specialty is children with reading difficulties, and, with characteristic modesty, she says she 'continues to do her best' to learn from them in the assessment and intervention process. In A17, she explores issues around teacher–clinician communication.

Q17.   Roslyn Neilson: Collaboration between clinicians and school teachers

Although it is firmly established that the most important factors associated with literacy difficulties in children include histories of speech-language delay and current weaknesses in phonological skills, literacy teaching (including 'remedial reading') is a traditional province of school teachers, and not SLTs/SLPs, especially in the eyes of teachers. Meanwhile, it can be argued that speech is our business, especially in the eyes of SLPs/SLTs. In your clinical, research, publishing (Neilson 2003a, b), and academic teaching roles, you have spent more time than most engaging with teachers around the topic of children's SSD, phonology, PA, and early literacy. Some of these teachers have been your clients' parents or your clients' teachers. Others have been graduate students in your university classes or participants in continuing education and in-service events. You also talk at SLP/SLT student and CPD/CEU gatherings about the key points to consider in engaging collaboratively and co-operatively with teachers. What role can teachers play in the screening and management of speech disorder? What are the inter-related speech and language weaknesses that place children in an at-risk category for literacy difficulties? What can be done to help, and what are the implications for the collaborative classroom? Are there regularly recurring issues of epistemology, terminology, ethos, and culture that need to be addressed before SLPs/SLTs can best support the knowledge base that teachers bring to literacy teaching and place themselves in a good position to receive support from them?

A17.   Roslyn Neilson: Teachers and speech language professionals: Communicating at the chalkface

Like many practising SLPs/SLTs, I have had my share of ups and downs when communicating with the teachers of school-age clients. Although collaborating at the chalkface isn't always easy, I do feel that working constructively with teachers is one of the most important clinical goals we can set ourselves.

I specialise in therapy with school-age children. Their Speech Pathology referral often relates to just one part of the school's and/or family's wider exploration of a classroom-based problem. My clients, that is, are usually experiencing serious literacy difficulties, with the core of their problem involving word recognition and spelling. For most of these children, their weakness involves laborious and inefficient handling of the alphabetic code. Many of these children were diagnosed with speech and/or language difficulties as preschoolers, but have reached the stage where they 'sound normal to the naked ear' (Paul 2007, p. 429). However, their phonological difficulties have often not entirely resolved, despite their generally intelligible speech—and as Nathan, Stackhouse, Goulandris, et al. (2004) point out, children who still have even mild speech sound difficulties past the age of 6;9 are at risk for complications in literacy development. Usually, however, these children's phonological difficulties have, as Paul (2007) expresses it, gone 'underground' (p. 436). There are hundreds of empirical studies to be cited to demonstrate the relationships between underlying phonological difficulties and problems with literacy, and a good starting point for the interested reader is Stackhouse (1996). The term 'underlying' phonological difficulties is a challenging one that can only be explored briefly here. For children with these phonological difficulties, their most obvious speech symptom in casual conversation involves difficulty, at a phonetic or phonemic level, or both, pronouncing and remembering complex words (e.g., *ask* and *twelfth*) or words of three or more syllables (e.g., *congratulations* and *extinguisher*). Weak syllable deletion is common, and consonant sequences are often confused. Assessment of more formal expressive language typically shows slow, inaccurate word retrieval, with the children's sentences getting lost in 'mazes' (Dollaghan and Campbell 1992). These children struggle to hold sequences of sounds in their working memories. Many of them have difficulty with the rapid automatic naming of known words and will show characteristics of word finding difficulty under pressure. Stackhouse (1996) and many others have posited that the core of all these symptoms involves the quality of lexical representations, where the phonological specifications for the representations are unstable, coarse-grained, or imprecise. Importantly, these phonological difficulties seem to permeate many aspects of higher-level language functioning, including those functions upon which literacy development depends.

The flow-on effects of underlying phonological difficulties include weak phonological awareness, with children having difficulty segmenting, blending, or manipulating sounds in words. Mastering written language is difficult for this group of children because the English alphabetic code, with its complex and often opaque system of mapping letters onto sounds, places extraordinary demands on the phonological system. Children with underlying phonological weakness do not develop orthographic lexical specifications along typical lines. They do not, that is, develop a database of easily retrievable and generalisable word knowledge in which sequences of letters are mapped precisely on to the sounds or syllables in words.

It is important to mention that this is not the only aspect of literacy difficulties with which SLPs/SLTs may be involved. Children who have decoding difficulties (and some who do not) may also have primary language comprehension problems affecting reading comprehension (Nation and Norbury 2005). Language comprehension problems require collaboration between SLPs/SLTs and teachers, too—but that is, in a sense, another story.

When children with reading difficulties show underlying problems at the phonological level, we SLPs/SLTs naturally feel that this is our business. Our sense of involvement and connectedness is particularly strong if we have engaged with the individual children as preschoolers with phonological disorders and have seen literacy problems looming as they headed towards school. Professional demarcation issues are inevitable once formal schooling commences, because teaching children to read and write is traditionally teachers' business. Furthermore, by school-age, the main concern of the children and their parents is literacy development and not the finer points of speech acquisition. Accordingly, to serve our clients well, the delicate interface between SLPs/SLTs and teachers requires careful thought and negotiation.

SLPs/SLTs can play a useful role in alerting teachers and parents to both the presence and relevance of phonological difficulties, and it may be necessary to assume a degree of naivety on teachers' part. Overby, Carrell, and Bernthal (2007) report that half of a group of teachers listening to recordings of moderately intelligible second graders (in their third year of school) judged that the children were not at risk for literacy difficulties. This finding suggests that, although the social repercussions of expressive phonological difficulties may be recognised by teachers, large numbers of them may be oblivious to the associated learning implications.

Pleasingly, teachers usually find information sessions on the connections between phonological difficulties and literacy quite interesting, reporting increased confidence in referring children for speech and language assessment. Atypical speech patterns, difficulties with word retrieval, mazes, and stumbling over polysyllabic words are easily recognisable once a teacher, or a parent for that matter, knows what to listen for.

What are the implications for therapy? There has been a general move in most English-speaking countries towards explicit instruction in alphabetic code in the early years of literacy instruction (*National Enquiry into the Teaching of Literacy* 2005; Rose 2006), and many schools now use systematic phonics programs. This is a welcome break-through for children experiencing difficulty with the alphabetic code, but questions about our Speech Pathology clients remain. Should SLPs/SLTs be suggesting adaptations to teaching practices to help children to compensate for phonological weaknesses, and should we be offering to work with the children ourselves? Are we really needed in the management of these children's learning, or is the business of remedial reading best left to schools?

I would argue that SLPs/SLTs currently have a key role to play. The problem from my perspective is that most school reading and spelling programs work on the assumption that the learners have normal underlying phonological skills. Teachers assume that children know what they mean when they are asked to 'sound out' words. Fortunately, most children actually manage the task, or learn to, with minimal modelling. When things go wrong, as they do for our clients with subtle phonological difficulties, it is difficult for teachers to pinpoint the exact problem, let alone work out ways to scaffold the children's attempts.

I believe this gap in teaching practice exists because the phonemic level of language is surprisingly inaccessible to individuals who, because of their training, are unattuned to it. Phonemic awareness easily gets subsumed into thinking about spelling patterns in words (Ehri 1989). Teachers, and writers of programs such as *Jolly Phonics* (Lloyd 1998), actually think that, when children are asked to sound out and blend /æ/ and /s/, the word *as*, rather than *ass*, will emerge. SLPs/SLTs may shake their heads at teachers' apparently poor phonemic awareness, but we must remember that teachers are quite 'normal' in their tendency to think of letters rather than phonemes. It is our own mindsets that were transformed as we attended our undergraduate phonetics classes! Teachers do, generally, have all the implicit phonemic awareness they need to be able to read and spell unfamiliar words themselves, but they become confused about distinctions we draw between orthography and speech, and are unaware of issues relating to allophones and coarticulation. Given that phonetic analysis is such a useful tool in working with SSD *and* with early reading and spelling (Fielding-Barnsley and Purdie 2005), I predict that teacher-training undergraduate curricula will eventually include basic phonetics.

Until then, however, SLPs/SLTs *can* usefully provide in-services about phonetics to help bridge the gap in teachers' knowledge bases (Moats 1994). The depth of in-servicing offered must depend on the enthusiasm of the teachers and the time available to them. I have an untested hypothesis to offer here: how effective might it be to teach teachers how to use *The Quick Screener* (Bowen 1996b) and then have them test a few young children with mild to moderate SSDs? My hope is that teachers would emerge from such an experience sensitised to phonetics, allowing them to understand better the analytical, multi-sensory approach that best helps children with phonemic awareness difficulties learn to read and spell.

There is also, I think, a role for SLPs/SLTs to work directly with school-age clients who have literacy-related problems, complementing what they receive at school. Therapy can usefully target the remnants of the phonological difficulty in the child's oral language, developing strategies for sharpening the child's phonological representations and providing individual support with reading and spelling that the teacher cannot offer in the whole-class setting. It can be rewarding to join forces and plan remedial strategies with teachers, parents, and the children themselves as part of the therapy process. Collaboration must be an ongoing process, however, because the child is part of a classroom context where the curriculum, not the child's rate of learning, drives the content of what is being taught. When collaboration succeeds, it involves regular meetings at which current concerns and achievements are discussed, goals are set or revised, strategies are reinforced, and, perhaps most importantly, ways for the teacher to adapt regular classroom and homework activities to suit the child are negotiated.

And the ups and downs mentioned in the opening paragraph? These have included disputation with a client's teacher, involving strong disagreement on how to program for the child. Inter-professional disputes of this kind are disconcerting for both the child and the parents. I invariably find that the teacher's disagreement with my recommendations is a salvo from the 'Whole Language' (Fox 2001) side of the so-called 'Reading Wars', with the teacher reacting against anything that begins with 'phon' (Scarborough and Brady 2002). The teacher is typically convinced that any strategy that draws attention to the phonological level of the alphabetic code will automatically prevent the child from gaining meaning from print (Goodman 1976). In such circumstances, in order to provide useful therapy without making the child and family feel they have to choose sides, I can usually work on the spelling side of literacy, rather than on reading, without antagonising the teacher.

There tends to be another interesting difference between myself and teachers that manifests when we collaborate in my Australian work context, and it involves terminology. The term 'dyslexia' draws at best a mixed reception from teachers, and they seem unwilling to use the label. I gather from discussion and from the education literature that this reluctance is largely on the grounds that the term connotes unwanted medical baggage; reading difficulty is seen by teachers as a teaching problem, not a 'medical' one. By contrast, SLPs/SLTs accept that children may bring their own physiological processing difficulties to the language learning task, although we naturally expect that their literacy progress will be moderated by environmental factors. We are therefore more disposed to use labels like 'dyslexia'. I often feel, however, that our labelling tendency brings vulnerability with it—a vulnerability that we share with parents, who are not willing to leave any stone unturned in their efforts to find help for their children. We are often tempted, that is, by the thought of treating the underlying processing difficulties, and we can be distracted by cures ranging from the glossy procedures and gizmos that crop up so often in the popular media (Rosen and Davidson 2003), to more subtle and apparently physiologically plausible procedures claiming to rewire the child's brain. SLPs/SLTs and parents do well to take a leaf from the teachers' book, I feel, and remind ourselves that there is, so far, little evidence for the effectiveness of anything other than careful, analytical, systematic, and motivating experience with reading and writing for helping children with phonological difficulties to come to grips with the alphabetic code.

Children with speech impairments in culturally and linguistically diverse settings

Our final 'special' special population comprises children with speech impairments in culturally and linguistically diverse settings. There is a reciprocal relationship between culture and communication, each influencing the other. One of the effects of population migration, relocation, and dislocation throughout the world has been to add a new dimension to SLPs/SLTs attention to the individual differences of our clients, and most clinicians need to take diversity and multi-culturalism into account to ensure that clinical management leads to functional and meaningful outcomes for *all* the clients we see. The International Affairs Association (IAA) is an ASHA-related professional organisation that has been promoting humanitarian and international networking opportunities since 1990. Its mission is the globalisation of the professions of Speech Pathology and Audiology, partly through humanitarian work in under-served areas and in developing countries. IAA and other organisations, including some universities, have given SLP/SLT professionals and students unique opportunities to experience different cultures, expanding their professional horizons.

Dr. Ken Bleile is an internationalist, a professor in the Department of Communicative Disorders at the University of Northern Iowa, and the author of several practical child speech publications, including *The Late Eight* (Bleile 2006) and the *Manual of Articulation and Phonological Disorders* (Bleile 2004), among many scholarly publications. Passionately interested in the impact of communication impairment on people living in the non-industrialised world, he has taken students on field trips to places as diverse as New Zealand (which is industrialised) and Nicaragua—and that's just the Ns! As well, he is vitally interested in the SLP issues that affect culturally and linguistically diverse populations in the United States.

Q18.   Ken M. Bleile: Humanitarian SLP/SLT outreach and the ICF-CY

The International Classification of Functioning, Disability and Health–Children and Youth (ICF-CY; WHO 2007) is a classification system to be used throughout the world to support the health and wellness of all people (McLeod and Bleile 2004). In Bleile (2002), you outlined an assessment procedure for speech you would use if time was short. How would you tackle the same exercise with culturally and linguistically diverse test subjects, taking into account the ICF-CY criteria?

A18.   Ken M. Bleile: A Nicaraguan experience

How would I tackle an assessment for speech with culturally and linguistically diverse test subjects if the time were short, taking into account the ICF-CY criteria? For reasons given shortly, the quick answer is: with humility.

I have provided speech-language services in six different countries. Most recently, students and I spent a good portion of summer preparing for and then providing services (including many short speech and language assessments) to children with communication disorders in Nicaragua. Nicaragua is a beautiful country of volcanoes, lakes, and widespread poverty surrounding small islands of great wealth. It is the second poorest country in Latin America, second only to Haiti, and 4-hour electrical blackouts, armed guards, and emaciated animals are part of daily life. We worked in the outskirts of Managua in a school and an orphanage for children with developmental disabilities, the country's only orphanages and schools for such children. Many children we assessed were from families that were impoverished even by Nicaraguan standards.

On assessment days, we saw children as long as there were children to see, which usually meant from early morning to late afternoon. Assessments typically lasted approximately 30 minutes and were undertaken by a team that included a Nicaraguan special educator (the professions of communication disorders are only beginning to be developed in Nicaragua), the child, a caregiver, a translator, several American students, and myself. The assessment location typically was an area set off from a noisy play area, and, because it was the rainy season, the room was hot, steamy, and buggy, even during those rare occasions when the electricity and fans were on and working simultaneously. The children typically had severe developmental disabilities. Injuries from head trauma and malnutrition were present, though less prevalent.

Although chronologically many children were between five and ten years old, this was the first communication assessment most had received. Much of what the team did would seem familiar to individuals trained in our profession. First, a case history was obtained to determine what factors in the child's past might influence present functioning and prognosis for future development. Current functioning in speech and language was obtained through a combination of observation and parent report. Because no standardised assessment instruments exist for Nicaraguan children, 90% of whom speak Central American Spanish, only non-standardised testing was performed. However, this was not much different from procedures in countries in which normative speech and language information is available, because children with such severe levels of disability typically are unable to perform on standardised tests. In addition to assessing speech and language development, we listened for voice and fluency problems and screened for feeding and oral motor difficulties. A hearing screening was performed separately.

The most challenging assessment task was determining long-term prognosis and developing therapeutic recommendations. Among other factors, prognosis depends on the nature of the developmental disability and availability of services. Many times the nature of the developmental disability was unknown, stated in vague terms ('brain problems'), or involved a disease for which little or no information on developmental disorder exists (for example, what is the developmental outcome in speech and language for Dengue Fever?). Limited medical care and poor health conditions also impacted prognosis. To illustrate, most children were observed to cough and show other signs of aspiration after feeding, and caregivers reported frequent episodes of pneumonia. Even for children with well-studied disabilities, prognosis could be difficult to determine. What, for instance, is the prognosis in speech and language for a ten-year-old orphan with Down syndrome in a country in which the professions that treat communication disorders are scarcely older than the youngest children they serve, where developmental services for adults are virtually non-existent, and where most children leave an orphanage at 18 years to enter the community, where life for the homeless often is brutal and short?

Most caregivers wanted their child to receive a speech and language assessment for the therapeutic recommendations they hoped to receive. This critical aspect of the assessment would have been impossible to provide were it not for our Nicaraguan special educators and for the caregivers themselves. Our Nicaraguan team members knew the children, their families, and the types of available services. They were our leaders in turning general recommendations into plans of action. Caregivers in conjunction with the special educators identified aspects of communication about which they wanted additional information. One highlight of our experience in Nicaragua was a meeting with approximately 30 parents and their children in a school for children with disabilities. Prior to the meeting, family members selected topics about which they wanted information, and, during the meeting, guided us further with questions and ideas. We provided the information orally and demonstrated techniques and approaches.

Why 'with humility'?

Because performing a speech evaluation in another language and culture is challenging work. Because often we were aware of the difference between providing the 'best service' and providing the 'best service possible under the circumstances'. With humility because we often worked hand-in-hand with professionals, both Nicaraguan and from other countries, providing excellent services, year in and year out, with a positive spirit under challenging conditions. With humility because many families, though living sometimes in dire poverty, give their children lives that are rich, nurturing, and filled with love. With humility because the world is an uneven playing field for a person with a communication disorder, and the extent to which disability isolates socially, educationally, and limits access to medical care in large measure is determined by the accident of where one is born.

ICF-CY

The ICF-CY is the acronym for the *International Classification of Functioning, Disability and Health–Children and Youth* (McLeod, A1), a classification and diagnostic system developed by the World Health Organization for use with persons who experience developmental disabilities (WHO 2001). The ICF-CY is intended to serve the needs for professionals from many different disciplines, including those who assess and treat children with speech, language, swallowing, and hearing disorders. Within the field of communication disorders it has found some use both as a general orientation and as a specific diagnostic system and the ICF (the adult version) has been especially relevant for adults who have experienced strokes and voice disorders.

The ICF-CY provided a general mindset for our work in Nicaragua. Because the ICF-CY was developed by an international organisation (the World Health Organization) for professionals from many different countries and cultures, it did not impose an American system on our Nicaraguan colleagues. Use of the ICF-CY was in accordance with the view that international work is collaboration between colleagues from different cultures and countries on topics of mutual concern, rather than an imposition of the perspective of one country on the care provided in a different country.

The ICF-CY system distinguishes between biological, psychological, and social aspects of health. This distinction is critically important in international work in communication disorders, because culture plays an enormous role in determining consequences of a deficit [see Louw, A28 for a discussion of the Developmental Systems Model (Guralnick 2001), taking an ecological systems perspectives (Bronfenbrenner and Morris 1998) in a South African context]. For example, two children may be born with similar hearing deficits, one in a country with well-developed hearing services and another in a country without such services. In the country with well-developed hearing services, a child may elect to enter the deaf community or receive a cochlear implant, whereas in a country without such services, a child may effectively be denied access to education, health services, and community (Jewett 2003). When performing international work, the ICF-CY also provides a useful mindset for considering degree of impairment. This is because whether a communication disorder is 'milder' and 'more serious' depends in large measure on cultural and economic factors. To illustrate, in many developed countries, a seven-year-old who mispronounces /s/ is considered to have a mild communication disorder. In a country with limited economic and educational resources, the same communication disorder may result in serious consequences, including early death. This is because in countries with intense poverty, a family may need to select among its children who is allowed to attend school. A child with a communication difficulty, even one as seemingly minor as difficulty pronouncing /s/, may not be deemed by the family to be the best educational candidate. A disability that limits a person's educational and vocational opportunities, including those in communication, contributes to poverty and, consequently, to higher childhood mortality (UN Millennium Project 2005). In recognition of the importance of education and disability on childhood mortality, the Millennium Project's five-point agenda includes improving human development services by rapidly increasing the supply of skilled workers in health and education (UN Millennium Project 2005).

A case study

The child described in this brief case study will be called 'Olaf', after a poem by E. E. Cummings (Cummings and Firmage 1994), which begins, 'I sing of Olaf glad and big'. In the poem, Olaf is undone in part because he is glad and big, and the same may prove true for the child described here. The case study is offered to illustrate some of the challenges that may face a child with communication disorder in a country with limited financial resources.

When we met Olaf, he was 14 years old and living in an orphanage, in a room apart from the main group of children. His room was attached to the outside of an outlying building, and was a cage-like structure with a dirt floor, a barred glassless window, and a cement ceiling over one-half of the room and open sky over the other half. At that first meeting, Olaf was naked from the waist up, a large thickset boy with short cropped hair. An attendant stood nearby, encouraging him to dress. When Olaf saw us, he half stumbled, half ran over to give us welcoming hugs, nearly knocking us over.

Olaf was evaluated and was found to communicate largely through grunts, eye gaze, and reaching. He spoke no words. Olaf appeared to have a severe cognitive impairment, though no standardised testing was available to confirm this impression. Olaf's nearly constant movement was consistent with hyperactivity. Hearing could not be assessed. The staff reported that Olaf received medications to reduce his restlessness, though they believed none of them were effective. Trials of sign language and picture communication systems were undertaken, without effect.

In a country with greater financial resources, a child with similar apparent intellectual disabilities and attention difficulties might have received extensive therapy and effective medications to maximise his learning potential. These were not available to Olaf. Instead, what Olaf had was a home away from the dangers of the streets and freedom from abuse and malnutrition. He lived through the care and sometimes heroic efforts of the orphanage staff. Discussions with orphanage caregivers revealed that Olaf was housed in his cage-like room because he frequently wandered, and the orphanage had no other structure that might hold him. Because Olaf was big and affectionate, he posed a significant threat to the many much smaller children in the orphanage, and so was largely kept apart under the care of an aide, who provided for his daily needs and watched carefully when Olaf interacted with other children.

Olaf's future is unknown. The orphanage keeps children until age 18, and no settings exist for adults with Olaf's level of disability. The orphanage, recognising the need to work quickly, is attempting to develop and build a setting for adults with disabilities. The hope is that the setting will exist when Olaf turns 18. If it does not, Olaf will likely live on the street or in the Managua city dump among the approximately 5,000 people who make their home there.

Special issues and concerns

This chapter has canvassed some of the issues and concerns associated with several special groups of children. Included have been children with concomitant speech and language issues, co-occurring speech and literacy difficulties, and low levels of stimulability; children with cleft palate, craniofacial anomalies, and velopharyngeal dysfunction; and those who have been internationally adopted. As well we have thought about self-efficacy and motivation (so important to the five populations just mentioned), and the factors involved in humanitarian outreach in serving speech-impaired infants, children, and youth in the developing world. To varying degrees, the interventions described in the following chapter will have a place in the management of the special populations considered here.

Chapter 4

Intervention approaches

In this chapter, brief allusions to evidence-based approaches to intervention with children speech sound disorder (SSD) that *have* been covered elsewhere in this book are included, along with more detailed accounts of those that have not. The reader is referred to Mirla Raz (A4) for information about Traditional Therapy (Van Riper 1978); Barbara Hodson (A5) regarding Cycles (Patterns) Therapy; Karen Golding-Kushner (A13) and Dennis Ruscello (A42) on craniofacial anomalies and speech; Watts Pappas (A25) for a discussion of family-centred practice, and Brenda Louw (A28) for the closely related Assets-based Approach; and B. May Bernhardt and Angela Ullrich (A32) for constraints-based non-linear phonology approaches. Additionally, in Chapter 3, Karen Pollock (A14) discusses the intervention needs of children adopted from overseas, and Adele Miccio (A15) talks about Stimulability Therapy; and, in Chapter 7, Pam Williams (A41) describes the Nuffield Programme. Each account contains sufficient information for clinicians to implement the methodologies and/or to locate relevant literature. Meanwhile, in this chapter, the minimal pair approach called Multiple Oppositions therapy is presented by A. Lynn Williams (A19), Auditory Input Therapy by Gwen Lancaster (A20), a Psycholinguistic Model by Hilary Gardner (A21), Phoneme Awareness Therapy by Anne Hesketh (A22), Vowel Therapy by Fiona Gibbon (A23), and Perceptually-based Interventions by Susan Rvachew (A24). What a line-up! The author turns her hand to providing summaries of the phonetic, Grunwell, and *Metaphon* approaches; three further minimal pair approaches: Conventional Minimal Pairs, Maximal Oppositions, and Empty Set; and the Imagery, Patterns, Whole Language, and Core Vocabulary approaches. Therapy for Childhood Apraxia of Speech (CAS) and Phonotactic Therapy (applicable to both phonological disorder and CAS) are in Chapter 7, and Parents and Children Together (PACT; Bowen and Cupples 1999a, b) is presented in Chapter 9.

Phonetic approaches

Phonetic approaches focus on discrimination and production of articulatory targets. Motor-skills learning techniques (Schmidt and Lee 2000) are used to teach individual error phones to preset criteria. Therapy that targets the phonetic level has its roots in traditional articulation therapy, and as Van Riper (1978, p. 179) wrote, 'The hallmark of traditional therapy lies in its sequence of activities for: (1) identifying the standard sound, (2) discriminating it from its error through scanning and comparing, (3) varying and correcting the various productions until it is produced correctly, and finally, (4) strengthening and stabilizing it in all contexts and speaking situations.'

When it is used as a stand-alone intervention (Raz, A4) to address one or a few sound substitutions, omissions, distortions, or additions in cases of functional articulation disorder or persisting residual errors in children with articulation disorder, phonological disorder, CAS, or structural anomalies, target selection usually incorporates the traditional criteria displayed in Table 8.1 (p. 282) of (1) proceeding in developmental sequence, (2) favouring targets that are socially 'important', (3) prioritising stimulable phonemes, (4) using minimal feature contrasts, (5) selecting unfamiliar therapy-target words, (6) preferring inconsistently erred sounds, (7) opting for sounds most destructive of intelligibility, and (8) addressing errors most deviant from typical development (e.g., affricates produced with lateral air emission).

Phonetic placement techniques are routinely incorporated into the treatment of children with phonological disorder and children with CAS; even children with 'pure' developmental phonological disorder (DPD) or CAS. Of course, co-occurring error-types are a frequent clinical finding with children experiencing more than one type of problem, concurrently. In an individual, some errors may have a phonetic basis, whereas some may have a phonological basis, a perceptual basis, a motor planning basis, or a motor execution basis. In principle, separating phonetic approaches from phonemic approaches helps us think clearly about the level at which we are working. In practice, though, 'phonemic/phonological therapy', 'phonetic therapy', and even 'auditory discrimination training' are not always completely distinct. Ruscello (A42) describes phonetic techniques suitable for children with compensatory errors associated with cleft palate.

Phonemic intervention

Selecting targets for phonemic (phonological) intervention begins with describing the child's error patterns, and this can be done in at least two ways: by identifying phonological processes or by identifying phoneme collapses. Working from a natural processes perspective, the therapy targets are the correct productions, meaning that the correct adult form (the target) is contrasted with the sound the child usually produces. For example, in working on velar fronting, with a child who replaces /ŋ/ with /n/, the therapist might choose *fan, run, pin, gone,* and *thin* to contrast with *fang, rung, ping, gong,* and *thing,* respectively. On the other hand, when working from a phoneme collapses perspective, there are two steps. The first is to look for lost contrast, for example, *funny* → /tʌni/ *shell* → /tæw/ *cup* → /tʌp/ *cheese* → /tid/, where four phonemes have been collapsed into one: /t/. The second step is to decide how to present the minimal contrast in therapy: will the therapist choose a Minimal Opposition (as in Conventional Minimal Pairs), Multiple Oppositions, a Maximal Opposition, or an Empty Set? No matter how targets are selected, in minimal pair therapy, activities are designed to demonstrate to the child how changing sounds in words, or how changing the structure of syllables, results in changes in word meaning, and that this affects communication. And no matter which approach is chosen, feature contrasts are central to the child's learning.

Feature contrasts in English

Phonemes are not 'contrastive' but their features are. Featural distinctions serve to create an 'opposition' between phonemes (see Table 2.5, p. 58). The Non-Major Class Distinctions are in place: differentiating labial, coronal, and dorsal consonants; manner: differentiating stops, fricatives, affricates, nasals, liquids, glides; and voice: differentiating the voiced–voiceless cognate pairs, /p b, t d, k g, f v, s z, ʃ ʒ, tʃ dʒ, θ ð/. Major Class Features distinguish between the main groupings of sounds in a language, namely, consonants versus vowels, glides versus consonants, and obstruents (stops, fricatives, affricates) versus sonorants (nasals, liquids, glides, vowels). For example, *bake–make* illustrates a major class distinction between obstruents and sonorants; *make–wake* illustrates the major class distinction between consonants and glides. In the minimal pair *silly* versus *Billy*, the contrast is not *quite* maximal, but it is 'maximal enough' to be highly salient for a child receiving intervention. In *silly* versus *Billy* is labial /b/ versus coronal /s/, stop /b / versus fricative /s/, voiced /b/ versus voiceless /s/, and unmarked /b/ versus marked /s/. It cuts across many featural dimensions, but /s/ and /b/ are both obstruents so there is no obstruent versus sonorant opposition (i.e., no Major Class Feature distinction).

All phonological (phonemic) approaches focus on teaching children the function of sounds, and all rest on the principle that, once it is introduced to a child's system, a featural contrast will show generalisation to other relevant phonemic pairs (Barlow and Gierut 2002). Four stand-alone minimal pair therapies—Conventional, Multiple Oppositions, Maximal Oppositions, and Empty Set—are described below. Other phonological approaches incorporate minimal pair therapy, and these include Grunwell's approach, *Metaphon*, Imagery Therapy, Auditory Input Therapy, Patterns (Cycles) Therapy, the Psycholinguistic Model, and PACT, whereas minimal pair treatments are used in tandem with perceptually based interventions, such as SAILS (Rvachew, A24).

Grunwell's approach

British Linguist Pamela Grunwell proposed a treatment that was based on the principle that homophony motivates phonemic change, challenging the clinician to, 'Expose the child systematically to the dimensions of the target system absent from his or her speech in a way in which both their form and communicative functions are made evident' (Grunwell 1989). Grunwell saw four main types of phonological change that could become the clinician's focus for target selection and intervention:

1. Stabilisation: the resolution of a variable pronunciation pattern into a stable pattern;
2. Destabilisation: the disruption of a stable pattern, resulting in variability;
3. Innovation: the introduction of a new pattern; and
4. Generalisation: the transfer of a pronunciation pattern across four possible contexts: phonological, lexical, syntactic, and socio-environmental.

In selecting targets, Grunwell advised therapists to work in developmental sequence where possible, giving priority to patterns most deviant from normal phonology, and/or to those most destructive of communicative adequacy. Systemic feature contrasts were minimal (e.g., *pull* vs. *bull*; *nip* vs. *nib*) and structural contrasts near-minimal (e.g., *team* vs. *steam; bell* vs. *belt*) on the basis that, with small feature difference between the target and the error, there was nothing else to get in the way. There was no attempt to increase the saliency of contrasts.

In Grunwell's approach, procedures are system-based (metalinguistic) or word-based (manipulative). Minimal pair therapy is a metalinguistic procedure, in Grunwell's terms, demonstrating to the child that sound differences signal meaning differences. A manipulative activity might involve listening to, and eventually saying in context, words that shared common phonological features (e.g., all with fricatives in onset). The approach is suitable for children with mild to severe phonological disorder (or 'phonological disability' to use Grunwell's term), and procedures incorporate auditory discrimination, minimal pair and near-minimal pair games, homophony confrontation, phoneme–grapheme correspondences, and metaphonological skills training. The far-reaching influence of Grunwell's pioneer research, pedagogy, and phonological principles can be seen in Multiple Oppositions Therapy (A19), Auditory Input Therapy (A20), Phoneme Awareness Therapy (A22), and the contrastive Vowel Therapy proposed by Gibbon and Mackenzie Beck (2002) [also see Gibbon (A23), PACT (Bowen and Cupples 1999a, b), and *Metaphon* (Dean, Howell, Waters, et al. 1995)].

Metaphon

Metaphon (Dean and Howell 1986; Dean, Howell, Hill, et al. 1990; Dean, Howell, Waters, et al. 1995) is also based on the principle that homophony motivates phonemic change. Phonological analysis is performed by using the assessment materials in the *Metaphon Resource Pack*, and errors are described in terms of phonological processes. Target versus substitute sound pairs are selected for treatment as in conventional minimal pair therapy. For example, to eliminate palatal fronting, the target /ʃ/ might be contrasted with the substitute (error) /s/ in word-pairs such as *ship–sip, shine–sign, show–sew, shell–sell, shower–sour, push–puss, mesh–mess, gash–gas,* and *ash–ass*. Feature contrasts are usually minimal or near-minimal. The essence of *Metaphon* is in two overlapping treatment phases followed by a discrete final phase. Metaphonetic skills are trained to improve a child's 'cognitive awareness' of the properties of the sound system, whereas metalinguistic tasks are implemented to develop communicative effectiveness through more successful use of repair strategies.

Metaphon Phase 1

In phase one, the child is taught that language is used to communicate and that language which is normally opaque can be made transparent or tangible. Phase 1 comprises Concept Level, Sound Level, Phoneme Level, and Word Level. Phase 1 is the most important phase of *Metaphon*, and the one most distinct from other published phonological intervention programs. The aim is to capture the child's interest in the phonology of the target language, to alert the child to the properties of sounds and their contrastive potential, to show that contrasts between sounds convey meaning, and to facilitate the child's knowledge that these features can be manipulated to increase the likelihood of being understood.

At Concept Level, individual speech sounds are *not* contrasted, and the child learns a conceptual vocabulary to use later for PMV awareness. Metaphors associated with voicing features are employed, such as Mr. Noisy or Mr, Growly to denote voiced consonants and Mr. Whisper or Mr. Quiet for voiceless ones. Other concepts, such as Long Sound versus Short Sound (denoting fricative vs. stop) and Back Sound versus Front Sound (velar vs. alveolar) are introduced, with the aim of having children identify sounds by their properties with 100% accuracy. The Metaphon team reported that it may not take long for children to achieve this level of accuracy. The next step is different depending whether substitution processes (e.g., fronting, stopping, and gliding, where one sound replaces another) or syllable structure processes (e.g., cluster reduction, final consonant deletion, or weak syllable deletion, where the structure of the syllable changes) are being targeted.

Substitution processes

For *substitution processes* at Sound Level, the vocabulary the child has learned (Mr. Growly, Short Sound, etc.) is transferred to describing non-speech sounds: castanets, whistles, the therapist's vocalisations, and animal and vehicle noises. The aim is to show the child that environmental sounds and vocalisations can be classified as long-short, front-back, and noisy-whisper (growly-quiet). Then, at Phoneme Level, entire sound classes are contrasted, using visual cues. For example, all fricatives versus all stops are presented to the child, still referring to the sound properties (long-short, etc). Next, the child enters Word Level, and minimally contrasted word pairs are introduced for *listening* (not production). The child judges whether a word has a long-short, front-back, or noisy-whisper sound in it. Again, visual support is provided in the form of gesture cues and pictures.

Syllable structure processes

For *syllable structure processes* at Sound Level, concepts such as beginning (as a preparation for working on Initial Consonant Deletion) and end (preparatory to tackling Final Consonant Deletion) are introduced, as well as imagery and concrete demonstrations. For example, for Cluster Reduction SIWI, imagery coupled with a concrete demonstration might involve a train with one locomotive versus a train with two locomotives in preparation for a near minimal pair such as *rip–trip*. At Syllable Level/Word Level, nonsense syllables and words are contrasted (e.g., *hot* has an engine, *ot* does not).

Metaphon Phase 2

In Phase 2, metaphonological tasks involving minimal pairs (introduced in Phase 1) and homonymy confrontation are emphasised, and the focus shifts to developing communicative effectiveness by giving the child feedback about success or failure to convey meaning, through behavioural responses, prompting him/her to review output. Dean and Howell (1986) postulated that, in the short term, such feedback would improve production by triggering the use of repair strategies based on the new knowledge of sound contrasts learned in Phase 1, and that the long-term effect would be a change in central phonological processing. Phase 2 is concerned with developing phonological and communicative awareness, and the link between phases one and two is achieved by incorporating Phase 1 activities into Phase 2. Phonological awareness and awareness of the properties of speech sounds must be well developed before the *core activity* of Phase 2 can be successful.

Core activity

In the Metaphon core activity, the clinician and child take turns to *produce* and *select* minimal pair words (e.g., *pin* vs. *fin*) pictured on cards or worksheets. If the child says a target word, such as *fin*, correctly: (1) The therapist selects the correct word; (2) feedback is given, and (3) guided discussion occurs; for example, 'Yes. That was a long sound. I guess you know lots of other long sounds.' If the child says the target word *incorrectly* (e.g., *bin* for *fin*): (1) The therapist selects the incorrect word (the one the child actually said); and (2) no feedback is given directly to the child, but the child's attention is drawn to the sound property; for example, 'That was a short sound. Should it have been a long sound?' The aim of the core activity is to have the child revise incorrect productions 'spontaneously'.

Metaphon Final Phase

In the final phase of *Metaphon*, minimal pair sentences are introduced. The therapist and child take turns, each instructing the other to, for example, 'Draw a *pin/fin* on the fish'; 'Draw a *pan/fan* in the box'; 'Draw a *pole/foal* in the stable'. Emphasis is still on guided discussion of sound properties ('I think that should have been a long sound') aimed at facilitating the spontaneous use of repair strategies.

Minimal pair approaches: Conventional Minimal Pairs

The Conventional Minimal Pair model (Weiner 1981a) rests on the principle that homonymy motivates phonemic change, and its foundation, according to Fey (1992a), is to:

(1) Modify groups of sounds produced in error, in a patterned way.
(2) Highlight featural contrasts rather than accurate sound production.
(3) Emphasise the use of sounds for communicative purposes.

Rewarding the use of contrast: (1) encourages a reduction in homophony, which (2) evokes an improvement in phonological organisation, and (3) facilitates phonological restructuring. Selecting minimal pairs (e.g., win vs. wing for velar fronting) or near minimal pairs (e.g., *up* vs. *pup* for initial consonant deletion) is predicated on the idea that Grunwell (1989) shared, that of making the difference between the target and the error as small as possible so that there are no interfering featural factors. Within intervention activities, a sound used in error (e.g., /v/) by the child is paired with its substitute (e.g., /b/). The approach may be suitable for children with mild and moderate phonological disorders. In the therapy activities, the child says the name of a picture or object, and the adult responds to what the child actually says. Only miscommunications (errors) attract feedback in the form of challenge or feigned listener confusion, and non-homophonous productions are rewarded by successful communication. For example, if the child says *bet* for target word *vet*, the therapist would hand him/her *bet* (listener confusion) or challenges it ('you take your puppy to the bet?'). If the child produced a different (non-target) voiced fricative in attempting *vet*, perhaps saying /zɛt/, then he/she would be rewarded by being handed the *vet* picture, because *bet-zet* is not homophonous and /v/ and /z/ are in the same sound class and are both voiced. Similarly, if the child said /fɛt/ for *vet*, then the non-homonymous production would be rewarded. In this way, the intervention is around homonymy, ambiguity, 'pretend' listener confusion, and effective communication (making meaning). As a conceptual approach, phonemic manner and place cues and production drill do not occur in Conventional Minimal Pair Therapy in its pure form, but in practice they are usually incorporated (see, e.g., the video clips in Williams 2006a).

Minimal pair approaches: Maximal Oppositions

The Maximal Oppositions approach (Gierut 1992) is not based on homophony. The guiding principle is that heightened saliency of contrasts increases learnability, thereby facilitating phonemic change. The word pairs are still 'minimal pairs' in the sense that one sound changes, but the feature contrasts are 'maximal' or 'nearly maximal' (as in the 'nearly maximal' *silly* vs. *Billy* example used above). Gierut applies feature geometry in the explicit creation of pairs that are high and low on the feature tree. She called the contrastive pairs in Maximal Oppositions Therapy (and in its close relation, Empty Set Therapy) 'non-proportional pairs'. Because non-proportional pairs do not share many features in common with other minimal pairs, they are highly perceptually salient, and, according to Gierut's findings, therefore more learnable. In Maximal Oppositions and Empty Set, the clinician aims to present a target and contrasting word that have many feature differences: in place, manner, and voice; major class; and markedness. It might be opportune to remind the reader here that the marked consonants in English are /p t k f θ ð s z ʃ ʒ tʃ and dʒ /. The contrasting sound is independent of the target sound, is produced correctly by the child, and is maximally distinct. As in the Conventional Minimal Pairs approach, only one contrast is presented at a time. Take for example Xing-Fu, 4;5 who had a severe SSD. He exhibited velar fronting, replacing /k/ with /t/ in all contexts, whereas /n/ was one of only eight consonants he produced correctly in all contexts. The nasal /n/ differed from /k/ in place, manner, voice, major class, and markedness, and minimal pairs used in Xing-Fu's therapy included: *key–knee*, *cat–gnat*, *coat–note*, *cow–now*, and *cot–knot*. This Maximal Oppositions approach is suitable for children like Xing-Fu who have severe phonological impairment, as is the Empty Set approach.

Minimal pair approaches: Empty Set (Unknown Set)

Empty Set (Gierut 1992) is a variation of Maximal Oppositions also using non-proportional pairs, and is also not based on the idea of homophony motivating phonemic change. Again, the principle behind it is that heightened perceptual saliency of contrasts increases learnability, facilitating phonological restructuring. In Empty Set Therapy, two targets are addressed concurrently. An *error* the child has (the first target) is contrasted with *another* erred sound (the second target) that is maximally distinct from the first.

Probably the better name for this is 'Unknown Set' as it signals that the child 'knows' neither sound and is 'learning two *new* sounds'. So, error is contrasted with error—but not just any error pair! For example, Vaughan, 5;8 was from a monolingual South African-English background, and was a recent migrant, with his family, to Australia. He had a severe SSD, a percentage of consonants correct (PCC) of 41%, he replaced /f/ with /b/ (stopping) and /r/ with /w/ (gliding), and both /f/ and /r/ were absent from his repertoire. Recognising the severity of his impairment, and wanting to use the Unknown Set approach, his speech-language pathologist (SLP) needed to find a contrasting sound for his minimal-pair–maximally-opposed treatment set that was maximally distinct from /f/, remembering that the sound had not only to be maximally distinct but also *absent* from Vaughan's repertoire. The /r/ for which he was non-stimulable was a perfect choice. Accordingly, Vaughan's Minimal word pairs (non-proportional and maximally contrasting) included *rind–find*, *reel–feel*, *red–fed*, and *rocks–fox*, which he produced at the outset of therapy as: [waɪnd-baɪnd, wil-bil, wɛd-bɛd, wɒks-bɒks,]. As it happened, Vaughan's error productions were also maximally distinct (non-proportional), but not homonymous. The procedures used in Empty Set are the same as for Conventional Minimal Pair Therapy and Maximal Oppositions, and may include the provision of phonemic place and manner cues, suggestions, and 'instructions' to the child.

Drawing on the results of several elegant experiments, Gierut (1992) determined that therapy was most effective, promoting the greatest generalisation, if two new maximally opposed phonemes representing a major class feature difference were targeted, as in Vaughan's case. By contrast, targeting one new maximally opposed phoneme representing a non-major class distinction was effective, but less effective than the preceding option. Between these two were two further equally effective alternatives. The first was to target two new maximally opposed phonemes representing a non-major class distinction; and the second was to target one new maximally opposed phoneme representing a major class feature difference.

Minimal pair approaches: Multiple Oppositions

Unlike the Conventional Minimal Pairs approach, in Multiple Oppositions Therapy it is not assumed that minimal *feature* contrasts will be formed, because, of course, the phoneme collapses (or homonymy) in which several targets are realised the same way determine which oppositions will be used. In therapy, several targets are presented to the child at once, all contrasting simultaneously with what the child usually produces. For example, if a child collapsed the voiceless velar stop /k/, the voiceless affricate /tʃ/, the voiceless alveolar fricative /s/, and the consonant cluster /tr/ to /t/ so that *cap*, *chap*, *sap*, and *trap* were all realised homophonously as /tæp/, his/her treatment sets (in the first two columns below) and their corresponding untreated set to use as a generalisation probe (shown in the third column) might look like this:

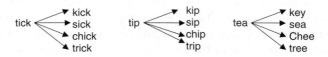

Any non-words would be made meaningful by using it as the name for a fantasy creature or object, so you might have a picture of a character called *Chee* for the probe set above. Two further examples of 'phoneme collapses', the term Williams uses to denote the simplified one-to-many correspondence between the child's customary (error) productions and targets, are: *lick*, *wick*, *rick*, and *flick* all realised homophonously as /jɪk/; or *beat*, *been*, *beak*, and *beach* all produced as a CV /bi/.

As noted above, in the Multiple Oppositions approach, it is *not* assumed that minimal feature contrasts will be formed because the contrasts are based on a child's error relative to the adult target. A further difference between Multiple Oppositions and the Conventional Minimal Pairs paradigm is that it is not based on the assumption that a child's sound system is organised according to phonological processes. A phoneme collapse describes a child's phonological organisation more broadly, employing a child-based and systemic perspective. Accordingly, a phoneme collapse would be considered one rule, rather than several phonological processes. From this, it is clear that Multiple Oppositions is not only distinguished by having more targets in training than the other minimal pair approaches, but also by the way in which those targets relate to each other as 'members' of one rule set.

Multiple targets are treated simultaneously across a child's rule set. These multiple targets are contrasted as a group with the child's error substitute, creating the so-called multiple oppositions. The activities themselves are as for Conventional Minimal Pair therapy. Therapy occurs in four phases.

1. Familiarization + Production
2. Contrasts + Naturalistic Play: Phase 2 begins at an imitative level and moves to spontaneous when the first training criterion of 70% accuracy is achieved.
3. Contrasts within Communicative Contexts
4. Conversational Recasts

With regard to production accuracy in connected speech, Williams uses a structured and systematic treatment paradigm to program for generalization at all phases of intervention, aiming for high response rates in each treatment session (about 60–80 responses in a 30-minute session). In the early phases of treatment, she commences a session with focused production practice of the contrasts and ends the session with a conversation-based naturalistic activity. She believes that this conversation-based activity bridges the focused practice and allows the child to hear and practice his/herr sound(s) in a more naturalistic activity (Phase 2). These brief naturalistic activities include sound-loaded conversational activities in which the child can hear and have opportunities to produce a large proportional frequency of their target sound(s). The approach is geared to children with severe phonological disorders.

Sound contrasts in phonology

From the 1970s onwards, clinically applicable developments took place in Generative Phonology and Natural Phonology. Linguists turned their attention, in great detail for the first time, to the plight of children with speech impairment. Although there were obvious clinical applications for this work (see Grunwell's approach above), the hard task of converting it into therapy that was practical, efficient, effective, and acceptable to practitioners and clients required adequately funded, concentrated research effort from the SLP/SLT side. In an environment of often inefficient service delivery, and overstretched services within the SLP/SLT profession, with most therapists only dimly aware of how the new knowledge from linguistics could inform practice, Lynn Williams responded by developing, implementing, and successfully testing the efficacy of her Multiple Oppositions treatment approach, for children with severe speech intelligibility challenges. Knowing that it is all too likely for important clinical research to receive wide publication in the peer-reviewed literature (which it has) while remaining virtually undiscovered by grass roots practitioners, Williams devised ways of bringing her own, and, quite remarkably, *other* evidence-based speech sound treatments (Conventional Minimal Pairs, Maximal Oppositions, and Empty Set) to the world's workplace. A major outcome of her extraordinary endeavour has been the *Sound Contrasts in Phonology (SCIP)* intervention software, published in 2006.

Commenting on the effects and efficiency of a Multiple Oppositions approach, Williams (2000a) wrote, 'The use of larger treatment sets in multiple oppositions may lead to several new phonemic contrasts being added to a child's system. Thus, multiple oppositions has a potential advantage over singular contrastive models of phonological intervention in terms of shortened length of treatment, improved intelligibility, and more efficient intervention.' But implementing Multiple Oppositions through the use of use *SCIP* is not just a question of client plus clinician plus software with a dash of homework! Whether it is done with the aid of the software or without, the success of the intervention rests on up to 2 hours of detailed assessment, which allows the clinician to map the child's sound system onto the adult system and determine the extent of the child's phonological knowledge and what he/she needs to learn before establishing a treatment plan with highly specified goals aimed at expeditious restructuring of the child's disordered system in order for it to match age-expectations.

Dr. Lynn Williams is a Professor of Speech-Language Pathology in the Department of Communicative Disorders at East Tennessee State University (ETSU) in Johnson City, Tennessee. She is a Fellow ASHA, and she served as an Associate Editor of the journal *Language Speech and Hearing Services in the Schools* from 2004 to 2007. Lynn is the author of *Speech Disorders Resource Guide for Preschool Children* (Williams 2003b), and she has published and presented extensively on her research with children who have SSD. Lynn has received several grants from the National Institutes of Health in support of her translational research, resulting in the development of a software program called *Sound Contrasts in Phonology* (SCIP; Williams 2006a). Embedded in SCIP is her own approach to speech therapy called *Multiple Oppositions*. In her response to Q19, she addresses a question about assessment and a multi-part question about this powerful therapy.

Q19.   A. Lynn Williams: The multiple oppositions approach

The SCIP software includes clinical training videos that show, with helpful commentaries, snippets of four contrastive therapies in action, namely: Conventional Minimal Pairs, Multiple Oppositions, Maximal Oppositions, and 'Empty' or Unknown Set. Specifically in relation to Multiple Oppositions, what assessment process is typical for a suitable candidate for this therapy? And in terms of the therapy itself, can you give us a case example that describes the aspects of the therapy not shown in the videos?

For example, how long are the treatment sessions, how frequent are they, are families involved in sessions or in homework, what procedures and activities are incorporated, and at what stages of the child's progress?

A19. A. Lynn Williams: Assessment and intervention from a systemic perspective

What assessment process is typical for a candidate for this therapy?

In order to implement the systemic treatment approach of Multiple Oppositions, it is important to describe the child's speech disorder systemically. A systemic approach is a system-based approach that compares the child's system with the adult system by mapping the two sound systems to each other using phoneme collapses. For example, a child might produce [t] for several sounds in the adult target system, such as /s ʃ k tʃ st/.

Systemically, this is viewed as one rule involving a phoneme collapse of voiceless obstruents and a cluster (adult system) to the voiceless obstruent, [t] (child system). This broader system-to-system comparison provides a more holistic description of the child's speech than is possible with a sound-based approach that uses a narrower sound-to-sound comparison of the child's production relative to an adult target. Using this example, a sound-to-sound comparison employing phonological processes would describe the phoneme collapse as four separate and independent error patterns (i.e., stopping, fronting, deaffrication, and cluster reduction).

In addition, a systemic analysis is child-based rather than adult-based, as is common in many traditional assessment approaches that are based on a pre-determined and finite number of rules (or processes) to describe the child's error patterns. As a consequence, the broader system-to-system comparison and child-based aspects of a systemic analysis allow the clinician to describe idiosyncratic errors that are common in unintelligible speech, as well as gain insight into the organizational structure the child has developed to compensate for a smaller sound system relative to the adult sound system. As Grunwell (1997) stated, we can discover the 'order in the disorder'.

To complete a systemic description of a child's speech, I administer the Systemic Phonological Analysis of Child Speech (SPACS), which provides information on the child's phonetic inventory (Word Initial and Word Final), distribution of English consonants relative to the ambient sound system, and mapping of child:adult sound systems using phoneme collapses. For a more detailed description of the SPACS approach, readers can refer to Williams (2001, 2003b, 2006b). In my clinical research, I use a 245-item single-word elicitation probe (Systemic Phonological Protocol; Williams 2003b) and a 15- to 20-minute conversational sample. Clinically, however, this sample is likely to be too time-consuming for practicing clinicians who have large caseloads and severe time constraints. Clinicians can complete a SPACS on smaller databases, such as the Goldman-Fristoe Test of Articulation-2 (GFTA-2; Goldman and Fristoe 2000) or other sound inventory tests that are commonly used. Phoneme collapses can be constructed by word position by mapping the adult sound targets that are replaced by the error production in the child's system. Using the GFTA-2, the clinician can look down the word-initial column on the response matrix 'to diagram' (or construct) phoneme collapses of frequently occurring error productions.

For example, a case study of 'Adam' indicated that he produced [g] for adult targets /b d f v ð s z ʃ tʃ dʒ dr fr gl gr kw st tr/ in word-initial position on the GFTA-2. This represents a 1:17 phoneme collapse between Adam's sound system and the adult sound system. A closer examination of the adult targets reveals that they are obstruents and clusters. Thus, Adam collapsed obstruents and clusters to [g], which is also an obstruent. This SPACS was completed easily and quickly, and it represents Adam's logical and systemic organization more clearly than if a phonological process analysis had been completed on his GFTA-2 responses.

What specific procedures are involved in the Multiple Oppositions approach?

After the child's system has been described, a systemic intervention approach using Multiple Oppositions can be implemented in order to facilitate phonological restructuring with the greatest amount of change occurring in the least amount of time. I structure intervention using a treatment paradigm that I described in detail elsewhere (Williams 2000b, 2003b, 2005). There are four phases; all are data-based with the exception of Phase 1, which is time-based. Basically, Phase 1 involves Familiarisation (of the rule, the sounds, and the vocabulary) + Production of the contrasts. This initial phase creates a meaningful context that lays a foundation for the feedback and work that will be carried out in the following treatment phases. Phase 2 encompasses focused practice of the contrasts at an imitative level with a dense response rate (about 60–80 responses in a 30-minute individual session or 20–40 responses in a 30-minute small group session). Although Multiple Oppositions has larger treatment sets of target sounds, the contrasts are practiced one at a time. For example, *tip–sip*; *tip–ship*; *tip–kip*; *tip–trip*. The focused practice is followed by a short (5-minute) naturalistic play activity. These are brief, sound-loaded activities that bridge the focused practice that occurs on a narrow training set and the communicative use of the contrast within meaningful play activities. An example might be *I Spy* using objects or pictures of items that have the target sound in untrained words. The clinician and child take turns giving hints for the other to guess the item. I typically use the naturalistic activity for one sound per session and generally choose the sound with which the child is having the greatest difficulty. The focused practice continues at an imitative level until the child achieves training criterion (70% accuracy across two consecutive treatment sets; 1 treatment set = 20 responses). Once the criterion is met, Phase 2 continues with focused practice + naturalistic play, but at a spontaneous level of production. Intervention continues at the spontaneous level of Phase 2 until the second training criterion is met (90% accuracy across two consecutive treatment sets). At that point, treatment moves to Phase 3: contrasts within communicative contexts. This treatment phase intertwines the focused practice and naturalistic play so that the child plays games with the contrasts (such as *Go Fish*). Although most children achieve the generalization criterion (50% accuracy in conversational speech) in Phase 3, some children need additional intervention at a conversational level to attain generalization (see Williams 2000b for longitudinal data from an intervention study with 10 children). For those children who are doing well in Phase 3 at a spontaneous response level in communicative contexts but not reaching generalization, movement to Phase 4 would occur. Phase 4 involves conversational recasts that encompass Stephen Camarata's Naturalistic Speech Intelligibility Training (Camarata 1993, 1995). In this phase, treatment switches from the contrasts in games to using the contrasts communicatively in conversational scenarios, such as ordering food at a family restaurant that includes food items containing the target sounds.

The treatment paradigm provides a structure, or blueprint, for intervention and the child's progression through the treatment phases. As noted earlier, the child is in the driver's seat, so to speak, and matriculation through the treatment phases is based on the child's performance data. The paradigm structures intervention to address two important aspects of phonological intervention: (1) the duality of sound learning: phonetic and phonemic aspects; and (2) programming for generalization. In the early phases of treatment, greater emphasis and support are placed on helping the child learn the production aspects of the new contrast (the imitative response level, plus the focused practice with dense response rates). The early phases also control for extraneous distractors by avoiding activities such as playing board games. This allows the child to engage intensely with the SLP/SLT, with a tight focus on the physical, visual, and auditory cues that the SLP/SLT provides in a rich context, and to achieve the required levels of practice and responses rates. Yet, I program for generalization from the outset by pairing the focused practice with the bridging activities of naturalistic play involving the new contrast in sound-loaded activities. I want to quickly bring in the phonemic aspects of sound learning (moving from imitation to spontaneous with a lower training criterion level) and gradually and systematically re-introduce the distractors (playing games with the contrasts in Phase 3 or conversational recasts in Phase 4). A summary of the treatment phases and activities is provided in Table A19.1. As you look at the treatment phases, activities, and response levels, you will notice the systematic and gradual programming for generalization, as well as the shift in intervention focus from phonetic learning to phonemic learning.

Regarding the intervention 'dosage' (Dodd, A43), I generally see children twice weekly for 30-minute sessions. Although in my research lab I often see children in individual treatment sessions, I have recently begun to do small group therapy with two to three children in 30-minute sessions twice weekly. The modifications I make to the treatment paradigm include the following: (1) in Phase 1, which is time-based, I see the children individually for that first treatment session in order to familiarize them to their rule, sound, and vocabulary; and (2) reduce the response rate to about 20–40 responses per child in a 30-minute group session.

Engaging families in the intervention process is an important component of treatment and can take many different forms from active to passive involvement. The particular way that I involve families reflects my philosophy that (1) learning a sound system is similar to learning language—it involves communication; and (2) parents are not trained therapists. As a consequence, I ask parents to leave the focused practice of facilitating new sound contrasts to me as the trained professional, and I ask them to extend the work the child and I are doing in the clinic at home through fun, play-based, sound-loaded activities that involve models and recasts. I interview the parent(s) to find typical routines they share with their child through the week, and then I develop naturalistic activities that they can implement within those routines. I know that many families live full and hectic lives with dual careers and frequent after-school activities, so the naturalistic activities I send home have a greater chance of being completed (and enjoyed!) if I can ask them to do them within their normal routines. For example, at the grocery store, play a game to see who can identify the most items with the /k/ sound (coffee, candy, cauliflower, carrots, etc.). I teach the parents how to use set-ups (e.g., asking the child if s/he would like corn or cabbage

Table A19.1 Summary of Multiple Oppositions treatment phases

Treatment Phase	Intervention Focus	Response Rate	Response Level	Example of Activities	Criterion
Phase 1: Familiarization + Production EXAMPLE: s ʃ k tr ← t k	Create a meaningful context that lays foundation of work the child will be doing	1 treatment set = 20 responses (5 contrastive word pairs of 4 target sounds = 20 responses)	Imitative	Familiarization of: • Rules (long versus short [t ~ s, ʃ]; front versus back [t ~ k]; buddy sounds [t ~ tr]) • Sound (ticking clock sound versus flat tire sound and quiet lady sound; coughing man sound; sounds that go together) • Vocabulary	First treatment session
Phase 2: Contrasts + Naturalistic Play	Initial focus is on the phonetic aspects of sound learning (imitative) and then moves to phonemic aspects (spontaneous)	60–80 responses (individual session); 20–40 responses (group session)	Imitative then Spontan-eous	Produce contrasts [5 contrastive word pairs] with imitative model (control distractors and get high response rate); give tokens for each response regardless of accuracy—when child gets 20 tokens, s/he has completed one treatment set and s/he gets a sticker; switch order of presentation of contrasts to prevent child developing articulatory set. Naturalistic Play (e.g., I Spy)	70% accuracy across two consecutive treatment sets (move to Spontaneous); 90% accuracy across two consecutive treatment sets (move to Phase 3)
Phase 3: Contrasts within Communicative Contexts	Rule Learning (phonemic)	60–80 responses (20–40 responses for group session)	Spontan-eous	Go Fish; Concentration; Memory; Teacher	90% accuracy across two consecutive treatment sets (if generalization criterion of 50% accuracy in conversation speech not met, move to Phase 4)
Phase 4: Conversational Recasts	Incorporate new contrast into conversational rule	60–80 responses (20–40 responses for group session)	Spontan-eous	Communicative Scenarios, such as Family restaurant/McDonald's	50% accuracy in conversational speech

for dinner), protests (e.g., identifying 'beans' so the child can say that doesn't have their coughing man sound; or saying *torn* for *corn* to see if the child can correct them), models, and recasts in the activity. I give the parents two to three activities each week, along with a questionnaire they complete about the number of times they used the activities, how well the activities worked, what questions they had, etc. The questionnaire structures the home activities and communicates to the parents an expectation that they will carry out these activities on a regular basis. Occasionally, I give the parents a tape recorder to take home and record an activity that we will review together.

Auditory input therapy

Not to be confused with Auditory Integration Training (AIT) (ASHA 2004d), Auditory Input Therapy (Lancaster and Pope 1989; Flynn and Lancaster 1996) has the advantage of being suitable for younger children, and it encourages the active participation of their caregivers (Lancaster 1991). In essence, the approach involves setting up interesting and attractive games and tasks, called 'thematic play' in some literature, during which the client is exposed to multiple 'repetitions' of particular sound targets, spoken by the adult, with no requirement for them to practice saying words or sounds. It incorporates minimal pair therapy and metalinguistic activities.

Gwen Lancaster is a British SLT working in a community setting in Bristol. She was a lecturer at City University in London for 10 years, where she taught in the area of child speech at Master's level. Ms. Lancaster is the surviving co-author of *Working with Children's Phonology* (Lancaster and Pope 1989) and *Children's Phonology Sourcebook* (Flynn and Lancaster 1996), and author of *Phoneme Factory: Developing Speech and Language Skills* (Lancaster 2007), the companion book for the *Phoneme Factory* and *Phoneme Factory Sound Sorter* software (Roulstone, A8). She is involved in professional development teaching to SLT colleagues in the South West region of England, mentoring and providing second opinions. In her response to A20 she talks about Auditory Input Therapy.

Q20. Gwen Lancaster: Implementing Auditory Input Therapy

Has Auditory Input Therapy evolved since the first half of the 1990s? And, if so, what does it look like now? Can you outline the specifics of the planning approach to adopt in assessment, treatment goal-setting, therapy delivery, caregiver training, and outcome measurement with unintelligible three or four year olds? How is feedback about his/her performance provided to the child, and what does it comprise?

A20. Gwen Lancaster: Auditory Input Therapy

Developed in the mid-1980s in the UK, Auditory Input Therapy (AIT) evolved from clinical practice with children with speech impairments aged three to six years. AIT was inspired in part by the *auditory bombardment* component of the Cycles or Patterns approach (Hodson and Paden 1983), more recently called *focused auditory input* (Hodson 2007), and takes into account the unconscious or implicit level that is fundamental to learning first and additional languages (Velleman and Vihman 2002). It focuses on the child *listening to* rather than producing speech, helping build up the information he/she needs about the speech sound system from repeated, intense auditory models delivered naturalistically. Similar to the suggestions of Ellis Weismer and Robertson (2006), it is usually employed as a *component* of an eclectic approach to intervention for children's SSDs (Lancaster and Pope 1989) and is not conceptualised as a total 'therapy package'.

Velleman and Vihman (2002) explain how typical language learners unconsciously register, and implicitly acquire, the features of their ambient language or languages. In keeping with this, the theory proposed for the effects of AIT is that at least some children with speech impairment benefit from receiving repeated exposure to carefully selected targets that are relevant for them. This intense exposure facilitates their acquisition of new syllable structures, speech sounds, and contrastive phones. AIT activities are based around *topics* (e.g., things seen on a walk, such as *stick*, *rock*, and *bike* to target SFWF /k/), *semantic groups* (e.g., foods, such as *bean*, *burger*, and *banana* to target SIWI /b/), and *stories* (e.g., a story about a 'sad seal' to target SIWI /s/) and can be used to address language and/or speech goals (Ellis Weismer and Robertson 2006). With regard to *speech* activities specifically, materials for most consonants are provided in Flynn and Lancaster (1996), but of course, ingenious clinicians and caregivers can invent novel activities to target consonants, vowels, and syllable shapes according to the individual child's intervention needs and interests.

Individuals and groups

For an individual child, or for groups of up to six children, in the age range of three to six years, grouped by error-type, the clinician selects games, activities, and stories that will allow a particular speech sound or syllable structure to be repeated often by an adult for the children to hear. Treatment targets are selected relative to independent and relational analysis (Stoel-Gammon and Dunn 1985), including contrastive assessment (Grunwell 1985a).

The activities are portrayed to the children as 'listening games', and while they are urged to listen, they are not actively encouraged to say the words. This means that AIT can sometimes be used with clients who are unwillingly to talk, or where compliance is difficult, including children who sit outside the therapy room door refusing to enter, and those who can't, won't, or 'don't want to' co-operate. AIT can be incorporated into *any* appealing pursuit, so the creative adult is often in a position to follow the child's lead in the choice of materials and activities (Girolametto and Weitzman 2006).

Implementing AIT

If, for example, a child's current target is /s/ SIWI, an appropriate game could be creating a collage with silver paper cut-outs of *scissors*, *saws*, and *circles*. While making the collage, the SLP/SLT would produce utterances that included /s/ SIWI, frequently repeated but without hyperarticulation, such as 'Let's make some silver circles.' Another activity could be a story involving characters such as a *superhero*, *Sara*, and *Surjeet*, who have favourite foods that are collected for them by the child in response to the therapist's input. The therapist might say, 'Sara wants some sauce', 'Give Surjeet a sandwich', and so on. The target sounds can receive *slight* emphasis, but the aim is for the child to hear natural-sounding speech.

When using AIT with children of any age, it is necessary to include objects or items that can be easily illustrated (with pictures) or demonstrated by showing (e.g., for nouns and adjectives) or enactment (e.g., for verbs), so that unfamiliar vocabulary does not get in the way of enjoying the activities. The actual words used can include some that are unfamiliar to the child, potentially building their semantic knowledge. This suggests a possible additional reason for using AIT with preschoolers, since Rvachew (2006a) concluded that maximising children's vocabulary and speech perception skills prior to school entry may be an important strategy for ensuring that children with SSDs start school with age-appropriate speech *and* phonological awareness abilities. Targets are *cycled*, in that a child, or children, grouped because they have similar error patterns, listen to a target (e.g., /s/ SIWI) in therapy sessions or at home, for 1 or 2 weeks, and then perhaps other initial or final fricative will be introduced. The same cycles may be repeated later in therapy, depending on progress. AIT activities provide a relatively easy way for many parents and caregivers, including education staff, to work with children. The clinician should make it clear to these adults that children involved in the activities are not expected to *say* the words themselves, and they may need demonstrations of how to play the games so that they don't feel self-conscious about the repetitiveness of their input.

In the implementation of AIT, I follow the treatment principles of Grunwell (1985a) and Hodson and Paden (1991). Target selection is largely based on typical developmental expectations (e.g., those proposed by Dodd, Holm, Hua, et al. 2003), so that early sounds, such as /p/, /b/, and the nasals, are selected before later developing sounds, like the affricates. In acquisition of languages other than English, order of acquisition may differ, so appropriate normative expectations (McLeod 2007a) should be applied. I recommend that the activities be carried out daily at home or in educational settings for 5 or 10 minutes, once a day or more. Different people can play the games with the child, and siblings, friends, and peers can be involved.

A comparative study

In my MSc research (Lancaster 1991; Lancaster, Keusch, Levin, et al. in revision), I compared the speech progress of groups of children receiving (1) parent-delivered AIT, (2) no treatment (the children in this control group later received therapy), and (3) clinician-delivered eclectic intervention with full parental participation. The research was conducted in a National Health Service (NHS) centre with 15 three- and four-year-old clients on my caseload, referred by health or education professionals. The participants had moderate to severe speech impairments (Hodson and Paden 1983) and were randomly assigned to the three groups. Intervention took place over 6 months and was followed by reassessment. The parents assigned to the parent-delivered AIT group received 2 hours of group training using materials later published in Flynn and Lancaster (1996). They were then supplied with materials to carry out AIT activities for 6 weeks. These addressed each child's speech targets determined via contrastive assessment (Grunwell 1985a). At the end of each 6-week period, I met with each child's parent(s) to discuss their child's progress and set new therapy targets. In order to evaluate the possible effectiveness of parental intervention *alone*, the child was not included in these meetings but was seen for reassessment after the 6-month treatment phase. It was found that the children in both intervention groups improved significantly more than those in the no-treatment control group, in terms of their percentage of occurrence of speech error patterns in a citation naming test of 55 single-words: 41 from the Edinburgh Articulation Test (Anthony, Bogle, Ingram, et al. 1971) plus 14 additional words. From the results of this and other studies, it appears, however, that therapy that directly involves both clinicians *and* parents or caregivers is the most effective (Lancaster, Keusch, Levin, et al. in revision).

Although intervention by caregivers alone may not be the most *effective* therapy, it can be used *efficiently*. My small study (Lancaster 1991) demonstrated that the children who received AIT made significantly more progress than children who received no therapy, suggesting that AIT may provide a partial solution in situations where long waiting lists, unmanageable caseloads, or gaps in provision exist. Between 1997 and 2000, clinicians working in a busy community clinic in Essex, UK used AIT with all newly referred children with speech impairments. During the initial appointment, clinicians carried out a speech assessment and explained to caregivers how to conduct AIT. The clinician analysed the child's speech after the session and then mailed relevant AIT activities, including written instructions for how to carry out AIT, to the parents. This meant that, while waiting for 2 to 4 months for therapy, parents could start the intervention themselves.

Small groups in community settings

The following is a typical example of how I implement AIT in community settings. In 2007, I saw four boys aged from three to four years, in term-time for weekly therapy in their state nursery school in Bristol, UK for 16 weeks. One of the boys received support from an adult who attended the groups and continued the activities throughout the week at nursery. Parents attended for at least 1 of the 16 group sessions and were provided weekly with homework activities. The children's needs differed, but there was overlap. For example, they all needed intervention for fricative targets. One deleted all fricatives, one was stopping, one replaced /f/ with [s], and the fourth boy replaced /s/ with [f]. Their first cycle of AIT, conducted over 6 weeks (i.e., 6 treatment sessions), included voiceless fricatives SFWF and SIWI, changing phonemes each week: /f/, /s/, and /ʃ/ SFWF then /f/, /s/, and /ʃ/ SIWI. The boys' needs included increasing their awareness of velar stops, so in the ensuing 4 weeks, /k/ and /ʃ/ were the focus of therapy (4 sessions in all) and caregiver-administered activities.

The duration of each session was 45 minutes, and included three or four activities, at least one of which would be sent home. The first activity was usually a story. For example, when inputting /f/ SFWF, a story was told about 'Jeff the giraffe' (Flynn and Lancaster 1996, pp. 148–149) that included pictures of *Jeff* and his *wife*, *scarf*, *wolf*, *roof*, *knife*, and *shelf*. The children took the pictures and the story home. A related game involved the objects *leaf*, *wolf*, *elf*, *knife*, *calf*, and *giraffe*, which were covered in turn with a *scarf*. The support teacher whispered an instruction to a child like, '*Hide the knife under the scarf*', putting the other items into a bag. The clinician then 'guessed', saying perhaps, '*I think the leaf is under the scarf*', and a child took that object from the bag to indicate that the clinician's guess was incorrect. In these sorts of activities, the therapist seizes opportunities to say the objects' names repeatedly or to 'muse aloud' on what the object might be (e.g., *It can't be the leaf or calf, we only have elf, giraffe, and wolf*) to increase the children's exposure to the sound target in the particular syllable or word position. Another enjoyable game involved the clinician placing objects and toys for each sound target on a table for a bean-bag-throwing game in which the adult told a child which object to aim for and knock to the floor. Alternatively, the adult hid something under an object and instructed the children, via a puppet, where to look for it (under the *leaf*, under the *knife*, etc.).

By week 6, other therapy methods were incorporated into the boys' sessions. Sets of minimal and near-minimal pair pictures and/or objects representing words that addressed speech input and output goals for *all* the children were introduced. One set of objects and pictures included *tea, key, sea, ski, eat, beat, feet, seat, wheat,* and *sweet* to target several of the speech error patterns used by the boys (including fronting, stopping, and deletion patterns). These were used for auditory *input* and then in auditory *discrimination* activities, where the children had to find objects named by an adult. Towards the end of 16 weeks, the children were able to say some of these words using newly emerging contrasts, so they were presented with opportunities to say the words more accurately using Minimal Contrast Therapy (Weiner 1981a).

In AIT, as soon as any child achieves success in signalling a new contrast, he/she is encouraged to produce the particular target sound or structure in words. For some children, this happens faster than for others, so the short-term goals for each child in a group will not be the same and will change as they progress. For this reason, it is advisable to use a range of procedures and activities to address phonological awareness, auditory discrimination, and speech production within the same session, especially in group work.

Imagery Therapy

In Imagery Therapy (Klein 1996a, b), error and target are contrasted and the feature difference is usually minimal, so *Sue-zoo, sue-shoe,* or *Sue-soon* would be more usual oppositions for the therapist to introduce than more perceptually salient contrasts, like *Sue-moo* or *Sue-roo*. Labels and images of phonetic characteristics are used to aid the child's learning of new phonological rules, and once again, the rational for the approach is that homonymy motivates phonemic change. Klein (1996a) says that the approach is suitable for 'children with one or many phonological processes' with mild to severe SSD. Therapy proceeds in three steps.

Step 1: Identification and production of the contrast in nonsense syllables

An imagery term or imagery label is assigned to the 'intruder' (Klein's term for error) and 'sound class' (target class). For example, if the child stops fricatives, the stops (intruders) may be called poppies, and fricatives (the target sound class) may be called windies. These are combined with vowels to make CVs, representing the intruders (e.g., *pah, pee, paw; tah, tee, taw*) and target sound classes (e.g., *fah, fee, faw; sah, see, saw*). The therapist produces a syllable (e.g., *paw*), and the child indicates the associated imagery term on a poppies poster or a windies poster (if the therapist *has* said *paw* then the child should choose the poppies poster). The child is then asked to produce a syllable containing a sound from each imagery class (e.g., *Give me a poppy sound* or *Give me a windy sound*). If the child is confused at this point, the therapist provides a choice, usually with the target produced first: 'which one is windy—*paw* or *faw*?' Printed captions accompany all picture-and-object stimuli to support literacy acquisition. Bear in mind that the child is required to produce CVs and not isolated phones.

Step 2: Identification, classification, and production of the contrast in single words

Next, the therapist *shows* a picture or an object representing a real word containing either the intruder or target, *says* the word, and asks the child to indicate the imagery term associated with the word. For instance, the therapist says '*sail*', and the child should respond correctly by placing the picture on the poster for 'windies' because he/she knows that /s/ is 'windy'. Then the therapist *silently* shows a picture or object with either the intruder or target, and the child indicates the associated imagery term on one or other poster. By now, the clinician's production has been eliminated. The child is drawing on his/her own internal representation in order to make the classification, and each treatment word is classified thus.

Following classification of a word, the child is asked to *produce* the word, keeping in mind the classification. For example, the child is shown a picture of *sail* and classifies it as a 'windy'. The clinician responds, 'That's right. Now make it with a windy sound.' Note that the child is instructed to say the target word but *no model* is provided. The clinician responds to any errors in production by referring to the classification the child provided. For example, if the child said *tail* for *sail* the therapist might say, 'Tail? You said it was a windy word, but you made it with a poppy sound. Can you try it again and put in the windy sound that you said it should have?' Conventional Minimal Pair activities (Weiner 1981a) that include communicative consequences for using both the intruder and target are *also* used at this level.

Throughout Step 1 and Step 2, isolated sounds are not elicited and the clinician does not overtly model how to say the treatment words. For example, when eliciting g-words, the therapist might say, proffering a picture, 'Can you say this one with your throatie?' Natural feedback is given if the child errs, perhaps by producing /d/ in place of /g/: 'But you said it was a throaty and you said it with a tippy. Try it again with your throatie?'

Step 3: Production in narratives and conversational speech

The procedures from this point on are quite 'traditional' and include activities such as story telling, games incorporating target sound classes, and 'controlled conversation tasks'.

The Patterns Approach ('Cycles Therapy')

This approach is widely used in the US, where it is popularly referred to as 'Cycles' (Almost and Rosenbaum 1998; Stoel-Gammon, Stone-Goldman, and Glaspey 2002), and is discussed by one of its originators in Chapter 1 (Hodson, A5). It combines traditional and linguistic approaches and was devised for SLPs/SLTs working with highly unintelligible children. According to the authors, 'processes' are not targeted in therapy, but they are used to describe error patterns and to guide target selection. Patterns that have a percentage of occurrence of 40% or more are targeted. Although Cycles is a word-based approach, it does not include contrastive pairs until late in therapy when secondary patterns are targeted. Fey (1992a) was hesitant to classify Cycles as a 'phonological' therapy, except for the fact that it aims to promote system-wide generalisation and change. It is 'phonological' in other ways, too. The therapy 'works' at word level and above, and establishing phonemic contrasts, as opposed to perfecting phonetic accuracy, is emphasised. Techniques include focused auditory input as well as production practice. All of these things are characteristic of phonological therapies.

Somewhat confusingly, because 'phonological therapy' and 'phonemic therapy' are often used quite properly as interchangeable terms (see for one of many examples Williams 2003b), Hodson (2005) emphasises that Cycles is 'not a phonemically oriented therapy', meaning that it is not a therapy that proceeds in a Van Riperian phoneme-by-phoneme hierarchy (as described by Klein 1996a, b). Cycles targets phonemic organisation, with the aim of fostering the development of a child's phonological system, thereby enhancing intelligibility. The four guiding concepts, their rationales and implementation, and target and contrast selection within Cycles are summarised in Table 4.1.

Whole Language Therapy

Whole Language Therapy (Hoffman 1993; Tyler 2002) is intended for children experiencing moderate to severe phonological issues and expressive language impairment concomitantly (McCauley, A12). A typical treatment session targets might include question forms, personal pronouns, and /h/ SIWI. The clinician might read to the child a book such as *Are You My Mother?* from the Berenstain Bears series, modelling the question form, pronouns, and /h/ SIWI, especially in *he*, *his*, and *her* that occur frequently in the story. Then the therapist would re-tell the story, stating with short utterances and gradually increasing their length. As the story is re-told, the child repeats each brief utterance and then, if able, tells the story again (perhaps to a puppet or doll). Therapy takes place via conversational interactions and story contexts, incorporating cues, cloze sentences, rebus stories, story reading (to the child), and story telling (to the child and by the child) with no picture- or object-naming per se.

Core Vocabulary Therapy

The Core Vocabulary Approach (Crosbie, Holm, and Dodd 2005; Crosbie, Pine, Holm, et al. 2006) is intended for children with Inconsistent Speech Disorder (Broomfield and Dodd 2004a; Dodd 2005). Hypothetically, the underlying deficit of inconsistent speech disorder is a phonological planning deficit, not a cognitive–linguistic deficit, and most affected children probably fall in the severe SSD range. The rationale for the approach is that different parts of the speech-processing chain respond differently to therapy targeting different processing skills, and that treatment that targets the speech-processing deficit underlying the child's speech disorder will result in system-wide change.

Table 4.1 Summary of Patterns or Cycles Therapy

Four Guiding Concepts	Rationale	Implementation
1. **Cycles**	The cycles mirror gradualness in normal phonological acquisition.	One of several phonological patterns is targeted within a time period called a cycle. Specific sounds within an error pattern are targeted for about one hour per cycle. Several error patterns can be addressed within a cycle. One cycle equals 6 to 18 hours. Phonological assessment (Hodson 2004) is performed at the end of each cycle. Typically, six cycles are required for intelligible speech to be achieved.
2. **Focused Auditory Input** (Formerly 'Auditory Bombardment' or 'AB')	Acquisition occurs through listening. AB 'tunes up' the child's sound system in order to maximise the effect of production practice.	The child listens to 15–20 words, spoken by an adult, through headphones at the beginning and end of each session and once daily at home without amplification.
3. **Facilitative Contexts** **Active Involvement** **Self-monitoring** **Generalisation**	In a drill-play format, the child does production practice of individual words involving facilitative phonetic contexts. This promotes the development of new kinaesthetic and auditory images. These are internalised through practice, so facilitating the child's self-monitoring skills.	A small set of production practice words (target words) is included in each session. Models and tactile cues are used to help the child consistently produce the targets *correctly*, to facilitate new auditory and kinaesthetic images. Four or five words with captions are drawn on index cards. The child actively participates in drill-play for 7 to 8 minutes. At home, the caregiver reads the 'AB' words once daily to the child, and the child names the words on the cards in a 2-minute-a-day homework activity.
4. **Optimal Match**	This means matching the child's current phonological level with a corresponding treatment level facilitates learning.	Treatment is geared to 'one step higher' than the child's current phonological level to (1) challenge the child, and (2) encourage success.
Target selection	Phonological process analysis (Hodson 2004) is performed in order to identify treatment targets: the affected sounds and sound combinations. Target selection follows developmental expectations of the suppression of processes: primary patterns first: early syllable structure patterns, anterior–posterior contrasts, /s/ clusters, and liquids; then secondary patterns: other clusters, and palatals; then advanced patterns: multi-syllabic words.	
Contrasts	Phonemic contrasts (minimal pairs) are not included in therapy until 'secondary target patterns' are introduced. Hodson (2004) writes, 'Potential secondary target patterns need to be reviewed to ascertain if any of these need to be targeted after the following three criteria are reached: (a) All early developing patterns (e.g., syllableness) are established; (b) /s/ clusters are emerging in conversation; and (c) anterior and posterior consonants are used contrastively. Although a number of these Secondary patterns may have been evidenced during the initial evaluation, many will have "normalized" during the time that the client was working on the Primary patterns.'	

Following Independent and Relational Analysis, an Inconsistency Assessment (Dodd, Hua, Crosbie, et al. 2003) is administered. In this assessment, 25 pictures are named on three separate occasions in one session, ensuring that the same lexical items are elicited within an identical context. The productions are compared in order to calculate an inconsistency score. Children are deemed to have Inconsistent Speech Disorder if 40% or more of the words are produced variably, and Consistent Speech Disorder if they exhibit two or more atypical patterns and an inconsistency score below 40%.

The Core Vocabulary Therapy procedure begins with the child, parents, and teacher selecting, with the therapist's help if required, 50 words that are functionally 'powerful' for the child and 'mean something' to him/her, such as names of family, friends, teacher, pets; places like school, library, a park, swimming, McDonalds; functional words like please, thank you, toilet; and favourite things like a sport, superheroes, games, and characters. Ten words are selected from the list and best production is drilled in twice-weekly sessions. At the end of the week, the child produces the 10 words three times. Words produced consistently are removed from the list of 50 words. Words that are inconsistently produced remain on the list, from which the next week's 10 words are randomly chosen. Crosbie, Holm, and Dodd (2005) reported that children with inconsistent speech disorder benefit most from Core Vocabulary Therapy in terms of increased consistency and PCC, whereas children with consistent speech disorder make the most change in PCC when error patterns are targeted. These results, for children aged 4;8 to 6;5, provide *support* for the hypothesis that the underlying deficit of inconsistent speech disorder is phonological planning and not a cognitive–linguistic deficit. By improving the child's ability to form or access phonological plans, the phonological system was self-corrected and operated successfully. An inexpensive resource CD that includes an explanatory video of a child and therapist engaged in Core Vocabulary Therapy is available from the authors at The University of Queensland and an order form is in the links area of Bowen (2001).

A psycholinguistic framework

'Comprehensive' and 'British' are the words that immediately occur when thinking of the psycholinguistic framework developed, and developing, in the hands of researchers and clinicians in London and the north of England. The psycholinguistic approach (Stackhouse and Wells 1997; Stackhouse, Wells, Pascoe, et al. 2002; Stackhouse, Pascoe, and Gardner 2006) provides an inclusive means of investigating, describing, and profiling children's speech and literacy difficulties through the application of a speech-processing model and a developmental phase model of speech and literacy. A child's spoken and written language-skill strengths are identified and used as a foundation for selecting intervention targets that build on a child's existing abilities. For a child with speech-processing and production difficulties, these targets would be selected not only in relation to speech data but also in relation to linguistic, educational, medical, and psychosocial factors, according to individual need, thereby optimising the prospect of across-the-board case management.

Dr. Hilary Gardner is a practising SLT and a lecturer and researcher in the Department of Human Communication Sciences at The University of Sheffield in England's north. Her research interests include conversation analysis of therapy interactions and other adult/communication-impaired-child dyads, the nature of specific language impairment (SLI), the interactional strategies of children affected by SLI, and collaborative practice. Among her publications are two chapters on assessment (Gardner 1997, 2006). Dr. Gardner has been closely acquainted with the development of the psycholinguistic framework, and she discusses its practical implementation in A21.

Q21.   Hilary Gardner: Psycholinguistic profiling and intervention

Joffe and Pring (2008) reported that one of their UK clinical practice survey respondents said that she and other therapists she knew were 'terrified' by psycholinguistic models. Can you produce for the reader, who may not have heard of this approach before, what might be called an 'unterrifying' Psycholinguistic Approach 101, emphasising its implementation in assessment and management of children with SSDs?

A21.   Hilary Gardner: Finding the psycholinguistic model in everyday practice

The 'psycholinguistic' models of speech and language assessment and intervention *can* seem rather scary, with their boxes, arrows, terminology, and many manifestations (Baker, Croot, McLeod, et al. 2001). They can make the assessment process seem unduly complex and less intuitive, especially for experienced clinicians working in established ways. As I came into the profession when linguistic approaches to speech disorders were gaining ground, I can empathise with this. Less considered at that time were the underlying cognitive 'psycholinguistic' skills that might explain why certain types of linguistic errors occur. Some of the first publications (Hewlett 1990; Ingram 1989a; Locke, 1980) about these issues made me wary, too. After due consideration, however, it became apparent that actually I was already 'psycholinguistic' in my approach, as were most of my SLP/SLT workmates. We just didn't realise it!

What is a psycholinguistic model?

Baker, Croot, McLeod, et al. (2001) provide a comprehensive review of theory to practice relationships across various psycholinguistic models of speech processing, one of which is the framework considered here. Proponents of the psycholinguistic approach to speech disorder developed at University College London and The University of Sheffield (Stackhouse and Wells 1997, 2001) have constructed a cohesive model, coordinating all aspects of speech input and output processing: the same components clinicians have implicitly attended to for years. The speech-processing abilities and deficits, which underlie children's speech production difficulties, are mapped onto a speech chain from ear to mouth. In the case of Stackhouse and Wells' framework (Stackhouse and Wells 1997, 2001; Pascoe, Stackhouse, and Wells 2006), this is done quite literally (see Figure A21.1). Underlying skills such as the child's ability to discriminate targets from other sounds, to imitate nonwords and real words, and to respond appropriately to their own errors are included. As my understanding of the model grew, it became less threatening, and by mapping my own behaviours into it, I grasped its intricacies and advantages.

Representations

In this approach, it is assumed that a child listening to oral language perceives auditory and visual stimuli. This information is analysed, remembered, and stored in various forms, called 'lexical representations' (Stackhouse and Wells 1997, p. 8) in the word-store or 'lexicon'. The stored information includes aspects of the word's meaning (semantics), its place in the sentence (grammar and syntax), and written forms. Phonological information about a word includes its sound-sequence (syllable structure), voice, place, and manner of articulation. All of this is retrieved when the child wants to say a word.

Here our primary focus is on how therapists can recognise a child's ability to process, store, and retrieve knowledge about sound segments in words. Sound segments in this framework are consonants and vowels, combined according to the sound pattern of the language(s) in question, to produce meaningful word contrasts. In other paradigms, these sound segments would be called phones or phonetic realisations (Grunwell 1997; Ingram 1989a).

How does the 'psycholinguistic model' reveal itself in the everyday work of an SLP/SLT?

From the moment we start taking a case history, we attend to a child's psycholinguistic profile. For instance, we ask whether the child can hear well, whether they can distinguish speech in a noisy room, or attend to environmental sounds. Thus, we deal with the first level on the input side, that of peripheral hearing and perception.

Input processing

Having ascertained the speech errors and immaturities a child has, we begin work on improving his/her intelligibility, possibly going straight to intervention without additional assessment. Most intervention approaches start by asking the child to listen and sort pictures that show the difference between speech sounds used erroneously and correctly, or between minimal meaningful contrasts where the target sound makes the difference. In so doing, the SLP/SLT moves up the speech chain, increasing the difficulty of the tasks in psycholinguistic terms. So the child may be expected to perceive a target sound in isolation or in a nonsense word, without needing to access his/her lexical knowledge-bank and then, to link sound to meaning, where phonological information in the lexical store is utilised.

Output processing

On the output side, it is perhaps easier to see how processing difficulty might equate to a traditional view of increasing task difficulty. Routinely, we start with the child saying the sound in isolation, and/or in real words, progressing from CVs to more complex combinations, in phrases and sentences, perhaps supported by the written form with school-aged clients. With phonologically disordered children, many therapists recognise that using syllables or nonsense words as an interim stage in production can be helpful (Meyer 2004;

Stackhouse, Vance, Pascoe, et al. 2007). They know that this will probably be easier for the child, who can practice articulating new sound combinations without interference from their habitual, faulty phonological patterns that are stored in the lexicon. This does not imply an articulation difficulty per se. Therefore, within a single task, a child might imitate a word, without recourse to stored knowledge, and say it correctly with the target sound in place: for example, saying *fin* correctly when he/she typically says [pɪn]. Yet, in the next breath, that same child will return to the stored incorrect version, saying /pɪn/, when cued to produce *fin* spontaneously.

The same *outward* feature might have very different *underlying* weaknesses, and this is what 'psycholinguistic profiling' seeks to disentangle, discovering whether those processing weaknesses lie in input and/or output. Imagine struggling to greet your child's new teacher, Mr. Copperthwaite. His unfamiliar name is on your tongue-tip and you may know how many syllables it has, even some of the vowels and consonants. Your initial perception of the word was poor and your memory of the name is fuzzy. So the next time you meet, you say something rather approximate: 'Hello Mr. Potherway'. Nothing is wrong with your speech muscles or motor programming, as you can say the necessary sound combinations in a different context. By contrast, a young child may produce it incorrectly, simply because they cannot construct a motor program to say /θw/, so, excusably, they correct you with, 'No, it's Mr. Copperfaite!'

Recognising children's processing skills 'online'

Much of a child's ability is revealed by responses during therapy. The consummate skill of an experienced SLP/SLT includes monitoring a child's performance at each turn. This vigilant monitoring leads to subtle alterations of the task, and the models and feedback provided, all based on this clever 'online' assessment of the child's processing skills. For instance, whenever clinicians respond to an error, we ask the child to think about speech sounds at a particular level of the speech chain, perhaps recognising his/her habitual error and matching it against the target: for example, the clinician says, 'Did you say *fin* or *pin*?' (where the target production is /fɪn/). The child cannot just parrot the answer but must process the error, *pin* (realising that, in his/her lexical store, it means something sharp, not part of a fish), and make a choice as to the contrasting form *fin* and finding the appropriate motor program. If a child actually has difficulty *articulating* a sound, the SLP/SLT helps by giving placement models, cues, and instructions: for example, 'That's it, put your teeth on your lip and say /f/.' This is at the lowest level of speech processing, literally at the mouth, with no recourse to the lexical store (until the child is asked to produce it spontaneously, from memory). Thus, the SLP/SLT has assessed different levels of cognitive processing whilst working on the target, simply by doing the job the way they have always done.

I hope I have persuaded any 'scared' clinicians to take heart and be confident that they are *already* using a psycholinguistic approach in interactions with children with speech impairments. What they might need to do, though, is target assessment of the cognitive processes involved more explicitly, supplementing what they do already within tasks. These skills are summarised in the Stackhouse and Wells (1997) speech processing model displayed in Figure A21.1.

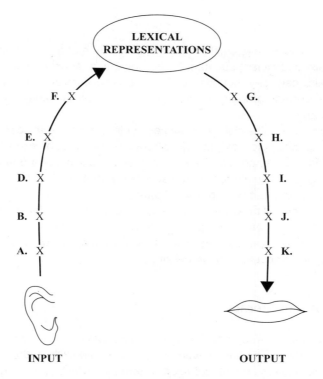

Figure A21.1 Crosses A-K on the simple speech processing model mark levels at which tests cluster. Reproduced by kind permission of Wiley Publishers, from Stackhouse and Wells (1997)

Input

A. Tasks may involve discrimination between isolated speech sounds, for instance by choosing between pictures representing /f/ and /p/. They are not in word or word-like contexts, so simple perception or 'bottom up processing', without reference to lexical representations, is assessed.

B. The child's task is to discriminate between a series of non-words or to identify rhyming syllables without accessing stored word knowledge (lexical representations).

D. Higher up the processing pathway, the child has to access the lexicon (top down processing), demonstrating whether he/she can discriminate between spoken real-words, recognising segmental change: for example, from *pin* to *fin*, signalling meaning differences.

E. A child detects whether an adult's production of a word is correct and identifies any unusual variations as being 'incorrect'. If a child's phonological information is unclearly stored, he/she may respond as though, for example, *poon*, *spoon*, and *soon*, were interchangeable.

F. At the highest level, children manipulate sound segments in patterns that change the word and the meaning by generating the information required independently: for example, sorting pictures of words beginning with the same sound 'mentally' or with sub-vocalisation, according to their phonological similarity, without hearing them spoken by another person.

G. At this level the child accesses accurate motor programs from the lexical store and names pictures spontaneously, without a spoken model. It may be found that the child can say sounds in non-words accurately but that entrenched patterns prevent correct production of real words when habitual lexical representations are accessed.

H and I. Here, the child manipulates or plays around with sound segments. These levels relate to phonological output skills where the child has some ability to create novel rhymes, or perform consonant deletions, immediately after hearing a word. The child can imitate ('parrot') and articulate real words accurately, that is, with no motor difficulty without really thinking about the meaning of what they say.

J. Here, output tasks involve non-words, building, or repeating modelled syllables. There is no recourse to the lexical store *because* these are non-words.

K. Physical or articulatory difficulties preventing accurate target production are found here, at the lowest level of processing.

Speech and literacy

The addition of literacy to the equation has stimulated a huge difference to the way clinicians in the UK think. The link between oral and written skills further justifies the work of SLTs with preschoolers and school-aged children. Previously, relating speech to literacy (even 'dyslexia') was 'out of bounds', with literacy seen as the educationalist's remit, within the UK system at least. Nowadays, speech and literacy are inextricably linked, with the latter more dependent on the former than first realised (Gillon, A27; Hesketh, A22; Neilson, A17). SLPs/SLTs can be confident that, by profiling and working with children's processing strengths and weaknesses, they target more than 'intelligible speech' (as if that wasn't enough), helping them achieve their educational potential. What has been added to the speech-language clinician's battery is the focus on tasks at the meta-level, helping children perceive and manipulate sound segments, very much at the higher end of the speech chain. This sounds quite sophisticated but of course refers to phonological awareness tasks like recognising and creating rhymes, consonant deletions, and even recognising jokes based on playing about with word structure.

Conclusion

The psycholinguistic approach, therefore, can be seen as explicating and enhancing, but not replacing, 'traditional' ways of working. With growing confidence in newly discovered, 'psycholinguistic' skills, clinicians may be tempted to read more about the *intervention* applications of this approach in a range of work settings. There is much to read in the Stackhouse and Wells series, where several practitioners have explained their work with great clarity. Rees (2001), for instance, describes many tasks and 'stand alone' assessments at each discrete skill level, and the fourth book in the series (Stackhouse, Vance, Pascoe, et al. 2007) offers a CD-ROM of materials for use in clinics and schools.

Phoneme Awareness Therapy

There are many reports in the literature of diverse, evidence-based therapies for child SSDs that incorporate metalinguistic techniques in general, and phonetic awareness and/or phonemic awareness in particular. For example, we find: Blache (1982); Bowen and Cupples (1999a); Gillon (2006); Grunwell (1985b, 1992); Dean and Howell (1986); Dean, Howell, Waters, et al. (1995); Dodd, Holm, Crosbie, et al. (2006); Flynn and Lancaster (1996), Hesketh, Adams, Nightingale, et al. (2000); Klein (1996a, b); Moriarty and Gillon (2006); Weiner (1981); and Williams (2000a), among others. To varying extents, these approaches specifically target and use *phoneme* awareness in therapy with pre-literate children, sometimes with the aim of improving the child's intelligibility and sometimes with the aim of enhancing literacy acquisition or pre-empting reading and spelling difficulties in at-risk populations.

Dr. Anne Hesketh qualified and worked as an SLT before joining the University of Manchester, and now has over 26 years of experience encompassing clinical practice, teaching, and research. Children with developmental speech disorders are the main focus of her clinical work and teaching; and her research includes both speech disorder and a broader interest in effective practice in speech and language therapy. In A22, she talks about phoneme awareness therapy.

Q22. Anne Hesketh: Working with phonemic awareness and speech

You have said that SLPs/SLTs 'can be confident about the early literacy achievement of most children with isolated speech disorder, but should undertake assessment of phonological awareness to identify those children whose phonological awareness skills after speech intervention continue to be low' (Hesketh 2004). Going on to talk about phonological awareness (PA) assessment, you cited earlier work (Hesketh, Adams, Nightingale, et al. 2000) in which you found that your early PA tests of rhyme-and-onset awareness and segmentation were possible for preschool children to complete. Starting with your definition of PA, can you clarify the terminology for the reader? How can SLPs/SLTs working in busy clinical settings efficiently and effectively identify the low PA performers, and when and how should they step in? Can you provide a glimpse of what PA intervention for these preschool children might entail and who should be implementing it? Do any of the therapies mentioned above particularly lend themselves to early PA work, and how can clinicians best integrate it into their therapy without compromising speech intelligibility progress (if that is indeed a possibility) or overloading the child?

A22. Anne Hesketh: PA intervention for children with speech disorder: Who, when, and how?

Phonological awareness (PA) is an umbrella term for conscious knowledge about the sound structure of words, from syllables to phonemes. *Phoneme* awareness is a sub-type of PA, restricted to the awareness of individual phonemes within a word, and is the level I'm interested in. It covers a range of levels of skills, for example, identification of the word onset, matching, counting, or manipulation (movement or exchange) of phonemes.

In this contribution, I will be considering the relationship between PA and *speech* rather than PA and literacy. Almost everyone agrees that PA is important in the early stages of literacy development, and there is much written about PA work for literacy purposes in older children with speech disorder. In contrast, we know much less about the levels of PA necessary for speech change, and there is less research involving the four- and five-year-olds we often see for assessment and intervention.

Continuing research has highlighted the distinction between large-unit (syllable and rime) and small-unit (phoneme) awareness. Whereas in Hesketh (2004), rhyme awareness was treated as an archetypal PA component, further results and experience in Hesketh, Dima, and Nelson (2007) suggested that rhyme was a somewhat *separate* skill, very hard for some children to grasp and not an essential pre-requisite for the first steps in phoneme awareness. Small-unit awareness is generally seen as the important predictor in literacy acquisition (Hulme, Hatcher, Nation, et al. 2002) and intuitively seems more relevant than rhyme to typical speech sound errors. Note that other people disagree; Anthony and Lonigan (2004) argue that rhyme and phoneme awareness are highly correlated facets of a single underlying phonological ability. Mann and Foy (2007) agree that rhyme and phoneme awareness are somewhat separate skills, but argue that phoneme awareness is linked to literacy and rhyme to speech.

Most children have only limited phoneme awareness before they start to read. As a rough guide, the literature reports that many four-year-old children have syllable awareness and the majority develop rhyme awareness during their fifth year. Approximately half show some sensitivity to word-initial single consonants by five years, but this is likely to vary with the exact nature of the task; for example, children may be able to say the first consonant of a word but be unable to identify which of a series of words begin with the same phoneme. Very few can deconstruct consonant clusters or delete, add, or move consonants in words at this age (Carroll, Snowling, Hulme, et al. 2003).

So, are children not cognitively ready for phoneme level awareness before five or six years, or could it be triggered earlier by focused teaching? In Hesketh, Dima, and Nelson (2007), children with speech disorder, aged 4;0–4;6, were allocated to either a PA or a language stimulation program. Significantly more children improved in the PA group on phoneme awareness tasks. Improvement on phoneme isolation was very marked in the PA group; it was the most easily learned skill and one that appears very relevant to speech and language therapy. For the two most advanced tasks (segmentation and addition/deletion of consonants), however, only a small minority of the more cognitively able and older children showed improvement. We concluded that is possible to teach *some* phoneme awareness skills to *some* pre-literate children.

So we have a conundrum. We frequently work with children between four and five years of age to improve their speech. Many therapists want to include PA in their intervention and indeed feel that working on speech *requires* some awareness of individual sounds. But, it's perfectly normal not to have phoneme awareness at this age, and most children can only acquire the easier stages of it. Clearly, we need further research into the level of PA that is necessary for speech change and the degree to which it is necessary to address it directly and separately. But for now, what follows is my current perspective based on clinical experience and the published research evidence.

How to identify low performers

Standardised assessments show how children are performing relative to their peers and are designed to identify problems. Preschool children are below the age range of many standardised tests of PA, but the *Pre-school and Primary Inventory of Phonological Awareness*: PIPA (Dodd, Crosbie, MacIntosh, et al. 2000) is appropriate for UK and Australian children. Among even typically developing four-year-old children, there is a considerable range of ability in PA, as shown by the wide confidence intervals for standard scores; therefore, it can be hard to know if there is actually a problem. Because of my clinical belief that speech intervention of whatever kind *itself* involves PA and can trigger further PA development (Hesketh, Adams, Nightingale, et al. 2000; Stackhouse, Wells, Pascoe, et al. 2002), I would be more confident diagnosing a significant PA problem based on the assessment of a five-year-old child at the end of therapy than I would for a four-year-old child prior to intervention. Such diagnosis is important, though, because the prognosis for those children is different. Children who are worse at PA tend to do worse in speech intervention (Hesketh, Adams, Nightingale, et al. 2000) and are more at risk for literacy difficulties (Hesketh 2004).

When and how to step in

Although there is a lack of strong evidence for the necessity of tackling PA for the purposes of speech change, most clinicians include PA in intervention to some extent. Further, there is no clear answer to the question of when, how, and whether to step in and tackle PA; these decisions must depend on ongoing assessment of the individual child's abilities. There is evidence that it *can* be taught or incorporated into therapy: for example, Warrick, Rubin, and Rowe-Walsh (1993); Bowen and Cupples (1999a, b); Roth, Troia, Worthington, et al. (2002); Laing and Espeland (2005); and Gillon (2005) have all demonstrated gains in the PA of preschool children following intervention. As in Hesketh, Dima, and Nelson (2007), the highest level skill described was phoneme isolation of word-initial consonants (i.e., the earliest step into phoneme awareness).

My intervention principle is to incorporate PA-type activities in support of speech change using stimuli relevant to the child's target processes, syllable structures, contrasts, or sounds, rather than seeing PA skills as a target in their own right. A typical intervention session will involve the child in listening to, thinking about, and producing sounds; but the balance between these three elements varies enormously across children and across sessions.

I have seen two children in my clinical practice recently with whom I have taken different approaches. 'Ricky', a slightly immature little boy with a very strong preference for velar plosives, has attended for several blocks of therapy since he was just five. Although his awareness of word structure was not a strong point, neither were his speech motor skills and he responded well initially to a fairly traditional approach that gave him lots of production practice and used some PA activities in support. Now, at six years, Ricky is more confident with letters, and we have begun to work more explicitly on awareness of word structure, backing up his school literacy work and using graphemes to reinforce the phoneme distinctions we are asking him to make. In contrast there is 'Luke', whose ignorance of phonological structure at 4;8 is too severe to ignore. Lacking fricatives, he is easily stimulable for /f/ and /v/ word-initially, but has no idea *when* to use them. On any suspicion of being tested, he uses /f/ on every word he is asked to produce and, at phrase level, simply inserts /f/ at the beginning of the utterance, wherever the target word falls. Further assessment showed that he was unable to grasp the concept of the beginning and end of a word or even to say which was the first, middle, or last word in a short phrase (yes, he did understand the vocabulary). Surprisingly, he is able to categorise words by their initial phoneme, assigning pictures correctly to a /d/ or a /f/ pile as I speak the words. For Luke, it feels necessary to address PA more specifically and immediately, although it is hard to know the appropriate level to tackle.

What should PA intervention be and who should be doing it?

I start with a general expectation that PA work in my speech intervention will be directed at a small unit level (i.e., awareness of phonemes) and will be linked to graphemes or supported by sound symbol pictures (e.g., those suggested by Lancaster and Pope 1989), depending on the child's familiarity with letters. Activities will highlight the specific current speech targets for that child. Our work in Hesketh, Dima, and Nelson (2007) suggested that competence in large units is not a necessary pre-cursor to awareness of phonemes. Rhyme games may well be included in sessions, but if they cause a child difficulty, I will normally omit them rather than backtrack to spend time on rhyme. The program given in Hesketh, Dima, and Nelson (2007) was devised as an exercise in teaching PA as an end in itself and does not reflect my approach to speech intervention.

Both the Gillon (2005) and Hesketh, Dima, and Nelson (2007) studies show that phoneme isolation is a skill that is mastered by many children around 4;0–4;6 years and which can be triggered by relevant activities (i.e., the kind of games and tasks that are a natural part of speech intervention focusing on single consonants at the beginning or end of words). Games that require children to judge presence/absence of a phoneme, to identify a phoneme in a particular word position, or to match words that have the same (initial or final) phoneme can be adapted to a range of structural and systemic processes and to a range of phonological approaches. Such activities develop a child's phoneme awareness even as they use it to drive speech change. Awareness of consonants within multisyllabic words and within consonant clusters will be more difficult. Children do need hooks on which to attach and stabilise their knowledge of abstract phonemes, for example, coloured blocks (for phoneme presence and change) and symbolic sound linkage pictures (for phoneme identification). I use letters alongside, but unreliable letter knowledge and the irregular sound-letter correspondence of English mean that other supportive cues are also necessary in young children.

When, in the activities above, the therapist says the stimulus words aloud, a child is carrying out PA activities and deconstructing what they hear but not necessarily accessing their own lexical representations for those words (Gardner, A21). Carrying out the same tasks without the spoken model from the therapist requires a child to use his/her own lexical representations as the data source. Such tasks can yield a lot of information about internal phonological representations but are beyond the capability of most preschool children. Phonological representations are a relatively recent topic in SLP/SLT, but research has begun into their assessment and use in therapy (Rvachew, Nowak, and Cloutier 2004; Sutherland and Gillon 2007).

Where PA is used as an integral part of a speech intervention, using the sounds, word positions, and contrasts relevant to the specific child, then an SLP/SLT should be doing or planning the work. It can be written into a program for home or school practice in carefully explained tasks.

How to integrate PA into speech work without compromising speech progress

Integration is the key word here. By embedding PA work into sessions that also include speech production practice, and by tailoring the PA tasks to highlight the concurrent speech targets, there should be no negative effect on speech progress. Gillon has successfully incorporated PA work (and has improved children's PA skills) without detriment to speech progress in two studies (Gillon 2000, 2005), the latter with preschool children.

In summary, my approach is to use a variety of earlier-developing phoneme-level awareness tasks in support of the target change in speech. It is impossible to do any work on speech without drawing a child's attention to word form, and so PA is likely to progress even in a predominantly production-based program. If PA skills remain weak at the end of speech intervention, then a more direct focus on PA with more explicit reference to letter sounds and names will be necessary.

Vowel Therapy

Fiona E. Gibbon, PhD, FRCSLT, is a Professor and Head of Speech and Hearing Sciences at Queen Margaret University, Edinburgh, UK. Her research and clinical interests include the use of instrumentation to diagnose and treat speech disorders in children. She has published over 70 papers in professional/scientific journals and book chapters, and has been awarded numerous research council and charity-funded grants. This research was awarded the Queen's Anniversary Prize for excellence in 2002. She is a Fellow of the Royal College of Speech and Language Therapists.

Q23.   Fiona E. Gibbon: Vowel assessment and remediation

There is a commonly held SLP/SLT view that if you, 'work on the consonants, the vowels will take care of themselves'! You touched on this point in 2003 when you made an invited contribution to the 'Ask the Expert' column for the Apraxia-Kids Monthly Newsletter on the topic of vowel production (and possibly vowel perception) difficulties experienced by children with CAS. You wrote, 'At the moment there is a lack of research evidence to guide the SLP about the most efficacious therapy approach for vowel errors in CAS.' Can you expand on this, please? What is the current research suggesting that clinicians do in terms of vowel assessment and intervention? Might vowel intervention have a side-benefit in the form of improved prosody in children with CAS? And should we be giving consonants priority over vowels? Would you tackle vowel assessment and intervention differently for a child with CAS than you would with a highly unintelligible child of the same age with a developmental phonological disorder? Is there a role for stimulability training (Miccio, Elbert, and Forrest 1999; Miccio 2005) within vowel therapy?

A23.   Fiona E. Gibbon: Vowel errors in children with speech disorders

It is undoubtedly true that SLPs/SLTs who work in clinical contexts tend to focus primarily on identifying and remediating abnormal consonants, rather than vowels, in children's speech. However, as we will see in the sections that follow, available evidence does not support neglecting vowels in the belief that these errors will necessarily 'look after themselves'. Indeed, expert opinion suggests that the opposite is true, at least for children with CAS. Based on their extensive clinical experience, Hall, Jordan, and Robin (1993) say that 'some children self-correct vowel errors, but not many children with DAS [developmental apraxia of speech] have this experience' (p. 160).

The lack of attention to vowels is surprising when one considers what is now known about these types of errors. For example, children with CAS and children with moderate and severe phonological disorder (Flipsen, A10) frequently experience difficulties producing vowels. Studies show that at least some vowel errors may occur in as many as 50% of children with these diagnoses (Eisenson and Ogilvie 1963; Pollock and Berni 2003). Vowel errors are also considered of diagnostic importance, with these errors posited as a potential diagnostic marker for CAS (Davis, Jakielski, and Marquardt 1998). Difficulties with vowels are additionally significant because they have a detrimental impact on speech intelligibility, and they often have serious consequences for consonant production. For these reasons, it is important that SLPs/SLTs are familiar with the types of vowel difficulties that occur in children's speech and are aware of different approaches to their remediation.

So why do clinicians, and indeed researchers, often ignore vowels? A combination of factors may explain this situation. Even skilled listeners, such as SLPs/SLTs, find vowel errors more difficult to detect through perceptual analysis compared with consonant errors. As a result, vowels are less reliably transcribed than consonants (Stoel-Gammon 1990). Another important factor is that the normal dialectal differences that exist in vowel systems make listeners more tolerant of vowel distortions. As a result, vowel errors can remain undetected in a transcription-based speech analysis. More is known about patterns of abnormalities affecting the consonant system compared with the vowel system, and consequently, most standard assessment procedures are devised primarily to identify abnormal patterns of consonant production. Many assessment procedures therefore do not allow for a full range of vowels to be elicited, so vowel errors are not always recorded in routine clinical evaluations. Finally, even when vowel errors are identified as occurring in a child's speech, there is a lack of literature about therapy approaches specifically for these types of difficulties. As Hall, Jordan, and Robin (1993) state, 'much has yet to be learned about strategies and techniques for vowel remediation' (p. 160).

Diagnosis and therapy for vowel errors

Despite the difficulties in identifying vowels, outlined above, real progress has been made over the past 20 years in our understanding of normal and abnormal vowel systems in children's speech (see Davis, Jacks, and Marquardt 2005 for an overview). For example, in relation to children exhibiting vowel errors, studies show that children often have complete or near-complete vowel inventories, at least for nonrhotic monophthongs (Gibbon, Shockey, and Reid 1992). Furthermore, studies show that some vowels are more likely to be produced as errors than others. Diphthongs (e.g., /aɪ/, /ɔɪ/), rhotic vowels (e.g., /ɪɚ/, /ɜ˞/), and the midfront vowels /e/ and /a/ are particularly problematic. A number of recurring patterns of vowel difficulties, usually described in terms of phonological processes (e.g., lowering/raising, fronting/backing, diphthong reduction) have been documented in studies by Davis, Jacks, and Marquardt (2005); Reynolds (1990); Pollock and Hall (1991); and Bates, Watson, and Scobbie (2002). It is now recognised that articulatory difficulties in positioning and sequencing of articulators, particularly the tongue and lips, affect vowel quality and accuracy. Timing difficulties also affect vowels, so that in some cases they may be excessively long. Vowels may also be distorted, for example, partially voiced due to difficulties controlling vocal fold vibration or with excessive nasality due to difficulties controlling velopharyngeal closure. These co-ordination difficulties are core features of CAS (Campbell 2003; Hall, Jordan, and Robin 1993; Rosenbek and Wertz 1972) and often cause difficulties affecting vowels.

Unfortunately, advances in our knowledge about abnormal vowel systems are not mirrored in increased knowledge about therapy for these types of errors. Our understanding about therapy for abnormal vowels comes primarily from studies that focus on the remediation of abnormal consonants. SLPs/SLTs have to understand and then apply underlying principles of a particular therapy approach when targeting vowels. There is a remarkably wide selection of approaches available, however. Baker and McLeod (2004) recently described 12 therapy approaches that are currently used in clinical contexts. As well as having a wide choice of approaches, the evidence base for treating abnormal consonant systems in children with phonological disorder is strong, and there is now a substantial literature demonstrating beneficial effects of phonological therapy (Gierut 1998; Law, Garrett, and Nye 2004; Almost and Rosenbaum 1998).

Therapy for vowels that has been adapted from an approach intended for consonants may prove useful but may also present with additional difficulties. Any therapy approach that requires a child to focus on his/her own articulatory activity is more difficult with vowels than it is with consonants. The high degree of vocal tract constriction involved in consonant production generally results in a high level of tactile feedback, which enhances speakers' awareness of articulatory placement. With the exception of close vowels, such as /i/ (as in *heat*) and /ɪ/ (as in *hit*), this tactile feedback is greatly decreased during vowel production. As Hall, Jordan, and Robin (1993) state, these difficulties mean that, for some SLPs/SLTs, 'vowel therapy is elusive, frustrating, and often appears to be avoided' (p. 161).

Indirect versus direct focus on intervention targets

Despite good evidence that therapy is beneficial for abnormal consonant systems, it is not known whether therapy that focuses on improving the consonant system has an indirect, but equally beneficial, effect of improving the vowel system. Some support for the view that targeting consonants has an indirect and beneficial impact on vowel production comes from a study by Robb, Bleile, and Yee (1999). They adopted an indirect approach to treating vowels in a four-year-old girl with a phonological disorder that affected both consonants and vowels. Consonants were selected as targets in therapy, and no emphasis was placed on accurate vowel production during the course of therapy. By the end of her therapy program, however, the size of her vowel inventory and overall vowel accuracy had improved. Robb, Bleile, and Yee (1999) commented that, although therapy did not focus on vowel accuracy, it was nevertheless possible that the activities undertaken in therapy facilitated improvements in both consonant and vowel production.

Early researchers into CAS recommended that vowels are selected for direct remedial efforts because vowel errors have a detrimental effect on speech intelligibility (Chappell 1973; Yoss and Darley 1974). A handful of more recently published studies have reported therapy that directly focused on vowel error patterns in children with phonological disorder (for a review, see Gibbon and Mackenzie Beck 2002). The tentative conclusion that emerges is that direct therapy for vowels can have a positive outcome in some cases. The studies were limited, however, to reporting only small numbers of cases, so it is not possible to generalize the findings. Another limitation of these studies is that some did not report adequate baseline data, making it difficult to know whether the progress reported was a result of therapy or due to some other factor, such as spontaneous development.

Clinical implications

Turning now to the implications of current research, the finding that children with moderate to severe phonological disorders or CAS have a high risk of abnormal vowel systems means that it is necessary to screen all such children for vowel errors. There are various procedures that SLPs/SLTs can use for this purpose. Clinical assessment of vowels in CAS is usually based on phonetically transcribed speech samples, which SLPs/SLTs analyse and interpret alongside other routine clinical examinations. There are now readily available resources that SLPs/SLTs can use to assist in describing, transcribing, and classifying normal and disordered vowel systems (Howard and Heselwood 2002; Pollock and Berni 2001; Watts 2004). Speech samples usually include spontaneous and imitated speech consisting of single words/phrases of increasing phonetic complexity. Analysis of speech samples may involve identifying a child's vowel inventory, which in CAS may be restricted, with certain 'difficult to produce' vowels, such as diphthongs and rhotic vowels, absent.

An important component of an assessment of vowel systems is identification of error patterns of vowel substitutions, distortions, and phonological processes. SLPs/SLTs are very familiar with phonological process analysis when applied to children's consonant systems. It is possible to apply this type of linguistic description to show how vowel errors are not separate, unrelated phenomena, but are instead systematic and rule-governed. These patterns allow SLPs/SLTs performing relational analyses to compare children's pronunciations with an adult's correct productions and with typically developing young children's productions. Another feature of vowel systems that is relevant to assess is the nature and degree of variability in production. In children with CAS, there is often a high degree of token-to-token variability. As with consonants, it is important to assess vowel stimulability in isolation and in a range of syllable structures because targets that can be elicited through modelling are a potential focus in therapy.

A final area to assess is the effect of surrounding consonants on vowel accuracy. Vowels may be produced correctly in some words, but not others, because the vowels are 'conditioned' by the surrounding consonants. The most frequently reported context-conditioned error pattern in typically developing infants is the co-occurrence of alveolar stops /t/, /d/ and high front vowels, such as /i/, /ɪ/, and the co-occurrence of velar stops /k/, /g/ with high back vowels such as /u/ (Davis and MacNeilage 1990, 1995). Bates, Watson, and Scobbie (2002) underline the importance of identifying such context-conditioned error patterns in children with speech disorders in order to focus therapy in the most effective way. For instance, accurate identification of such contexts will avoid wasting therapy time on practising targets in contexts that are unproblematic for the child. Bates, Watson, and Scobbie (2002) provide a comprehensive description of consonant–vowel interactions and how these can be assessed in clinical practice. These analyses will allow the SLP/SLT to make a diagnostic statement about a child's vowel production, and to formulate goals of therapy in relation to any vowel difficulties highlighted during assessment.

Gibbon and Mackenzie Beck (2002) discuss general principles of vowel therapy and a range of therapy approaches that are of potential, although as yet unproven, value for increasing vowel production accuracy. In their view, a prerequisite for effective treatment is that clinicians should have good perceptual skills to analyze vowels. SLP/SLPs also need to formulate therapy goals in the light of a clear description of the adult target vowel system, that is, if and how the target system differs from standard systems (see Wells 1982a,b, c, for an outstanding description of how English vowels vary across the world). SLPs/SLTs should also consider children's overall speech and language processing skills (Stackhouse and Wells 1997), as well as relevant information gathered as part of routine clinical assessment. This profile will suggest what aspect(s) of speech processing to focus on in intervention and which approach is most likely to result in improved speech intelligibility. Some children have demonstrable auditory perceptual deficits, for instance, whereas others have cognitive/linguistic deficits associated with the phonological structure of the language. A third possibility is that motoric/articulatory deficits, including dysarthria, affect the movements and co-ordination necessary for normal speech production. Gibbon and Mackenzie Beck go on to describe a variety of approaches that focus on vowel errors in each category. In many cases, different approaches are not mutually exclusive, and the SLP/SLT will often select a combination of multisensory techniques that will meet each child's specific needs.

Due to the lack of research evidence to guide the SLP/SLT about the most efficacious therapy approach for vowel errors, SLPs/SLTs need to select therapy techniques based on the most complementary matching between a child's specific speech difficulties and the strategies employed in a particular approach. SLPs/SLTs own vowel production skills are vital because they may need to model a full range of vowel qualities during therapy activities. Reid (2003) has developed a framework based on phonetic features of vowels, which also incorporates links to written vowels. This may be particularly useful for improving children's phonological awareness of vowels, for literacy teaching, as well as for targeting spoken vowel production difficulties. The framework has been specifically devised for the vowels of Scottish English, but it may be adapted for other varieties of English.

Perceptually based interventions

Dr. Susan Rvachew is an Associate Professor in the School of Communication Sciences and Disorders at McGill University, Montreal, Canada. Her research interests are focused on phonological development and disorders with specific research topics, including: the role of speech perception development in sound production learning; speech development in infancy; efficacy of interventions for phonological disorders; and computer applications in the treatment of phonological disorders. Current projects include a longitudinal investigation of deficits in phonological awareness skills in preschoolers with delayed phonological development, relationship between auditory attention and babbling skills in infants with early onset otitis media, and cross-linguistic differences in the acoustic characteristics of vowels produced by infants. In her response to Q24, she discusses the role of speech perception development in sound production learning, and the use of the *SAILS* software and other therapy tools in the remediation of categorical misperception (Rvachew 2005a).

Q24.　Susan Rvachew: Speech perception training and its effects on speech production

'Children with expressive phonological delays often possess poor underlying perceptual knowledge of the sound system. . . ' (Rvachew, Nowak, and Cloutier 2004). What are the implications of this research finding for evidence-based clinical practice with children who have SSDs? When would you introduce the SAILS computer game to improve children's speech perception skills? What low-tech approach alternatives to the SAILS program exist?

A24.　Susan Rvachew: Perceptually based interventions

Many studies have shown that a large proportion of children with SSDs have difficulty with speech perception in comparison to children of the same age who do not have SSDs. The speech perception difficulties may not be obvious to parents or other people who are talking with the child. However, these difficulties with speech perception have been found in studies using a large variety of assessment techniques and speech stimuli (Cohen and Diehl 1963; Edwards, Fox, and Rogers 2002; Hoffman, Daniloff, Bengoa, et al. 1985; Hoffman, Stager, and Daniloff 1983; Munson, Baylis, Krause, et al. 2006; Munson, Edwards, and Beckman 2005; Rvachew 2007b; Sherman and Geith 1967; Shuster 1998; Sutherland and Gillon 2007). These findings imply that attention to children's speech perception abilities may be an important component of a speech therapy program, and indeed this hypothesis has been supported by intervention studies (Jamieson and Rvachew 1992; Rvachew 1994; Rvachew, Nowak, and Cloutier 2004; Rvachew, Rafaat, and Martin 1999). The Speech Assessment and Interactive Learning System (SAILS) is a computer-based tool that can be used to improve children's speech perception skills. SAILS targets commonly misarticulated consonant phonemes in the onset (initial) and coda (final) position of words. The program is based on recordings of naturally produced words. These words were recorded from English-speaking adult talkers with accurate speech, child talkers with accurate speech, and child talkers with a SSD. The child's task is to listen to each word and indicate whether it is an exemplar of the target word or not an exemplar of the target word. The child responds by pointing to a picture of the target word or to an 'X'. Visual feedback is provided after the child's response. Typically, the child engages with the SAILS task for 5–10 minutes at the beginning or end of each therapy session. In Rvachew (1994), the SAILS program was used as part of a traditional speech therapy program in which phonetic placement, modelling, and drill-play activities were used to help children master a single phoneme in syllables, words, and sentences. In Rvachew, Rafaat, and Martin (1999), SAILS was provided for three sessions concurrently with phonetic placement targeting three target phonemes, as a prelude to a 9-week course of group phonological therapy using the 'Cycles approach' (Hodson and Paden 1983). In Rvachew, Nowak, and Cloutier (2004), the child's speech therapist decided whether to use a traditional or phonological approach, depending on her perception of the child's needs. The SAILS intervention was provided after each therapy session. In all of these studies, children who received the SAILS intervention showed twice as much progress toward the achievement of age-appropriate articulation accuracy than children whose intervention programs did not include a speech perception component.

What are the conditions under which the program has been shown to be effective?

In the studies mentioned above, the intervention was provided for only 5 to 10 minutes at the beginning or end of the child's therapy sessions. In these studies, the intervention was provided by a communication disorders assistant or undergraduate student research assistant. These individuals, who had access to a procedural manual if required, received about 1 hour of training in administering SAILS, all demonstrating that it can be provided very efficiently by non–SLPs/SLTs with minimal training. The children in all of these studies were four to five years of age with moderate or severe SSDs, as determined by a standardized test of articulation accuracy. Other groups of children are known to have difficulty with speech perception and thus may benefit from the intervention (e.g., older children who have residual distortion errors, second language learners, and children with specific language impairment or dyslexia). However, no studies have investigated the effectiveness of SAILS with these groups. I have found that children younger than four years of age have difficulty with the SAILS identification task. Finally, the program was developed for use with children who speak Canadian English. It would not be appropriate to use it with other dialect and language groups without first developing stimuli that represent the local dialect or language.

Are there alternatives to the SAILS program?

It is not known whether SAILS will improve the effectiveness of live-voice procedures for presenting good quality speech input to children, such as focused stimulation or AIT. It is possible that these procedures are effective enough on their own. However, basic research on optimum procedures for perceptual training indicates that stimulus variability is very important. Therefore, SAILS includes multiple voices and a variety of good and poor exemplars of the target words. Thus, SAILS may be an effective adjunct to these live-voice procedures that usually involve the presentation of exaggerated speech models produced by one or two talkers (e.g., speech therapist and/or parent). If you do not have access to SAILS, you can still find ways to introduce multi-talker variability into your treatment. Many technologies exist that can be used to develop speech perception tasks for specific clients. For example, if you were working with a group of children who misarticulate /r/, you could use a computer with digital recording software to record the children's efforts to say words that contain this phoneme. If there is variability within the group and within children with respect to their production accuracy, you will have a perfect set of stimuli for teaching identification of correct and incorrect exemplars of the /r/ phoneme. You can insert the recordings and pictures of the target words into power point slides for presentation to your students. Arrange the slides so that there is a random ordering of correct and incorrect exemplars and ask the children to identify the words that are pronounced correctly.

Case example

Kenny commenced speech therapy for treatment of a moderate SSD at age 3;8, when he presented with unintelligible speech despite above average receptive language abilities, age-appropriate expressive language skills, and normal hearing and oral structure and function. His error patterns included backing of alveolar stops and nasals, backing of affricates, fronting of palatal fricatives, and gliding of liquids. Initially, his SLP employed a traditional approach to target /l/ in word initial singleton and cluster contexts during weekly 1-hour individual speech therapy sessions. When Kenny was 4;3, he was enrolled in a randomized control trial (Rvachew, Nowak, and Cloutier 2004) and was assigned to receive the SAILS intervention in addition to his regular speech therapy program for 16 weeks. His SLP continued with weekly sessions, targeting /t/, /d/, /ʃ/, and /tʃ/ using a traditional approach and a horizontal goal attack strategy. In addition to these sessions, he also received 15 minutes of the SAILS intervention, administered by his mother under the guidance of a student research assistant. Each week he learned to identify correct and incorrect versions of words that began or ended with a given phoneme, specifically /t p m k lr f s/ in the word initial position for the first 8 weeks and in word final position for the second 8 weeks of the study (see the published research report for details of the phonemic perception and phonological awareness activities that were implemented by computer for these phonemes). All treatment was discontinued when he was 4;7, and he received no further treatment as a preschooler. It is not know whether he ever received speech therapy in elementary school.

His speech accuracy was assessed at enrollment to the study just as the SAILS intervention was about to begin (pretreatment assessment), 6 months later (post-treatment assessment), and 12 months later (follow-up assessment). These assessments were conducted by an SLP who was blind to his assigned experimental treatment condition and who was not involved in the regular or experimental portion of his intervention. Obtained percentile rankings of 5, 10, and 32 on the Goldman-Fristoe Test of Articulation (Goldman and Fristoe 2000) during the pre-treatment, post-treatment, and follow-up assessments, respectively, revealed excellent progress. When examining total number of errors on this test, his improvement between the pre- and post-treatment assessments was almost twice as great as the improvement that was observed on average for children in the control group who did not receive the SAILS intervention, mirroring the results obtained for the experimental group as a whole. The clinical importance of this outcome is highlighted by the fact that he began first grade with age appropriate speech (w/r substitutions being the only remaining speech error), an outcome enjoyed by comparatively few children in the control group. These improvements in speech accuracy were also reflected in significantly improved speech intelligibility, as illustrated in brief excerpts from speech samples that yield Percent Consonant Correct scores of 65, 85, and 92 for the pretreatment, post-treatment, and follow-up assessments, respectively.

> *Pre-treatment Speech Sample Excerpt:*
> 'Karl's putting her in there where is all fishes.'
> [gɑɪz pʊgɪŋ hə ɪn gɛʌ wɛ ɪza fɪsəz]
> *Post-treatment Speech Sample Excerpt:*
> 'He is putting the baby in there. In . . . tank. There's fishies.'
> [hi ɪz pʊrɪŋ ə bebi ɪn dɛʌ . . .ɪn. . .tæŋ̊k..dɛɪz fɪʃiz]
> *Follow-up Speech Sample Excerpt:*
> 'And then he takes the baby to the fishtank and the baby swimming in the fishtank.'
> [æn ðɛn hi teks ə bebi tʊðə fɪʃtæŋk æn ðəbebi swɪɪmɪn ɪnðə fɪʃtæŋk]

More information about the application of perceptually based approaches to speech therapy can be found in Rvachew (2005a, b, 2007). Please contact the author at susan.rvachew@mcgill.ca if you wish to create new stimuli appropriate to a different dialect or language group.

Implications for service delivery

The availability of the smorgasbord of intervention options described in this chapter carries with it weighty implications for 'common', 'best', and evidence-based practice, the topic of the next chapter. In it, ten contributors from around the world reflect on pertinent issues in the transitions between theory and therapy, and research and ethical practice.

Chapter 5

'Common', 'best', and evidence-based practice

In Chapter 5, information, opinions, and reflections on clinical 'common', 'best', and evidence-based practice are presented by contributors working in Australia, Canada, Germany, New Zealand, South Africa, the United Kingdom, and the United States. Proceeding alphabetically by country, the questions that are put to them vary considerably, covering diverse issues and canvassing a range of views. In A25, Nicole Watts Pappas reviews several studies of SLP/SLT clinical 'common practice' in child speech, with an emphasis on family-centred practice in Australia. Megan Hodge (A26) follows with insights into clinical practice gained from a survey of Canadian SLPs' opinions and experience using non-speech oral motor exercises (NS-OME) in children's speech therapy. Next, Gail Gillon (A27) discusses effective practice and positive and enduring partnerships between SLT and Education in New Zealand. Then, in a context of unprecedented barriers to practice that few have experienced, Brenda Louw (A28) provides a fascinating exploration of issues in service delivery in Early Communication Intervention (ECI) situations with speech-impaired populations in South Africa. Drawing on the results of a survey of clinicians in the UK, Victoria Joffe (A29) examines minimalist assessment practices in one of the world's top ten richest nations. Mirroring Hodge (A26), Gregory Lof (A30) then talks about the puzzling situation wherein large numbers of US SLPs, who have been steeped, at Master's level, in scientific method and critical analysis of the evidence-base, continue to implement a therapy methodology with children with SSD that is anything *but* scientific (Arvedson, Clark, Frymark, et al. 2007). These six contributions are followed by discussion of four related issues. Karen McComas (A31) reflects on student preparation for professional practice; B. May Bernhardt and Angela Ullrich (A32) discuss the role of linguistic theory, particularly nonlinear phonology, in clinical problem solving; Karen Froud (A33) has interesting things to add about reading and critically evaluating the literature around the so-called 'terrifying therapies' (Gardner, A21; Joffe, A29); and Thomas Powell (A34) presents a multifaceted model for ethical practices.

Dr. Nicole Watts Pappas is actively engaged in research, publication, and SLP clinical practice in a community clinic in Brisbane, Australia, where she endeavours to use family-centred approaches in her work with young children and their families. In her PhD research, she explored the involvement of families in SLP/SLT intervention for speech impairment.

Q25.   Nicole Watts Pappas: Family-centered speech intervention in Australia

The distinction between involving parents in their own children's speech intervention, and involving them as collaborative partners in the assessment, intervention, and management process, is not always clear to the parties concerned: child, parent, therapist, and policy maker. Against a background of common practice (McLeod and Baker 2004), the nexus between therapists' beliefs and practice (Watts Pappas, McLeod, McAllister, et al. 2006), and what the evidence-base would encourage us to do (Baker 2006), what is the Australian experience of family-centred practice in the area of children's SSD?

A25.   Nicole Watts Pappas: The Australian experience of family-centred practice in intervention for speech impairment

History of parental and family involvement in speech intervention

What is considered to be 'best practice' in working with parents and families in paediatric intervention has undergone significant changes over time. Traditionally, parents were given limited opportunity to be involved in their child's speech intervention with services planned and delivered by the SLP/SLT in a therapist-centred approach to management (Crais 1991). In the late 1970s and 1980s, SLPs/SLTs and other allied health professionals were encouraged to increase parents' participation in intervention, primarily by requesting them to complete home activities with their child (Bazyk 1989). However, parental involvement in these activities tended to be expected rather than optional, and parents continued to have limited involvement in service planning and decision making.

More recently, a new philosophy of working with parents and families, family-centred service, has been recommended as best practice (Rosenbaum, King, Law, et al. 1998). Family-centred practice promotes the formation of collaborative parent/professional partnerships and acknowledges parents and families as the primary decision-makers regarding their child's intervention (Bailey, McWilliam, and Winton 1992). Additionally, based on the theory that change to one family member will affect all other family members, family-centred practice considers the whole family as client rather than just the child.

Typical practice of parental involvement in speech intervention

Although recommended models for working with parents and families in SLP/SLT practice have changed, the practices of clinicians may not have undergone a corresponding transformation. The well-documented researcher/practitioner gap highlights the fact that clinicians may take time to incorporate new models of service into their clinical practice (McLeod and Baker 2004). Two Australian studies have investigated how SLP clinicians involve parents in intervention for speech impairment. A survey conducted by McLeod and Baker (2004) of the speech intervention practices of 270 SLPs found that 88.2% of respondents reported they involved parents in their intervention for speech impairment. However, this involvement appeared to occur predominantly in intervention provision rather than planning; when asked about factors they considered when selecting treatment targets, only 49.6% of respondents indicated they considered parental preference as a high priority.

In a more comprehensive study, Watts Pappas, McLeod, McAllister, et al. (2008) surveyed 277 SLPs regarding their beliefs and practices of parental involvement in speech intervention. The results of the survey indicated that the vast majority of respondents involved parents in some way in their intervention for speech impairment. The most common form of involvement was the provision of home activities, with 95% of respondents indicating they always or usually provided home activities to parents. Other typical forms of involvement included parental attendance at assessment (84%) and intervention (80%) sessions. The SLPs reported using family-centred practices, such as considering parents' time and priorities, when providing home activities (94%). However, other family-centred practices were not used as frequently by the respondents. For example, only 44% of the SLPs indicated that they allowed parents to choose the extent of their involvement in the intervention, and only 17% always or usually gave parents an option regarding the service delivery format provided to their child. Parental involvement in intervention planning occurred less frequently than some other forms of involvement: 67% of the SLPs reported that they involved parents in goal-setting; however, only 38% always or usually allowed parents to make the *final* decisions about intervention goals and activities.

The results of these two studies of the typical practice of SLPs indicate that, although parents are usually involved in speech intervention services, the SLP retains primary control over the direction of the intervention, representing a therapist-centred rather than a family-centred approach to management. However, a gap may be present between SLPs' typical practice and their beliefs about what constitutes ideal practice, especially if barriers to using ideal practice exist.

SLPs' beliefs regarding parent and family involvement in speech intervention

Two studies have investigated Australian SLPs' beliefs regarding parental and family involvement in intervention for speech impairment. The previously described study conducted by Watts Pappas and colleagues (2008) also investigated the SLPs' beliefs with regard to parental involvement. This study found that the overwhelming majority of respondents (98%) agreed or strongly agreed that parental involvement is essential for speech intervention to be effective. The SLPs also believed that parents should be present at (78%) and participate (97%) in intervention sessions. However, 40% of respondents indicated they were not happy with the level of parental participation in their service or aspects of their service. In open-ended questions, the SLPs reported the presence of various barriers that they believed prevented them from giving what they considered 'ideal' practice to the parents they worked with. These included workplace barriers (such as working in a school setting), parent barriers (such as parent time, skills, and inclination to be involved), and personal barriers (such as a lack of knowledge and confidence in working with parents in intervention for speech impairment).

Similar to the findings of other studies of professionals' perceptions of working with families (Bruce, Letourneau, Ritchie, et al. 2002; Litchfield and MacDougall 2002; Minke and Scott 1995), although the SLPs held a strong belief in the importance of parental involvement in intervention *provision*, they generally supported a more therapist-centred (as opposed to a family-centred) approach to management in the area of intervention *planning* and decision making. For example, only 42% of the SLPs indicated that they agreed that parents should have the final say on the content of intervention goals and activities.

Why did the SLPs' reported beliefs and practice support a more traditional approach to working with parents and families than is encouraged by the literature? A second, more in-depth study of the beliefs and practices of Australian SLPs addressed this issue. Watts Pappas and McLeod (2008) conducted a focus group of six SLPs working with children with speech impairment. The focus group discussion centred on parental and family involvement in speech intervention and parent/professional relationships. The findings of the analysis of the group interview indicated that the SLP participants believed strongly in the importance of parental involvement in speech intervention and attempted to engage parents and families in their child's intervention as much as possible. They also believed in providing respectful and supportive service to families. However, similar to the results from the survey, although the SLPs felt that parental involvement in intervention was critical, they also held a strong belief that the professional should make the final decisions regarding intervention planning and provision.

Several factors may have contributed to this belief. The SLPs considered themselves as the specialists in intervention for speech impairment. As the specialists, they felt it was their role and responsibility to take the lead in the management of speech intervention. Additionally, the participants in the focus group believed that parents both wanted and needed guidance from their SLP. Considering the complexity of intervention for speech impairment, the SLPs felt that parents did not have the skills to have the final say about intervention. Indeed, adopting parents' choices for goals was postulated as an ethical issue if parents requested goals or activities that were contraindicated for the child.

With the current focus on efficiency and accountability in paediatric intervention services, SLPs are under pressure to ensure that their intervention is evidence-based and effective (Reilly 2004). Most evidence-based speech intervention approaches require specific choices regarding treatment targets or intervention activities (Baker 2006). These approaches may be difficult to provide if parents insist on other, alternative goals and activities. Although family-centred practice has been promoted in the literature and by policy makers as best practice in intervention for young children (Crais, Poston Roy, and Free 2006), little evidence of its impact on speech intervention outcomes or its acceptability to parents is available. Considering the lack of evidence for this approach, SLPs may be reluctant to use family-centred practice when it contravenes other demands of their workplace, such as providing service that is evidence-based and efficacious.

Parent's beliefs regarding parent and family involvement in speech intervention

Contrary to the recommendations of best practice, the three studies that have investigated parental involvement in speech intervention in Australia have indicated that SLPs' beliefs and practice are not supportive of a truly family-centred model of service, particularly in relation to decision-making. However, a progressive in-depth study of the views of seven parents accessing speech intervention for their child (Watts Pappas and McLeod 2008) indicated that Australian parents may not necessarily want a family-centred approach to intervention for their child with speech impairment. The analysis of the interviews indicated that the parents believed that it was the SLP's role and responsibility to both work with their child in the intervention sessions and provide guidance about intervention goals and activities. If the parent trusted their SLP, they felt the best thing they could do for their child was to follow the SLP's lead in the intervention process. Similar beliefs and expectations about parent/professional roles have been reported in other studies of parents' perceptions of paediatric allied health intervention (Glogowska and Campbell 2000; Leiter 2004; MacKean, Thurston, and Scott 2005; Mirabito and Armstrong 2005; Thompson 1998). Although the parents felt that their involvement in their child's intervention (particularly the provision of home activities) was important, they wanted their SLP to take the lead role in intervention provision and planning, and preferred intervention to focus on their child rather than their family.

Summary

SLPs believe strongly in parental participation in speech intervention and, against a background of various barriers to family involvement, strategise to engage families as much as possible in the process. They also attempt to provide respectful and supportive care to families and consider their needs and wishes in intervention planning. Allowing parents to take the lead in intervention planning and delivery, however, poses a dilemma for SLPs, especially when parents' wishes are at odds with the demands of evidence-based practice. Although SLPs consider the child within the context of their family, both clinicians and parents appear to prefer a SLP-led and predominantly child-focused approach to intervention for speech impairment.

A Canadian survey

In a survey of SLPs (Hodge, Salonka, and Kollias 2005), clinicians in Alberta, Canada were asked about their use, and the roles and benefits as they saw them, of NS-OME in the treatment of children with speech disorders. Like Lof and Watson (2008), who analysed survey responses from 537 US SLPs and found that 85% used NS-OME to target speech, the Canadian researchers found that 85% of 535 Albertan respondents used NS-OME for the purpose of changing speech sound production.

Dr. Megan Hodge is a Professor in the Department of Speech Pathology and Audiology at the University of Alberta, where she teaches in the areas of anatomy and physiology of the speech mechanism, speech science, and motor speech disorders. Dr. Hodge's research interests include developmental aspects of normal and disordered speech perception-and-production, perceptual-acoustic correlates of speech intelligibility, and linking theory with practice in evaluating and managing children with neurogenic communication disorders. In her response to Q26, Dr. Hodge discusses the survey results and their implications, providing an informed view of common practice in at least one Canadian province, and effective practice as it is taught in Canadian universities.

Q26.   Megan M. Hodge: A Canadian perspective on non-speech oral motor exercises

What insights do the results of the 2004 survey of Albertan SLPs' use of NS-OME in children's speech therapy reveal about common clinical practice, compared with effective practice as taught in Canadian universities?

A26.   Megan M. Hodge: What can we learn about clinical practice from SLPs' experiences using NS-OME in children's speech therapy?

Information about the survey conducted by Sophie Kollias and Robin Lester (2004) under my supervision is followed by conclusions from our research. After each conclusion, I comment on: (a) what it might reveal about clinical practice for childhood SSD, (b) how this relates to my knowledge about effective practice as taught in Canadian universities, and (c) what I see as the implications for action to address the evidence-to-practice gap for SLPs serving Canadian children with SSD.

The survey results represented responses from approximately 28% of SLPs registered with the Alberta College of Speech-Language Pathologists and Audiologists who provided speech therapy to children (0–16 years of age) during June 2004. The survey involved collecting information about respondents' opinions and experiences using NS-OME. We do not know how representative the sample is of Albertan or Canadian SLPs who use NS-OME, so these results cannot be generalised to all SLPs. However, they represent a range of responses from a substantial sample of SLPs. It is also important to understand that the purpose of this survey was not to describe common practice for children with SSD; rather, it addressed use of NS-OME in children's speech therapy. Eighty percent of survey respondents served children between birth and eight years; 30% worked in schools, 25% in community health centres, 18% in private practice, 16% in early education settings, 8% in hospitals, and 3% in other settings. The majority of respondents (67%) had more than five years of clinical work experience.

Conclusion 1

For the 85% of respondents who reported using NS-OME with at least one child in the past five years, the most common practice was to use NS-OME in therapy as warm-up activities, as part of a speech goal (i.e., stimulability for consonant and vowel sounds), and/or assigned for home practice. The three most common therapy objectives identified for using NS-OME were to increase articulator strength and coordination, facilitate stimulability for consonant and vowel sounds, and improve speech intelligibility. Respondents' reasons for using NS-OME were their belief that NS-OME were effective or that no other technique had worked. When NS-OME were used, 56% of SLPs reported spending between 5 and 15 minutes performing these exercises in therapy, whereas 31% spent less than 5 minutes. However, some SLPs reported using NS-OME for an entire treatment session and, in a few cases, not as part of a speech goal (e.g., to decrease drooling, improve feeding skills, and strengthen muscle groups unrelated to a specific articulation goal).

Comment

'Warm-up' activities in speech therapy sessions, assigning NS-OME as home practice activities, and training articulator strength are not presented as evidence-based practices for childhood SSD in Canadian university training programs. The rationale, nature, and cost/benefit of these practices and why some SLPs believe that these are effective require further study. Information that is available in NS-OME materials appears useful to SLPs (beyond what they receive in their training) in stimulating production of difficult-to-elicit sounds. Publications such as Secord, Boyce, and Donohue, et al.'s (2007) *Eliciting Sounds: Techniques and Strategies for Clinicians* may be useful resources for student training and continuing education programs.

Conclusion 2

In general, developers of NS-OME strongly advocate that they are a useful tool for improving speech intelligibility in individuals with various communication disorders (Chapman Bahr 2001; Rosenfeld-Johnson 2001). Published peer-reviewed original research does not exist to substantiate or unequivocally discredit these claims (Hodge 2002; Lof 2007). Not surprisingly, survey respondents reported using NS-OME most often for children with phonology/articulation delay/disorder (37%), suspected CAS (33%), and dysarthria (15%). Answers to open-ended survey questions suggested that: (a) respondents have children on their caseloads with these diagnoses that they are experiencing difficulty treating and NS-OME seem to be helpful in some cases, and (b) the prescriptive treatment offered by NS-OME allow SLPs to be 'time efficient'. Many clinicians stated that they use whatever technique works for them (including NS-OME), or they don't know what else to do and NS-OME are a place to start. NS-OME appeared to be used most commonly for syndromic, neurological or medical conditions that typically result in concomitant difficulties producing intelligible speech, such as Down syndrome and cerebral palsy. Possible reasons for the higher frequency of NS-OME with these conditions include: (a) developers of NS-OME often 'market' their use for these children, (b) NS-OME provide a step-by-step approach for children with more complex speech disorders and challenging speech intelligibility problems, and (c) intuitively it may make sense to SLPs to use motor exercises in therapy because children with these conditions have difficultly controlling the oral musculature as part of their impairment (see Clarke 2003, 2005 for discussion about why this 'intuition' needs careful examination).

Comment

SLPs appear most likely to use NS-OME in treatment for children who: (a) appear to have a motor component to their speech disorder and do not benefit from traditional articulation therapy approaches, and/or (b) present with a severe and complex SSD. Canadian university training programs are heterogeneous in how they teach students to diagnose and treat children with SSD that have a suspected or known motor component (i.e., CAS, dysarthria, mixed CAS-dysarthria). ASHA's (2007a) position statement should standardise information provided to students about CAS. It also provides guidelines for treatment that explicitly excludes NS-OME and highlights the need for treatment research. As observed by Love (2000) and demonstrated by Pennington, Goldbart, and Marshall (2003), there is also a paucity of research about effectiveness of speech interventions for children with dysarthria. Hodge and Wellman (1999) provided guidelines for practice for childhood dysarthria based on a review of available literature. Joffe and Reilly (2004) described the evidence base for evaluating and managing motor speech disorders in children as minimal and largely reflective of advice from 'clinical experts'. My experience is that most Canadian universities provide minimal information about speech therapy practice for this population of children. Development and dissemination of current best practice guidelines and development and evaluation of therapy programs for children with motor speech disorders, which include clinicians as collaborators, are obvious needs in Canada.

Conclusion 3

Users of NS-OME indicated that they were influenced by the high degree of exposure to NS-OME products and materials (predominantly Sara Rosenfeld-Johnson's programs: *Oral Motor Exercises for Speech Clarity and TalkTools^{TM}*) and clinical success (self and reported by colleagues). Other popular NS-OME products used included those marketed by SuperDuper and LinguiSystems and Pamela Marshalla http://www.pammarshalla.com. Sara Rosenfeld-Johnson and Pamela Marshalla have made several presentations in Canada and Alberta in the past 10 years, some as invited speakers at conferences hosted by professional associations. SLPs have ready access to NS-OME products marketed commercially in North America through catalogues, Web sites, and conference exhibitors.

Comment

SLPs' responses reveal the weight put on knowledge of products gained through 'marketing' exposure and that of their own and colleagues' experience in influencing their practice. All Canadian training programs aspire to graduate SLP professionals who can think independently and critically. Concerted, focused efforts are needed to foster and develop these skills so that graduates are informed, judicious consumers of products in the marketplace and colleagues' advice. Sara Rosenfeld Johnson (2001) states 'remember that the exercises in this manual do not replace anything that you are using now. They are a piece of the pie that we did not get in our education.' (p. 1). One might conclude that, for whatever reason(s), she and SLPs who use her materials do not have useable knowledge or skills gained from their university training to apply to treating some children with SSD. As noted in the comments for Conclusion 2, for many survey respondents, these children appeared to have a motor component to their speech disorder and/or presented with a severe and complex SSD. It would appear that we need to increase the number of graduates who are knowledgeable and confident about practice for these subgroups of children. There also appears to be a disconnect between what is presented as effective practice in Canadian training programs (see summary by Rvachew 2006b for an example) and what information is presented by invited speakers and marketed by exhibitors at professional conferences. Greater communication and collaboration between Canadian academic training programs and national and regional professional conference committees to promote and debate best practices in SSD appear warranted.

Conclusion 4

Survey respondents were asked whether they have seen significant changes in clients' speech because of NS-OME and, if so, to describe the changes observed. Those who answered 'yes' typically stated that NS-OME improved the strength/coordination of articulators as well as overall speech intelligibility or resulted in stimulability of speech sounds and improved production of particular sounds classes (i.e., rhotics and sibilants). Respondents who reported variable results stated that NS-OME helped with stimulability/awareness or strength/coordination of the articulators, but were ineffective with certain children and that some NS-OME programs were not as effective as others. A strong theme that emerged was that NS-OME are useful with certain children and that they are not meant for everyone. Many respondents explained that NS-OME have a small role in a therapy session and are not the sole treatment strategy. Other treatment approaches mentioned were traditional articulation therapy, Hodson's cycles, phonological processes, minimal pairs, phonetic placement, auditory discrimination, visual feedback, multiple opposition, maximal opposition, nonlinear, PROMPT, rate reduction, whole language, and a total communication that incorporates some form of AAC. However, a small sub-group of respondents appeared to use NS-OME for many clients and disorders and believed that NS-OME produce effective changes in multiple areas. The majority of respondents rated the evidence base for NS-OME as minimal or nonexistent (64%). Surprisingly, 36% of the 137 respondents rated the evidence as adequate or extensive. Whereas only 36% of respondents thought there was evidence to support NS-OME in SSD, 50% claimed that NS-OME have an important role in children's speech therapy. Obviously, some clinicians who do not think there is evidence to support the use of NS-OME still believe that they have an important role in speech therapy. Many respondents commented that they would like to see research investigating the benefits of NS-OME.

Comment

The survey results revealed that Canadian SLPs are heterogeneous in their beliefs and practices about using NS-OME for treating children with SSD and use an eclectic and pragmatic approach to speech therapy. Experience/exposure, training, and available resources were common responses for why SLPs do or do not use NS-OME. Some SLPs firmly believe that NS-OME are effective in improving children's speech and their clinical experience is much more meaningful than existing empirical research. Other SLPs do not see any benefit from NS-OME and will not use them without research-based evidence. The majority of SLPs surveyed fell between these two positions. In summary, the role of NS-OME in children's speech therapy is an example of a complicated issue for which Canadian SLPs need and desire clearer guidance.

The survey results provide a basis for further research about clinical use of NS-OME in SSD and several hypotheses to test in treatment studies. For example, 'Do NS-OME improve strength and coordination of the articulators and do these improvements increase speech intelligibility?' and 'Are NS-OME more effective at increasing speech intelligibility than treatment approaches where NS-OME are not used?' Because many respondents indicated that they use NS-OME in combination with other therapy approaches, this question has high priority. The results of this project also revealed that there are gaps in the existing evidence to answer questions that SLPs have about treating certain children with

SSD. However, progress is being made, and Canadian researchers are playing leading roles in generating and disseminating research evidence (Almost and Rosenbaum 1998; Rvachew 2006b) and providing tutorials about finding and translating evidence to practice for children with SSD (Johnson 2006). Our training programs and professional associations advocate and support evidence-based practice, and SLP managers and policy makers are starting to express their desire to do so (Robertson 2007). Major continuing challenges in the Canadian context include scarce research dollars for treatment research for SSD and scarcity of services due to the shortage of SLPs (Brown 2007).

SLT and education in New Zealand

Dr. Gail Gillon (Ngāi Tahu iwi) is Pro-Vice-Chancellor of the College of Education at the University of Canterbury in Christchurch, New Zealand, and an Associate Professor in the Department of Communication Disorders at the University of Canterbury. In 2007, she was involved in writing best practice documents for the New Zealand Ministry of Education. Professor Gillon discusses effective practice within a New Zealand context and issues facing new graduates from SLP/SLT university programs as they blend into the reality of the workplace.

Q27.   Gail T. Gillon: Collaborative relationships between speech and education in New Zealand

What is the relationship between the SLT academic community and Education community in New Zealand given the profession's historical development from an educational context? What are some of the challenges facing SLTs working in educational contexts in New Zealand in terms of meeting 'best practice', and how may these challenges best be addressed?

A27.   Gail T. Gillon: New Zealand SLT: Partnerships between the academic and educational community

The successful management of childhood speech and language disorders has been a dominant theme in the history of speech and language therapy within New Zealand. The education of New Zealand SLTs grew from a teacher education context. Christchurch Teacher's College established the first tertiary education course for SLT in 1942, with a 1-year intensive diploma course that followed a 2-year training programme in teacher education.

Over time, the education of SLTs in New Zealand expanded to reflect the increasing scope of practice in the discipline and to ensure that graduates could serve the needs of both adults and children with communication and swallowing disorders. The University of Canterbury in Christchurch first offered a 4-year Bachelor of Speech and Language Therapy degree in 1989 and continues to offer this degree alongside Masters and PhD research degrees in speech-language therapy. Recently, Massey University began a 4-year

Bachelor of Speech-Language Therapy degree programme at its Auckland Campus, and the University of Auckland now offers a 2-year Masters Degree in Speech and Language Therapy Practice.

All three providers of SLT education in New Zealand are committed to ensuring that graduates are well qualified to manage communication and swallowing difficulties across the lifespan, and their graduates readily gain employment with a variety of employers in the health, education, and private sectors. However, the relationship with the Education sector and the profession of SLT and, in particular, the New Zealand Ministry of Education continues to be robust.

The Ministry of Education is one of the main employers of SLTs in New Zealand. Through its Special Education Division, its SLT services concentrate on children who have significant communication impairments. In its endeavours to ensure that this population is well served, the Ministry commissioned a 'best practice' report of SLT assessment and treatment practices for children aged five to eight years with speech and language disorders in 1998 and commissioned updates in 2001 and 2006 (Gillon and Schwarz 1998, 2001a; Gillon, Moriarty, and Schwarz 2006). Policy makers and budget holders in education rightly asked fundamental questions about the delivery of SLT services for children in New Zealand Schools, including:

- What are the most valid and reliable assessment methods for identifying children who are in need of SLT services?
- What is the best method to treat a particular type of childhood speech and language disorder?
- How much treatment time is required to resolve a particular disorder?
- What are the most cost effective methods to address the needs of young children with communication disorders?
- How can the needs of young Māori (New Zealand indigenous population) be best met, particularly for those children with speech-language needs who are being educated in a Māori immersion education environment?

Addressing the last question has been particularly emphasised in recent years. New Zealand Ministry of Education statistics indicate that 21.4% of school students are Māori, and in 2004, close to 30,000 students (over 27,000 Māori students) were being educated in Māori medium education programmes (i.e., either all or some curriculum subjects were taught in the Māori language).

Answering questions regarding best practices, cost efficient practices, and culturally appropriate practices is not straightforward. The complexities of communication development and cultural influences from diverse populations result in there being no single assessment tool or intervention programme that is recognised as universally effective for all children with speech or language impairment. Rather, SLTs must use a range of assessment measures and plan intervention that is specific to a child's needs, including educational needs, and sensitive to the child's cultural and family environment. The intervention approach selected needs to be appropriate to the type and level of severity of the child's communication impairment and must foster both spoken and written language abilities and the prerequisite skills for successful reading and writing development.

Understanding effective or best practices for children based on research evidence is of fundamental importance to the advancement of the SLT profession. The claim made by some practitioners that an intervention method is adopted clinically 'because it works' has been challenged (Gruber, Lowery, Seung, et al. 2003). More powerful justification for an intervention decision than clinical perception is required (Powell, A34). The many confounding variables that influence the perception of intervention effectiveness necessitate the use of well-designed research studies to demonstrate an intervention method is causing the positive changes observed in children's communication development.

Thus, the profession of SLT is being challenged to be more accountable for the services provided to children with communication impairment and to ensure services are educationally relevant and culturally and linguistically appropriate. Service providers need to have confidence that assessment and treatment methods implemented with children are grounded in research and theory, validating their use. Therapists need to demonstrate the effectiveness of their services for diverse populations, and within a limited resourcing funding model for SLT, the cost efficiency of the services must also be considered.

The challenges of providing effective, cost-efficient services for children with communication impairment occur in a context of increasing demand for services. The need for childhood SLT services in New Zealand is undeniably high. The New Zealand Government's educational strategy places a strong emphasis on enhancing literacy success and improving academic achievement for all New Zealanders. A core element of literacy and academic success is proficient reading ability. Although New Zealand continues to enjoy a high overall reading standard at an international level, there are areas of significant concern that warrant urgent attention. For example, children in New Zealand who enter school at five years of age with low 'literate cultural capital' (low levels of phonological awareness, grammatical sensitivity, receptive vocabulary, and letter knowledge), frequently children from low socioeconomic areas, continue to demonstrate poor reading achievement in Year 7 (Tunmer, Chapman, and Prochnow 2006). Tunmer et al. concluded from their longitudinal study, which followed 76 children from 5 to 11 years of age, that the current language curriculum and standard reading interventions provided in New Zealand schools do not adequately address the needs of children who enter school with low language abilities. This suggests that either the curriculum and methods of reading instruction require modification or new interventions to enhance these children's development in the early school years are necessary. SLTs' expertise and scope of practice suggest that they have a critical role in supporting and collaborating with teachers to ensure that the language needs of young children are being enhanced within their classroom learning (Neilson, A17).

Of fundamental importance to literacy and academic success is strong oral language development. Gillon and Schwarz (2001b) developed and administered a screening test to explore critical spoken language skills for academic success in six-year-old children in New Zealand. The screening test measures articulation, receptive and expressive language, and phonological awareness. A total of 952 children were screened across the country, with children with any type of diagnosed disorder that would influence speech or language development excluded from the study. The results indicated that as many as 18% of the children warranted in-depth assessment of their spoken language skills. Consistent with Tunmer et al.'s (2006) findings, the study indicted that children from schools in low socioeconomic areas and Māori children were over-represented in the at-risk group.

Provision of SLT services needs to expand to ensure adequate resourcing for SLTs to work with educators in early intervention and preventative roles. Subsequent reading and writing difficulties experienced by young New Zealand children identified as being at risk due to delayed or disordered spoken language development can be prevented with appropriate intensity levels of intervention and intervention focused on building underlying skills critical for literacy success (Gillon 2000, 2002, 2005). Funding of SLT services must be at a sufficient level to ensure that research-based interventions can be implemented when appropriate to meet individual children's needs.

A further challenge for the educational community is raising literacy achievement for boys. A recent international literacy report documenting reading and writing performance of 10- to 11-year-old children in over 30 countries (PIRLS report 2005/2006) indicated that boys are achieving significantly lower than girls in literacy at an international level. In New Zealand, the difference between boys' and girls' literacy underachievement was more marked than in many other western countries. Mirroring this finding clinically, SLTs typically have many more boys on their caseloads than girls, and the relationship between early speech and language difficulties observed in boys and their academic achievement needs to be further explored.

Challenges are frequently best addressed through collaborative efforts. The current challenges in meeting the needs of children with speech and language impairments require enhanced meaningful relationships between various communities. Partnerships between universities (or the providers of SLT and teacher education), school and family communities, government bodies in policy and funding services, and appropriate cultural and ethnic groups need to be well established. Such collaborations must be directed towards a common goal of ensuring that every child meets his/her educational, social, and cultural potential and can contribute to their society in positive ways.

Meaningful partnerships between universities and the education community is an area of particular importance. In New Zealand, all providers of SLT are in universities that have a strong research orientation. Academics teaching in SLT programmes are expected to conduct research in areas of relevance and importance to their discipline. Robust, scientific models of research using both quantitative and/or qualitative designs are embraced. Effective partnerships between the academic community of SLT (as well as other relevant academic disciplines, such as education, linguistics, and psychology) will help facilitate the transfer of knowledge from research to the practice of SLT.

As with all good partnerships, trust and respect between the academic community of SLT and the educational community are vital. The knowledge of the researcher and the knowledge of the practitioner need to be understood and equally respected. Ethical responsibilities in conducting research must be of paramount importance, yet a balance between protecting children, families, and school communities and potentially restricting most forms of science-based research needs to be reached. The practitioners must trust the researcher to act in an ethically responsibly manner and adopt methodological procedures approved via robust ethical clearance processes. The researchers need to trust practitioners involved in research studies to implement research protocols as agreed, to maintain confidentiality, and to adhere to standard research procedures. Developing vigorous partnerships in research where both practitioners and researchers in SLT and teacher education are contributing to the advancement of knowledge is essential to address the challenges faced by our profession.

Through partnerships, the practical implications of the research can be more adequately addressed. Consideration of a number of factors is important in deciding whether it is appropriate for latest research findings to be immediately integrated into clinical or teaching practice (Ingram 1998). The depth of the research body, the quality of the research methodologies employed, the relevance of the findings to a specific clinical population, the practicalities of implementing an assessment or intervention technique explored under ideal research conditions into a school setting and the appropriateness of the intervention to a child's cultural, family, and educational environment all influence the transfer of research knowledge to practice.

The small population base and geographical size of New Zealand is conducive to facilitating relationships at regional and national levels. Indeed, historically, there have always been strong and close affiliations between the academic and professional community in SLT and New Zealand educational communities both from a teaching and research perspective. Maintaining and further enhancing these partnerships will be critical as we move forward in the 21st century in successfully addressing the needs of individuals with communication impairments.

The rainbow nation

The 'rainbow nation' holds unique challenges to the provision of effective and accountable speech assessment and intervention services to young children with cleft lip and palate (Louw, Shibambu, and Roemer 2006) and craniofacial anomalies, and even more extreme obstacles to overcome in working with HIV/AIDS-infected or -affected children and their families (Louw 2006).

Dr. Brenda Louw is Professor in Speech-Language Pathology and head of the Department of Communication Pathology at the University of Pretoria. Her interests include cleft lip and palate and family-focused, community-based early childhood intervention in South Africa, where the incidence and prevalence of HIV/AIDS has reached pandemic magnitude (Louw and Delport 2006). The most vulnerable groups requiring ECI are the numerous infected or orphaned infants and young children who are placed in care centres. Working with these children in skilled multicultural teams, clinicians and consultants need to sustain their energy and motivation to accommodate issues of multilingualism, cultural variation, grief, and loss in order to facilitate client empowerment.

Q28.   Brenda Louw: Building on families' strengths in early intervention in South Africa

How do you implement an 'assets-based approach' in ECI, and what special strengths, knowledge, and capabilities do families bring to the tasks of supporting their children and participating comfortably and productively in trans-disciplinary teams? Do SLPs/SLTs make valid contributions with these particularly at-risk children, and what steps can they take to improve their cultural competence and deliver in ways that are contextually relevant?

A28.   Brenda Louw: An asset-based approach to ECI

Speech and language professionals adopt clearly defined, theoretically sound, evidence-based approaches to assessment and intervention (Dodd 2007) within which they can organise ECI with children in the zero-to-three age range. The asset-based approach

(Kretzmann and McKnight 1993) is a broad framework within which both *ecological systems perspectives* (Bronfenbrenner and Morris 1998), and the *Developmental Systems Model* (Guralnick 2001) can be applied. Guralnick's model is guided by developmental, integrative, and inclusive principles, providing structure for community-based early intervention *services* and *support* for vulnerable children, like 'Tumi' in the following case illustration. Her management incorporated ecological and developmental systems theory, drawing on the 'assets' of all concerned. It is a 'given' in this framework that child, family, and the social ecology (including professionals) all have 'positives' to contribute. The SLP/SLT shows caregivers and families that they are valued team members, and through sensitivity to family culture(s), needs, concerns, and priorities, outcomes may be improved (Rivers 2000).

The basis of intervention planning is that a family system must function as a whole, within the wider social milieu, and be viewed broadly in order to find a stimulus for change (Klein and Gilkerson 2000). Recognising the *status quo*, the SLP/SLT pinpoints the family's capacities, skills, and social resources (Daniel and Wassel 2002). Incorporating the concept of *resilience* into practice promotes positive perspectives, maximising the likelihood of improved outcomes by building support networks from existing resources, permitting necessary professional input. To determine individual resilience, *risk* and *protective* factors are identified, remembering that environmental risk factors can be mediated by protective factors only if they are in balance (Werner 2000). Protective factors support positive outcomes, despite adversity.

Tumi and the asset-based approach in action

Tumi, aged 13 months, with a repaired left, complete unilateral cleft, was referred for developmental and communication ECI-team assessment by a Cleft Palate Team (CPT). Tumi's 18-year-old, Zulu-speaking mother, Sophie, and her maternal aunt Miriam accompanied Tumi to the assessment. Sophie had previously completed a case history questionnaire, assisting preparations for the assessment as an informant and partner (Ebersohn and Eloff 2006). Sophie's responses revealed that Tumi was delivered at term but was small for gestational age at 2.3 kg. Her cleft was diagnosed at birth, formal CPT evaluation occurred on day 7, and a feeding obturator was provided. Tumi experienced frequent otitis media and was hospitalised at 6 and 10 months for a successful two-stage cleft lip and palate repair. Tumi sat at 9 months, crawled at 12 months, was not walking, and sucked her bottle with difficulty. She babbled, and communicated with vocalisations and eye contact.

Assessment

In assessment, the asset-based approach sees a shift away from emphasising deficits, towards valuing capacities and strengths of child, family, and community. Accordingly, the ECI interview began with Sophie sharing what was special about Tumi and her expectations of the assessment, without having her explain 'problems' (Kretzmann and McKnight 1993). Unlike traditional interviews, this was a 'family conversation' with Sophie and Miriam, assisted by an experienced interpreter, engaged to lessen barriers of language and culture (Iglesias and Quinn 1997). A genogram (displayed in Figure A28.1) facilitated

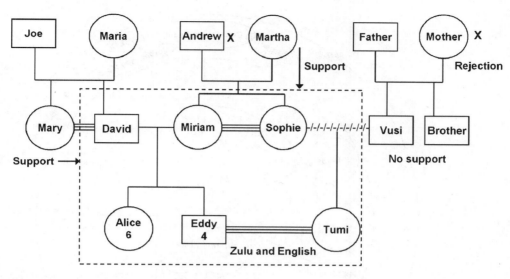

Figure A28.1 Tumi's family genogram

a life-cycle perspective (Carter and McGoldrick 1999; Thomlison 2002), providing insight into Tumi's family structure and system over three generations (Thomlison 2002). Such active family involvement promotes ownership of issues, shared responsibility, capacity building (Ebersohn and Eloff 2006), and empowerment, allowing professionals to ascertain a family's perspective (Hammer and Weiss 2000).

An eco-map (Figure A28.2) was also created, identifying household members, their relationships with each other, and their relationships with the wider world (Bronfenbrenner and Morris 1998; Irwin 1993).

We learned that Sophie was an unemployed single parent, residing in a two-bedroom house with Miriam, her husband, and their two children. The family's support network included individuals, a traditional healer, their church, and the CPT. Tumi's father lived elsewhere, providing inconsistent financial and emotional support. The healer's role was accepted as integral to the family's approach to illness and health (Louw and Avenant 2002). Our advice that Mary and Vusi were HIV/AIDS-infected remained unconfirmed by Sophie, possibly because of the social stigma associated with the illness. South Africa's HIV/AIDS pandemic burdens and stresses families and the community at large. They have constantly to cope with *infected* and *affected* community members, including many orphans.

Identified protective factors were Tumi's extroversion; Sophie's motivation, commitment to Tumi, and co-operation with the CPT; and her family and community support-network. Risk factors were Tumi's cleft, low birth weight, otitis media, hospitalisations, and poverty (potentially limiting access to treatment). Optimistically, the medical risks were treatable and the protective factors offered hope (Werner 2000). We responded to the family's request for techniques to stimulate Tumi's development, facilitating access to speech-language intervention, other specialist services, and eventual school placement.

We then focussed on Tumi, conducting a transdisciplinary, arena-based assessment, following the Carter, Lees, Murira, et al. (2005) guidelines for ensuring cultural appropriateness. With our guidance, Sophie and Miriam participated, identifying assessment

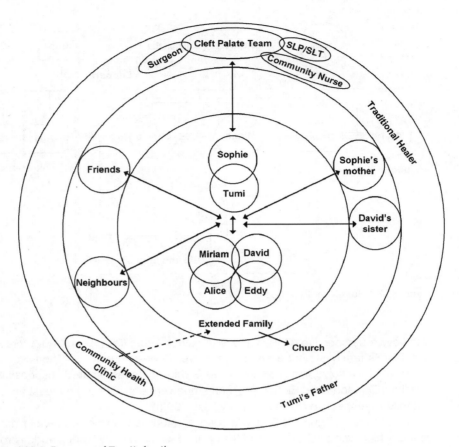

Figure A28.2 Eco-map of Tumi's family

strategies, eliciting behaviour, and telling us whether observed behaviours were typical of Tumi (Crais, Roy, and Free 2006). Assessment results were communicated via an interpreter, relating strengths first and then areas requiring attention (Kretzmann and McKnight 1993). Strengths included mother–child communication and Tumi's age-appropriate play, personal–social skills, and communicativeness.

Areas for ECI planning were feeding, middle ear functioning, auditory skills, communication functions, verbal expression, sound repertoire, and motor development. Referrals were made to public sector otorhinolaryngology and physical therapy. Without discounting Tumi's or her family's problems, strengths were emphasised and incorporated into intervention planning (Kretzmann and McKnight 1993).

Intervention

Approaching intervention, the SLT rejected deficit-oriented, needs-driven, medical models, favouring social, eco-systemic methodologies and a positive approach. The challenges of poverty and Tumi's developmental functioning were reframed and incorporated to make positive contributions to the ECI process. Rather than the ECI team 'leading', a dynamic partnership and collaborative empowerment were fostered (Ebersohn and Eloff 2006). Turnbull, Turbiville, and Turnbull (2001) believe that the asset-based approach holds the best promise for growth of children, families, and professionals. Within this approach, the SLP/SLT acted sensitively and collaboratively when Tumi's family prioritised motor development for intervention (Louw and Avenant 2002). The SLP/SLT also liaised with the CPT's community nurse regarding feeding. Communication intervention was family-centred, and the SLP/SLT, through an interpreter, provided family education and direct intervention, also guiding parent-implemented intervention. Techniques and strategies were explained, discussed, demonstrated, and monitored. Empowered, Sophie shared these with significant others, strengthening her support network and involving the family.

Outcomes

One year later, positive outcomes were evident for Tumi, 2;1, the extended family, and the community. Following physiotherapy, Tumi's motor development was age-appropriate; she was feeding herself and had gained weight. With the insertion of grommets, otitis media had reduced in frequency, and her auditory comprehension and listening skills had improved. Although her phonetic repertoire remained limited, she had a 60-word expressive vocabulary, imitated 2- and 3-word combinations, and followed 2-stage commands.

Sophie's confidence as a parent and communication facilitator had flourished, and she actively participated in the annual CPT evaluation of Tumi, perceiving herself as the expert on her child and more knowledgeable about cleft lip and palate. The extended family took pride in Tumi's development, *volunteering* to educate their church congregation about clefts and to support families of new babies with clefts. The family were also enthusiastic about the ECI team's support. The community had benefited indirectly, having been mobilised through education regarding clefts, treatment options, and the impact of a cleft on families, so that their societal understanding of such a disability was changing (Louw, Shibambu, and Roemer 2006).

Reflection

Reflection (Klein and Gilkerson 2000) is a valuable technique that SLP's/SLT's can employ to examine their ECI practice. It allows them to understand their own values and beliefs, cultural practices, and professional biases, while increasing self-awareness of professional styles, actions, reactions, and responsibilities. Tumi's outcomes *were* mainly positive, but reflection suggested that the ideal would have been for: (1) the SLP/SLT to have proficiency in Tumi's home language, Zulu (Lynch 1998); (2) the family to have made their own observations of Tumi's behaviour during the assessment; (3) the family to have participated more actively in determining communication goals (Crais, Roy, and Free 2006); and (4) financial assistance to have been sourced to alleviate travel expenses between home and ECI. An additional, broader goal, not of particular benefit to Tumi's management, would have been for the SLP/SLT to have expanded her role to implementing a community programme for the primary prevention of communication disorders (Popich, Louw, and Eloff 2007).

Families are the unit of ECI service delivery that provides a natural, collaborative, and enabling context for intervention. They impart essential information on non-verbal and verbal communication styles in the family, enabling better understand of their perspective and the growth of trusting relationships (Bennet, Zhang, and Hojnar 1998). Optimally, families play a constant role in the ECI process, providing continuity for the child as he or she develops, whereas professionals and educational contexts may change. Families, therefore, are ideally positioned to advocate for their children through active collaboration with professionals (Crais, Roy, and Free 2006). Family capabilities contribute to the outcomes of intervention by three interactional patterns: parent-child transactions, family-orchestrated child experiences, and nurturing behaviour (Guralnick 2001).

Cultural competence

One of the guiding principles for ECI practice formulated by Guralnick (2005) is that true partnerships with families cannot occur without sensitivity to cultural differences and close understanding of their developmental implications. Cultural competence may be achieved via a four-step process (Louw and Avenant 2002):(1) the *development of self-awareness* of the clinician's own cultural heritage and values, behaviours, beliefs, and customs (Lynch 1998); (2) the *acquisition of knowledge* of the facets of the specific culture that influence communication development, such as the dynamic interaction among cultural beliefs, family values, expectations, experiences, and child-rearing practices (Louw 2004); (3) *becoming cognisant of cultural factors* that impact ECI (Hughes 1992; Bennet, Zhang, and Hojnar 1998), which may include health beliefs and practices, views of family and professional roles, help-seeking styles, and time orientation; and (4) *by gaining experience* in actually providing cross-cultural ECI services and reflective practice.

By collaborating with parents and caregivers, SLPs/SLTs implementing asset-based approaches to ECI develop a range of skills. Their listening and observational skills improve, and they develop help-giving styles that empower family participation in intervention. By emphasising strengths, they help families build their capabilities, reinforcing their networks (Bennet, Zhang, and Hojnar 1998). They become knowledgeable about adult learning styles and skilled in imparting knowledge for skills training (Popich, Louw, and Eloff 2007). They also become adept at monitoring both child progress and family change to determine whether intervention goals are being met and the impact of any goals and changes on the family as a whole.

In line with the asset-based approach, Lynch (1998) proposed that the SLP/SLT should consider value sets that are common across cultures, viewing each as a continuum. This process reduces stereotyping and leads to a better understanding of cultural influences. But of course, cultural and family diversity mean that there is no blueprint or formula for a culturally appropriate ECI programme (Iglesias and Quinn 1997). Moreover, they mean that, wherever they are in the world, SLPs/SLTs are challenged by cultural mismatches between themselves and client, and the effects they have on ECI interrelationships and the way in which families and professionals interrelate and participate in ECI (Madding 2000). Within the asset-based framework however, cultural mismatch is viewed not only as a source of *risk* but also as a developmental *resource* (Garcia Col and Magnuson 2000). Attaining cultural competence empowers the SLP/SLT because it allows for the development and improvement of contextually relevant and culturally sensitive ECI services, maximising and enhancing the prospect of optimal outcomes for children.

Phonological assessment and intervention practices in the UK

Dr. Victoria Joffe is a specialist speech and language therapist and senior lecturer in developmental speech, language, and communication impairments in the Department of Language and Communication Science at City University, London. She is program director of an MSc degree in *Joint Professional Practice: Language and Communication* run in conjunction with the Institute of Education, London (http://www.talklink.org). Victoria obtained her DPhil degree in the Department of Experimental Psychology, The University of Oxford, exploring the relationship between oral language ability, metalinguistic awareness, and literacy in language-impaired children. Her areas of clinical and research interest include specific language impairment, speech disorder, the interface between education and SLT, the relationship between language and literacy, narrative therapy, and language impairment in secondary school age children. Victoria is currently involved in a large-scale intervention project funded by the Nuffield Foundation on enhancing language and communication in secondary school children with language impairments (http://www.elciss.com). In recent research with a colleague at City University (Joffe and Pring 2008), Dr. Joffe investigated the methods of assessment and remediation of 'phonological problems' used by therapists working in the UK. The surveyed therapists comprised 9 who were in their first year of practice, 25 with 1–3 years, 13 with 4–6 years, 13 with 7–10 years, and 38 with more than 10 years of experience. They reporting using a variety of therapies: auditory discrimination, minimal contrast therapy, and phonological awareness were the most popular and were often used in combination. Most respondents reported involving parents, and, in planning therapy, clinicians were more influenced by children's language and cognitive abilities and the motivation of parents than by the nature of the impairment. Probably the most striking outcome of this research was the information about assessment practices. Dr. Joffe talks about this in her response to Q29.

Q29.   Victoria Joffe: Barriers to EBP in child speech intervention in a UK context

Reporting on a survey of child speech practice in the UK (Joffe and Pring 2008), you wrote: 'Constraints upon clinicians make it difficult for them to convert research findings to practice. In particular, assessments that allow more individualised and targeted interventions appear little used. Clinicians are aware of research but there is a danger that clinical practice and research are diverging.' Of your 98 respondents, 83 (85%) used the South Tyneside Assessment of Phonology (STAP; Armstrong and Ainley 1988) as a primary data source for planning speech intervention. Although it is promoted as a 'phonology test' that 'gives a profile of a child's phonological system' and permits 'phonological analysis', the STAP is a 3-position citation-naming articulation screener in which 27 pictures are used to elicit production of 78 words, sampling all singleton consonants and 19 consonant clusters word initially, and by default, some vowels. Whereas assessment with the STAP would provide only one small, non-standardised fraction of the relational analysis component of phonological assessment (Baker 2004; Stoel-Gammon and Dunn 1985), 77% of the respondents rated themselves 'very confident' or 'confident' in their ability to select therapies. Can you comment on this remarkable finding and reflect on the possible barriers, in the British context, between pedagogy, research findings, and evidence-based practice?

A29. Victoria Joffe: A survey of clinical practice in the UK

Around 6.5% of all UK children have a SSD in the absence of any other cognitive, sensory, or physical impairment (Broomfield and Dodd 2004b). Such children typically dominate SLP/SLT paediatric caseloads (Gierut 1998), and in Britain, most receive treatment in community clinics or schools. Except for anecdotal accounts, little information exists about the practices of SLTs, and a dearth of information around the relationship between practice and outcomes constitutes a serious gap in our knowledge-base (Kamhi 2006a). Accordingly, we surveyed, via a carefully constructed questionnaire, paediatric SLT clinicians across the UK (Joffe and Pring 2008), seeking to build a detailed picture of clinicians' routine practices, experiences, and opinions regarding children's SSD.

Completed questionnaires came from a representative sample of 98 clinicians from the health, education, and private sectors. The proportion of children with SSD ranged from 40% or more of their caseloads (44% of participants) to 70% or more (10% of participants). The respondents' clinical experience extended from 1–3 years (35%), 4–10 years (26%), and more than 10 years (39%). Only 7% specialised exclusively in SSD, whereas 42% identified it as one of several specialist areas.

Assessment

Between them, the participants identified 21 assessments they used most frequently to identify and assess SSD, with the overwhelming majority (85%) nominating the *South Tyneside Assessment of Phonology: STAP* (Armstrong and Ainley 1988, 1992). A clear picture emerged of clinicians opting to use this quick screening tool, supplemented by other non-standardised assessments, including personally designed assessments and informal observation. In some respects, the popularity of the small, easily transportable *STAP* with its quick administration and scoring is understandable. It is, however, unlikely that the *STAP*, assessments like it, or informal observations provide sufficient detail to permit comprehensive description and diagnosis and optimal therapy planning; and there is a danger that incomplete or insufficient assessment protocols may promote inadequate intervention practices (Bernhardt and Holdgrafer 2001).

Alternative, detailed linguistic analyses, such as psycholinguistic profiling (Stackhouse and Wells 1997) and non-linear analysis (Bernhardt and Stemberger 2000), enable more precise identification of the nature and levels of speech impairment (Bernhardt and Ullrich, A32; Gardner, A21; Froud, A33). These analyses take more time than *STAP*-type measures and perhaps more time than many working clinicians are likely to have. They also require specialist knowledge, sometimes necessitating ongoing training. The current financial climate sees restrictions placed on the CPD/CEU events clinicians may attend, exacerbating this problem. Moreover, anecdotally, UK SLTs fear implementing in-depth speech analyses, sometimes acknowledging their own lack of expertise, like one respondent who claimed that she and some of her colleagues were 'terrified' by psycholinguistic models (see Gardner, A21 for reassurance!).

Respondents noted dissatisfaction with their limited assessment options, wishing to try others that were currently inaccessible, often due to financial restrictions. For example, we found that some workplaces can afford to purchase just one copy of an assessment, rendering its routine use throughout an agency impossible. The *Diagnostic Evaluation of Articulation and Phonology: DEAP* (Dodd, Crosbie, Zhu, et al. 2002) retails for over £250, so that most clinic budgets can only permit the purchase of one or two copies. A consequence of clinicians using screening measures over comprehensive phonological analysis is that they provide insufficient information upon which to select the most appropriate therapy *and* identify treatment targets most suited to the individual child's intervention needs, and order them appropriately (Stoel-Gammon, A9).

Therapy, clinician confidence, and the evidence-base

Our survey suggested that SLTs were aware of research, and that this awareness reinforced their confidence in choosing between therapies, but this was not necessarily so. Some respondents expressed confidence although unimpressed by or unaware of the evidence, whereas some *were* aware of the evidence but reported a lack of confidence. In the analysis, confidence was particularly high, especially among experienced clinicians, with 79% of all respondents confident or very confident in their ability to select an appropriate therapy. Only 3 of the 98 rated themselves as 'not very' or 'not at all' confident. Asked whether they felt there was sufficient evidence for the effectiveness of therapy with these children, 72% agreed or strongly agreed that strong evidence supported their clinical practice.

Confidence and knowledge of the evidence appear closely related. Whereas 60% agreed or strongly agreed that sufficient evidence existed and were confident or very confident about selecting therapy, a substantial minority disagreed, with 19% of respondents confident in their therapy choice but ambivalent about the evidence for its effectiveness, and 11% agreeing that there was sufficient evidence while reporting low confidence in choosing a therapy. So, very intriguingly, on one hand, therapists appear to know about the available research evidence, and this knowledge improved their confidence in selecting therapy; but, on the other hand, a sizable minority, who expressed confidence, were either unimpressed by or unaware of the evidence. This suggests that their confidence emanated from clinical experience rather than from their reading of research findings, exemplifying the research–practice gap (Duchan 2001; Joffe 2008; McLeod and Baker 2004), discussed in detail in Chapter 1.

Choosing a therapy

We explored the factors that drove the SLTs' therapy choices. They appeared most concerned about general factors that might affect therapy, particularly the child's age (57%) and parental 'attitude' (56%), including the parents' motivation, awareness of the problem, and level of concern. Then, they were interested in general indicators of children's ability, specifically: attention and listening (30%), language performance (21%), and cognitive ability (17%). The child's own awareness of his/her problem was important to 15% of respondents. The child's phonological characteristics were given far less prominence than the considerations itemised above. Here, the severity of the disorder was the *only* frequently mentioned factor (40%) followed by information about delay/disorder (16%) and stimulability (11%). Strikingly, and undoubtedly due to time and expertise constraints, few therapists said they would conduct more detailed phonological analyses or investigate phonological knowledge as a basis for choosing a therapy.

From a list of 14 readily identifiable therapies drawn from published sources, participants reported their frequency of use as just over 2 therapies all the time, 4–5 most of the time, and 8–9 sometimes, indicating SLTs' eclecticism in choosing and combining approaches across clients and SSD types. They also had clear favourites, with 50% always or often using *auditory discrimination*, *minimal contrast therapy*, and *phonological awareness*, and 84% employing all three at least some of the time. Apparently, therapists combine them as a core (or 'standard package') method of treatment, targeting different levels of input and output processing (Pascoe, Stackhouse, and Wells 2005). The popularity of the conventional minimal pair approach (Weiner 1981a), one of the most commonly cited interventions for SSD (Joffe and Serry 2004), is confirmed by McLeod and Baker (2004). The prevalent use of phonological awareness (PA) activities was unsurprising given PA's prominence in the SLP/SLT, psychology, and education literature (Hatcher, Hulme, and Ellis 1994; Hulme, Hatcher, Nation, et al. 2002). Reports of the effectiveness of PA training in remediating speech disorders are equivocal (Hesketh, Adams, Nightingale, et al. 2000; and Gillon 2000), and its customary adoption with all speech-disordered children should be viewed with extreme caution (Dodd and Gillon 2001). The inclusion of auditory discrimination is quite remarkable, as some children with SSD have robust auditory discrimination skills alongside severe output difficulties (Stackhouse and Wells 1997), and for them, work on auditory discrimination may be redundant, time-wasting, and unjustifiable.

Parents and intervention

Three-quarters of respondents reported always or often involving parents in therapy, with 43% in the 'always' category. Seeing parents as a useful resource in SSD management may have been encouraged by research accounts of their use (Bowen and Cupples 1999a, 2004; Lancaster, Keusch, Levin, et al., in press). It is difficult to determine the expectations that SLTs have of parents and whether they select their treatments with parental involvement in mind. Parents' variability in their ability to assist their own children may affect therapy outcomes unpredictably. In fact, it may be a *concern* if SLTs are so accustomed to engaging them routinely as 'co-therapists' that they are reluctant to treat children whose parents are unable, unavailable, or unwilling to participate in therapy sessions or homework. There is a hint that this may *indeed* be the case, with over 50% of respondents emphasising the importance of parental attitude or motivation in making decisions about treatment (see Watts Pappas, A25 for discussion).

Eclecticism and intervention

Curiously, therapists are confident in selecting therapies and are convinced that they work. Support for the view that 'therapies work' comes from research demonstrating that a variety of different therapy approaches are effective for a substantial number of children with

SSD (Hesketh, Adams, Nightingale et al. 2000; Gillon 2000; Rvachew, Ohberg, Grawbyrg, et al. 2003; Rvachew, Nowak, and Cloutier 2004). But this evidence may be confusing for practitioners wanting to apply it clinically, and little advice is available to tell them which therapies to use for what and with whom! These different therapies may all appear effective because of careful research-subject selection and because they each consti-tute an optimal approach for certain children (or certain speech disorders). If this is so, then even greater gains may be achieved if clinicians eschew eclecticism, incorporating explicitly principled, evidence-based matching between children and therapies into their practices.

Alarmingly, the eclecticism that, from our study, appears to be *usual* in clinical prac-tice is unsupported by recent SSD research, which more typically examines the effects of specific therapies, for example, phonological awareness (Hesketh, Adams, Nightin-gale, et al. 2000; Gillon 2000) and core vocabulary (Crosbie, Holm, and Dodd 2005; Dodd, Holm, Crosbie, et al. 2006). Although the therapies in the evidence-base for SSD treatment foster optimism, they are not the therapies of choice for our 98 representa-tive UK clinicians, and little is known about the effectiveness of their preferred (audi-tory discrimination plus minimal contrast therapy plus phonological awareness) eclectic approach.

By the same token, eclecticism seems reasonable in relation to the heterogeneity of children with SSD (Dodd 2005). The chances are relatively good that one area of focus of a 'catch all' eclectic approach will meet the needs of particular individual clients. At least one small-number study (Lancaster, Keusch, Levin, et al., in press) shows promising outcomes from an eclectic therapeutic approach. An eclectic approach may work because it targets a variety of levels, and therefore may benefit a wide range of children. But, although *effective*, such an approach may not be the most *efficient*, and, as discussed above, more powerful *effects* may be achieved by matching specific therapies to different types of SSD.

Implications of the survey

In conclusion, this survey provides direction for both researchers and therapists. It is no longer sufficient to ask whether a therapy for SSD is effective, but rather, we now need to address questions of which specific therapy, or therapy mix, is most effective for which group of children with SSD. Additionally, ways must be identified for clinicians to routinely incorporate detailed phonological analyses into their workaday assessment protocols. This has important resource implications, and discussions need to involve not only SLTs and SLT managers but national health and education managers and policy makers. Further-more, researchers and therapists need to co-operate in diminishing the research–practice gap. Once clinical researchers have investigated the efficacy of specific treatments, SLTs should be encouraged to evaluate their effectiveness in 'real' clinical contexts, as part of routine clinical practice. Researchers should be encouraged to focus more attention on issues that directly reflect, and impact upon, clinical practice, like the differential impact of service delivery models (including dose, schedule, and agent of therapy) on outcome (Dodd, 2008; see also Dodd, A43). As work partners, researchers and therapists can succeed in identifying the most effective, efficient, and efficacious therapies for this client group.

NS-OME

Dr. Gregory Lof is an Associate Professor and the Associate Director in the Graduate Program in Communication Sciences and Disorders at the MGH Institute of Health Professions in Boston, Massachusetts. His research, teaching, and clinical work primarily involve children with articulation and phonological disorders, and he is also interested in professional issues. Recent research and writing has been in the area of the lack of efficacy of using NS-OME to change speech sound productions. Dr. Lof was the 2004 topic coordinator for phonology for the ASHA Convention and served on the 1995, 1998, 2002, and 2007 ASHA Convention Program Committees for phonology and the 2008 committee for multicultural issues. He is also an editorial consultant for the journals *American Journal of Speech-Language Pathology*, *Contemporary Issues in Communication Sciences and Disorders*, and *Language, Speech, and Hearing Services in Schools*. He has presented workshops at ASHA conventions, at local universities, in school districts, and at numerous state conventions. He is a member of the ASHA National Center for Evidence-Based Practice Committee, formed in 2006. The committee has already conducted an evidence-based systematic review (EBSR) to determine the state of the evidence surrounding OME. The main objective of this EBSR was to determine the impact of OME on swallowing/speech outcomes, swallowing/speech physiology, secretion management, and sensorimotor function.

Q30.   Gregory L. Lof: A US perspective on NS-OME

Controversy surrounds the range of therapy activities and techniques categorised as NS-OME or 'oral motor activities' that are implemented in an effort to address speech sound production problems. Nevertheless, they are commonly used by SLPs in North America, often in conjunction with 'tools and toys', including bite blocks, straws and tubes, toy wind instruments, and chewable objects and thickened drinks. What exercises are used and why? What is the evidence and logic against using these exercises? Is there evidence and logic in their favour? Why do clinicians continue to use them? What is the responsibility of ASHA and other continuing education providers and sponsors in ensuring that therapy techniques that are presented to CEU/CPD participants adhere to the principles of EBP?

A30.   Gregory L. Lof: The NS-OME phenomenon in speech pathology practice

It is puzzling to think that the controversial therapy technique of NS-OME to change speech sound production problems is a common practice among SLPs in North America. Indeed, NS-OME is used by approximately 85% of SLPs in the United States (Lof and Watson 2004, 2008) and Canada (Hodge, A26; Hodge, Salonka, and Kollias 2005). Why puzzling? Because convincing evidence for their use is lacking, and the motor and linguistic theories do not support them. My exploration of the issues surrounding NS-OME begins with a series of questions, some of which I can answer. How can NS-OME be defined? What exercises are used and why? What is the evidence and logic against using these exercises? Why do clinicians continue to use them? What is the responsibility of ASHA and other organisations supplying continuing education (CE) opportunities in ensuring that the therapy techniques that are presented follow the principles of EBP?

One of several possible definitions of NS-OMEs provided by ASHA's *National Center for Evidence-Based Practice in Communication Disorders* (Arvedson, Clark, Frymark, et al. 2007) is: *'Oral-motor exercises (OMEs) are non-speech activities that involve sensory stimulation to or actions of the lips, jaw, tongue, soft palate, larynx, and respiratory muscles which are intended to influence the physiologic underpinnings of the oropharyngeal mechanism and thus improve its functions. OMEs may include active muscle exercise, muscle stretching, passive exercise, and sensory stimulation'.* The term 'oral motor' relates to movements and placements of the oral musculature. Although the existence and importance of the *oral motor* aspects of speech production are not in dispute, the use of *non-speech* oral motor *exercises* is. Such exercises, aimed at directly changing the performance of the articulators for speech production, typically include: blowing; tongue wags, curling, and push-ups; tongue-to-nose-to-chin, pucker-smile, and big-smile movements; cheek-puffing; and kiss-blowing (Lof and Watson 2008). SLPs who use them believe their clients' speech will benefit relative to: enhanced tongue elevation and lateralisation; better oral–kinaesthetic awareness; stronger tongues, lips, and sucking; and improved jaw stabilisation, lip/tongue protrusion, control of drooling, and velopharyngeal competence (Lof and Watson 2008).

Theoretical issues

Many scholars and clinicians have questioned the use of NS-OMEs on theoretical grounds (Clark 2003, 2005; Forrest 2002; Lof 2003; Lof and Watson 2008; Ruscello 2008b), raising issues of: (1) part-whole training and transfer, (2) strengthening of the articulators, (3) task specificity, (4) relevancy, and (5) awareness.

Part–whole training and transfer

Part–whole training and transfer implies breaking a task (in this instance, speaking) into smaller parts; for example, working on isolated sounds rather than linguistic units. Researchers and clinicians have demonstrated repeatedly that segmental production will not transfer to the syllable or word levels (Bernhardt and Stemberger 1998; Hodson 2007; Ingram and Ingram 2001). But curiously, NS-OME breaks the speaking task into even *smaller* gestures than sounds-in-isolation, when, for example, tongue tip-to-alveolar ridge movement gestures are practised in order to teach alveolar stops, or lip puckers are elicited repeatedly in hopes of helping mid-back vowel production. Criticising this compartmentalisation, Forrest (2002) says, '. . . tasks that comprise highly organized or integrated movements will not be enhanced by learning the constituent parts; rather training on parts of these organized behaviors will diminish learning' (p. 18). She reminds us that, 'Fractionating a behavior that is composed of interrelated parts is not likely to provide relevant information for the appropriate development of neural substrates' (p. 19). Applying this reasoning, it appears there is inadequate theoretical justification for training disconnected 'components' of speech gestures on the assumption that it will transfer to speech.

Strengthening of the articulators

'Strength needs' is a frequently stated reason for conducting NS-OMEs (Lof and Watson 2008), raising four pertinent questions: (1) How do clinicians verify that oral musculature strength *is* diminished in children with SSD? (2) How much strength does speaking require? (3) Do NS-OMEs increase articulator strength? (4) Do children with SSD have weak articulators? Clinicians typically measure articulator strength subjectively, for example, by feeling the force of the tongue pushing against a tongue depressor, gloved finger, or cheek, or by simply 'observing' weakness (Solomon and Munson 2004). But seasoned clinicians are less accurate in their 'guesstimations' of reduced strength than are student clinicians (Clark, Hensen, Barber, et al. 2003). This means that SLPs/SLTs probably cannot initially verify whether strength is diminished, so they cannot *then* report an increase in strength following an NS-OME regimen. But how much strength is needed for speaking? The answer 'not much' prompted Wenke, Goozee, Murdoch, et al. (2006) to state, '. . . caution should be taken when directly associating tongue strength to speech' (p. 15). For example, lip muscle-force for speaking is only about 10–20% of the maximal capabilities for lip-force, and the jaws use only about 11–15% of their potential force (Bunton and Weismer 1994; Forrest 2002).

Even if strengthening were necessary, the question remains, 'Do NS-OMEs *really* increase articulator strength?' Answer: 'probably not'. In order to strengthen *any* muscle, exercises must be done repeatedly, against resistance, to the point of fatigue. . . again and again. This standard and empirically supported muscle-strengthening paradigm, relevant to *all* muscle groups, is used whenever someone adheres to a weight-training program. Armed with this indisputable evidence, let's pose a three-part question about a commonly used NS-OME. How many tongue-wag repetitions do most clinicians require clients to perform, how often, and are the wags done against resistance? If the answers are 'not many', 'not often', and 'seldom', respectively, probably *no* transient or lasting strength gains accrue from tongue-wag exercises. Finally, do children with SSD have oral weakness? Definitely not, according to Sudbery, Wilson, Broaddus, et al. (2006), who demonstrated objectively that preschool-aged children with SSD had *stronger* articulators than their peers with age-typical speech.

Task specificity

Thinking about task specificity leads to the truism: 'speech is special' (Liberman 1996). The anatomical structures used for speaking and other 'mouth tasks', like swallowing, sucking, and breathing, function in different ways, each mediated by different parts of the brain. In other words, although identical structures are involved, organisation of movements within the nervous system is not the same for speech gestures as it is for nonspeech gestures; and the neural basis of motor control is different for speech and non-speech oral movements. Weismer (2006) summarises 11 studies showing that speech and non-speech neuromotor processes are different for numerous structures, including facial muscles, the maxilla, mandible, tongue, lips, and palate. Furthermore, Bonilha, Moser, Rorden, et al. (2006) used functional magnetic resonance imaging (fMRI) to demonstrate that non-speech movements activated different *parts* of the brain than did speech movements. Evidence from task specificity studies therefore indicates that working on non-speech activities will fail to change speech.

Relevancy

NS-OMEs usually lack relevance. Because isolated articulator movements do not constitute or even resemble the actual gestures used for the production of *any* sounds in English, their value in improving phonetic production is highly questionable. It seems ridiculous to contemplate, but no speech sounds require tongue-tip elevation towards the nose, puffed-out cheeks, blowing, or tongue-wagging! Oral movements that are irrelevant to speech movements will not be effective as speech therapy techniques.

Awareness

Some NS-OME programs centre on a 'metamouth' assumption of children developing, via the exercises, metacognitive awareness of articulatory place, manner and movement, alongside a process of 'waking up' or 'warming up' the speech musculature (Lof and Watson 2008). Muscle warm-up may be appropriate prior to exercise regimens, like distance running or weight-training, designed to maximally tax the system (Pollock, Gaesser, Butcher, et al. 1998). Conversely, muscle warm-up is superfluous for less strenuous tasks, below the maximum, like walking, handwriting, or lifting a spoon to mouth. As speaking does not *approach* the oral muscular maximum, warm-up is quite unnecessary. Besides, children up to and including seven year olds are probably unable to use the mouth cues provided by NS-OME to make themselves more aware of their oral structures (Klein, Lederer, and Cortese 1991; Koegel, Koegel, and Ingham 1986). Because of this lack of 'metamouth' awareness, no transfer to speech occurs from the NS-OME movements and 'mouth awareness cues'.

The research evidence

The *theoretical* underpinnings for using NS-OME to improve children's speech are not strong, but might a literature search reveal *research* supporting their widespread use by clinicians who wish their work practices to be guided by the principles of EBP? Answer: 'no'. Following scientifically rigorous procedures, all available published research studies were scrutinised by members of an ASHA committee (Arvedson, Clark, Frymark, et al. 2007), who reported that only 17 suitable articles were available for evaluation with *none* meeting the minimum criteria to render them scientifically sound. Accordingly, the only possible conclusion drawn from this exhaustive review on the effectiveness of NS-OME for speech is that *no* studies exist showing that they are or are not beneficial.

On the other hand, several unpublished research studies that have been presented at peer-reviewed ASHA national conventions are available for review (Abrahamsen and Flack 2002; Colone and Forrest 2000; Roehrig, Suiter, and Pierce 2004). Although not necessarily as rigorously peer-reviewed as publications in high-quality, refereed scholarly journals, most of the studies provide some level of evidence that NS-OMEs are ineffective. In fact, only 1 of the 10 available presentations (Fields and Polmanteer 2002) shows any positive effects of NS-OME, and that study is methodologically flawed.

Clinicians' and associations' responsibilities

Given the weak theoretical underpinnings and the absence of evidence that might support the use of NS-OMTs, why do clinicians persist in using this technique? And what is the role of ASHA and other organisations that are providing a mechanism for presenting CE events that encourage and facilitate the use of NS-OME?

SLPs probably continue to use NS-OME for a range of reasons: the procedures constitute an easy 'cookbook' approach that can be followed in a step-by-step fashion; the exercises give the appearance that something tangible is being 'done' in therapy; various techniques and tools have been heavily and attractively promoted in self-published materials and workshops; many practicing clinicians do not read the peer-reviewed professional literature; occupational and physical therapists on multi-disciplinary teams encourage exercises; and frequently other clinicians persuade their colleagues to use these techniques (Lof and Watson 2008). This final reason reminds me of Kamhi (2004), who said, '. . . no human being is immune to hearing a not-so-good idea and passing it on to someone else' (p. 110).

In the US, many CE events are offered to clinicians so they can maintain their certifications/licenses. Most of them are offered with ASHA authorisation; however, ASHA's explicit policy is that, '. . . *approval of continuing education sponsorship does not imply endorsement of course content, specific products, or clinical procedures'* (ASHA 1994). This means that the plethora of workshops on NS-OME (Clark 2005) is *not* validated for content or for their adherence to EBP through any peer-review process. Therefore, clinicians alone have the responsibility to evaluate the claims made by the presenters, and this is definitely an arduous task (Bernstein Ratner 2006).

Professional organisations like ASHA can play a role in fostering scientific environments enabling clinicians to become more knowledgeable consumers of new, innovative, and controversial treatments. But, ultimately, the SLP/SLT him/herself must be able to critically evaluate the logic used and the evidence claimed by CE presenters, because it is only through adherence to scientific methodologies (Kamhi 2004) that our field can progress.

NS-OMEs are used by many well-meaning, caring, and conscientious clinicians to change the speech sound productions of children with disorders. They use them for clients with diverse diagnoses: linguistic, structural, motoric, sensory, cognitive, genetic . . . the list goes on. Although it would be most advantageous to have one efficient, effective treatment procedure to correct all types of problems, it must be conceded that the likelihood of the existence of such a magical procedure is improbable. One of the reasons for EBP is not only to promote the use of proven effective treatments, but also to delay the adoption of unproven ones (ASHA 2004c). At this time, it seems that this delay in using NS-OME is most prudent.

The student experience

In their clinical placements for child speech, student clinicians may encounter practices that they have never heard of in class. Conversely, they may learn of therapy methodologies in lectures and in their readings that they never encounter in clinics.

Speech-Language Pathologist Karen McComas is an Associate Professor of Communication Disorders at Marshall University in Huntington, West Virginia. She holds the ASHA Certificate of Clinical Competence in Speech-Language Pathology and Audiology. McComas began her career with 8 years as an SLP in the public school system and has 23 years of experience in higher education. She teaches in the areas of articulation and phonological disorders, clinical principles, and technology, emphasising the use of

21st century technologies in professional contexts. McComas' current research is on identity development, specifically research identity, and her response to Q31 emphasises the ways in which educational programs can support students in the development of professional identities as SLPs/SLTs.

Q31. Karen McComas: Student preparation in a changing world: A view from the States

Given appropriate support and guidance in the process of easing into professional practice roles, students absorb and embrace the language, literature, issues, and modes and methods of enquiry of their chosen discipline. The support comes from people: peers, instructors, mentors, and clinical supervisors, and formal guidance comes from documents: codes of ethics, standards of practice, and expected competencies. Throughout the process, students are encouraged to think, evaluate, question, challenge, know, understand, and make sensible connections between what they are taught as best practice and what they observe to be common practice in formal clinical placements, in anecdotal discussion list offerings, and on Web sites that promise client and clinician the earth. Specifically, in the topic areas of articulation and phonological disorders, how can students, CFY practitioners, and new graduates be prepared to uphold the value of qualitative research that is reliable and valid and will stand up to peer review, in environments where they are very 'junior' and in which these tenets of scholarship are not well regarded or even derided?

A31. Karen McComas: Developing professional identities: A goal for educational programs

In a very short period of time, society has moved from predicting an information explosion to coping—or at least trying to cope—with that explosion. On top of that, the rate at which information is generated and replaced is increasing at an alarming pace, so quickly that, in many cases, some of what students learn during their freshman year of college is obsolete before they graduate 4 years later. It's hard to imagine the implications for society, much less for university programs scrambling to respond to these unstoppable changes in an efficient and timely fashion. But, in order to remain viable and relevant, educational programs must respond creatively and strategically.

I teach in the Department of Communication Disorders at Marshall University in Huntington, West Virginia. My own program, one my colleagues and I describe as having a clinical focus, serves as my point of reference. I am fully aware, however, that, although there are many programs that are similar to mine, there are just as many that are considerably different. Even so, I suspect that all programs struggle to keep up with a changing world and expanding Scope of Practice. Our success relies on our ability to change how we think about education. Successful programs will undoubtedly have to revise their goals and modify their methods. Quite simply, programs will have to decrease their emphasis on information and increase their emphasis on processes.

Goals

One process, specifically the process of socialising students into the culture of the discipline, offers promise as a goal for educational programs. This socialisation process fosters the development of a professional identity in learners as they acquire and refine the habits of mind and practice that will be required of them throughout their professional careers. The German psychoanalyst, Jacques Lacan, described this identification process as a '... transformation that takes place in the subject when he assumes an image...' (Lacan 2005, p. 549). Johnston (2004) further elaborated on this identification process:

> *Building an identity means coming to see in ourselves the characteristics of particular categories (and roles) of people and developing a sense of what it feels like to be that sort of person and belong in certain social spaces... [students] involved in classroom interactions... build and try on different identities.* (p. 23)

Developing a professional identity is an essential pre-requisite for success as an SLP/SLT. Hewitt claimed that the understanding of a discipline that comes from developing a professional identity '... allows entry into its [discipline's] knowledge and practice...' (Hewitt 2006, p. 110).

What is the culture of our discipline? Disciplines are generally recognised as distinct from one another in at least four ways: their issues (i.e., the problems the discipline seeks to solve or resolve), their modes of inquiry (i.e., ways of knowing), their literature (i.e., publications such as journals, texts, and tests), and their language (i.e., the vocabulary, ideas, and concepts). Through their academic and clinical coursework, students must learn to identify the central issues of concern to the discipline and the issues that emerge from their own clinical experiences; understand and experience the accepted modes of inquiry used to solve such problems; identify and utilise the extant literature of the discipline; and understand and use the language of the discipline. Such experiences should begin with students' first class, growing more complex as they move through a program. Additionally, these experiences must reflect the interactive and interdependent relationship of the four disciplinary components, recognising that one cannot functionally exist without the others.

Issues

The significant issues, or problems, that are central to a discipline contribute to defining the disciplinary culture, *and* they direct the work and resources of the discipline. Disciplinary leaders appoint Task Forces, or committees, to study particular issues and problems and develop position statements, guidelines, and technical reports; fund research to generate understanding and solutions to difficulties; sponsor meetings to disseminate the scholarly work of members; and publish journals to increase access to the discipline's work. In other words, the disciplinary issues form the foundation for conversations among the members of the discipline, the research agendas for scholars, programs for disciplinary meetings, and provide the substance for the public record of the discipline's work.

Most often, students take courses that are organised around informational topics, but without explicit examination of the disciplinary issues associated with those topics. For instance, introductory courses might include units of study that provide overviews of the profession, including the Code of Ethics, Scope of Practice, SLP/SLT qualifications, and employment opportunities; disorders; and assessment and treatment principles. Advanced graduate courses, generally designed for participants to examine specific disorders, are often organised around units of study related to aetiology, characteristics, assessment, treatment, and prevention. In many courses organised around topics, students passively receive information in a de-contextualised manner, preventing them from seeing the ways in which information becomes available as a result of asking questions about important issues.

On the other hand, coursework that is organised around questions and issues, instead of information, provides students with a context for understanding the value and relevance of particular pieces of information. For example, teachers could ask beginning students to answer this question: *What disorders can an SLP/SLT treat?* This would lead students into a study of the Scope of Practice. Graduate students might investigate more specific issues around which there exists professional disagreement and uncertainty. Examples of issues in phonology that students could study might include the issues of: what measures constitute a thorough assessment of the phonological system, the value of stimulability testing in assessment and treatment, what target selections result in the most efficacious treatments, or what constitutes clinically significant change.

Inquiry

Modes of inquiry, or accepted ways of examining the disciplinary issues and solving problems, also define the culture of a discipline. SLPs/SLTs employ a variety of forms of inquiry, from informal to formal. They explore ideas in writing, debate issues orally and in writing, and conduct various kinds of research. This research may be empirical or theoretical; quantitative, qualitative, or mixed; or basic or applied.

Instead of viewing the outcomes of these inquiries as answers to questions, students often understand these outcomes as facts when presented by a teacher, a supervising clinician, or a synoptic text. Consequently, students are denied the opportunity to appreciate the complexity of the disciplinary issues and to undertake their own investigations. For undergraduate students, research often takes the form of reporting about assigned topics, primarily a summarising task. Graduate students sometimes design and conduct their own studies; however, this practice is not universal. And, for those who do complete a study, they often do so with a limited understanding of research as a process by which questions can be answered. Coursework that examines disciplinary issues naturally supports learning about the ways a discipline inquires into, and attempts to solve, disciplinary problems. Beginning students learn that information is more than facts; it is the product of inquiry and is uniquely situated within particular social, cultural, historical, and philosophical contexts. Unless fledgling students interact with primary sources, these contexts will remain invisible to them. As students progress through their programs, and as they continue to interact with primary sources, they develop an appreciation for the relative value and contributions of the various kinds of inquiry methods SLPs/SLTs use to generate knowledge. By learning about the principles of evidence-based practice and using these principles in their own theoretical studies, students will develop the ability to draw on, and benefit from, the inquiries of other professionals. Consequently, when the time comes for graduate students to conduct their own research, they design experiments consistent with the quality expected within the discipline.

Literature

The culture of a discipline is also characterised by its literature. This literature includes historical texts that chronicle the development of the discipline and represent its central theories; diagnostic tests or tools; synoptic texts; and journals published by professional organisations. Some of these publications are primary sources, or those that represent original work, and some are secondary sources, or those that interpret original work. Each type of publication has specific advantages and disadvantages, and throughout their academic careers students should use a variety of these texts.

The prevalent practice of relying on secondary sources, such as synoptic texts, as a main resource in academic coursework brings to light two problems. First, unless students are explicitly taught the difference between primary and secondary sources, they rarely question the veracity of secondary sources. In other words, they consume information without questioning the inherent biases, contexts, or motivations of the authors. Second, unless students are explicitly taught how to utilise primary resources, they often struggle with reading and understanding texts of this kind. These struggles often compel students to revert to using more accessible secondary sources at times when they should be interpreting information for themselves.

Academic programs must be deliberate and strategic about introducing students to the discipline's literature. Beginning students will benefit from knowing about the various publications associated with the discipline as well as using primary sources, such as a key historical document, to supplement their learning about the discipline. Upper level undergraduate students will benefit from using diagnostic tests and tools to better understand principles of assessment. As well, these same undergraduates should use additional primary source materials as well as synoptic texts and learn how to critically analyse all of their resources. By the time they reach graduate school, they should be skilled at processing, and rely more heavily on, primary sources. Developing proficiency in using primary sources as students makes it more likely that they will turn to the literature to guide their clinical practice after their education.

Language

A specialised form of discourse, or language, is another characteristic of a disciplinary culture. This language, generally agreed on by members of the discipline, is composed of specific vocabulary and terminology, ideas, concepts, and conventions for written and spoken communications. In addition to acquiring vocabulary, students must understand the discipline's ideas and concepts. Furthermore, students must develop the skill of using this language to communicate effectively, in both oral and written forms, with other professionals as well as broader audiences.

Educational programs, by and large, excel in teaching students the language of the discipline. Through coursework, teachers transmit the major ideas and concepts to students and assess student learning. Undergraduate students, in particular, are rarely required to use these ideas and concepts beyond course assessment activities. Consequently, students rarely have opportunities to make decisions about what language, ideas, and concepts to use in order to solve particular clinical problems or to communicate solutions to others.

Students, especially those at the undergraduate level, must be given opportunities to demonstrate their understanding of the language of the discipline as well as opportunities to use that language in contextually appropriate activities. These activities should correlate with the students' levels of training. Beginning undergraduate students might develop informational pieces, such as brochures or Web sites, concerning communication disorders in general. Upper level undergraduate students can develop pieces concerning prevention activities or information about particular disorders. All undergraduate students can write an annotated bibliography, a literature review, or a scholarly paper. Graduate students, who have opportunities to use the disciplinary language in both academic and clinical work, must write scholarly papers and clinical documents.

Methods

Instructional methods can also socialise students into the culture of the discipline by teaching them the specific ways that professionals think about and conduct their work. Specifically, programs must use teaching methods that require students to ask questions; collect, select, and analyse resources; and publish their findings. By capitalising on the intra-relationships between the issues, modes of inquiry, language, and literature of the discipline, these methods contribute to the development of a professional identity. As a result, students are transformed from passive learners to independent and ethical practitioners capable of keeping pace with a rapidly changing and growing discipline.

Clinical problem solving

It probably goes without saying that certain linguistic principles can help us in devising evidence-based therapies that are conducive to treatment efficacy. Dr. B. May Bernhardt has been a clinical SLP since 1972 and is a professor at the University of British Columbia in Vancouver, Canada. Her major areas of research are in phonological and phonetic development, assessment, and intervention. Other interests include general language impairment in children and implications of First Nations English dialects for SLP. Angela Ullrich, MA, has been working as a research associate at the University of Cologne in Germany since 2005, and she also works as a clinical SLP in a private clinic, mainly with children with protracted phonological development. Currently she is writing her PhD thesis under the co-supervision of Drs. Roswitha Romonath and Dr. B. May Bernhardt, in which she has developed a phonological assessment tool for German-speaking children (NILPOD), based on constraint-based non-linear phonological theories.

Q32.   B. May Bernhardt and Angela Ullrich: A German–Canadian connection around constraints-based non-linear phonology

A striking finding that arose from non-linear phonological intervention studies in British Columbia (Major and Bernhardt 1998; Bernhardt, Brooke, and Major 2003) was the relationship between therapists' academic preparation and children's speech production outcomes. An analysis of factors such as educational background, years of experience, confidence level in the nonlinear approaches, and general treatment style (drill, play, or both) revealed that therapists with undergraduate linguistics degrees achieved superior results to therapists with SLP masters degrees and no linguistics undergraduate training. As Bernhardt (2004) points out, there is much yet to learn about practitioner training and intervention outcomes. What in particular would you both encourage SLPs/SLTs who do not have a strong linguistics background to pursue in their CPD/CEU endeavours, and how can goal-setting based on constraints-based non-linear phonological analyses expedite intelligibility gains?

A32. B. May Bernhardt and Angela Ullrich: Constraints-based non-linear phonology: Why and how to start

Primary sources of CE for SLPs/SLTs are on-the-job training from other SLPs/SLTs, workshops, conferences, and readings, the majority of which are focused directly on the clinical practice of SLP. Given an option between a workshop demonstrating some new clinical procedure and a conference on the latest developments in linguistics or psychology, the vast majority of SLPs/SLTs will choose to attend the former educational opportunity. The gap between research in psychology and linguistics and therapy with 'Susie' at 10 AM on Friday may seem insurmountable for clinicians without a strong university preparation in psychology or linguistics. Yet, as noted in the preamble to this question, one small study (Bernhardt 2004) has suggested that there may be a good reason for clinicians to be well-informed in linguistics. Goal-setting based on constraints-based non-linear phonological analyses may expedite gains in intelligibility. The following section provides an overview of studies supporting that perspective, before we return to the question of CE for SLTs/SLPs.

Constraints-based non-linear phonological theories have arisen over the last three decades in linguistics. Many of the basic tenets of the theories are assumed currently: that there are many levels of phonological form, from the phrase to the word to the syllable to the consonant or vowel to the feature, and that, in terms of phonological patterns, these levels can act independently ('constraints on pronunciation' affecting specific features or syllable positions) or interactively ('constraints' affecting features in specific contexts only). A description of current phonological theories is beyond the scope of this contribution, but the following short overview of clinical studies may provide some motivation for readers to learn more about these theories.

Table A32.1 lists the major British Columbia studies of non-linear phonological intervention for children with moderately to severely protracted phonological development (PPD). The single-subject design studies included from 2 to 20 children each, with durations of 16–18 weeks.

Although there was considerable variation in how the projects were implemented, four types of goals were generally targeted (see Table A32.2) that addressed word structure or segments (consonants and vowels) as either 'new' elements or elements in new combinations. SLPs/SLTs used both familiar activities and new ones that fitted the particular words for treatment (which did not include words for test probes). Caregivers were involved in the sessions and conducted home activities.

Table A32.1 Field studies conducted in nonlinear phonological intervention in British Columbia

Year	Investigators	Type	Number, ages of children	Project Duration
1990	Bernhardt (1990)	Dissertation	6: 3–6 yr	18 wk, 3×/wk
	Von Bremen (1990)	Master's thesis	Twin boys: 5 yr	18 wk, 3×/wk
1993–1994	Field SLPs across BC B. M. Bernhardt -Introductory workshop -Rigid design direction (Major and Bernhardt 1998; Bernhardt and Major 2005)	Quasi-experimental alternating conditions, rigid single subject design	20: 3–5 yr	16 wk, 3×/wk
1995	Edwards (1995)	Flexible single-subject design	2: 4 yr	16 wk, 2×/wk
1997–	Field SLPs Bernhardt, Major, Edwards -Introductory workshop -Minimal direction (Bernhardt, Brooke, and Major 2003)	Flexible single-subject design	17: 3–6 yr	16 wk, 2×/wk

Two major results pertain particularly to this question. The first concerns the goal type, and the second, clinician effectiveness. Concerning goal type, it was found that word shape goals (CVC, CVCV, CCV, etc.) were attained significantly faster than segmental goals in the first half of each study. Although intelligibility studies were not conducted, it is clear that an increase in use of within-word and word-final consonants and clusters would have an immediate positive effect on intelligibility.

The second result concerns clinician effectiveness. The 1994 and 1997 studies differed in that, for the former, Bernhardt did the analyses, chose goals, and provided stimuli and treatment strategies for the clinicians. In the 1997 study, clinicians were given the transcripts

Table A32.2 Types of goals addressed in non-linear phonological intervention studies

Phonological level in the hierarchy	New form	New combinations or interactions of existing form
Phrase and word structures	New word shapes, e.g., CVC	Establishing an existing segment (consonant or vowel) in (a) an established word position new to that segment, or (b) in a new sequence by word position
Segments (consonants or vowels) and their features	New features, e.g., [Dorsal] (velar)	New combinations of features already in the system, e.g., combining the 'fricative' features of an existing [f] with the coronal (alveolar) features of a /t/ to target [s]

of the assessment tapes. In accordance with what they had learned in a workshop, they did their own data analyses and goal-setting (which were briefly confirmed by the investigator). Principles of goal-setting and sequence were the same, but there was more flexibility, with the treatment being individualised. Another difference was that the 1997 study had twice-weekly therapy compared with thrice-weekly for the 1994 study. In terms of overall gains in Percent Consonant Match (PCM), there was no significant difference between the studies across children: a 16.4% gain in 1994 and 18.6% in 1997. These outcomes demonstrate that clinicians can learn to implement new ideas in treatment with minimal supervision. Comparing the results with other studies *not* based on non-linear phonology, Tyler and Lewis (2005) reported PCM gains of 7–20% for a longer (24-week) study, and Erickson (2007) a 7% mean gain for a 12–16 week study. Thus, non-linear phonological intervention for English has had observable benefits for clients in clinical field research studies of 16–18 weeks' duration. But what can be expected after single-weekend workshops? We turn now to a recent project by Angela Ullrich on this topic.

Non-linear phonological theories in clinical assessment have been mainly applied in Anglo-American countries. For Angela Ullrich's dissertation project, a nonlinear phonological assessment tool (*Nichtlineare phonologische Diagnostik,* NILPOD; Ullrich 2007) was developed for German-speaking children. NILPOD is conceptually based on Bernhardt and Stemberger's (2000) non-linear scan analysis in its application of constraint-based non-linear phonological theories (as shown in Table A32.2).

In order to evaluate effectiveness and clinical applicability of NILPOD, and also importantly, the effectiveness of knowledge transfer concerning a complex linguistic theory like non-linear phonology, an evaluation study was conducted in Cologne. Fifty-seven clinicians were trained in a 3-day weekend workshop to apply the assessment tool NILPOD. The group included German SLPs and logopedists with a range of 2 to 35 years of clinical practice experience. The linguistics background of most participating clinicians was rather limited, because linguistics coursework has been under-represented in the SLP curriculum in Germany. The first and second days of the workshop thus outlined basic concepts of phonetics and constraint-based non-linear phonology before the demonstration of phonological analyses using NILPOD. On the third day, a hands-on session was conducted, in which participants were given a transcribed data set of a child with PPD. They performed a non-linear analysis of the data alone or in groups, including identification of therapy goals. Ullrich assisted them as required and reviewed results at the end of the day.

At the end of the workshop, clinicians were asked to complete an evaluation form covering questions about their professional background, the structure and content of the workshop, and how the knowledge gained about non-linear phonology might affect their assessment and treatment of phonological impairment. Every clinician also received background information and transcribed data from four German-speaking children with PPD for home practice and NILPOD evaluation. Clinicians were asked to analyse the data by using the NILPOD analysis and select three short-term therapy goals. Clinicians were also asked to complete a final questionnaire, which included rating scales concerning the analysis sheets, the applicability and the efficiency of analysis, and the relevance of therapy goals, plus a set of open-ended questions inviting their suggestions for improvements to NILPOD.

The workshop evaluation form showed that 86% of the clinicians wanted to learn more about non-linear phonology and NILPOD; 70% stated that they understood the theoretical background; and 67% found the workshop, including the linguistic theory, relevant for their clinical practice. A lower percentage (39%) indicated that the workshop clearly changed their perception of phonological impairment. A number of key themes arose in response to an open-ended question set: (1) the importance of word structure for work in phonological intervention, (2) the importance of considering strengths and needs of the phonological system in goal selection, and (3) the relevance of the concept of phonological hierarchy for understanding phonological difficulties. After performing the four NILPOD analyses at home, similar results were observed in the 30 clinicians who returned the analyses. Additionally, 67% found that NILPOD gave detailed information to derive useful therapy goals. A lower percentage (29%) stated that they realised the necessity of doing detailed phonological analyses that are based on complex linguistic theories. Five clinicians wrote explicitly that they had already noticed the positive effects of the workshop training in their clinical work. As a negative open-ended comment, 42% noted that the analysis was both too time-consuming and complex in its current (workshop) version. Others stated that they did not feel confident enough yet to implement NILPOD themselves. Clinician's suggestions are being incorporated in the final (pre-publication) revision of NILPOD, especially ideas to improve time efficiency, avoid redundancy of analysis steps, and streamline and clarify analysis sheets. The comments regarding the NILPOD resonate with many of those offered in evaluation forms for Bernhardt's workshops on nonlinear phonology: 'I'll never look at an artic test the same way again'; 'I will pay far more attention to word structure than I ever did before' (very frequent comment); 'The idea of identifying both strengths and needs of the phonological system makes sense'; or 'The concept of "default" was useful and interesting'. Overall results show that a workshop can improve a clinician's basic understanding of phonological impairment and positively influence his/her clinical practice, through application of some of the major principles of constraint-based non-linear phonology: that is, taking phonological hierarchy into account, paying attention to word structure, considering strengths and needs of the phonological system when choosing therapy goals, and using constraints to explain underlying phonological difficulties.

The results of the studies in Canada and Germany suggest that clinicians can learn to incorporate more current versions of phonological analyses into practice with short-term training. If there are no available workshops or university courses in the clinician's immediate area, however, what options are there for CE? A book or journal club may be a useful solution, perhaps starting with the readings recommended below. Another suggestion might be for a clinical agency to form a partnership with a university linguistics program. Through ongoing case study, readings, and dialogue, the linguists could provide current theoretical perspectives, and the clinicians could provide data for the linguists to consider when developing theories. The Bernhardt studies suggest a more formal possibility: university researchers and students are often looking for clinicians to participate in evaluation studies of assessment or therapy approaches. Such partnerships can help close the gap between research and practice and, in so doing, enhance outcomes for the clients: one of the main objectives of CE.

Recommended readings

For English, an introductory article that may be easy to locate is Bernhardt and Stoel-Gammon (1994). For German, Ullrich and Bernhardt (2005) includes an introduction to non-linear phonology. For more in-depth learning, the Bernhardt and Stemberger (2000) *Workbook in Nonlinear Phonology for Clinical Application* has exercises for practice, case examples, and treatment method suggestions. Other case-based articles provide more examples of analysis and goal-setting, for example, Bernhardt (1992), Bernhardt and Gilbert (1992), Baker and Bernhardt (2004), Bernhardt (2005), and Bernhardt, Stemberger, and Major (2006). Advanced readings include Bernhardt and Stemberger (1998, 2007), Bernhardt, Gilbert, and Ingram (1996), and Dinnsen and Gierut (2008).

For SLP/SLT readers who want to begin their own clinical application of nonlinear phonology, Bernhardt and Holdgrafer (2001a, b) give information on word list construction for speech samples that facilitate nonlinear analyses. Computer programs that provide quantitative support for nonlinear analyses are Masterson and Bernhardt's (2001) *Computerized Articulation and Phonology Evaluation System (CAPES)*, and Long's (2007) *Computerized Profiling* shareware http://www.computerizedprofiling.org/downloads.html).

Reading and critically evaluating the literature

Assuming that the reader had covered phonological theory 101, and no more, Bernhardt and Stemberger (1998) provided an introduction to non-linear phonology and to its constraint-based implementation in Optimality Theory, explaining how this framework can describe and explain data on protracted phonological development (PPD), and the interface of their work with speech processing and connectionism. Then, helpfully switching focus to address SLP/SLT clinicians, Bernhardt and Stemberger (1998) produced a plain-English workbook in non-linear phonology for clinical application. These publications were predated by accessible tutorial articles for clinicians, for example, Bernhardt and Stoel-Gammon (1994), and Stemberger and Bernhardt (1997), and followed by case based accounts, such as Baker and Bernhardt (2004). Rather than regularly turning to these works and others like them for elucidation and help with difficult phonologies, clinicians shy away, regarding non-linear approaches in general as something new and difficult. Similarly, the author has seen many experienced, committed clinicians in CPD/CEU events tune out at the very sight of syllable trees in the context of phonotactic therapy (Velleman 2002), and as mentioned previously Joffe and Pring (2008) even report that one of their respondents said that she and other therapists she knew were 'terrified' by psycholinguistic models (Stackhouse and Wells 1997).

Q33 is addressed to Dr. Karen Froud, the director of the Neurocognition of Language Lab, and Assistant Professor of Speech-Language Pathology in the Department of Biobehavioral Sciences at Teachers College, Columbia University, in New York. She holds a PhD in Linguistics from University College London, and her research is concerned with the neurological underpinnings of linguistic processing and representation in normal and disordered language. She teaches Neuroscience, Adult Language Disorders, and Language Development to graduate students in the SLP program at TC, while maintaining a wide range of collaborative research projects in linguistics and the neurosciences, including work on the neural correlates of child speech disorders.

Q33.   Karen Froud: A Transatlantic spin on the theory to practice gap

There is an immediate and striking applicability to our understanding of children's phonological disorders and approaches to their assessment and treatment of non-linear models and psycholinguistic frameworks. Why do you think it is that clinicians are apparently so unambitious in tackling the research literature, and so conservative in applying and evaluating for themselves new, and not-so-new, theories and findings?

A33.   Karen Froud: Understanding and addressing the theory-to-practice divide in clinical training and practice

Why do we need theoretical models and frameworks? It has long been understood that there is a kind of 'disconnect' between sensory percepts (like acoustic signals) and the mental representations with which we associate them (like the mental image of an object or a situation in the world). In the domain of speech and language, this disconnect is particularly evident, and particularly vexing. There is nothing in the properties of an acoustic signal which biases that signal to be interpreted by the human mind as having referential properties; for example, auditory coding of frequency, intensity and phase in the cochlea is not directly related to retrieving the semantic properties of a real-life object or situation (but see Smith and Lewicki 2006, for suggestions that cochlear coding mechanisms may have adapted to maximise efficiency when processing speech sounds). The relationship between mental representations and speech signals, either for production or for comprehension, is quite opaque.

The traditional way to bridge this divide has been to develop models of cognitive processes, to help us understand the separate sub-processes that must be involved in relating sensory phenomena (like sounds) to mental representations (like concepts). Such models are useful because they permit a breakdown of the ways in which complex mental operations may occur, at the same time as abstracting away from complicating factors like individual differences, contextual effects, or psychological states.

Developing models that provide step-by-step breakdowns of the sub-processes and different levels of representation involved in speech and language processing has been very fruitful for clinicians, and has led to the development and testing of various approaches to assessment and treatment. For example, Hodson and Paden (1981), in their well-known *cycles* (or patterns) approach, take the view that stimulability (and hence perception) for a particular speech sound should be in place *before* that sound is targeted for production (Hodson, A5).

Linearity (and non-linearity) in models of speech and language

Such step-by-step views of speech sound development and remediation can be thought of as linear, in the sense that they conceive of speech and language as involving several processes that succeed each other in a predictable sequence. We are used to thinking of speech and language in a linear way, largely because the first step in any kind of fine-grained analysis is to chop up the signal into 'slices' (or segments) of information, the better to examine each segment independently of other factors (this is a standard approach in all kinds of linguistic analysis and was detailed very early in the history of generative linguistics (Harris 1951). However, this view of the linguistic signal as having a linear nature is quite problematic and really only comes from this way of segmenting complex signals and looking at them in a step-by-step manner. It's clear that speech and language are not really linear at all—such complex signals are multi-dimensional in nature, and different aspects of the speech stream overlap one another in processing and representation (Goldsmith 1972). Especially since it has become standard to examine cognitive operations from the perspective of their neural correlates, in experimental investigations utilising EEG, fMRI, and other brain-imaging techniques, it has become ever more apparent that the mapping between sensory stimuli and mental representations cannot be one-to-one, and does not unfold in a stepwise fashion over time. The involvement of various brain regions—and by hypothesis, various cognitive operations—in any given mental process is complex, multilayered, and not sequential in nature. Activations overlap in time and space, and even on an intuitive level we 'know' that we do not wait to build the syntactic structure of a whole phrase—or the phonological structure of a whole word, or the metrical structure of a whole syllable—before we begin to engage other systems, such as those required to identify semantic or pragmatic or prosodic properties of the same incoming signal. Even in the acoustic signal itself, the lowest-level sensory input, there is no discreteness of phonemes, syllables, or words; rather these units overlap, and are not perceived independently of one another (Fowler 1995). Nonlinear theories can be thought of as a response to this kind of problem with linear analyses. Rather than simplifying everything into a series of linearly associated representations, non-linear approaches try to take account of multiple levels of processing and representation occurring simultaneously (Goldsmith 1972; McCarthy 1988; Liberman and Prince 1977).

What's so hard about non-linearity?

Given this situation, what is it that makes non-linear approaches so apparently unappealing to those of us working in clinical professions? Is it just that the non-linear theoretical frameworks are somehow too 'difficult' for us, so we prefer not to concern ourselves with them and work instead within the 'simpler' linear approaches? The problem with that is, of course, that linear approaches are not necessarily 'simpler'. New theoretical developments are typically aimed at simplifying the amount of theoretical machinery required to gain the same (or a greater) degree of empirical coverage as earlier versions, and the shift from linear to non-linear approaches in phonology, like the move towards a Minimalist framework for syntax (Chomsky 1995), shares this goal. Most of the recent developments in relating linguistic theory to SLP have been motivated by simplification, too. For instance, before distinctive feature theory (Chomsky and Halle 1968) was widely accepted, the typical approach to remediation of phonological or articulation disorders was to take each 'error' individually, classify it as substitution, omission, or distortion (Van Riper 1978), and treat it separately from any other errors with no expectation of generalisation (Bernhardt and Stoel-Gammon 1994). With the widespread acceptance of phonological features (rather than segments) as the units of analysis and treatment, generalisation within classes of sounds could be expected, and was documented (Costello and Onstine 1976). Theoretical advances, far from being complications, actually resulted in simplification of remediation approaches, *and* in greater generalisation of therapeutic gains.

It has been argued that non-linear approaches have the potential to do the same. For instance, feature geometry clearly outlines how change at one level could be expected to filter throughout the entire system for speech sound representation. Feature geometries (McCarthy 1988; Bernhardt and Stemberger 1998) attempt to show how the relations between phonological features are hierarchically organised. Targeting speech sound intervention at higher levels in such a hierarchy is predicted to result in 'trickle-down' effects, meaning that careful choice of intervention targets can have widespread effects on the child's representation of many speech sounds. Supporting evidence has even been provided, in the form of several studies examining children's phonological disorders within non-linear frameworks, developing intervention strategies based on constructs of such frameworks and evaluating efficacy in clinical cases (Bernhardt 1992; Gierut 1989; Bernhardt and Stoel-Gammon 1994; and see Bernhardt and Ullrich, A32). Examples are proliferating: within the field of SSD, theoretically motivated interventions based on non-linear frameworks include minimal contrast approaches (e.g., *PACT*: Bowen and Cupples 1999), maximal oppositions (Gierut 1992), and approaches designed to increase metaphonological awareness (*Metaphon*: Howell and Dean 1994).

So, it's not apparent that linear approaches are 'simpler' than non-linear frameworks. It's not true that the non-linear approaches have been ignored in the field. It's not even the case that we have no evidence for the efficacy and generalisability of non-linear approaches to speech sound remediation. So what is going on? Why is there such resistance in our profession to staying abreast of theoretical advances that have great potential to enhance our understanding and remediation of phonological (and other) disorders?

What can we do about the theory-to-practice divide?

I think that this situation is very circular in nature. At least in part, it arises because clinicians are too busy, and lacking in the necessary background, to read and critically evaluate the research literature. Most students still do not encounter the newer theoretical approaches during their academic training, and most clinicians (there are notable exceptions, of course) do not use any recognisable theoretical framework to inform their interventions. The direct effect of this is that even students who do care about theoretical frameworks and their utility in clinical investigations will have, at best, only limited opportunities to explore these, in or out of the classroom—yielding another generation of clinicians who lack the confidence and background to implement shifts in thinking about representation and process in speech and language. The frustration gets compounded on all sides: clinicians feel that the research is lagging way behind their own intuitive thinking for treatment planning and implementation; and researchers think that clinicians simply ignore or don't use the work that goes into elucidating questions with deep relevance for clinical practice.

I believe it's time for a sea change. A large part of the solution to this ongoing problem lies with the educators and researchers working in universities where clinicians are trained; we have to take that bold step, start teaching the newer theories, make sure that we are also up to date, and instil into students that reading the literature is not just another commitment to fit in around field placements. We are also obligated to provide students with the tools to approach the relevant research independently, and critically. This means teaching rigorous courses in research design, evaluation of research, statistics, even philosophy of science. For instance, the processes of hypothesis formation and testing should be basic, consciously available tools in the repertoire of *every* clinician. Furthermore, it seems to me essential that every SLP/SLT program provide a fair degree of training in linguistics, including phonology. SSDs are not just articulatory disorders; we are speech and *language* pathologists, and the training should support this duality (Nunes, A3). This is the first step in taking theory into practice: we must provide the theoretical frameworks and the tools for evaluating them.

The second step, of course, is moving the theoretically driven approaches into the clinical arena. It's no good if a new emphasis on research and theory comes only from the academic programs. Students need to see this rigorous and inclusive approach being implemented in their field placements, too. They need to recognise that the theoretical frameworks are not simply things one has to learn in order to pass the final. Clinicians and supervisors can shift their mindsets and their practices; they can assimilate new theoretical developments and discuss these with colleagues; they can develop and implement strategies for assessment and intervention that have a firm theoretical grounding. By doing so, not only do we stand to provide better training for our students and better care for our clients, we also stand to contribute data and experience that can guide the development of ever more fine-grained theories of the mental representations and processes involved in speech and language.

In summary, theoretical frameworks serve a purpose: they are there to help us understand complex processes at a level of abstraction which renders the complexities at least somewhat transparent. In clinical fields like SLP, this should have the advantage of permitting a more detailed understanding of the mechanisms underlying a disorder, and hence motivating approaches to assessment and intervention. In linguistics, there have been logarithmic advances in recent years in our understanding of linguistic rules and representations, at every level from speech sounds to mapping between language and cognition. Better understanding leads to better approaches to assessment and remediation. We are speech-language professionals: we have a responsibility to understand and disseminate advances in our field. It's simply not possible to effectively remediate a language disorder if we don't know anything about language. The challenge to our field, then, is to keep abreast of theoretical advances and take real, bold steps to incorporate them into our practice. This holds for everyone, from students to clinical fellows, clinical supervisors, senior professionals, researchers, and the professors providing the academic training; and it's a necessary step, to maintain ethical, efficacious, well-motivated approaches to assessment and remediation in our field.

A model for ethical practices

Dr. Thomas W. Powell is Professor of Speech-Language Pathology in the Department of Rehabilitation Sciences at Louisiana State University Health Sciences Center in Shreveport. He serves as a co-editor of the international journal *Clinical Linguistics and Phonetics*. His professional interests include phonological disorders, aphasia, clinical phonetics, multilingualism, and ethics.

Q34.   Thomas W. Powell: Professional ethics and NS-OMEs

In a nationwide survey of 537 SLPs in the United States, Lof and Watson (2004) determined that 85% used NS-OME to change speech sound productions, and a similar study of 535 SLPs across Canada by Hodge, Salonka, and Kollias (2005) yielded exactly the same finding. Your multi-faceted Model for Ethical Practices in Clinical Phonetics and Linguistics, presented at the 11th Symposium of the International Clinical Phonetics and Linguistics Association (ICPLA) in Dubrovnik, Croatia, in 2006, delineates six ethical domains. They are: beneficence, non-maleficence, competence, compliance, integrity, and respect; and they apply across four levels of interaction with peers, students, participants, and the general public. Can you provide the reader with an account of the model, and explain how it could be applied to the decision-making process of to be or not to be an oral motor therapist?

A34.   Thomas W. Powell: NS-OMEs: An ethical challenge

As speech and language professionals, we enjoy certain rights and privileges. We make decisions and provide services that impact the lives of others. In return, we receive compensation for our expertise, as well as the satisfaction that results from helping another human to communicate more effectively. As professionals, we also share a responsibility for providing the highest possible quality of service and for protecting our clients from exploitation. Ethical codes empower us to monitor and evaluate our own conduct; they help us to maintain professional autonomy and reduce the need for external regulation (Irwin, Pannbacker, Powell, et al. 2007).

The model of ethics in Figure A34.1 is adapted from a previous work (Powell 2007). This model was inspired by an international sample of ethical codes from professional SLP associations. Codes from related disciplines (e.g., linguistics, forensic phonetics, acoustics) were considered as well, and several common principles were identified during this review process:

- **Beneficence:** We seek to do good by acting in the best interest of others.
- **Non-maleficence:** We pledge to do no harm and to minimize risks to others.
- **Respect:** We agree to respect differences, as well as the rights of others.
- **Integrity:** We promise to be honest and to avoid conflicts of interest.
- **Compliance:** We agree to work within established rules and laws.
- **Competence:** We accept responsibility for ensuring a high quality of service, including appropriate delegation and referral.

Most ethical standards for professional and scientific associations are linked to one or more of these six principles.

Principles of ethical behaviour may have somewhat different implications as we interact with different groups. Specifically, this model differentiates among four levels of interaction: with other professionals (peers), with students and/or assistants (subordinates), with clients, and with the general public.

Our ethical imperative to act in the best interest of our clients includes the responsibility for selecting treatment approaches that are in the best interest of our clients (i.e., beneficence). Accordingly, we should avoid treatments that carry a degree of risk

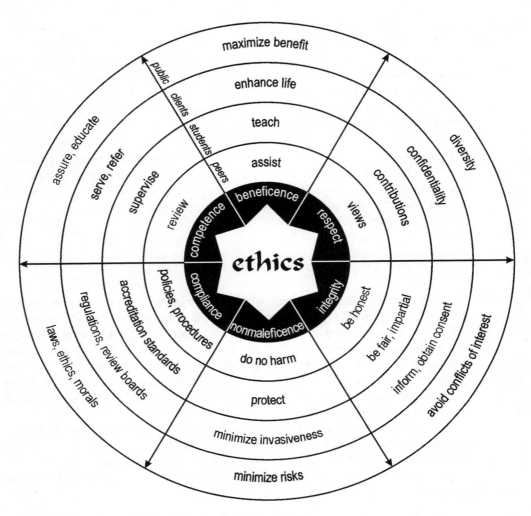

Figure A34.1 A six-factor model for ethical practice in SLP.

(non-maleficence). We must be respectful of differences and affirm others' right to privacy (respect). We seek to be honest and to provide information accurately and impartially (integrity). We recognise the limits of our knowledge and skills, and we refer appropriately (competence). Finally, we agree to observe and obey policies, procedures, guidelines, and laws (compliance).

I believe that the resourcefulness and creativity of speech and language clinicians is a strength of our profession. Our education encourages critical thinking and independent problem solving (McAllister and Lincoln 2004); consequently, we tend to be sceptical of generic 'one size fits all' treatments. Instead, we tend to value intervention plans that address the specific needs of our clients (Kamhi 2006b). When faced with difficult clinical challenges, we may put on our 'thinking caps' and develop novel treatment approaches to help our clients. But are good intentions sufficient in an ethical sense? Sadly, history shows that many dubious treatments have been developed by well-intentioned people in the helping professions (Jacobson, Foxx, and Mulick 2005).

Although innovation is desirable, we must be mindful of our ethical responsibilities as we introduce novel treatments into the clinical setting (Lum 2002). Professional associations advocate unbiased scientific evaluation of new treatments before widespread clinical application, and currently the most commonly employed framework is that of evidence-based practice (ASHA 2005; Dollaghan 2007; Reilly, Douglas, and Oates 2004; Taylor-Goh 2005).

Unfortunately, not all treatments are equally effective, and our field has perhaps been less systematic in assessing treatment efficacy than one might wish (Tharpe 1998). Recently, non-speech oral-motor treatments (NS-OMTs) have generated considerable controversy in this regard. Although non-speech exercises have been used for many years (cf. Nemoy and Davis 1937; Swift 1918), there have been few controlled studies of their effectiveness (Lass and Pannbacker 2008). Nevertheless, many clinicians use NS-OMTs as part of their treatment regimen (Lof and Watson 2008).

In theory, NS-OMTs are designed to establish improved articulator control during non-speech activities, with the expectation that gains in oral function will enhance speech production (Bahr 2001; Marshalla 2004; Rosenfeld-Johnson 2001; Strode and Chamberlain 1997). In practice, the use of NS-OMTs has not been limited to motor-based speech movement disorders (dysarthria). Proponents have recommended oral-motor exercises to treat phonological disorders (Marshalla 2004, p. 109; Rosenfeld-Johnson 2001, p. 1), as well as speech disorders associated with hearing impairment (Loncar-Belding 1998, p. 5; Orr 1998, p. 1). The diversity of presenting diagnoses is perhaps most strikingly illustrated in a retrospective study by Beckman, Neal, Phirsichbaum, et al. (2004), who described the use of NS-OMTs with children representing more than 75 different diagnoses, including Trisomy 21, ankyloglossia, cleft lip and palate, ear infections, heart problems, spina bifida, and bruxism. Larroudé (2004, p. 139) described how the use of oral-motor exercises has been incorporated into a multicultural–multilingual group programme designed to improve functional communication. Clearly, NS-OMTs are being used to treat a wide range of conditions, aside from primary motor speech disorders.

Although many speech and language clinicians employ NS-OMT approaches (Lof and Watson 2008), there has been considerable controversy regarding the adequacy of the underlying theory (Lof 2003; Ruscello 2008b) as well as a disconcerting lack of experimental evidence (Forrest 2002; Lass and Pannbacker 2008). Concerns about the widespread adoption of such methods have been voiced by many authorities on SSD in children (Baker and Bernhardt 2004; Bankson and Bernthal 2004; Bowen 2005; Clark 2003; Davis and Velleman 2000; Forrest 2002; Hodge 2002; Kamhi 2006b; Lof 2002, 2003; Lof and Watson 2008; Powell 2008a; Ruscello 2008b; Rvachew 2005a; Shelton 2005; Shriberg 2003; Tyler 2005; Weismer 1997; Williams 2003b).

Ethical considerations can help us evaluate our treatment decisions, and this process is especially important when one is considering a controversial approach such as NS-OMTs. The principle of beneficence leads us to consider treatment options critically and to adopt procedures that are appropriate for the individual client. Factors to be considered include the nature of the disorder, the client's capability and focus, the clinician's knowledge and skills, the nature and evidence base of the treatment, as well as logistical considerations such as scheduling frequency (Baker and Bernhardt 2004; Kwiatkowski and Shriberg 1998; Powell 2008b).

Although the use of controversial or experimental treatments is not prohibited by most codes of professional ethics, certain conditions should be met to ensure their ethical use. First, treatment methods and outcome measures must be clearly defined, and these procedures must be evaluated by an institutional ethical review board (compliance). Treatment should be provided only if the clinician possesses the appropriate knowledge and skills (competence). Potential contraindications and safety issues (e.g., infection control) should be considered carefully (non-maleficence). Additionally, we have an obligation to provide the client (or responsible adult, in the case of minors) with honest information about the procedure, including potential risks and cost-to-benefit ratios (integrity). Informed consent must be obtained (compliance). To experiment on a client who is unaware of the controversial nature of the treatment would represent a serious infraction of basic ethical standards (Irwin, Pannbacker, Powell, et al. 2007).

Although ethical models provide guidelines for ethical problem solving, ultimately professionals must make decisions on the basis of available information. Duchan, Calculator, Sonnenmeier, et al. (2001) provided a useful framework for clinicians who elect to provide controversial treatments (such as NS-OMTs). This framework encourages a thorough understanding of controversial practices, including how they relate to more accepted treatment options. Procedures for obtaining informed consent should be developed, as well as for adapting treatment procedures to reflect the needs of individual clients. Clinicians are well advised to be scrupulous in their documentation (Duchan, et al. 2001). The use of single-subject methodologies, for example, can be an effective means of demonstrating accountability (Lum 2002). Finally, it is important to anticipate professional and/or legal challenges and to be prepared to resolve them (Duchan, et al. 2001).

In summary, although NS-OMTs are widely used, they continue to generate considerable controversy. Carefully designed studies are needed to evaluate NS-OMTs systematically across target populations; however, such studies must comply with generally accepted ethical practices, including informed consent. Until such data become available, speech and language clinicians are encouraged to utilise treatments with stronger scientific support (Forrest 2002; Gierut 1998). Aggressive marketing, at any rate, should never be mistaken for scientific evidence.

The last say

Best practice guidelines for SLP/SLT services require clinicians to act in accordance with the evidence and ethics of their own profession while keeping a larger framework of knowledge, principles, philosophies, and beliefs in mind (see Leitão, A48 and Powell, A34 for discussion). The bigger-picture framework grew out of years of collective research, practice, and client/family experiences across disciplines, settings, and cultures. Reflecting on the big picture, Bernstein Ratner (2006, p. 257) wrote, 'EBP is a valuable construct in ensuring quality of care. However, bridging between research evidence and clinical practice may require us to confront potentially difficult issues and establish thoughtful dialogue about best practices in fostering EBP itself.' Bernstein Ratner stresses the necessity for us to establish robust communication at all points, from laboratory to clinic. That is, between the funding bodies and researchers who develop the evidence, the academics who spread the word, the administrators who regulate change, the employers charged with maintaining beneficial workplaces, the practitioners who implement the evidence, and the client who, in egalitarian speech intervention in everyday practice, may have the last say.

Part II

Speech Intervention in Everyday Practice

Chapter 6

Symptomatic management of moderate and severe disorders

In Chapter 6, we look at issues in counselling, dynamic assessment, and differential diagnosis of children with moderate and severe SSD, including childhood apraxia of speech (CAS) or suspected CAS, sometimes called sCAS. The chapter also addresses intervention goals, approaches, and techniques for these children. Developmental Phonological Disorder (DPD) and CAS have at least six inter-related characteristics in common that, when it gets right down to it in everyday practice, we find ourselves treating symptomatically, while still taking the primary diagnosis into account. In this sense, we 'treat the symptoms and not the label'.

Six speech characteristics that CAS and DPD may have in common

The characteristics that can be evident in either disorder, or that may be present when CAS and DPD co-occur in the same child, are:

1. Consonant (C), vowel (V), and phonotactic inventory constraints;
2. Omissions of segments and structures: that is, omissions of consonants, vowels, and syllable shapes already in the child's repertoire;
3. Vowel errors including vowel replacements and distortions;
4. Altered suprasegmentals, that is, atypical prosody;
5. Increased errors with utterance length and/or complexity; and,
6. Use of simple, but not complex, syllable and word shapes.

In Box 6.1, the characteristics and signs of DPD are listed in the left column and suggestions for how to test and what to look for are in the right column. Similarly, Box 6.2 shows the characteristics of CAS, how to test, and observations.

Therapy goals in common in DPD and CAS

The six characteristics are listed in the left column of Table 6.1. Reading across Row 1, we see that the first characteristic is consonant and vowel inventory constraints, or in

Box 6.1 Testing for and observations of DPD

DPD Characteristics	Testing for/observations of DPD characteristics/signs
1. Static speech sound system	Look for stable PCC and stable percentage of occurrence of processes over time (6 to 12 weeks). Test: Relational Analysis
2. Variable production without gradual improvement <u>DEAP Inconsistency Assessment</u> 25 pictures named three times in one session. Productions are compared to calculate an inconsistency score (same lexical items within an identical context). <u>Inconsistent speech disorder:</u> Children with at least 40% of words produced variably. <u>Consistent speech disorder:</u> Children with at least two atypical patterns and an inconsistency score below 40% (Holm, Crosbie, and Dodd 2007)	'Inconsistent' has three distinct meanings in child phonology (Seddoh, Robin, Sim, et al. 1996): A. Variable production of a particular phone (e.g., [b]) or a sound class (e.g., voiced stops) in different word positions. For example, /b/ is produced word initially but replaced with a glottal within word. This type of inconsistency is attested in typical development and in children with phonological delays or disorders. B. Variable production of a particular phone (e.g., [b]) or a sound class (e.g., voiced stops) in the same word position. For example, a child may use [b] and [d] interchangeably in the word initial position. This type of inconsistency is seen in very young, typically developing children usually in the first 40 to 60 words they acquire. In some children, a few of these early word productions will persist as frozen forms (child can say chocolate but says /trɛə/ for chair). C. Variable production of a particular phone (e.g., [b]) or sound class (e.g., voiced stops) in multiple repetitions of the same word. In measures of the frequency of an error type that occurs in multiple repetitions of the same word, this type of variability is sometimes referred to as 'token-to-token variability'. Test: DEAP Inconsistency Assessment (see #2 in the left hand column)
3. Persistence of phonological processes	Persistence of phonological processes (natural processes, phonological patterns – call then what you will!) beyond typical age-expectations. Test: Relational Analysis: Study the norms.
4. 'Chronological Mismatch'	In this phenomenon, children with DPD acquire later 'more difficult' sounds, apparently bypassing early 'easy' sounds. Test: Observe CS.
5. Idiosyncratic rules	Non-developmental patterns; idiosyncratic patterns Test: Observe CS; look for patterns that are never produced by adults.
6. Restricted use of contrast	Look for constraints and homophony Test: Observations of speech data and contrastive assessment.
7. Puzzle phenomenon	Look at phonetic mastery relative to phonemic organisation Test: Observations of speech data.
8. Unusual errors	Look for unusual error-types: systematic sound preference; 'favourite sound'; 'favourite place' of articulation; 'favourite manner' of articulation Test: Observations of CS if possible.
9. Marking	Some children give us hints that their difficulties are phonological, not phonetic, by 'marking' the presence of the correct sound, indicating that they 'know' more than they can produce. Test: Look for marking with nasality or marking with vowel length.
10. Stimulability	Look for comparatively 'ready' stimulability. If the child is stimulable for a sound, even if only in isolation, but is not using it systematically, it may be that his/her difficulties are essentially phonological. Test: Stimulability testing to two syllable positions.

Box 6.2 Testing for and observations of CAS

Characteristics	Testing for/observations of CAS characteristics/signs
Receptive–expressive gap (Receptive performance outstrips expressive)	**Language Testing** Use any language test procedure(s) the child can manage. We may be unable to test in the formal sense. Testing may range from a simple Structural Analysis (MLUm and Brown's Stages), through to procedures like the RAPT (Renfrew 1997) or PPVT-3 (Dunn, Dunn, and Williams 1997), right up to demanding formal language batteries (CELF, CASL, etc.).
Delayed development of syllable and word structures	**Relational Analysis** Look for syllable structure processes: FCD, CR, WSD, Reduplication, Consonant Harmony. **Independent Analysis** Look at the phonotactic inventory and phonotactic constraints. **Test Instruments** Use the phonological process analysis of the DEAP, HAPP-3, QS, etc., and/or a CS Sample.
Deviant syllable structures and word structures	**Relational Analysis** Look for deviant (disordered/idiosyncratic) syllable structure errors (particularly ICD and schwa insertion/addition). **Independent Analysis** Look at phonotactic inventory (repertoire) and phonotactic constraints. **Test Instruments** DEAP, HAPP-3, Quick Screener, and/or a process analysis of a speech sample.
Sequencing difficulties	**Relational Analysis** Look for metathesis, word reversals, and unusual sequencing; especially uncommon examples: matdoor (doormat), Peeker Parter (Peter Parker), yoomsli/yoombleese (muesli). **Test Instruments** Motor speech examination; DEAP, NDP (Williams and Stephens 2004), TSSS (Kirkpatrick, Stohr, and Kimbrough 1990a, b), VMPAC (Hayden and Square 1999); or make informal observations of polysyllabic words. Caregivers often recount frequently used 'big words' and word combinations a child has difficulty sequencing. These may be useful later as 'power words'.
Word and syllable stress errors	**Relational Analysis** Look for excessive and equal stress (EES) and WSD. **Independent Analysis** Make a syllable stress patterns inventory (W for weak syllable; S for strong syllable). **Test Instruments** Use data from the process analysis; speech sample; informal polysyllabic word task.
Vowel constraints and deviations	**Relational Analysis** Look for vowel replacements and distortions that do not match the adult target system. **Independent Analysis** Look for vowel inventory and constraints and calculate PVC, if applicable. **Test Instruments** Use process analysis; speech sample; informal polysyllabic word task (e.g., NDP: Williams and Stephens 2004); observations of CS; vowel summary (Watts 2004).
Prosodic differences	**Independent Analysis** Subjective impressions of prosody. Does prosody affect intelligibility? **Test Instruments** Speech sample (CS); listener judgment, eventually PEPS-C (Peppe and McCann 2003).
PA difficulties	**Phonological Awareness Tests** Look particularly at rhyme awareness, syllable awareness, and blending. **Test Instruments** TOPA (Torgesen and Bryant 1994), SPAT-R, and AIST (Neilson 2003a, b).

Table 6.1 Speech characteristics and therapy goals in DPD and CAS*

Characteristics that CAS and DPD may have in common	DPD typical errors	CAS typical errors	DPD and CAS typical therapy goals
1. Consonant (C), vowel (V), and phonotactic inventory constraints	Simplification: systemic processes, e.g., stopping, gliding	Simplification *and* increased segmental complexity, e.g., affricates replacing stops; clusters replacing singletons; diphthongs replacing vowels	• C inventory expansion • V inventory expansion
2. Omissions of consonants, vowels, and syllable shapes already in the inventory	Simplification: syllable structure processes and phonotactic errors, e.g., initial consonant deletion (ICD), final consonant deletion (FCD), cluster reduction (CR), and weak syllable deletion (WSD)	Simplification *and* increased structural complexity, e.g., epenthesis (schwa insertion) /bə/l/u/ for 'blue'	• Syllable shape inventory expansion • Word shape inventory expansion • Increased accuracy of production of target structures
3. Vowel errors	Vowel errors are less common in children who don't have CAS.	Vowel errors are more common, and more persistent, in CAS.	• More complete V repertoire • More accurate V production
4. Altered suprasegmentals	Weak syllable deletion	Excessive and equal stress	• Production of S and W syllables • Differentiation of S and W syllables
5. More errors with longer and/or more complex utterances, including the so-called 'SODA' errors of substitution, distortion, and addition	SODA errors and errors that can be described in terms of phonological processes occur more frequently in more complex contexts, reducing intelligibility.	SODA errors, process errors, and segmental complexity errors with increasingly challenging contexts sees even more obvious difficulties in children with CAS, than in those with DPD.	• Generalisation of new sounds (Cs and Vs), syllable structures, and word structures to more challenging contexts
6. Use of simple, but not complex, syllable shapes and word shapes	Syllable structure processes: ICD, FCD, CR), WSD, and reduplication.	Syllable structure processes are more prevalent and persistent, even when phonetic repertoire is apparently adequate.	• More complete phonotactic repertoire • More varied use of phonotactic range within syllables and words • Improved accuracy

*Adapted with the authors' permission from an unpublished short course handout by Flahive, Hodson, and Velleman (2005).

other words, missing vowels and consonants. In DPD, this manifests as systemic simplifications (or substitution processes), such as stopping of fricatives and affricates, gliding of liquids and affricates, velar fronting, palatal fronting, and deaffrication. For consumer-friendly descriptions of some of these error-types, see Table 2.4 (p. 47). In, CAS consonant and vowel inventory constraints manifest as the same sorts of *simplification* errors that are found in DPD, but in addition to these, errors that involve increased *complexity* are found. Complexity errors might include affricates replacing stops (e.g., *top* pronounced as [dzɒp] or [dʒɒtʃ]), clusters replacing singletons (e.g., *rabbit* pronounced as [bræbɪt] or [dræbrɪt]), and diphthongs replacing vowels (e.g., *bed* pronounced as [bæɪd]) (these are real examples from clients). In the right column for Row 1, we see that the typical therapy goals in common are consonant and vowel inventory expansion to give the child 'more to work with'. The same format is used in the following five rows of Table 6.1. The clinician then has to determine how best to address these goals given the overall presenting picture. This question of 'how' is addressed towards the end of this chapter, and the reader who cannot bear the suspense is referred to Table 6.4!

A difficulty associated with this commonality of characteristics is that, when families who do not have a background in SLP/SLT seek out information without professional guidance, suspecting or even convinced that their child has CAS, they will often recognise enough 'features' of CAS to be certain that they 'know' what their child's speech problem is. Clinical experience suggests that they often do this without realising that those same symptoms are *far* more likely to signal DPD, given the low incidence of CAS. Compounding this difficulty, when lay people turn to the Internet for elucidation, they find a glut of Web sites dealing with CAS, the less frequent SSD. These sites often present unsubstantiated opinion and supposition as fact in order to sell products and services. By contrast, few sites deal explicitly and accurately with DPD, the more common SSD. It may not be obvious to them that SSD affects about 7 children in every 100, with approximately 86% of *these* children having articulation and phonological difficulties (if we combine SD-GEN and SD-OME), or 98% if we combine SD-GEN, SD-OME, and SD-DPI, whereas the CAS-affected children (SD-AOS) represent a miniscule <1% of the SSD population.

An exemplary Internet source of trustworthy CAS information for consumers and clinicians is the Apraxia-KIDS Web site (Gretz, A7). A positive effect of the growth of Apraxia-KIDS and CASANA has been increased accuracy of information about speech development and disorders circulating on the Web, and with it enhanced communication concerning CAS between consumers and professionals, especially on the Apraxia-KIDS listserv. For some clinicians, this has undoubtedly enabled a 'more equal' relationships with clients and a keener appreciation of the effects of communication disorders on affected individuals and their families, perhaps with the added benefit of improving their skills as counsellors, or recognising when to refer to a professional counsellor or prompting them to seek advanced training and supervision in this important area.

Among the issues and concerns that arise in parent and family counselling, and in counselling 'older' children and youth with persisting SSD, are the potential long-term consequences of these conditions. Gierut (1998) provides a concise summary of likely repercussions, indicating that some individuals can expect life-time challenges in terms of their retrieval, manipulation, and comprehension of linguistic information; their expressive language capabilities; and their education and work choices. Discussing these ramifications, Gierut takes the view that, 'research calls for both retrospective and prospective studies of the etiology of phonological disorders and the identification

Table 6.2 A 10-point CAS assessment prompt

1. Hearing
Audiology Report

2. Developmental History

Perinatal History

Milestones
Suspected/confirmed
cognitive delay?
Psychometric/paediatric
evaluation. Motor
development.

Feeding
Latching issues, fighting the breast, sucking, lactation consultant,
other professional intervention re: feeding and/or sleep pattern,
drinking from cup, chewing, gag reflex, vomiting, reflux, failure to
thrive, holding food in the mouth, breast or bottle, diet, mouth as
a sensor, mouth stuffing, variety of foods, preferred foods.

Health/Wellbeing
Illnesses, accidents, injuries,
ear infections, seizures,
'separation', hospitalisations,
operations, fatigues easily,
sleep pattern.

Babble
Quiet baby, no babbling, late
babbling; lots of babbling,
lots of vocal play (always
gurgling and blowing
raspberries), undifferentiated
babbling (all sounded the
same); few or no consonants
in babbled utterances;
'babble' mainly squeals and
grunts (i.e., not true
babbling).

Sounds/Words
Is independent phonetic
inventory larger than relational
(as it should be)? How many
intelligible words; how many
word approximations; first words
(when?), limited vocabulary for
age (parents' judgement),
comparison with other children
in the family and/or age-peers;
one word for many meanings
('big' for all machines/vehicles).
Only says words at home.

Social Development
Wants to communicate;
solitary; aloof; 'separation
issues' (clingy, why?), play
(with whom?).

Gesture/Grunts
Uses gesture instead of
words; uses vowels and
grunts instead of words.

Imitation
Little attempt to imitate sounds;
disinterested in imitating words;
refusal to imitate; upset if asked
to imitate. Does/does not imitate
play.

Frustration
Frustrated when not
understood (or passive,
unhappy, 'resigned'/used to
it/'adjusted' to not being a
talker?)

Lost Words
Says a word and it is never
heard again; keeps a word for
a while and then 'loses' it;
words come and go.

Groping/Struggle
Silent posturing?

Intelligibility
Ask parents, can you put a
percentage on it? Who
understands? Does another child
'interpret'? Does the other child
make mistakes in interpreting?
Does intelligibility vary? Worse
when tired? Worse/better in
certain situations? Worse with
longer utterances?

Comprehension
'Understands everything'/'very bright': essential to test receptive skills; parent report may be
positive but testing tells you about co-operation, attention, and may reveal subtle deficits in
comprehension (this can come as a shock to parents; don't assume they 'know'). Be alert to the
possibility of a receptive–expressive gap (comprehension higher than output suggests).

Any theories? Family history?
Ask parents what they think the problem might be (or might be 'called'). Have you wondered about
a particular 'label'; done a Web search; joined an e-mail discussion; received 'suggestions' and
advice from family, friends, and others? Thought about family history? What brought you here?

3. Language
Ask parents; formal tests.

4. Cognition
Ask parents; formal tests.

5. Phonological Awareness/Literacy
Ask parents; formal tests. With younger children, ask if they like stories.

Table 6.2 (*Continued*)

---

6. Neuromuscular Examination
- Gait
- Posture (sitting/W-sitting?)
- Muscle examination
- Muscle strength
- Muscle tone
- Coordination
- Reflexes
- Sensory function
- Involuntary movements (if yes, query dysarthria)
- Physiotherapist or Occupational Therapist report?

7. Motor Speech Examination (Table 6.2) and Structural–Functional Examination (Skinder-Meredith, A37)

8. Speech and Non-Speech Characteristics (Davis, Jakielski, and Marquardt 1998)
Non-speech characteristics:
1) Impaired volitional oral movements
2) Reduced expressive compared to receptive language skills (RLS-ELS gap)
3) Reduced diadochokinetic rates

Speech characteristics:
1) Limited C and V repertoire
2) Frequent omissions
3) High incidence of vowel errors
4) Inconsistent articulation errors
5) Altered suprasegmentals
6) Increased errors with output length
7) Difficulty in imitation (groping or refusal)
8) Use of simple, but not complex, syllable shapes

9. Speech Assessment
Standardised Articulation and Phonology Test (e.g., DEAP, HAPP-3)
Independent and Relational Analysis
Consistency Assessment
Compare SW and CS PCC and PVC
Intelligibility ratings
Use CS sample for MLUm and structural analysis if formal language testing is not possible
Look for silent posturing/groping
Is prosodic contour of utterance / sentence intact on imitation?
Contrastive stress (I want MY teddy/I want my TEDDY)
Rule dysarthric component out or in
Rule phonological component out or in

10. Speech Characteristics Rating (Skinder-Meredith, A37)

---

of integrated causal relationships and their outcome on a speaker's daily life.' Such implications impact the assessment and intervention process, right from the opening moments of the initial consultation or case history interview.

Case history interview

Table 6.2 provides an 'assessment prompt' in note form, developed over many years, that clinicians can use, and potentially add to, in case history-taking and initial assessment when they suspect CAS. Procedures and observations will vary with the child's age and stage; there is overlap between the 10 sections, and not every section will be needed for every child.

Table 6.3 Motor speech examination worksheet designed by Edythe Strand (used with permission)

Motor Speech Examination
A: Observations during connected speech:

	Vowels	Consonants	Typical/Maximum word length (any 'long words' of more than two syllables?)	Syllable Shapes C, CV, VC . . .	MLU
Conversation					
Picture Description					
Narrative					

B: Observations during elicited utterances
Example for a child with very severe impairment

	Immediate repetition	Repetition after delay – no cues	Needs simultaneous production	Needs gestural or tactile cues
Vowels				
CV				
VC				
CVC				

B: Observations during elicited utterances
Example for a child with very severe impairment

	Immediate repetition	Repetition after delay – no cues	Needs simultaneous production	Needs gestural or tactile cues
Vowel errors Note the different co-articulatory contexts tested				
Words of Increasing Length				
eat eating eating it				
cow cowboy cowboy hat				
me meat meeting				

Table 6.3 (*Continued*)

B: Observations during elicited utterances
Example for a child with very severe impairment

	Immediate repetition	Repetition after delay – no cues	Needs simultaneous production	Needs gestural or tactile cues
bye bite biting				
Long Words				
banana animals potato kangaroo Saturday lemonade				
Sentences of Increasing Length				
Examples: I ate the cookie. I ate the cookie yesterday. I ate the chocolate chip cookie yesterday.				

Motor speech examination worksheet

In working through the motor speech examination worksheet, displayed in Table 6.3, the tasks chosen and the order or presentation depend on the severity of the particular child's difficulties and any predictions the clinician makes regarding his/her probable performance. The worksheet is intended to help the investigator confirm or reject CAS as a diagnosis, bearing in mind that any determination of oral apraxia would have been made during the structural functional examination (Skinder-Meredith, A37). As with the assessment prompt (Table 6.2), the procedures overlap, and not all will be done with every client. There is no particular order of presentation of these tasks, other than the logical hierarchy that the clinician deems appropriate for the particular individual.

With regard to the long words, *banana, animals, potato, kangaroo, Saturday,* and *lemonade*, it is fascinating to see that James (A44) identified the following 10 words as being the most 'clinically useful' or most revealing diagnostically: *ambulance, hippopotamus, computer, spaghetti, vegetables, helicopter, animals, caravan, caterpillar,* and *butterfly*, in her study of long words and words containing consonant clusters.

Counselling and 'educating' families and significant others

Despite relevant academic and clinical preparation, our counselling and information-sharing capacities are often tested when issues of severity of involvement and complex co-morbidities arise, and Dr. Ruth Stoeckel has thought about this deeply. Dr. Stoeckel is an SLP engaged in clinical and research work. For her PhD at the University of Minnesota, she investigated how specific work on the listening skills of children with cochlear implants may or may not contribute to a child's overall speech-language development. She is also employed at the Mayo Clinic in Rochester, Minnesota, where she evaluates and treats young children with a range of speech-language difficulties, including motor speech disorders. She presents her work at professional conference and CEU events locally and nationally in the US and is strongly identified with CASANA (Gretz, A7) through advisory board, workshop, and other contributions. Dr. Stoeckel is known for her theoretically unassailable and evidence-based postings to the Apraxia-KIDS listserv, and for her skill as a writer in e-mail and message board discussion in expressing complex, technical, and potentially disquieting information unambiguously and supportively. It may be that the empathy she brings to these sometimes delicate exchanges is a product not only of her professional experience but also of her personal insight as a parent of an adolescent struggling with aspects of speech-language processing, and with the way she is perceived.

Q35.   Ruth Stoeckel: Communicating with families

For SLPs, fundamental aspects of child-centred dynamic assessment (Stone-Goldman, A39; Strand, A40) and therapy delivery within family-centred practice frameworks (Watts Pappas, A25) are the provision of accurate and timely information. There is also an obligation for us to communicate sensitively in a manner that 'fits' with the needs, capacities, cultures, value systems and beliefs, levels of acceptance, and emotional landscapes of the family and their significant others (see McLeod, A1; Bleile, A18). In each unique and changing situation that arises around minimally verbal or highly unintelligible children with major SSDs, such as severe CAS, we have both an educative and a counselling role. Many of our families, endlessly striving to do the best they can for their children, are influenced by information about the nature and management of their children's issues that is variously unscientific, misleading, time-wasting, worrying, or downright dangerous. This is of particular concern in cases of children who may indeed have CAS, and for whom its treatment becomes a raison d'être for their parents, but who have a range of other challenges impacting progress. It is also of concern with regard to parents of severely communicatively impaired children who do not have, and may never have, a definite speech-language disorder or other diagnosis. Misinformation can come from the immediate and wider circle of family and friends, where inevitably there will be a self-styled, often critical or denying, child development expert at hand! It can also come from our SLP/SLT and other professional colleagues and friends, and from faceless but ostensibly authoritative Internet 'experts' and 'e-friends'. There are no easy answers, but how would you educate the educators and counsel the counsellors charged with these important and demanding SLP/SLT educative and counselling tasks?

A35.   Ruth Stoeckel: Discussing appropriate treatment options for children with SSD and co-morbid conditions

Mrs. Smith brings in her 4-year-old son 'Bobby', who runs around the room, opens every door and drawer, impulsively picks up toys then drops them, and produces a constant stream of unintelligible jargon. He does not look at you or his mother, even when you are trying to get his attention so that you can begin the evaluation. Attempts to have him sit quietly for a moment result in screaming and squirming away. Mrs. Smith reports that Bobby was seen by a local speech pathologist who made a diagnosis of verbal apraxia and probable sensory issues. She is concerned that Bobby is making very slow progress in speech therapy. You are being asked for a second opinion about diagnosis and appropriate treatment strategies. Mrs. Smith expresses an expectation that, if Bobby receives the right kind of therapy for his speech problem, then his behaviour will be much improved as well. Do you agree with Mrs. Smith? If not, how would you approach your concerns about Bobby's behaviour with her?

A 5-year-old girl with Down syndrome named 'Precious' is brought for evaluation by her father, Mr. Sanchez. Precious has approximately 15 recognisable word approximations and can produce most speech sounds in isolation. She expresses herself through a combination of vocalisations and signing. Her sign language vocabulary consists of approximately 50 single signs, used to label items in her environment and to make requests. Her only two-sign combinations consist of 'want' plus a noun. She follows one-step directions easily, but needs help to follow through on two-step directions. Precious can identify several letters of the alphabet and tries to count along with her teacher. Mr. Sanchez has heard about CAS from the parent of another child in his daughter's preschool program, and wants to know if that is the reason his daughter has so much trouble talking. He wonders if her delay in language is a result of how hard it is to say words clearly. How would you explain the relative contribution of cognitive issues, language impairment, and speech impairment to Mr. Sanchez? How you would approach teaching improved communication skills to Precious?

'Sigrid' is the 27-month-old daughter of Mr. and Mrs. Happel. She was born nearly 6 weeks premature and has been slow to achieve developmental milestones. Sigrid began walking at 19 months. She had difficulty sucking as an infant and now chokes easily on any foods other than thickened cereal. Babbling is limited to 'ah' either alone or repeated in syllable strings. Sigrid is just beginning to point to objects and manipulate toys rather than put them in her mouth. Her parents realise that she is delayed in some areas and have been searching the Internet for answers. They tell you that Sigrid 'fits all the signs' of CAS that they found at one site and want to know if you can begin intensive speech therapy immediately to help their daughter overcome this disorder. They are looking for someone to do *Demosthenic Rock Therapy* (DRT) because they have read testimonials on a Web site suggesting that correct use of the special rocks sold by the developer of this therapy will result in dramatic improvements in the speech of children with CAS. Will you reject the request for DRT as an unproven method? Or will you work with the family to understand the theoretical principles and practical application of this treatment so you can determine together whether this is the most appropriate intervention for Sigrid?

Ten-year-old 'Nadif' was given a diagnosis of CAS by his paediatrician when he was three years old because he was unintelligible. He is now speaking clearly, except for a mild distortion of /r/ that he continues to work on in speech therapy. Nadif has struggled with learning to read. Other children are reading at a much higher level, whereas Nadif is still working hard to read books designed for beginning readers. Nadif does well in mathematics and has no trouble understanding what is being taught by his teacher during class. He just can't seem to grasp information that he has read or sound out words that he doesn't already know. His parents are frustrated and want to know why he is having so much trouble with reading when he has done so well on his speech goals. Would you question the diagnosis of CAS made by someone other than an SLP/SLT? How would you broach the subject of a possible reading disability as a separate issue from the speech problem with Nadif's parents?

What the above scenarios have in common is the likelihood that there are additional developmental issues whether or not the child has a definitive diagnosis of CAS. Some parents may be well aware that their child has multiple challenges. Others may be focused on thinking of CAS as the core problem, which, when treated, will result in improvements in other areas. Our job as clinicians is to not only evaluate and treat a child's speech and language disorders, but to help parents understand the relative contribution of speech and language problems within the context of the 'whole child'. Reviewing the examples above, that means identifying to what extent each child's problem with speaking may reflect the effects of a more general developmental disorder.

When co-morbid problems exist, it is important for us to be empathetic listeners who are sensitive to what parents are ready to hear about the possibility of other problems (Luterman 2001). We need to invite parents to work *with* us in discovering their child's strengths as well as their needs. In some cases, intervention will need to address a child's other areas of need before a diagnosis of CAS can be confirmed or ruled out. When it is not possible to arrive at a confident differential diagnosis based on the child's current level of abilities, we can describe specifically how our proposed treatment will address the child's current communication needs and how it will be modified based on the child's progress.

Parents become aware of specific problems like CAS because information is so widely available through a variety of sources, including in-person professional workshops that allow parents to attend, publicity in the popular press, and Internet sites that run the gamut from general information sites to discussion lists and product advertisements. This ease of access to information is a double-edged sword. It is helpful when parents can independently learn about CAS and more actively participate in the process of assessment and treatment. However, without the ability to critically evaluate what they learn, parents may have misplaced confidence in their own ability to diagnose their child's communication disorder, or request specific treatments based on content that may be incomplete, incorrect, or even irresponsible. We need to help parents understand CAS and other speech-language problems by sharing information based on our own knowledge and experience, and accept the fact that they may want to seek additional information elsewhere. Instead of feeling threatened by parents' desire to educate themselves, we can demonstrate a sense of mutual respect and shared power for decision-making (Stone and Olswang 1989) by facilitating their efforts and avoiding the tendency to play the part of the expert. We encourage parents to become our partners when we respond to questions with evidence-based explanations for why we agree or disagree with what has been learned and when we demonstrate that we can keep an open mind about ideas that may be new to us.

Parents may realise that something is 'too good to be true', but when they are desperately seeking answers, it can be hard to set aside the desire to try those interventions, however unrealistic they may be and however hard friends and family might encourage them to try them out. The emotional aspects of dealing with a child's special needs should not be underestimated. We can acknowledge the parents' concerns and our own fallibility while trying to guide them towards choices that are most likely to benefit the child. Materials such as the ASHA brochure *Questions for Consumers to Ask About Products or Procedures for Hearing, Balance, Speech, Language, Swallowing, and Related Disorders* are helpful for facilitating discussion about treatment options. Resources such as the Apraxia-KIDS Web site (http://www.apraxia-kids.org) offer both a network of support and theoretically sound, evidence-based information for parents to review at their own pace. We can combine face-to-face education with directing them to credible alternate resources (print and electronic media or other professionals) so they will be prepared not only to work with us more effectively, but to be able to explain their child's communication disorder to family, friends, and the world at large. Parents will be better able to handle well-meaning but misguided advice or awkward questions if they are confident in their own knowledge about their child or children.

One important aspect of education is to clarify for parents that SLPs/SLTs are the professionals with the particular knowledge and expertise to diagnose speech and language problems. Other professionals, such as physicians, educators, and occupational or physical therapists, may contribute important observations and information, but it is within our scope of practice to evaluate and treat disorders of speech and language (ASHA 2001). In the sample cases of the children above, there would certainly be a need to include other professionals in the child's care to assure appropriate intervention for all their areas of need. Designing appropriate intervention means obtaining accurate diagnoses.

Educating parents should not be considered a one-time event, presented as part of an evaluation summary or prelude to initiation of therapy. It should be an ongoing, reciprocal process between clinician and parents, in which both parties come to appreciate and build on the child's strengths as well addressing areas of need. We can provide parents with a variety of resources, help them evaluate information that they obtain under our guidance or on their own, and be supportive and respectful even when we disagree. We can listen carefully for concerns that are difficult for parents to express, or discuss with each other and/or with family, friends, and others, and make a genuine effort to learn about this child and his/her place in the family, so we can be more effective in our interactions and treatment and make appropriate referrals to other professionals. Bobby, Precious, Sigrid, and Nadif are counting on us to help their parents understand that learning to speak clearly may not be all that is required to help them achieve their fullest potential.

Reading the literature

In order to adequately inform and support families, and to fulfil the requirements of evidence-based and ethical practice (Powell, A34), we must be *au fait* with the relevant literature, whether by reading it diligently ourselves, perhaps as part of professional self-regulation, or by absorbing it in 'distilled' form at CPD/CEU events, where it is often presented by individuals pursuing, or holding, doctoral degrees and who have seriously immersed themselves in a topic (Bernthal and Overby, A46). Among the first steps in the PhD process are choosing both a topic area and a research question or questions. This requires the identification of a 'do-able' (by one person) piece of *original* research, and then the development of a proposal: which is probably when the real work of the dissertation begins. Completing a focused literature review around the research topic and questions is an important aspect of this endeavour, with the review itself eventually becoming the essence of the introduction to the doctoral dissertation. In response to what is found in the literature, and in response to what emerges from discussion with advisors or supervisors (Deem and Brehony 2000), the potential doctoral candidate may reach a point of wanting to reformulate the topic and/or questions, abandoning some questions and honing and sharpening others. The aim of the review is to frame and shape the research, demonstrate that it will fill a crucial gap, and link it to the larger body of knowledge (Mullins and Kiley 2002). Ultimately, according to Sternberg (1981), the literature review tells readers that the candidate has grasped the subject, has connected the topic to larger historic and current themes, can demonstrate that the proposed contribution is unique, and that the candidate can produce and critically evaluate an astutely refined and focused bibliography.

Chantelle Highman is an Australian SLP working as a clinician at a child development centre in Perth. She is also a doctoral candidate in the department of Human Communication Science, School of Psychology at Curtin University in Perth, Western Australia, investigating potential early speech motor and language precursors in infants at risk of CAS, and looking for evidence for a motor specific core deficit for the disorder (Maassen 2002). Her methodology across three studies has involved a combination of retrospective reports by parents of children with CAS, case study analysis of retrospective CAS data, and a prospective longitudinal study of siblings of children with CAS, aimed to provide an insight into the potential earliest features of disordered speech motor control. One of the drivers of this research is a question often asked by parents of children with CAS regarding the 'early warning features' they should be watchful for in their younger children, an obvious one that most families probably think we would be able to answer quite easily.

By some quirky synchronicity, Ms. Highman completed her literature review just as the final draft of the ASHA Draft Technical Report on CAS (ASHA 2006b) was circulated for comment. In her response to Q36, she discusses the role and process of reading the literature as it relates to practice and the therapy and research implications of the ratified position statement (ASHA 2007a) and report (ASHA 2007b).

Q36.   Chantelle Highman: A clinician's strategies for keeping up with the literature

The ASHA (2007b) Technical Report on CAS is wide ranging and comprehensive, prompting more questions than it answers, and some of those questions will likely be answered by SLPs/SLTs as PhD research questions (see Bernthal and Overby, A46, for discussion of the doctoral need in SLP/SLT). The report also makes for absorbing reading for those with the interest and inclination. A recurring theme in discussion with clinical SLPs/SLTs is that, although they would like to, they rarely read the literature for a range of reasons that include lack of time and limited access to journals and other publications (like professional association reports and position statements). On the other hand, for SLPs/SLTs with a theoretical or research bent, reading the literature is routine, time is set aside, and new articles are eagerly awaited and consumed. Can you suggest strategies that clinicians might employ to make the task of keeping abreast with the published evidence base less challenging and more enjoyable; suggest what readers of the Technical Report might gain from it in a practical, clinical sense; and indicate the key areas for further CAS and other child speech research that it points to?

A36.   Chantelle Highman: Keeping abreast of the evidence base

The literature confirms practical issues faced by clinicians in attempting to implement evidence-based practice (EBP), including lack of time, lack of ready access to published literature, and lack of skill in evaluating the evidence (e.g., Bernstein Ratner 2006; Gosling and Westbrook 2004; Johnson 2006; Rose and Baldac 2004; Vallino-Napoli and Reilly 2004). Daunting though these barriers may appear to be, clinicians know from their professional associations' Codes of Ethics that keeping up to date with relevant literature is an integral part of an SLP/SLT's responsibilities. Indeed, when surveyed, most clinicians report placing a high value on the importance of research, and desire to keep up to date with the evidence base underpinning practice (Vallino-Napoli and Reilly 2004). By combining our clinical knowledge with new evidence and theories, we may be better positioned to provide more effective, efficient, and appropriate services (Reilly, Douglas, and Oates 2004).

Keeping up with the literature

Drawing on the suggestions provided by Johnson (2006) and Reilly, Douglas, and Oates (2004), and from my own experience as a clinician, post graduate student, and researcher, practical strategies to make keeping up with the literature less challenging and more enjoyable for the clinician might include:

- Identifying a particular area of interest or a current focus (e.g., diagnosis of CAS, or treatment approaches for phonological disorders). Allowing your focus to be directed by clinical cases and questions can be particularly motivating. For me, a question asked by a parent of a child with CAS about what to look out for in the younger sibling, and a current interest in infant vocalisations, prompted a literature search.
- Linking up with other clinicians and researchers. Tackling one focussed area as a 'team' will ensure that practical implications can be maximised. This may include joining (or forming) a relevant interest group or journal club, or extend to partnering with students and universities for joint benefits. My approach was to speak with colleagues and local specialists in the field.
- Making use of information available on reputable Web sites (Bowen 1998b; CASANA 1997; see Gretz, A7). Joining the associated discussion groups to receive posts (which often include relevant abstracts) is a time-efficient way of staying connected with clinical and research issues. Making use of the archives and files areas allows clinicians to

search for clinically relevant topics, articles, and associated discussions with ease. This continues to be one of the most important ways for me to integrate theoretical and clinical knowledge.

- Investigating your access to online journals. Setting up automatic alerts for particular topics and journals' table of contents will allow you to stay informed without having to repeatedly search for new information. Most databases and journals have instructions on their Web sites on how to do this, and it really does make keeping up with the literature easier.

- Checking association Web sites (e.g., ASHA, CASLPA, IASLT, NZSTA, RCSLT, SASLHA, Speech Pathology Australia) for information regarding EBP and continuing professional development, as well as for access to technical reports, position statements, and clinical guidelines. In my case, the ASHA (2007b) CAS Technical Report consolidated my understanding of the area.

- Utilising available published conference proceedings on topics of interest (Shriberg and Campbell 2002). This was an important step for me; The Proceedings of the 2002 Childhood Apraxia of Speech Research Symposium included not only the presentations, but also transcripts of frank discussions between the top researchers in the field! My understanding of the current state of the literature increased dramatically after reading these proceedings.

- Making use of sources that have already synthesised information for you, such as review articles, book chapters, and meta-analyses. Johnson (2006) provides a list of speech and language-relevant sources, as well as practical examples of how to apply such information to clinical problems.

- Attending relevant CPD/CEU events, especially those that present a synthesis of the available literature on a given topic. Much of my clinical knowledge in CAS came from attending events such as these.

- Utilising your professional association, by helping to identify areas of need (in terms of reviews and practice guidelines), and contributing to and/or accessing book and journal reviews that are often included in newsletters and journals.

There are other strategies, but an important first step is a commitment to becoming 'literature-active'. For me, keeping abreast of the literature in one particular interest area led to a proposal for a small clinically relevant project, which then led to a small grant, which ended up leading to enrolling in a doctorate! For clinicians who do not wish to actively engage in research at that level, starting with focussed clinical questions is still important in helping you stay up-to-date.

Practical, clinical applications of Technical Report and Position Statement

The ASHA Childhood Apraxia of Speech Technical Report (2007b) and associated Position Statement (2007a) are recent examples of readily available resources that synthesise the literature. The documents provide clinicians with an up-to-date review of CAS-related literature, referring often to typical development and other SSDs. As such, they provide the busy clinician with a current perspective on this controversial area. As indicated earlier, many questions remain unanswered. However, a number of directly relevant and clinically

applicable recommendations are presented in the report. These are su
terms of the four questions referred to previously:

Is it (CAS) a recognised clinical disorder?

The Technical Report and accompanying Position Statement clearly support the existence
of CAS as a recognised paediatric SSD. The literature suggests that CAS is a complex
disorder, characterised by particular speech production and prosodic features, warranting
clinical services and further research. However, the report also acknowledges the overlap of
features with other SSDs, and the present lack of a set of validated, differentially diagnostic
criteria for CAS. The committee suggest that the term CAS be applied to the idiopathic form
as well as those occurring in the context of neurological and neurobehavioural.

What are its core characteristics?

In the committee's proposed definition of CAS, 'a core impairment in planning and/or programming [the] spatiotemporal parameters of movement sequences' is described (ASHA
2007a, p. 1), highlighting the importance of skilled motor movements underlying speech
production. Such impairment results in speech production and prosodic errors. Despite
recognising the lack of a validated set of differentially diagnostic criteria that reliably distinguish CAS from other SSDs, the committee did report on features likely to be diagnostic.
Based on the reviewed research and consensus opinion, the following three segmental
and suprasegmental core characteristics were proposed (ASHA 2007a, p. 2):

1. Inconsistent errors on consonants and vowels in repeated productions of syllables or
   words;
2. Lengthened and disrupted coarticulatory transitions between sounds and syllables; and
3. Inappropriate prosody, especially in the realisation of lexical or phrasal stress

The committee acknowledged that an affected child's speech characteristics may change
over time, and that the three features 'are not proposed to be the necessary and sufficient
signs of CAS' (ASHA 2007a, p. 2). That is, as there is no set of validated criteria, one
cannot diagnose (or rule out) CAS on the presence (or absence) of these features alone.
A number of additional features often observed in CAS are discussed in detail within the
report. These include those features that often comprise clinical diagnostic checklists for
CAS (e.g., vowel errors, increased errors as syllable and word complexity increase) and
those also observed in children with other SSDs (Forrest 2003; McCabe, Rosenthal, and
McLeod 1998).

How should it be assessed?

The report does not describe definitive assessment guidelines or a single diagnostic test
for CAS, due to the lack of evidence supporting such specific recommendations (Caspari
2007). However, guidance for assessment, based on theoretical and research findings,
is presented. A key recommendation from the report was that SLPs/SLTs (and not other
professionals) are responsible for diagnosing CAS. Assessment should involve sampling

speech and language skills across a range of task difficulties and considering detailed case history information.

Of the available research reviewed, maximal performance tasks of multisyllable production (e.g. diadochokinetic tasks, non-word repetition, and multisyllabic word production) and observation of prosody (especially lexical stress) were reported to be the most informative. However, until validated protocols are identified, assessing CAS remains a cautious exercise, where the clinician must assess broadly and in detail, and usually over time. This is particularly the case for younger or less verbal children who are not yet able to take part in detailed speech assessments that sample speech production abilities across contexts (Davis and Velleman 2000). All areas of speech and language, including receptive language, expressive language, speech sequencing, phonological development (including inventory, independent, and relational analyses), oral-motor skills, communicative intent, compensatory strategies, facilitative techniques, and pre-literacy skills, need to be considered in identifying the strengths and weaknesses of the individual child.

The report documented assessment considerations from researchers with substantial clinical experience (ASHA 2007b, p. 54), which included the importance of differentiating performance on:

- functional/automatic versus volitional actions,
- single [speech] postures versus sequences of postures,
- simple contexts versus more complex or novel contexts,
- repetitions of the same stimuli versus repetitions of varying stimuli (e.g., sequential motion rates vs. alternating motion rates), and
- tasks for which auditory versus visual versus tactile versus a combination of cues are provided.

As is often the case clinically, a 'working' diagnosis may need to be considered, with diagnostic therapy (Davis and Velleman 2000) further informing us of the nature of the deficit and relative contribution of speech motor planning and phonological abilities to the child's communication impairment.

How should it be treated?

There were few treatment efficacy studies relating to CAS available to the committee (reflecting the state of the literature), and none that met the highest levels of scientific rigour (Reilly, Douglas, and Oates 2004). However, the report provides guidance on treatment approaches and supporting efficacy data (where available), including discussions on intensity (dosage) and funding issues. Descriptive and single-subject experimental designs provided preliminary support for the use of augmentative and alternative communication devices (AAC) to improve overall communicative competence in children with severely compromised speech production abilities (Bornman, Alant, and Meiring 2001; cited in ASHA 2007b). In addition, research describing intervention approaches that specifically target speech production has provided preliminary efficacy information and direction for practice. In particular, the integral stimulation approach (Strand and Debertine 2000), which incorporates principles of motor learning (such as the need for frequent, distributed practice), has reported positive efficacy data (Strand, A40). Clinicians can make use of the emerging treatment efficacy research, either to refine and support approaches they may already be using or to learn about these further. Importantly, the report contains discussion of issues surrounding treatment intensity and length of sessions, describing 'emerging support for the need to provide three to five individual sessions per week' (ASHA 2007b, p. 55). The need to acknowledge and treat the various associated deficits (e.g., pre-literacy skills) that often co-occur in children with CAS is also highlighted in the report.

All in all the Technical Report and Position Statement reflect the current literature, research, and clinical needs of this symptom complex. Clinically, they highlight the challenges involved in making differential diagnoses of SSD and provide the clinician with a theoretical and evidence-based platform for considering assessment and therapy issues. A document outlining clinical working guidelines based on the Technical Report is also available (Caspari 2007).

Key areas for further CAS and child speech research

Research on CAS is still in its infancy, with the lack of consensus about core diagnostic features presenting a significant barrier to progress (ASHA 2007a, b). As with SSD in general, there is much scope (and an urgent need) for research addressing areas such as:

- Diagnostic criteria
- Cross-cultural features and presentations
- Genetic and neurological factors
- Epidemiological factors (e.g., prevalence)
- Treatment efficacy
- Long-term outcomes
- Potential early markers

Perhaps after implementing strategies to keep up to date with the literature, *you* will be motivated to make a positive contribution to addressing some of these areas, and in doing so, improve the outlook for our clients.

Characteristics and general observations of CAS

Adopting the suggestions of Shriberg, Campbell, Karlsson, et al. (2003), the segmental and suprasegmental characteristics the clinician will look for with CAS as a suspected or working diagnosis are listed below. Then follows a guide to the general observations they might make during differential diagnosis. These are arranged under the overlapping section headings of: general characteristics, phonetic characteristics/phonetic error-types, sound sequencing difficulties, timing disturbances, disturbed temporal–spatial relationships of the articulators, contextual changes in articulatory proficiency, phonological awareness, receptive language, and expressive language.

ital characteristics of CAS

1. Articulatory struggle and silent posturing
2. Transpositional substitution errors
3. Marked inconsistency (especially token-to-token variability)
4. Sound and syllable deletions
5. Vowel/diphthong errors

Suprasegmental (prosodic) characteristics of CAS

6. Inconsistent realisation of stress
7. Inconsistent realisation of temporal constraints on both speech and pause events
8. Inconsistent oral–nasal gestures underlying the percept of nasopharyngeal resonance

General observations of CAS

1. Inability to imitate sounds and segments in the absence of structural or functional abnormalities of the speech mechanism.
2. Refusal or definite reluctance to imitate sounds and segments. Such refusal is often obvious and remarkable in otherwise biddable children and may be an indication of a child knowing his/her limitations, and it may sometimes signal that a child has been 'pushed' to imitate beyond realistic expectations.
3. Decreased proprioceptive awareness of where the articulators are and what they are doing.
4. Difficulty achieving and maintaining articulatory postures and configurations.
5. Silent posturing, groping for articulatory placement, mouthing utterances, or other trial-and-error articulatory behaviour. Although such behaviour may be a character-istic of CAS, it is probable for some children that it appears as an artefact of therapy or being instructed by therapist and parents 'how to' articulate.
6. Distinctive resonance, particularly hypernasality and nasality applied unexpectedly.
7. Prosodic disturbances, notably excessive or equal stress, or excessive and equal stress.

Phonetic characteristics/phonetic error types in CAS

1. Multiple speech sound errors that include: omissions (most common), substitutions, distortions, additions, voicing and aspiration errors, vowel errors, and errors related to complexity of articulatory adjustment.
2. Independent phonetic inventory (what the child can produce) is larger than relational phonetic inventory (what the child actually says).

Sound sequencing difficulties in CAS

1. Metathesis; for example, 'Brian' (26), an academically gifted comparative theol-ogy student and seminarian who was diagnosed at 4;1 and treated for CAS over a

7-year period, pronounced relevant as [ɹɛvələnt], evolution as [ɛləvuʃn], cavalry as [kæləvɹi], sepulchre as [sɛplʌkʌ], employee as [ɪmpɔli], Cathedral as [kɹəθɹidɹl], and Sydney as [sɪndi], while making typical, atypical, and variable errors when saying commonly mispronounced words, such as *ask, diphthong, espresso, et cetera, height, mischievous, nuclear,* and *percolate*. For example, the common errors for *ask, diphthong,* and *mischievous* are [aks], [dɪpθɒŋ], and [mɪstʃiviəs]; but Brian typically pronounced them as [atsk], [dɪθfɒŋ], and [mɪsvətʃəs]. His sister Bethany (11), also diagnosed with CAS, and who Brian called [bɛnəθi] unless he really concentrated, pronounced *tomato* as [mətatou] and *wattle tree* as [tɹɒtlwi] as did Daniel 6.7 (see point 5 below).

2. Difficulty with a particular phonotactic combination of sounds produced correctly in isolation or in CV or CVC combinations; for example, William (7;8) could say *tip, rip, tipped, ripped,* but not *trip*.
3. Sounds correct in some sequences are erred in other sound sequences, as in the case of Madison (7;0), who pronounced her name correctly as [mædɪsn] but called the *Radisson* Hotel near her home the [wætɪsn], replacing /d/ with /t/.
4. Producing clusters is more difficult than producing than singletons.
5. Transposition of sounds and syllables. Daniel (6;7) said [lʌndəwænd] for Wonderland.

Timing disturbances in CAS

1. Word and sentence durations may be longer due to lengthening of both speech events and pause events.
2. The slope of the 2nd formant may be shallower if the tongue is taking longer to get into position.
3. Longer duration of voice onset times may be present, and this can explain voicing errors.

Disturbed temporal–spatial relationships of the articulators in CAS

1. There may be imprecise, non-specific, 'wandering' speech gestures.
2. Palatometry data indicate that CAS children do not develop the fine-tuned speech movements with the same specificity and precision that typically developing children (and possibly children with other SSDs) exhibit.

Contextual changes in articulatory proficiency in CAS

1. Errors increase with increasing length of the word or utterance.
2. Imitation results in better articulatory performance than in spontaneous production. This is open to debate, with Ozanne's (1995, 2005) data suggesting the opposite.
3. Target sounds are easier to produce in single words than in conversational speech.
4. Errors vary according to the phonetic complexity of the utterance.
5. Errors are inconsistently produced (high token-to-token variability).
6. Articulatory accuracy increases if rate is decreased (e.g., if vowels are lengthened).
7. Articulatory accuracy increases with simultaneous visual and auditory models.

ical awareness (PA) and CAS

PA is an essential skill in literacy acquisition and a necessary aspect of making sense of an alphabetic script, and output phonology plays an important role in learning to read (Snowling, Goulandris, and Stackhouse 1994). Larrivee and Catts (1999) warned that SSDs *alone* are not strongly related to problems with early reading skills, but that when phonological disorders are accompanied by *another* speech or language impairment, such as CAS, reading and writing disabilities may emerge. Children with impaired phonological output are at increased risk for impaired phonological awareness skills. Many children diagnosed with CAS also exhibit PA difficulties; that is, difficulty reflecting on and manipulating the structure of an utterance as distinct from its meaning (Stackhouse 1997, p. 157).

Receptive language and CAS

A receptive–expressive (receptive higher than expressive) gap is often cited as a diagnostic characteristic of CAS. This gap is not necessarily across the board but may vary according to the particular language test task. Single-word (SW) receptive vocabulary on the PPVT-3 (Dunn and Dunn 1997) may be age-typical, whereas, at the same time, sentence comprehension may be impaired. Similarly, receptive skills for simple sentences may be age-appropriate, whereas comprehension of complex sentences is impaired. With these variations in performance in mind, Crary (1993) advocates testing, at a minimum, three areas: SW receptive vocabulary, semantic comprehension, and syntactic comprehension. Air, Wood, and Neils (1989) investigated 'older' children, finding that those who had apparently adequate language comprehension earlier on tended to have difficulty in language processing fundamentals involving categories, organisation, and abstract concepts in years (grades) 3 and 4 at school.

Expressive language and CAS

Pronoun errors are common in children with CAS. Morphemic and syntactic errors may be due to phonological simplifications (e.g., omitting /s/, /t/, /d/ word finally in tenses and plural markers). Word omissions are a frequent finding (Ekelman and Aram 1983), and speech may be telegrammatic. Speculatively, this may be an adaptive strategy to reduce linguistic load.

Rating speech characteristics

Following the case history interview and having worked through the motor speech examination worksheet and made pertinent observations, the clinician may wish to rate the child's speech characteristics systematically. A way of doing so is to use a procedure devised by Dr. Amy Skinder-Meredith, an assistant professor in the Department of Speech and Hearing Sciences at Washington State University. Dr. Skinder-Meredith's primary clinical and research interest is in children with motor speech disorders, and she has published and presented her research on CAS at conferences in the US and internationally. Currently, she is investigating PA and early reading skills of children with CAS. She is also looking at the role of visual feedback using electropalatography and real-time spectrography in treatment of children with persistent SSD, including CAS.

Q37. Amy E. Skinder-Meredith: Speech ratings in differential diagnosis

In implementing your speech characteristics rating (Skinder-Meredith 2000) in the differential diagnosis of children with sCAS, the clinician records, on a series of 5-point scales displayed in Table A37.1, quick but detailed observations of speech prosody, fluency, and rate; and, voice quality, loudness, pitch, and resonance. Can you lead the reader through this process, discussing these and other suprasegmental aspects of speech output, and the segmental aspects that you would include in your descriptive analysis? The nature of assessment for sCAS varies with the age, cognitive capacity, attention span, and compliance of the child. In general terms with a child who can cooperate well with testing, in an initial diagnostic workup at say, 3;0, 5;0, and 9;0 years of age, what procedures do you regard as essential components of a test battery? With children whose ability to cope with formal testing is compromised, what advice would you offer the clinician in terms of the observations he/she can make in the assessment process?

A37. Amy E. Skinder-Meredith: Speech characteristics rating form

Standardised tests are integral components of core test-batteries and necessary when qualifying children for services, but are limited in usually only addressing segmental (phonetic) performance and phonemic organisation. The errors of children with CAS are not exclusively segmental or phonological (ASHA 2007b; Highman, A36), posing an assessment challenge. The speech characteristics rating form (SCRF), shown in Table A37.1, was created in response to this challenge, allowing a thorough, more encompassing, *suprasegmental* view of a child's output. As clinicians, we know that some children progress well with phonetic production accuracy while remaining poorly intelligible due to some combination of atypical prosody, resonance, voice quality, and fluency. Moreover, disordered prosody in CAS is a prominent research finding (Shriberg, Aram, and Kwiatkowski 1997a, b, c; Velleman and Shriberg 1999).

Key elements of CAS assessment

The purpose of the assessment process is to understand the nature of the suspected motor planning deficit relative to any other deficits, such as cognitive, linguistic, and motor execution ones, so as to determine the relative contribution of the disorder to the child's overall communicative performance (Strand and McCauley 1999). Taking into account the age, compliance, and developmental status of the child, I typically obtain the necessary information in the following order, which can be varied: available test results (e.g.,

Table A37.1 Speech Characteristics Rating Form (SCRF)*

Speech Characteristics Rating
Circle the number that you judge, best correlates with the corresponding speech
characteristic: 1-never present 2-rarely present 3-sometimes present 4-frequently present 5-always
present

Speech characteristics	Rating scale				
PROSODY	never	rarely	sometimes	frequently	always
1 Monotone	1	2	3	4	5
2 **Hyperprosodic** e.g., sing-song, EES	1	2	3	4	5
3 **Dysprosodic** e.g., word/phrase stress errors	1	2	3	4	5
4 **Appropriate prosody**	1	2	3	4	5
Comment					
VOICE QUALITY / RESONANCE					
1 **Hoarse voice quality**	1	2	3	4	5
2 **Breathy voice quality**	1	2	3	4	5
3 **Glottal fry**	1	2	3	4	5
4 **Appropriate voice quality**	1	2	3	4	5
5 **Hypernasal**	1	2	3	4	5
6 **Hyponasal**	1	2	3	4	5
7 **Appropriate resonance**	1	2	3	4	5
Comment					
PITCH / LOUDNESS					
1 **High pitch**	1	2	3	4	5
2 **Low pitch**	1	2	3	4	5
3 **Appropriate pitch**	1	2	3	4	5
4 **Loud voice**	1	2	3	4	5
5 **Soft voice**	1	2	3	4	5
6 **Appropriate loudness**	1	2	3	4	5
Comment					
RATE/FLUENCY					
1 **Slow rate**	1	2	3	4	5
2 **Fast rate**	1	2	3	4	5
3 **Appropriate rate**	1	2	3	4	5
4 **Dysfluent**	1	2	3	4	5
5 **Appropriate fluency**	1	2	3	4	5
	never	rarely	sometimes	frequently	always
Comment					

*Adapted from Skinder-Meredith (2000).

audiology, psychology); developmental and family history; speech, language, PA and literacy assessment data as appropriate; observations of any groping, or silent posturing; oral musculature/structural–functional examination; physiological functioning; inconsistency assessment (Stoel-Gammon, A9; Betz and Stoel-Gammon 2005); and the motor speech examination (displayed in Table 6.3) and diadochokinesis. It is highly desirable, if possible, for the clinician to videotape the assessment so that they can make the necessary

Table A37.2 Comparison between dysarthria and CAS*

Characteristics	Dysarthria	CAS
Neurological	Decreased strength, coordination, and range of motion of the jaw, tongue, lips, and/or soft palate.	No weakness of the articulators.
Feeding	Potential long-term difficulty with tongue and jaw control for feeding.	Possible early history of feeding problems, but these typically resolve.
Physiological	Possibility of poor respiratory and phonatory control as noted by decreased subglottal pressure, weak cough, and poor ability to sustain phonation, breathy, or strained voice quality.	Respiratory and phonatory control are within normal limits.
Resonance	Hypernasality with nasal emission if there is flaccid dysarthria of the soft palate or hypernasality without emission for spastic dysarthria.	Disordered resonance is sometimes noted, but when it is observed, it is typically mild or inconsistent.
Language	Receptive language scores/performance may or may not be higher than expressive language scores/performance (i.e., RLS/ELS gap not typical of dysarthria).	Receptive language scores are typically higher than expressive language scores (RLS-ELS gap).
Prosody	Rate, rhythm, and stress are typically disordered, depending on the type of dysarthria (e.g., ataxic dysarthria is characterised by scanning speech; flaccid and spastic dysarthria are characterised by monotonous speech).	Excessive and equal stress (EES) sounding robotic. Reduced prosodic contours.
Speech	Consistently slurred and distorted in general regardless of the utterance length and complexity. No qualitative difference between automatic speech and novel utterances. Vowels may be distorted.	Errors increase with utterance length and complexity. Automatic speech (counting, saying the alphabet) is better than novel speech. Vowel errors are a frequent finding.

*Apraxia-kids.org (2004); Strand and McCauley (1999).

observations for differential diagnosis. For all children with suspected CAS, my *highest* priority is the motor speech evaluation, pinpointing best speech performance and where it breaks down. Applying the principles of dynamic assessment (Strand, A40), I also want to know whether varying tactile and temporal cues enhances output.

The SCRF is administered *after* the case history interview (see Table 6.2) and an initial core test-battery comprising the *key elements of CAS assessment*. The core battery will have included a structural–functional examination, identifying structural constraints (as in cleft palate), or physiological constraints (as in dysarthria) to speech production. Mixed resonance or inconsistent nasal resonance may indicate CAS, with the child struggling with timing velopharyngeal contraction, versus constant hypernasality suggesting structural (e.g., cleft palate) or cranial nerve damage (e.g., spastic or flaccid dysarthria) issues. Once dysarthria is ruled out (see Table A37.2 for a comparison of dysarthria and CAS), close inspection of prosody may help differentiate children with phonological issues only from those with CAS (or CAS plus phonological issues).

Working with the SCRF

Administration

Rapport with child and parent(s) is established, and a high-quality recording of a CS sample is obtained for independent and relational analysis (Stoel-Gammon, A9). Narrating a wordless picture book quickly yields a dense corpus, and reading ability is not a factor. With reticent children, I model the narrative and then have them try. Failing this, a CS sample is obtained through play. Preferably, listen to the sample once per speech characteristic being rated, including separate ratings for hyper- and hyponasality. Additional observations are recorded in the comments sections.

Comments sections

Observations might include groping (silent posturing); articulatory struggle; word retrieval difficulties; error consistency (suggesting phonological disorder) or inconsistency (suggesting inconsistent speech disorder) or inconsistency and consistency (suggesting CAS); dysfluencies; receptive language issues; and vowel neutralisation errors. In terms of comprehension, children with CAS may perform well on SW receptive vocabulary, but have difficulties with comprehending sentences, particularly as sentence length increases. With vowels, the child may be stimulable for isolated vowels, but unable to produce them in syllables or words.

Prosody

Speech may be hypoprosodic (monotone) *and* hyperprosodic (excessively inflected), making it essential to hear entire samples before rating in order to perceive any variation. Excessive stress (choppy, 'robotic sounding speech'), if present, may be due to the inherent nature of CAS (Shriberg, Aram, and Kwiatkowski 1997a, b, c) and/or the effects of speech therapy. For example, children focusing on the correct sequencing of syllables in multisyllabic utterances may be trained to compensate by speaking one syllable at a time, creating staccato, monotonous delivery (Meredith 2002).

Voice quality/resonance/glottal fry

The intelligibility of children with CAS may reduce when they use less than optimal voice quality. Some (not all) develop hoarseness secondary to vocal nodules, consequent to poor vocal hygiene. Interestingly, in a study by Skinder-Meredith, Lommers, and Yoder (2007), 60% of parents reported that their child with CAS often exhibited frustration. Those who express communicative frustration strongly and overtly are prone to hyperfunctional voice disorders. Glottal fry ('creaky voice' or 'pulse register'), a common physiological occurrence at the ends of sentences, manifests when a speaker is running out of air and attempting to vocalise at too low a fundamental frequency. Constant glottal fry greatly reduces intelligibility. *Some* children may be *more* at risk of going into glottal fry due to poor timing between respiration and phonation.

Boone and McFarlane (2000) determined that SLPs/SLTs can easily spot resonance disorders, but have difficulty distinguishing hyper- from hyponasal quality, so listening once for hypernasality and once for hyponasality is advisable. Children with CAS may have difficulty planning movements of the velum, as they do with other articulators (Hall, Hardy, and La Velle 1990; Weiss, Gordon, and Lillywhite 1987). Consistent with this assumption, researchers have found 50% or more of the children with CAS in their studies to have disordered resonance (Ball, Beukelman, and Bernthal 1999; Hall, Hardy, and La Velle 1990; Skinder 2000; Skinder-Meredith, Carkowski, and Graff 2004; Weiss, Gordon, and Lillywhite 1987).

Pitch/loudness

Many parents observe that their children with CAS have difficulty modulating loudness, and I have noted that they have similar problems with pitch. Speculatively, this might be due to poor speech monitoring or to difficulty in coordinating respiration and phonation sufficiently to allow appropriate pitch and loudness variation.

Rate/fluency

When observing rate, note the speed–accuracy trade-off. Children speaking at fast or normal rates may omit syllables and segments. Children using slow speech rates may be doing so deliberately to maintain segmental or structural accuracy. Skinder (2000) found that children with better segmental accuracy tended towards slower speech, whereas children with poor segmental accuracy spoke at either a normal or fast rate. Fluency is of considerable interest. Many parents report dysfluent periods as the phonetic repertoire of their child with CAS increases, and it is interesting to speculate about causes. Caruso, Ludo, and McClowry (1999) consider stuttering to be related to motor planning, and thus, dysfluency and apraxia of speech could be viewed as being related. But the dysfluencies of children with CAS may differ from those of children who stutter. For example, a client of mine only repeated word-final syllables (e.g., fish-ing-ing-ing), a perseverative pattern rarely attested in conventional stuttering.

Procedures to employ in structural–functional evaluation

Respiratory function

Use a *static blowing task* to evaluate adequacy of respiratory support. The child blows bubbles in a cup of water with a straw placed 10 cm below the surface. If bubbles are produced, the child can generate enough subglottal pressure for speech (Hixon, Hawley, and Wilson 1982). For children with VPI, occlude the nares, preventing nasal air escape.

Sustained phonation

Determine ability to imitate steady phonation for at least 5 seconds with adequate loudness and normal voice quality.

Velopharyngeal function and resonance

Employing a 'listening tube' (e.g., aquarium tubing) or straw about 45 cm long, position one end close to the child's nares and the other to your ear. Have the child repeat words and phrases (e.g., *sixty-six*, *Buy Bobby a puppy*) with high-pressure oral sounds and utterances with nasal consonants ('ninety-nine'; 'My mama makes lemonade'). If nasal emission is present, the examiner will feel the air, and if there is hypernasality, oral sounds will be amplified similarly to nasal sounds.

Comparison of resonance with nares occluded and open

Pinch and release the nares while the child says /pa/. Resonance should be the same in both conditions. If hypernasality occurs, structurally or neurologically based VPI warrants investigation.

Soft palate movement

Check that, when producing /a a a/ quickly and loudly, velar movements are forceful and quick.

Laryngeal function

Having the child cough provides an opportunity to listen for adequate vocal fold adduction. Eliciting even, sustained phonation allows observations of voice quality. Breathiness may indicate flaccid dysarthria, whereas strained, strangled quality may signal a spastic dysarthria.

Diadochokinesis (DDK)

Compare production rates of /pa/, /ta/, and /ka/ sequences and /pataka/ to developmental norms. Normative data are provided by Fletcher (1972) for ages 6–13, Yaruss and Logan (2002) for boys 3–7, and Williams and Stackhouse (1998) for ages 3–5. During DDK testing, note syllable sequencing, rhythm, voicing errors, and co-ordination of respiration, phonation, and articulation, and above all, any performance change between duplicated syllables (/papa/) and sequencing a variety syllables (/pataka/).

Cranial nerve (CN) examination

The functioning of cranial nerves V (jaw), VII (face and lips), and IX and X (pharynx and larynx) is addressed by default during DDK, phonatory, and resonance tasks. In addition, cranial nerves for speech can be quickly assessed by observing symmetry of movement, strength, range of motion, and co-ordination while doing the following:

- CN V: Observe jaw opening, closing, and side-to-side movements. Palpate the masseter and have the child bite down, feeling for (appropriate) bulging as the muscle contracts.
- CN VII: Observe the child smiling, eating, laughing, and puckering-and-smiling. Test resistance of the four quadrants of the lips, with either your finger or a tongue depressor, while the child keeps his/her lips closed tightly.
- CN XII: Check tongue protrusion, retraction, lateral movement, and elevation. Check strength by pushing against the tongue with a tongue depressor.

It is important to note that these tasks are only for evaluative purposes to assess whether there is a dysarthric component, not suggestions for treatment.

Assessing children with limited attention spans

Many two- to four-year-olds, and older children with a range of complicating issues, find it hard to stay on-task throughout a large test battery, so for them, formalised testing should be de-emphasised. Information can be gained from parents or caregivers, who may have video- or audio-recorded examples of their child talking. Most of the evaluation, however, has to rest on informal observations of play. Observations of the child's movement, play, and communication intent help predict cognition, motor skills, and language skills. Formal speech assessments that employ objects as well as pictures (Hodson 2004) or cute, colourful pictures (Dodd, Hua, Crosbie, et al. 2003) may tempt a young child to 'name' more readily. For the structural functional examination, clinicians can attempt to engage the child in making silly faces and observe closely as they chew and swallow a snack. I often have a candy stick or flavoured tongue depressors available to encourage compliance in testing tongue strength and resistance, as well as appealing reinforcers for cooperation with the *essential* motor speech evaluation.

Diagnosis and reporting

In reporting the diagnosis, the key symptoms that explain *why* a clinician believes a child has CAS should be clearly specified. Bearing in mind that these features may overlap with other child SSDs, these might include: token-to-token inconsistency, vowel errors, disordered prosody, increased errors on increased length of utterance, groping, and difficulty sequencing sounds and syllables. The speech characteristics that argue against alternative diagnoses should also be stated, for example, that structures have adequate range of motion, speed, strength, and coordination; age-appropriate language or a receptive–expressive gap; error types consistent with the CAS picture. Other speech issues or symptoms in a child with CAS should be specified, for example, symptoms that suggest a dysarthric or a phonological component, or that signal cognitive issues, or hypo- or hypertonicity (as in cerebral palsy and some syndromes). Lastly, the clinician must communicate clearly with caregivers about *all* of the factors contributing to the child's communication disorder (Stoeckel, A35). From my observations, it is a rare child who presents with pure CAS.

Overlapping symptoms and overlapping symptomatic treatments

As a motor speech disorder, CAS is a discrete diagnostic subtype of childhood (paediatric) SSD. There is a conservative consensus view that it is best characterised as a symptom complex rather than as a unitary disorder and that it may affect, to varying degrees, some combination of: non-speech motor behaviours; motor speech behaviours; speech sounds and structures (word and syllable shapes); prosody; language; metalinguistic/phonemic awareness; and literacy (ASHA 2007b). It is also generally agreed that many 'CAS characteristics' can be observed in children with other subtypes of SSD, including DPD, and that CAS and DPD can co-occur in an individual child. Little wonder then that Velleman and Strand (1994) declared that this, 'may result in a variety of motor, phonologic, linguistic, or neurologic signs or symptoms and in fact inconsistency among symptoms may be expected as typical'.

Current thinking in academia and in the field tends towards a focus on the overlap of symptoms, and the overlap of treatment methodologies, for children with CAS and children with moderate through to severe DPD. A common sense (to some) symptomatic approach to treatment is emerging. In this connection, Velleman (2005) wrote: 'CAS is different from 'regular' phonological disorders, but there are still patterns to be found and treated. There is a great deal of overlap in the symptoms of CAS and the symptoms of other phonological disorders, so it's often difficult to decide whether a diagnosis of CAS is appropriate. But, in a sense, that doesn't matter. Treat the symptoms, not the label.' But then, in an area that enjoys its spirited controversies, this idea does not appeal to all! In A38, Lynn Flahive, who *is* in agreement, elaborates this approach and what it means to her in practice. An instructor and clinic coordinator in the Department of Communication Sciences and Disorders at Texas Christian University, and *Past President of the Texas Speech-Language-Hearing Association, Lynn's areas of interest are* articulation and phonology, communication in the 0–3 age range, and augmentative communication and supervision.

Q38.   Lynn Flahive: Symptomatic manangement of SSD

Maassen (2002) reflects on a finding of Shriberg, Aram, and Kwiatkowski (1997) that, whereas late onset of speech and slow development are usual, neither a typical phonological developmental pathway nor a characteristic phonological profile for children with sCAS has been found, and that CAS has no phonological characteristics that are uniquely its own. That is not to say, however, that phonological processes (Ingram 1981), rules (Ingram 1974; Lowe 1994), or patterns (Hodson and Paden 1991) are not to be found in CAS. Can you explain and illustrate with a case example how a clinician might work with the 'treat the symptoms, not the label' directive that comes from much of the recent literature?

A38.   Lynn Flahive: Treat the symptoms not the label

In my university clinic work setting, I see an over-identification of CAS in preschool-aged children by speech pathologists in the surrounding community. For example, one Fall, 10 boys were admitted to our preschool programs and 9 of them had been diagnosed with CAS by other agencies. Shriberg, Campbell, Karlsson, et al. (2003) and Shriberg (2004) suggested that, if 10% of all children were on a speech pathology caseload at some time in their lives, only 10% of those children would have CAS, so that the incidence of children with CAS in a typical general paediatric caseload is less than 1%. By implication, this suggests that the proportion of children who actually have CAS is much lower than is indicated by the rate at which it is being assigned to speech-impaired children in my area.

One of the boys was 'Aidan', aged 3;8 when I first met him at my university clinic with his mother, 'Tina'. Aidan had been diagnosed with CAS at 2;2 by an SLP at a community agency, who noted that he had 'difficulty sequencing oral–motor movements, limited consonant inventory, limited vowel production, difficulty with volitional movements, and used only CV or V patterns', and that his phonetic inventory was restricted to [p, b, t, d, k, g, h, w, f, and s]. Administration of a standardised test of articulation or phonology was not reported. A review of Aidan's treatment plans with the treating clinician indicated that NS-OME comprised the bulk of the therapy, over 18 months. In addition to 'palate brushing', his exercises included imitation of kissing, blowing, tongue lateralisation, lip puckering, and cheek puffing, practised at home with Tina. Aidan was assigned the 'CAS label', without appropriate, detailed evaluation that might have revealed an alternative diagnosis. His presenting speech characteristics, as far as they were assessed, could have reflected CAS, or disordered phonology, or CAS plus disordered phonology. Features of Aidan's therapy at our clinic will be discussed in a subsequent section, but first, discussion of some of the points his case raises is presented.

Shared characteristics

It is critical that SLPs/SLTs look beyond the label when planning treatment goals and strategies because many of the characteristics of CAS are also seen in children with a profound phonological impairment (Hodson 2007). These children have a greater than 150 total occurrence of major phonological deviations on the HAPP-3 (Hodson 2004), with extensive sound omissions and substitutions. Children with both CAS and profound phonological impairment (Hodson 2007) may exhibit limited phonetic repertoires, reduplicated syllables, inconsistency in word production, vowel deviations, prosodic differences, and a gap between receptive and expressive language skills. Each of these characteristics, shared by both populations, requires careful assessment and treatment based on such assessment.

In my practice, I observe that children, like Aidan, diagnosed with CAS (but who may well have phonological impairment only) are treated, by speech-language professionals in the surrounding community, with therapies that do not take into account their presenting speech characteristics. Most often in our area, these children are treated with only NS-OME or with NS-OME plus traditional articulation therapy. This, of course, is worrisome given the lack of evidence for NS-OME's effectiveness (Lof 2003; A30; Hodge A26).

My strategy when working with highly unintelligible preschoolers is to take the route advised by Flahive, Velleman and Hodson (2005), and that is to treat the symptoms, taking suspected diagnosis into account. I begin by administering a standardised test of phonology, and my procedure of choice is the HAPP-3 (Hodson 2004). Based on the findings, I treat the child using the cycles approach (Hodson 2007), typically for a minimum of 1 year. In the cycles approach, the focus is not on individual phonemes, but rather on syllable structure and word productions (Hodson, Sherz, and Strattman 2002). If they were present, initial patterns that I would address would include syllableness, final consonant deletion, velar fronting, and /s/ cluster reduction. For children with limited phonetic inventories, working with a cycles approach will, by default, expand their inventories when these initial patterns become goals. It is also critical that PA tasks be incorporated into treatment regimens. Children with disordered expressive phonology are at risk for literacy difficulty. Early introduction of PA tasks, such as rhyming and syllable identification, may improve these skills and appears to benefit their expressive phonology (Rvachew 2006a; Gillon 2006). In response to research clarifying the relationships between expressive phonological abilities and PA, Hodson (2007) now advises the inclusion of a brief metaphonological (PA) activity within each intervention session.

As a child's intelligibility improves, and cooperation with speech imitation tasks grows easier for him/her, further evaluation is conducted, if indicated, to explore the possibility of CAS. The signs that might prompt me to undertake this further evaluation include continuing difficulties with suprasegmentals (prosody) and/or little progress. My assessment typically includes an oral mechanism evaluation and a prosodic assessment (Skinder-Meredith, A37; Strand, A40).

Case example

Returning to Aidan, now aged 3;8, we find that a HAPP-3 evaluation at my clinic revealed a Total Occurrences of Major Phonological Deviations score of 74, with a moderate severity rating. The percentages of occurrence of his significant phonological error patterns were consonant sequence/cluster reduction 59%, liquid deficiency 58%, gliding 50% and velar fronting 50%. He was able to produce, as singletons, all phones except for /ð/, /ʒ/, /j/, and no vowel errors were exhibited. He had difficulty in sequencing longer utterances, and his prosody, particularly word stress, was atypical with his speech sounding 'robotic'. In sum, Aidan's output had many of the characteristics of CAS as well as clearly defined symptoms of moderately disordered phonology. In terms of his phonology, it was noted that Aidan's phonological patterns had not been previously identified or addressed in his therapy between 2;2 and 3;8. Rather than intervening with an 'either-or approach' (i.e., either 'CAS therapy' or 'phonological therapy'), both were employed in our intervention in order to make the best use of his therapy time.

He entered our Early Childhood Speech and Language Program: Levels I and II, receiving both group and individual therapy. The Level I program consisted of 1.5-hours of group therapy one day per week with two, additional half-hour sessions of individual therapy over a 13-week period. The Level II program consisted of 1 hour of individual therapy and 2 hours of group therapy each week for 13 weeks. His Level I and II programs extended over two academic years, a total of four semesters. In total, he had 182 hours of group therapy and 104 hours of individual therapy. His therapy was provided by undergraduate and graduate students in our speech pathology program under the supervision of ASHA-certified and state-licensed speech pathology faculty. Once Aidan began therapy at the University clinic, he received no speech therapy intervention elsewhere.

Activities during group therapy involved the verbal routines suggested by Davis and Velleman (2000) for children with CAS. Tasks included rhythmic actions, such as beating on instruments in-time with speech (e.g., Aidan would beat on a toy drum while repeating a targeted syllable such as, *ba-ba-ba*), and multimodality activities, such as sliding down a slide while saying '*weee*' or drawing large circles/shapes on a board while saying sounds (e.g., Aidan would say, *ssss*, sustaining it while drawing circles). Also, sequential play activities were done with the children (e.g., Aidan would pretend to pour a drink into a cup and then feed it to a doll). Group therapy also incorporated various phonemic awareness tasks, such as simple rhyming activities (e.g., the student clinician would say a word such as *bat*, and Aidan and the other children would tell another word that rhymed) and syllable identification through hand clapping (e.g., Aidan would clap his hands three times, once for each syllable, when the student clinician said *butterfly*).

His individual therapy sessions during this time followed the cycles approach (Hodson 2007). Targeted patterns, over four semesters (2 years), included: syllableness, velars, /s/ clusters, and liquids for four semesters; and following Hodson's guidance, each of Aidan's sessions (group and individual) included a brief metaphonological (PA) activity. The HAPP-3 was again administered at the end of 2 years. Aidan, 5;8, now had a rating of mild, and his residual substitution errors were /f/ for /θ/ and /d/ for /ð/, both age-appropriate. He continued in therapy to work on mild difficulties with expressive morphology, particularly verb tenses and articles.

Aidan's previous SLP had applied the CAS label to him and treated him for 18 months with her agency's standard NS-OME approach without regard to his particular speech characteristics, failing to address his difficulties with acquiring the sound system of English. When I assessed him, I looked beyond the previously applied label and assessed his output in fine detail. With a combination of the cycles approach (Hodson 2007), CAS strategies (Davis and Velleman 2000), and PA activities (Gillon 2006), his speech sound system normalised within 2 years. Aidan's story provides a revealing example of the advantages of (1) adequate speech assessment; (2) not applying a 'standard' one-size-fits-all approach (especially not an NS-OMT approach) to poor speech intelligibility; and, most powerfully, (3) treating the symptoms, not the label.

Symptomatic overlap between DPD and CAS

Because DPD and CAS symptoms overlap, at times SLP/SLTs' assessment methods, treatment goals, therapy approaches, procedures, and activities will obviously be similar for both populations. As individual clinicians, our own individual theories of development, theories of disorders, and theories of intervention determine our assessment methods, the goals we prioritise, how we attack them, the strategies we use, and the therapy we select (Fey 1992b; and see Table 1.3, p. 31). Differential diagnosis between DPD and CAS is often lengthy and may be inconclusive. Box 6.3 displays the characteristics and signs of both, to guide the clinician's thinking in the process, and Boxes 6.4 and 6.5 provide a comparison between the treatment principles for DPD and CAS, respectively.

Table 6.1 displayed the typical errors found in DPD and CAS relative to each of the error types in common, as well as the typical therapy goals for both. Table 6.4 shows the error types and goals again, but this time with their corresponding approaches and techniques, or 'how to' address the goals. In the following section, these 18 approaches and techniques are either described briefly or the reader is directed to relevant sections in other chapters. Note that stimulability training, pre-practice, phonemic placement techniques, shaping, phonotactic therapy, progressive approximations, and techniques

Box 6.3 A clinician's prompt for differential diagnosis

DPD Characteristics

1. Static speech sound system
2. Variable production without gradual improvement
3. Persistence of phonological processes
4. Chronological mismatch
5. Idiosyncratic rules/processes
6. Restricted use of contrast

DPD Signs

1. Puzzle phenomenon
2. Unusual errors
3. Marking
4. Stimulability

Consider the possibility of DPD and a phonological intervention approach if:

● Puzzle phenomenon is evident*
● There are unusual errors
● The child is marking contrasts 'oddly'*
● Error sounds are readily stimulable

CAS Characteristics

(Davis, Jakielski, and Marquardt 1998)
In an individual child, speech *may* reveal:

● imited consonant repertoire
● Limited vowel repertoire
● Frequent omissions
● High incidence of vowel errors
● Inconsistent articulation errors
● Altered suprasegmentals (prosody)
● Increased errors with output length/complexity
● Difficulty in imitation (groping/refusal)
● Use of simple syllable shapes

and non-speech characteristics *may* include:

● Impaired voluntary oral movements
● RLS-ELS gap (receptive language better)
● Lower diadochokinetic rates

CAS Signs

● Speech motor sequencing difficulties
● Prosodic/suprasegmental differences
● Receptive language exceeds expressive language: 'the gap'

* examples are provided in Chapter 8

Six clinical characteristics that CAS and DPD may have in common:

1. Consonant, vowel, and phonotactic inventory constraints;
2. Omissions of segments and structures;
3. Segmental errors;
4. Altered suprasegmentals (prosody);
5. Increased errors with utterance length and/or complexity; and
6. Use of simple (but not complex) syllable and word shapes.

CAS: a 'symptom complex' rather than a unitary disorder of:

• Volitional (voluntary) movement
• Spatial–temporal coordination
• Motor sequencing
• Performing or learning complex movements
• Central sensorimotor processes
• Accommodation to context (co-articulatory, phonotactic, voice onset time, etc.)

Ask: Is it DPD? Is it CAS? Is it a dysarthria? Is it VPI? Or some combination of these? Or SLI plus?

Box 6.4 Treatment principles: DPD

Phonological Therapy

1. is based on the systematic nature of phonology;
2. is characterised by conceptual, rather than motor ('artic drill'), activities; and,
3. has generalisation as its ultimate goal.

Phonological therapy approaches are designed to nurture the child's system rather than simply to teach new sounds (Fey 1992a, p. 277).

Treatment Principles for DPD (based on the available literature)

- Work at *word* level.
- Work towards functional generalisation.
- Treat a pattern or patterns of errors.
- If using a three-position SODA test, transcribe entire words in order to see error pattern(s).
- Teach appropriate contrasts.
- Direct the child's attention to the way that different sounds make different meanings. Make this apparent to parents, e.g., give examples of their child's homonymy.
- Use naturalistic contexts that have *meaning* (hold interest) for the child, because this helps demonstrate to the child that the function of phonology is to make meaning.
- Stack the environment with several exemplars of each individual target word so the child can self-select activities, e.g., for work on eliminating Velar Fronting, for the target words: car, key, core, cow, have available several different cars, keys, etc.
- Select targets with an eye to their potential impact on the child's system.
- Carefully select exemplars of an error pattern/phonological rule. With clever exemplar choices, the rule is learned, and carries over to the other targets.
- In explicitly targeted therapy, it should be unnecessary to work on all possible targets.

Box 6.5 Treatment principles: CAS

Treatment Principles for CAS (based on the available literature)

- Use paired auditory and visual stimuli in intensive practice trials.
- Train sound combinations (CV VC CVC . . .) rather than isolated phones.
- Keep the focus in therapy (and at home) on movement performance drill.
- Use repetitive production trials/systematic drill as intensively as possible.
- Carefully construct hierarchies of stimuli, using small steps.
- Use reduced production rate with proprioceptive monitoring (child's self-monitoring).
- Use *simple* carrier phrases and *simple* cloze tasks.
- Pair movement sequences with suprasegmental facilitators: including stress, intonation, and rhythm.
- Use singing, whispering, and loudness judiciously.
- Establish a core vocabulary or a small number 'power words' (that make things happen) early in therapy, especially for non-verbal or minimally verbal children.
- Use sign/AAC to facilitate communication, intelligibility, and language development, and to reduce frustration. Reassure families.
- Be flexible. Treatment changes over time.
- Present regular, consistent, effective homework as a 'given', within reason.
- Expect 'good days and bad days' in terms of the child's performance.

Table 6.4 DPD and CAS goals, approaches, and techniques in common

Characteristics CAS and DPD may have in common	DPD and CAS typical therapy goals	DPD and CAS approaches techniques
1. Consonant (C), Vowel (V), and phonotactic inventory constraints	• C inventory expansion • V inventory expansion	1) Stimulability training 2) Pre-practice 3) Phonemic placement techniques 4) Shaping
2. Omissions of consonants, vowels, and syllable shapes already in the inventory	• Syllable shape inventory expansion • Word shape inventory expansion • Increased accuracy of production of target structures	5) CV syllable and word drills 6) Phonotactic therapy 7) Metalinguistic approach 8) Reading
3. Vowel errors	• More complete V repertoire • More accurate V production	• Stimulability training • Pre-practice • Phonemic placement techniques • Shaping 9) Auditory input therapy/thematic play 10) Minimal contrasts therapy
4. Altered suprasegmentals	• Production of S and W syllables • Differentiation of S and W syllables	• Phonotactic therapy 11) Melodic intonation therapy 12) Singing
5. More errors with longer and/or more complex utterances, including the so-called 'SODA' errors of substitution, distortion, and addition	• Generalisation of new sounds (Cs and Vs), syllable structures, and word structures to more challenging contexts.	13) Prolongation of vowels 14) Slowed rate of production 15) Progressive approximations 16) SW-production drill 17) Techniques to encourage self-monitoring
6. Use of simple, but not complex, syllable shapes and word shapes	• More complete phonotactic repertoire • More varied use of phonotactic range within syllables and words • Improved accuracy	• Phonotactic therapy • Progressive approximations 18) SW and CS production drill 19) Backward build-ups 20) Backward chaining • Techniques to encourage self-monitoring

to encourage self-monitoring are all mentioned in relation to more than one goal, and each is discussed under one heading below.

Approaches and techniques in symptomatic treatment

1. Pre-practice

Pre-practice is an early step in motor learning (see Chapter 7) that occurs prior to entering the practice phase. As Table 6.4 indicates, pre-practice, like stimulability training, phonetic placement techniques, and shaping, has an important role in consonant and vowel inventory expansion. This extends into pre-practice for new syllable shapes, words, and longer utterances. In treating SSD, pre-practice is usually inextricably bound up with stimulability training, phonetic placement techniques, and shaping.

2. Stimulability training

A rationale and a program for stimulability training are described by Miccio (A15; p. 97) (A15). Miccio's treatment (Miccio 2005; Miccio and Elbert 1996) was evaluated with children with phonological disorder and not CAS, but it has immediate relevance to all children with depleted phonetic and phonemic inventories.

3. Phonetic placement techniques

There are several excellent published sources of techniques for phonetic placement, particularly Bleile (1995, 2004, 2006); Secord, Boyce, Donohue, et al. (2007); Hanson (1983); Hegde and Pena-Brooks (2007); Ruscello (2008a); and Winitz (1984). Phonetic placement is precisely what it sounds like—the physical positioning of the client's articulators into the correct place of articulation and associating it with the correct manner of articulation (and of course voicing). Phonetic placement techniques may incorporate a variety of models provided by the clinician or other helper for immediate or delayed imitation. Imagery names, simple verbal cues and reminders, and iconic gesture cues, as displayed in Table 6.5, are also employed.

4. Shaping

Shaping involves altering a sound already in the child's repertoire to produce a new sound. For example, a prolonged, 'fricated' [t] might be shaped into /s/; or [t] closely followed by [ʃ] might be shaped into /tʃ/. An example of a shaping technique to address lateral and palatal fricatives and affricates is the Butterfly Procedure, available on the Internet at: http://www.speech-language-therapy.com/fsd-butterfly-procedure.htm.

5. CV syllable and word drills

CV-syllable drill and CV-word drill involve repetitive practice of spoken, chanted, or sung syllables, such as 'many repeats' of *bye-bye-bye*, or *bay-bee-bay-bee-bay-bee*, or rehearsal of a list of CV syllables with a common phonetic or structural characteristic, such as *fee-fie-foe-fum* or *ha-ha-hee-hee-ho-ho-hoo-hoo-hi-hi* or *up-up-up-up* or *off-off-off-off-off*. The term 'drill play' implies that syllable and word drills are performed in the context of games or other activities children like. Drill and drill play can be enjoyable for children with games such as *Go Fish*, *Snap*, and other card games, board games, and materials such as posting boxes, *Word Flips* (Granger 2005), commercially available, and home-made flip shoots, customised computer slide shows, and various speech therapy programs, notably the Williams and Stephens (2004) Nuffield worksheets.

Table 6.5 Information for families: Imagery names and verbal and gesture cues and reminders

Target in isolation, or CV or VC syllables modelled by parent or clinician	Imagery name provided by parent or clinician and possibly modified by the child	Verbal cue provided by parent or clinician	Gesture cue provided by adult (parent /clinician/'helper')
STOPS			
p b	Popping sounds Poppers Pop sounds	'Where's your pop?'* 'You forgot your pop.' 'Let's hear your pop.'	Adult puffs his/her cheeks up with air, and 'plodes' the /p/ or /b/ onto the child's hand for them to feel the 'pop'.
t d	Tippy sounds Tippies Tongue ready!	'Use your tippy.' 'Let's hear your tippy.' "Was your tongue ready?'	Adult touches his/her philtrum with straight finger.
k g	Throaty sounds Throaties Glug-glug sounds	'Where's your throaty?'	Adult makes a 'U' with thumb and index finger, so that they touch the angles of the mandible.
NASALS			
m	Humming sound Yum-yum sound	'Close your mouth and humm. . .' or 'mmm mmm'	Adult hums 'mmm' with lips shut, touching the larynx to feel vibration.
n	'N. . .' sound	'Tongue ready and buzz.'	Adult hums 'nnn' touching the larynx to feel vibration.
ADJUNCTS			
s + stop	Friendly sounds Twins	'You forgot your friend.'	Adult slides an index finger from left to right on the table top, or up his/her arm, while saying /s/, and ends by tapping the finger (silently) when the 'friendly sound' (the stop) is added. Or makes an arm movement that ends with the thumb and all fingers being snapped shut crocodile-style.
sp st sk		'Where's your friend?' 'You forgot his/her twin.'	
CLUSTERS 2-ELEMENT CLUSTERS	Two-step sounds Two-steps	'Let's hear your two steps.' 'Where's your other step?' 'And your next step?'	Adult 'walks' with fingers on a surface or up an imaginary ladder saying the first element on the first step and the second on the second step.
FRICATIVES			
h	Puppy panting sound Hot puppy sound Open mouth windy	'Where's your puppy? 'Where's your wind?' 'I didn't feel your wind.'	Adult places a flattened hand just in front of his/her or the child's mouth to feel the air.
f v	Bunny rabbit sound Biting lip windy Lip-up sound	'You forgot to bite.' 'You forgot your wind.' 'Where's your bunny?'	Adult brings his/her lower lip up to touch the teeth and blows, or makes a face like a rabbit.

Table 6.5 (*Continued*)

s SIWI	Smiley windy Snake sound Big snake teeth	'Show me your teeth.'	Adult makes a toothy smile and blows, indicating frontal air-flow with the fingers.
AFFRICATES tʃ dʒ	Chomping sound Munching sound Choo-choo train sound Elephant trunk sound	'Make those lips move!' 'Work your lips.' 'Where's the choo-choo?' 'Where's your trunk?'	Adult protrudes his/her lips (like an imaginary trunk) while making a chomping or choo-choo sound.
LIQUIDS l	Tower sound Up-down sound Tongue ready la-lal	'Open up - tongue up.' 'Tongue ready, and down.' 'Touch the top!'	Adult assumes a mouth open posture with the tongue up behind upper teeth, then lowers it to behind the bottom teeth, using a mirror to rehearse silently first.
r	'Rrr' sound Growly bear sound	'Push up on the sides and move back with your tongue.'	Adult demonstrates pushing up on sides of tongue in the butterfly position.
GLIDES w	Pouty face Puffy lips	'OOO-EEE sliding' 'OOO-WEE sliding'	Adult starts out in the 'oo' position with pouting lips then moves to 'ee'.
j	Sliding sound Eeyore sound Smiley-pouty sound	'EEE-OR sliding' 'EEE-YOR sliding'	Adult starts with 'ee' with a wide smile then moves to pouty face (or).
FINAL CONSONANTS All final consonants	Sticky sounds	'Where's your sticky?'	Adult moves his/her arm from left to right starting with an open hand and finishing with a closed hand.

* Refer to 'your' pop, 'your' windy, etc. so that the child 'owns' the target.

6. Phonotactic therapy

In a highly recommended article, Velleman (2002) adopted a non-linear framework noting that immature phonotactic patterns (immature word shapes and sound sequences) require us to focus on the syllable level, and that therapy that addresses syllable shapes has the potential to evoke generalisation well beyond the specific sound or sounds targeted in the particular syllable position. 'Phonotactic patterns' or syllable structure processes (see Table 2.4, p. 47) that may be problematic for children with DPD, CAS, or both diagnoses include initial consonant deletion, final consonant deletion, replacement of a VC with a diphthong, reduplication, weak syllable deletion, reduction of multi-syllabic words, and cluster reduction. These clients may also only ever produce monosyllables, and they may produce erroneous word stress patterns. Strategies to address these difficulties are suggested below.

Initial consonant deletion

In children with ICD, reinforce any initial consonants in CV syllables irrespective of accuracy, starting with consonants already in the child's inventory. VC combinations, repeated in strings, can be used to facilitate CV syllable shapes. For example, *oak-oak-oak-oak-oak-oak* might be repeated and gradually shaped into *coke-coke-coke-coke*, or *um-um-um-um-um* might be used to elicit *mum-mum-mum-mum*.

Final consonant deletion

FCD past about 2;10 is cause for concern (see Box 2.2, p. 57). Most consonants in English are mastered first SIWI with the exceptions being velars and fricatives, which are mastered first SFWF. English is a language with many final consonants and many CVC words and syllables. The most prevalent final consonants are velars, fricatives, and voiceless stops. To facilitate the development of final consonants, the clinician can reward *any* final consonant, irrespective of accuracy at first, focusing on sounds already in the child's inventory, and favouring prominent final consonants in the language—that is, fricatives, velars. and voiceless stops. It is helpful also to remember that, in typical development, children produce their first instances of final consonants (codas) after short (lax) vowels, so success may be optimised by target-word choices such as *buck*, *dove* (the bird), and *foot*, where the vowel is short, rather than *beak*, and *feet*, where the consonants are the same but the vowels are long, and to avoid CVCs containing diphthongs (e.g., *bake*, *dive*, *Dave* and *fight*).

Replacement of a VC with a diphthong

Due to a syllable weight unit constraint, some children with DPD or CAS will produce CVC words such as *bush* as [bʊə], *keys* as [kiə], and *walk* as [wɔə], evidently 'knowing' that something is needed after first vowel but making a mistake about its consonantal nature. This can be tackled by using repeated sequences of CVCVCV (which the child *can* produce) building up to the removal of the second consonant, for example, [pʌpʌ-pʌpʌ-pʌpʌ-pʌpʌ-pʌpʌ-pʌp]. Ideal early targets for this are pictured 'harmony words' with short vowels and the same initial and final consonants, such as *Bob, bub, cook, dad, kick, mum, nan, none, pip, pop, pup, sis,* and *toot*; these can be freely downloaded from http://www.speech-language-therapy.com/freebies.htm.

Reduplication

In reduplication, typical early language learners and older children with speech disorders repeat the first syllable of a two-syllable word or utterance so that *daddy* becomes [dædæ], *water* is pronounced [wɔwɔ], and *me too* becomes [mimi]. A natural phonological tendency is for toddlers to produce the high front vowel /i/ as the second vowel of CVCV babble of words (e.g., *blankie, cookie, dolly, doggie*). We can take advantage of this tendency by choosing two-syllable words with alveolar consonants and /i/ in the second syllable, noting that high front vowels actually tend to co-occur in the language. Early targets could include *buddy, busy, daddy, kissy, nanny, potty,* and *pussy,* and baby words like *nighty-night, mousie,* and *botty* that a given family actually uses in child-directed speech (or 'parentese').

Production of monosyllables only

To increase the number of syllables a child can produce, known vocabulary can be employed in a reduplication strategy. For example, *bye* might be repeated often in sung, chanted, or spoken sequences, and then the timing changed so that the child eventually finds that he/she is saying *bye-bye.* Not every family (or clinician) will be able to tolerate words like *poo, pee, foo-foo, kaka,* and *wee,* but where they are acceptable, they can be useful as early targets, not least because the children themselves are often fascinated by 'rude' words, and their siblings in the younger age group will often be quite delighted to reinforce them! Other useful early targets are *boo-boo, ho-ho, dah-dah,* and similar reduplicated combinations. Once a child is producing a range of these comfortably, a consonant or a vowel in one syllable can be changed to produce a new (meaningful) word or onomatopoeic sound effect. For example, *wee wee* might change to *peewee,* or *pee pee* might be changed to *pee paw* for a fire-engine sound effect.

Weak syllable deletion and reduction of multi-syllabic words

Some children only delete weak syllables if the word or phrase is iambic; that is, if the stress pattern is weak-strong as in *around* or weak-strong-weak-strong as in *a round-about.* So, for example, they can say the trochaic word *monkey* (strong-weak) but not *giraffe* (weak-strong). This tendency is exacerbated if a weak syllable precedes the iambic word or phrase, as it the following examples where the stress pattern is weak-strong-weak-weak-strong: 'I saw a guitar'; 'We got a balloon', which feed the tendency for the child to pronounce *guitar* as [ta] and *balloon* as [bun]. For carrier phrase in drill or drill play, these can be made easier for the child to say if the therapist makes the utterances iambic, with the insertion of a stressed word: 'I *saw* a *big* guitar'; 'I *saw* a *nice* guitar'; 'I *saw* a *red* guitar'; 'I *saw* a *great* guitar'; 'I *saw* a *strange* guitar'; and 'We *got* a *long* balloon'; 'We *got* a *round* balloon'; 'We *got* a *square* balloon'; 'We *got* a *weird* balloon'; 'We *got* a *good* balloon'. With the goal of increasing the number of syllables a child can produce, we can capitalise on the natural tendency in development for trochees (strong-weak) to be easier to say. To this end, we can target trochaic words and sequences first, gradually adding a few of the harder (iambic) sequences when the child is ready. Fun trochaic sequences that lend themselves to word play and promote repetition might include: *silly billy, polly wolly, dilly dally,* and *teeter totter*; and *water pistol, Peter Parker, Wonder Woman, Reader Rabbit, Buster Keaton, Mr. Fixit,* and *Lego Island.*

Cluster reduction

Remarkably, typical English-learning two year olds produce some combination of clusters SIWI, SFWF, or both, and by 3;5, full clusters are produced 75% of the time or better! The general trend in acquiring clusters is from complete deletion (which, like initial consonant deletion, is rare in English), such as [ɪm] for *swim*, then deletion of one element (e.g., [wɪm] for *swim*), substitution of one element (e.g., [fwɪm] for *swim*), to correct production (i.e., [swɪm] for *swim*). When an element of a two-element cluster is deleted, it is typically, but not always, the most marked one, that is, the one that is most *uncommon* in the languages of the world. For example, /s/ is deleted from *snail*, *small*, *swing*, and *squash*, and liquids are deleted from *blue*, *play*, *tree*, *cry*, *drop*, *flower*, and *slug*. Similarly, /s/ is deleted from the adjuncts /sp/, /st/, and /sk/. Note that for some linguists, /sm/ and /sn/ sit somewhere between 'true clusters' (complex onsets) and adjuncts. Baker (A11; p. 73) provides guidance on cluster target selection and a rationale for prioritising more marked clusters to evoke generalisation to less marked ones, inviting us to put three-element clusters (e.g., /spl, str/) or those with small sonority difference scores, such as /fl, sl, ʃr/, first. Morrisette, Farris, and Gierut (2006) postulate that initial /s/+ stop 'clusters' are adjuncts and not 'true clusters', and therefore are not subject to the implicational relationships amongst clusters with respect to sonority. Although Gierut (2007) advised against targeting adjuncts because they did not follow the sonority sequencing principle, and therefore did not lend themselves to promoting system-wide change, in clinical contexts, it may be tempting, and defensible, to 'break the rules'. Because /sp/ and /st/ are 'visible' or easily modelled for children, the clinician may target these early on in therapy for a child with no or few clusters, not with a view to system-wide generalisation, but with the intention of giving the child 'the idea' of a 'two-step sound' (see Table 6.5).

7. Metalinguistic approaches

In therapy for child speech, metalinguistic approaches involve the child talking about and reflecting upon: (a) the properties of phonemes (e.g., the features of place, voice, and manner displayed in Table 2.5, p. 58 expressed in age-appropriate language), (b) the structures of syllables, and (c) communicative effectiveness. They reflect on the functions of phonemes and syllable shapes in making meaning through a system of contrasts, actively revising and repairing their own error productions. If the child is able (this usually means 'old enough'), reading (see point 8 below) and/or Phoneme Awareness Therapy (Hesketh, A22; p. 143) are incorporated. Discrimination Training as a component of Traditional Articulation Therapy, Stimulability Therapy (Miccio, A15; p. 97), Auditory Input Therapy (Lancaster, A20; p. 129), Perceptuallybased Interventions (Rvachew, A24; p. 157), Metaphon (Chapter 4), the four Minimal Pair approaches and Grunwell Therapy (Chapter 4), Core Vocabulary Therapy (Chapter 4), Imagery Therapy (Chapter 4), the Psycholinguistic Framework (Gardner, A21), Vowel Therapy using a contrastive approach (Gibbon, A23), and PACT (Chapter 9) all rest to a greater or lesser extent on working actively at a metalinguistic level. Relevant activities and procedures include those described in Table 6.5 and under the heading *Multiple Exemplar Training* in Chapter 9.

8. Reading

In working on syllable shape inventory expansion, word shape inventory expansion, and increased accuracy of production of target structures, as sophisticated metalinguistic tasks, reading and spelling can contribute to speech progress whether the child is being read to or whether the child is doing the reading. Story reading and spelling and reading games can help young readers with speech impairment to increase their awareness of the structures of syllables, and the sequences in which sounds occur, and letters and words provide needed cues and prompts. Games that involve letter manipulation, word assembly and word building with concrete media such as letter-tiles, and similar activities are easily incorporated into therapy.

9. Auditory input therapy/thematic play

In this therapy, multiple exemplars of targets are provided in input, while the child *listens*, or better still *watches* and listens, during play activities with little or no requirement for the child to imitate or name words. Described by Lancaster (A20; p. 129) and an important ingredient of PACT, it has a twofold rationale: (1) homonymy motivates phonemic change; and (2) repeated exposure to a word target enhances saliency, thus increasing learnability. Figure 6.1 provides an example of a story a child might be told with word-final /f/ as the target. Once the story has been read, it is easy to pursue the goal of 'immersing' the child in final-f by developing games related to the story. For example, the child might make *scarves* for his/her soft toys, or play a game involving zoo animals crowding onto a *roof* one by one to be *safe* from a marauding *wolf*.

10. Minimal contrast therapy

The attributes of the four minimal pair approaches, or minimal contrast therapies (Conventional Minimal Pairs, Maximal Oppositions, Multiple Oppositions and Empty Set), are summarised in Table 6.6 and described in Chapter 4.

11. Melodic intonation therapy

Melodic intonation therapy (MIT) might be termed a 'prosodic approach' and perhaps called 'chanting therapy' and is based, according to Helfrich-Miller (1983, 1984, 1994) who developed it for children with CAS, on three elements of prosody: melody, rhythm, and stress. Although it has been validated as a short-term intervention demonstrating qualitative improvement in the speech of adults with Broca's Aphasia (Benson, Dobkin, and Gonzalez 1994), its efficacy with children with CAS is inconclusive. It was never intended as a stand-alone therapy (Helfrich-Miller 1994), and when used in conjunction with the kindred approaches of Integral Stimulation (Chapter 7), singing, and prolongation of vowels, it appears to have clinical utility. In MIT, an intoned utterance is lengthened and the rhythm and stress are exaggerated, while the pitch is held constant for several whole notes. In such intoned or chanted 'stylised' utterances, pitch typically varies by only one whole note. Its focus is not on the segmental level, but rather on prosody, and its role is in helping children to produce and differentiate strong and weak syllables and vary the length of notes (vocalisations) at will.

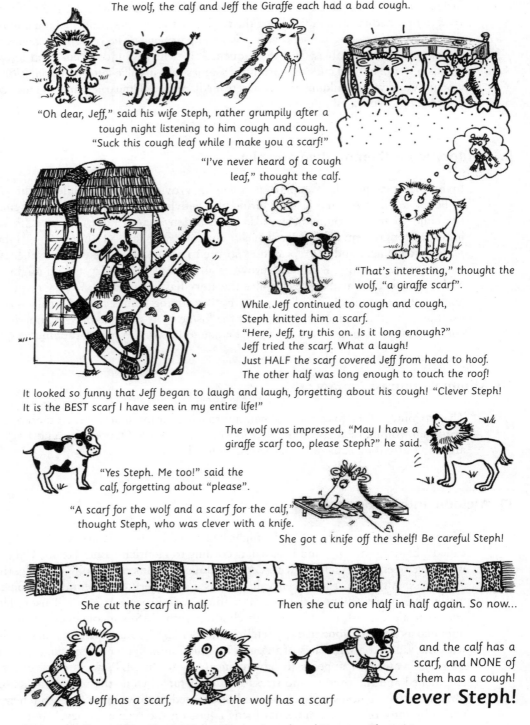

Figure 6.1 Jeff's scarf. Drawing by Helen Rippon, Speech and Language Therapist
www.blacksheeppress.co.uk

Table 6.6 Comparison of the minimal pair approaches described in Chapter 4

	Conventional minimal pairs	Maximal oppositions	Multiple oppositions	Empty set (unknown set)
Key Reference	Weiner (1981a)	Gierut (1989)	Williams (2003b)	Gierut (1989)
Contrasts	ERROR-TARGET The child's customary error is paired with the target.	CORRECT-TARGET The child's target sound (one that the child cannot say) is paired with a sound the child 'knows' (one that the child can say). The two sounds are maximally distinct.	ERROR-TARGETS Up to four of the child's targets (sounds they cannot say) are contrasted with an error. Target choices are based on phoneme collapses where the child replaces several sounds with one.	ERROR-ERROR Two errors (two sounds the child does not know) are paired as treatment targets. Not only does the child know neither of the sounds, but also the two sounds are maximally distinct.
Feature Difference	minimal or maximal, but usually minimal	maximal	minimal to maximal across a treatment set	maximal
Rationale	Eliminate homonymy by inducing a phonemic split.	Increased phonemic saliency facilitates learnability.	Eliminate homonymy by inducing multiple phonemic splits.	Increased phonemic saliency facilitates learnability.
	MILD-MODERATE	SEVERE	SEVERE	SEVERE
Severity of SSD	As a general guide, 'severe' SSD implies a PCC less than 50% at 4;0 years and above (see Table i.1; p. xii), and/or six inventory constraints across three manner categories and/or six sounds in error across three manner categories.			
Approach	LINGUISTIC	LINGUISTIC	LINGUISTIC	LINGUISTIC

12. Singing

Singing lends itself to decreased rate of production, so it may make proprioceptive monitoring easier for some children as well as allowing children who have difficulty 'keeping up' with the words of songs to cope better. 'Slowed down' versions of children's songs and nursery rhymes, such as *Time to Sing* from www.apraxia-kids.org, comprise an invaluable, fun resource for younger children, especially those who are minimally verbal. As well as facilitating self-monitoring, the clinician can run a 'visual check' to see that the child has optimal symmetry and the best possible articulatory configurations while producing the 'sung' words. For older children, slow karaoke is an entertaining vehicle for practice (e.g., http://perso.orange.fr/prof.danglais/animations/music/what_a_wonderful_world.swf).

Singing can be incorporated into several of the strategies listed above, particularly the reduplication strategy for increasing the number of syllables a child can produce, and auditory input therapy. With the reduplication strategy, a word sequence such as bye-bye can be repeated many times to the tune of a lullaby (e.g., Bye-bye baby, bye-bye-bye to *Doeler* the traditional tune for *Loving shepherd of thy sheep*; or to the tune of *There is a tavern in the town*. The latter lends itself to *Bye-bye bye baby, bye bye-bye*, *Mum Mum Mumma, Mumma Mum, Dad Dad Dadda Dadda Dad, Pop Pop*

Poppa Poppa Pop, *Nan Nan Nanna Nanna Nan*, and similar sequences) with a few tiddly-poms thrown in for amusement.

13. Prolongation of vowels

Clinicians can encourage generalisation of new consonants and vowels and new syllable structures and word structures to more challenging contexts by slowing children's utterance rate. It is more effective to prolong the vowels as in *Temporal and Tactile Cueing (DTTC) for Speech Motor Learning* (Chapter 7) (e.g., [sæː:ːt] for *sat* rather than consonants; e.g., [sː:ːæt] for *sat*). Vowel prolongation is a helpful strategy to apply when a novel word that is difficult for the child to produce is introduced, such as a significant name, like the surname of a new teacher that the child badly wants to say properly. Again, singing or chanting, as in MIT, can be incorporated into this technique and the three below.

14. Slowed rate of production

Within DTTC and in therapy generally when the aim is generalisation of newly acquired segments and structures to more difficult contexts for the child, it can be helpful to instate a 'slow talking time' as part of daily practice. This can be modelled by the clinician, and its purpose explained to parents and other helpers. It is important not to contrast 'slow talking' with 'fast talking'. It is rarely desirable to have a child with moderate or severe SSD to speak *rapidly*, and it is preferable to suggest to parents that they contrast slow rate with 'normal rate' or even 'ordinary rate'. This may prevent the child from getting the idea of talking quickly, a risky one for many of these children because their intelligibility may deteriorate as they gather speed.

15. Progressive approximations

The technique of progressive approximations, sometimes called successive approximations (Kaufman 2005), is used with shaping, cuing, and other feedback to 'convert' an utterance that the child can already produce into a new utterance. Usually the new utterance is not 'perfect' but rather a reasonable approximation to the intended target, intelligible to an interested or motivated listener. The following two examples are used by permission with the individuals' names changed. 'Simon', 19;0 was learning to travel independently by train and had to be able to ask for a ticket to Lindfield where his sheltered workshop was. *Lindfield* was beyond his capabilities, but he knew *Lynn* who helped at his school for many years, and associated *peel* with her name because one of her jobs was to assist students to peel and cut up fruit. He was trained to say *Lynn-peel* for *Lindfield*, and in the context of the railway station, this was fully intelligible to the ticket seller. In another example, 'Max', 6;0 needed to learn how to say the name of his school, *Leura Public*; the way that it happened can be found at http://www.speech-language-therapy.com/max.pps.

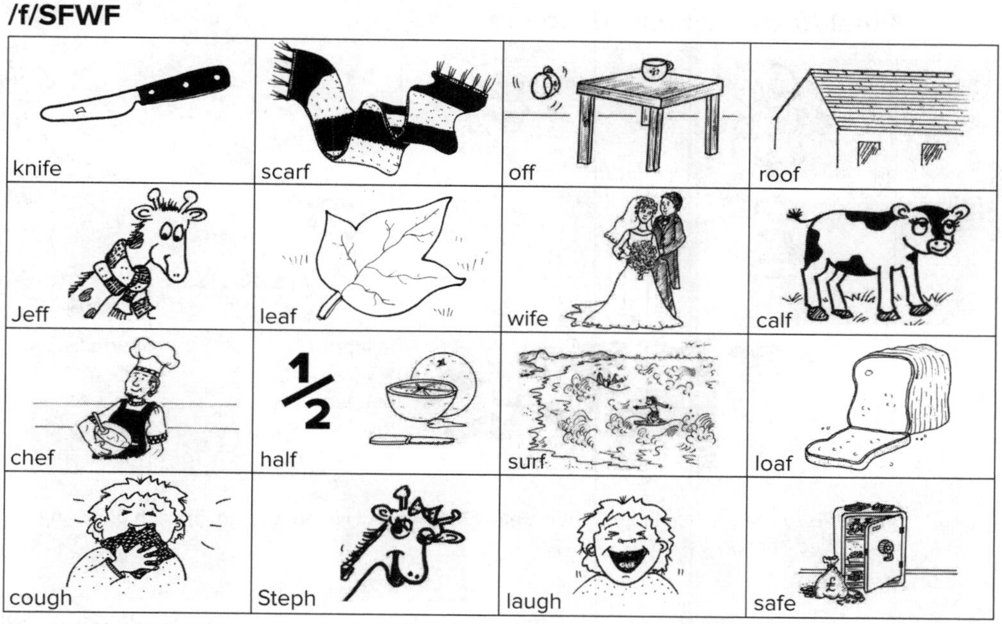

/f/ SFWF

Figure 6.2 /f/ SFWF – knife, Steph, off, roof, etc. Drawing by Helen Rippon, Speech and Language Therapist www.blacksheeppress.co.uk

16. Single word production drill

It is manifest in working with children with moderate and severe SSD, particularly children with CAS, that 'practice makes perfect' or at least 'practice makes good enough'. Production practice of single words containing target sounds or syllable shapes, or practice of 'difficult' or polysyllabic words, facilitates generalisation of newly-learned speech skills. The child might practice a few pictured words with a common phonetic feature, such as the final-f words displayed in Figure 6.2.

17. Techniques to encourage self-monitoring

Techniques to encourage self-monitoring are covered in Chapter 9 and in Lowe (A16, p. 102) in Chapter 3 and Ruscello (A42, p. 289) in Chapter 8.

18. Single word and conversational speech production drill

Production drill of single words, combined with production of the same words in phrases and sentences, and ultimately in controlled conversational contexts can facilitate a more complete phonotactic repertoire, more varied use of phonotactic range within syllables and words, and improved accuracy. For example, the words in Figure 6.2 might be used as the basis for a game in which the child has to use the words in short phrases, or the child might be asked to formulate short sentences with the words in Figure 6.3 to

Final /f/ vs. no final consonant

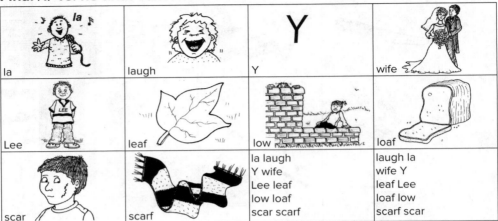

la	laugh	Y	wife
Lee	leaf	low	loaf
scar	scarf	la laugh Y wife Lee leaf low loaf scar scarf	laugh la wife Y leaf Lee loaf low scarf scar

Figure 6.3 /f/ SFWF – la laugh, Y wife, etc. Drawings by Helen Rippon, Speech and Language Therapist www.blacksheeppress.co.uk

highlight meaning differences. This could be something simple, such as the child saying, 'You can't say *la* if you mean *laugh*; You can't say *Y* if you mean *wife*; You can't say *Lee* if you mean *leaf*' etc., or the child instructing an adult to 'Point to *la*; Point to *laugh*'; etc.

19. Backward build-ups

Backward build-ups have long been used in foreign language teaching, and Velleman (2003) advocates them as a therapy technique for multi-syllabic words, especially with children with CAS. They are also useful for the shorter but 'tricky words', like *yellow*, which may exist as erred fossilised forms. The clinician starts with as much of the *end* of the word a child can say. This might even be all of the word except the first syllable. For example, to teach *dictionary*, the clinician might start by having the child rehearse and strengthen production of *arry*, then *shun-arry*, and finally *dick-shun-arry*, after which the stress and timing are adjusted until the child is saying *dictionary*. *California* might go like this: *yuh*, then *forn-yuh*, then *lee-forn-yuh*, then *callie-forn-yuh*, and ultimately *California*. An example of backward build-ups, showing how 'Jesssica' (5;4) learned to say *yellow*, can be found at http://www.speech-language-therapy.com/jessica.pps.

20. Backward chaining

Backward chaining is a technique that can be used to facilitate the production of two-syllable words in children who only produce monosyllables. The child produces the second syllable many times (e.g., the *king* in *making* or the *key* in *donkey*) until he/she can say it easily. Then, the highly rehearsed, habituated syllable is alternated with several potential 'first syllables'. For example, the child might practice *king-may-king-way-king-tay-king*, etc. At first, the child is actually saying *king-may, king-way, king-tay*, etc., but then the stress is gradually shifted so that he/she is saying, *making, waking, taking, looking, poking*, etc. It may be necessary to provide simultaneous models at first, and then 'fade' the model, Integral Stimulation style, using Dynamic Temporal and Tactile Cueing (DTTC) if required. DTTC is described in detail in Chapter 7. There are 'King Words' and 'Key Words' picture worksheets for backward chaining here: http://www.speech-language-therapy.com/tx-facts-and-tricks.html.

It is quite common in SSD to find children who can produce stops word finally (SFWF) and syllable finally within words (SFWW) but not word initially (SIWI) and at the beginnings of syllables within words (SIWW). This is particularly the case for /k/ and /g/. A variation of backward chaining can be used to address this difficulty using final velars that the child *can* already produce to facilitate initial velars. For example, using the 'King Words' and 'Key Words' worksheets mentioned above to elicit *king* and *key*, the chid rehearses *mong*-key, *dong*-key, *bling*-key, etc., emphasising the first syllable. The stress on the first syllable is gradually reduced and shifted to the second syllable, making it more prominent: mong-*key*, dong-*key*, bling-*key*, etc., and then a little 'gap' is inserted between the syllables. Moving at the child's pace, the clinician works towards just mouthing or cueing the first syllable of *monkey, Blinky, donkey*, etc. (silently), so that the child is saying *key* on his/her own with a strong onset /k/. Once *key* is well established, the child can be encouraged to practice strings of: *key-keep, key-keys, key-keen, key-keel, key-quiche*, etc., before introducing initial /k/ in combination with other vowels. There are pictures and therapy activity sheets for this here: http://www.speech-language-therapy.com/tx-facts-and-tricks.html.

Additional techniques

The available repertoire of approaches and techniques to apply in the symptomatic treatment of SSD does not stop here. There is more to come in Chapter 7, where the focus is on intervention specifically for CAS; in Chapter 8, which covers a range of 'tips' for target selection and intervention for phonological disorder; and in Chapter 9, which contains a detailed account of PACT in action.

Chapter 7

Treatment schedules, levels, and options

This chapter begins with a summary of the principles of motor learning defined as 'a set of processes associated with practice or experience leading to relatively permanent changes in the capability for movement' (Schmidt and Lee 2000). These principles are central to the dynamic assessment and treatment of CAS. Next is Judith Stone-Goldman's schema that allows the clinician to choose an appropriate level of intervention for a client relative to a specified therapy target. Although this chapter is essentially about CAS, it should be noted that Stone-Goldman's chart is applicable to articulation disorders and phonological impairment as well. We go on to explore more approaches to CAS therapy, and Edythe Strand from the Mayo Clinic and Pam Williams from the Nuffield Centre talk about 'their' assessment and therapy.

Motor learning principles

The precursors to speech motor learning are:

a) Motivation;
b) Focused attention; and
c) Pre-practice or phonetic placement training prior to entering the practice phase.

The clinician and parents may need to consider a behaviour management plan, implemented by a suitably qualified professional, for children who cannot focus or co-operate easily or who have motivation, attention, or compliance difficulties. It is important for parents (and us) to know that simply attending therapy will have little or no impact on the speech of children with CAS unless they engage adequately in the motor learning and other aspects of treatment.

The conditions of practice are:

a) Motivation;
b) Goal and target setting (what will be practiced, and how many times);
c) Instructions (how directions will be delivered);

d) Modelling (e.g., simultaneous production vs. immediate imitation vs. delayed imitation); and

e) Setting and with whom (e.g., where the practice take place and who will help).

Other factors may arise specific to a client. For example, the reinforcement (praise) used should not take up too much time, make too much noise, 'interrupt', or distract. It is usually necessary to guide parents in how to deliver reinforcement, providing explicit modelling and practice in sessions (with feedback to them). It is also necessary to choose and develop appealing activities for the child (and to an extent for the parents, too) that will facilitate and invite repeated opportunities for production of target behaviours or utterances.

Repetitive practice (motor drill)

The type of practice we aim for is repetitive practice, sometimes called motor drill. There *must* be sufficient trials ('repeats' of the target behaviour) within a practice session for any motor learning to take place and for it to become habituated. Habituation is a step towards more automatic speech output processing.

A comparison of practice schedules

There are four types of practice schedule, each with advantages and disadvantages. In the 'real world', we may not *have* much choice regarding practice distribution. We *must* decide, however, which targets to select and how many to address concurrently. The options are: massed practice vs. distributed practice; and random practice vs. blocked practice.

Massed practice vs. distributed practice

Massed practice involves fewer practice sessions, but the sessions themselves are longer. This promotes quick development of skills, but poor generalisation. Distributed practice, on the other hand, has the same duration (in aggregate) distributed across more sessions. Distributed practice takes longer, and can become tedious, but it has the advantage of promoting better motor learning and is potentially more motivating over time.

Blocked practice vs. random practice

In blocked practice, all practice trials ('repeats' of the behaviours) of a stimulus (target) are done in one time block before moving to the next target. This arrangement tends to lead to better performance. By contrast, in random practice, the order of presentation of all stimuli is randomised through the session, and this fosters better retention, better motor learning, and, in many instances, higher levels of motivation.

Feedback to the child

It is essential during motor drill to give a child frequent information about his/her movement performance, building his/her 'knowledge' of what the speech motor apparatus is capable of, what it is doing 'right now', and what it did a moment before ('just then'). Interestingly, there are reports in the cognitive motor literature that adults derive most benefit from finely specified feedback. Conversely, if feedback to children is too specific, their performance can decrease. Skilled observations by the SLT/SLP allow the frequency of feedback to be tailored to suit, bearing in mind that it can distract some children and that, for some, saving any 'reward' until the end of a session is the most effective way to proceed.

Rate of production trials

There is usually a trade-off between rate and accuracy. A slower rate of production will, up to a point, increase accuracy. *Varying the expected rate of production* can be an effective technique to incorporate into motor drill, using speech, chanting (Melodic Intonation Therapy) and singing, because it encourages habituation of articulatory movement accuracy while working towards automaticity, a natural rate, and natural prosody.

Finding the right level of intervention

Dr. Judith Stone-Goldman has recently retired from her post as a senior lecturer in the department of Speech and Hearing Sciences at the University of Washington, Seattle, where she taught in the areas of Child Speech-Language Disorders and Counselling. Qualified in SLP and counselling, she works as a clinician at a birth-to-three centre for children with developmental disabilities and their families. Her teaching commitments included assessment, counselling, and the treatment of, and clinical practicum for, speech and language disorders. In A39, she details a useful teaching tool she has created and enjoyed using in various contexts.

Q39.   Judith Stone-Goldman: Finding the right level of difficulty relative to the status of a therapy target

The grid in Table A39.1 is one of those deceptively simple-looking clinical nuggets! It allows a clinician to choose an appropriate level of intervention for a client relative to a particular therapy target. What prompted its development, and can you walk the reader through the process of using it, with real life examples? How would you suggest presenting the grid to carers and teachers, especially if more that one target and more than one level were involved simultaneously for a client?

A39.   Judith Stone-Goldman: Choosing where to start

- *A six-year-old touches his tongue tip with a tongue depressor and then says 'la'.*
- *A nine-year-old plays a game with hidden clues, using the words 'near' and 'far' to guide the clinician.*

Table A39.1 Choosing a level of intervention relative to the status of the therapy target*

Status of the therapy target → Clinical Decisions ↓	Absent → → Level 1	→ → Level 2	→ → Level 3	Mastered → → Level 4
Assessment: ↓ Current level of the target behaviour	a) Absent OR b) Beginning to emerge	Present but limited to certain activities and contexts. Inconsistent at different linguistic levels and/or in different activities.	Present across linguistic levels in familiar, practised, rehearsed tasks, but not produced naturally in a variety of situations.	Present in all linguistic contexts and environments, with a variety of child and adult communicative partners.
Goal: Desired ↓ treatment outcome	Establish the new behaviour or increase (reinforce) the emerging behaviour.	Make the behaviour more consistent, and establish it in varied linguistic levels, varied activities.	Generalise the behaviour to conversational speech, new communicative partners, and new situations.	Not applicable. Treatment not needed. Move on, but monitor the new behaviour.
Therapy contexts: ↓ Situations in which the client will produce the targeted behaviour	Under optimal, often contrived conditions (drill; drill-play), in simple linguistic forms, in a small range of activities.	In new linguistic forms and levels, in a variety of activities, with clear focus maintained on target.	In varied, natural interactions and activities, with different communicative partners, in different settings.	Not applicable; target is used in naturally occurring events and situations in the child's life.
Stimuli: Range of ↓ stimuli and materials **Cues:** Degree of clinician cues **Reinforcement:** Frequency, type **Responses:** Expected responses	A small set of familiar stimuli and predetermined target responses. Responses are tightly linked to treatment. Maximal cues, reinforcement.	An expanding set of practiced stimuli to evoke responses in varied linguistic contexts (naming, question/answer) and levels (phrase, sentence); frequent cues, reinforcement.	Less constrained stimuli and materials to allow practice of target responses in natural communicative contexts; overt cues are faded, reinforcement becomes natural, intermittent.	Not applicable; real events create opportunities for use of target.
Measurement: ↓ **Treatment:** Nature of the stimuli and expected responses as specified in behavioural objective	Practiced stimuli and responses; cues as needed.	Practiced stimuli and responses; limited cues.	Not practiced: Novel stimuli and unrehearsed responses (these may be sampled within familiar treatment activities); no cues.	Not applicable.

Table A39.1 *(Continued)*

Status of the therapy target → Clinical Decisions ↓	Absent → → Level 1	→ → Level 2	→ → Level 3	Mastered → → Level 4
Measurement: Generalisation: Probable generalisation measures	Probe/explore the next teaching level or new set of responses to see if the child is ready to move on.	Probe new, unpractised (unrehearsed) words containing the target or probe new linguistic levels.	Objectively probe generalisation beyond therapy activities (is the child using the target spontaneously?). Probe additional novel events and contexts (relay a message, tell a story).	Family and teachers may continue to monitor the target behaviour in everyday interactions outside the clinic.

*Adapted from 'Working at the Right Level', a handout by J. Stone-Goldman, October 2005.

- *A four-year-old takes turns with the clinician, rolling cars along a pretend road and saying phrases, such as 'car go!' and 'come on car!'*
- *A seven-year-old makes up a story from words containing /s/.*

Introduction

Activities like these are familiar to SLPs/SLTs who work with children with SSD. Although age-appropriate activities are important, they do not by themselves make up good therapy. What is important about the above activities for effective therapy? How might we evaluate their usefulness for a particular child?

A key factor that will affect an activity's usefulness is its *level of difficulty*. Activities that are too easy will not challenge the child sufficiently, but activities that are too difficult are frustrating and limit progress. Through my years of teaching and supervising, I have come to believe that zeroing in on the right level of difficulty, relative to the child's skill level, is critical for developing treatments that yield good outcomes. Finding the right level of difficulty is particularly important for choosing where to *start* intervention.

Determining level of difficulty raises many questions. Do you practise words or sentences? Should therapy stimuli be familiar and limited in number, or should they be novel and extensive? Is it better to keep an activity focused, or should activities be similar to natural communication? How do we know when it's time to make the work harder? We must ask and answer these questions repeatedly over the course of a client's treatment if we are to work at the right level and support the client's progress.

In my efforts to guide students in coming up with answers to these questions, I sketched out the ideas that are reflected in the chart displayed in Table A39.1. Creating the chart helped me organise clinical concepts that were second nature to me, and using it as a teaching tool brought these concepts to light for students. In our group case conferences, the chart helped us appreciate differences among clients' treatments. It gave students a way to be comfortable with clients who were 'just starting out' in therapy, as well as a way to imagine the future directions a client's treatment might take. Thanks to the initiative of one student, the chart subsequently became a tool for communicating with parents.

Orientation: Reading the chart

First, consider the top row, labelled *'Status of the therapy target'*. This describes how regularly a speech sound target (e.g., word initial /ʃ/) or syllable structure target (e.g., initial consonants) is produced correctly and the variety of contexts in which it is produced. A Level 1 target may be *absent* or just *barely emerging*, in which case it is never produced correctly or under rare conditions only. In contrast, a Level 4 target that is *mastered* is produced reliably in varying linguistic conditions, in different environments, with different communication partners. Levels 2 and 3 refer to targets that are produced with varying consistency, in varying contexts, on a progression towards mastery. The description of each level can be found in the row below the level numbers, labelled *'Assessment: Current level of the target behaviour'*.

Now examine the left-hand column, labelled *'Clinical Decisions'*. Each box in this column refers to an aspect of treatment that the clinician specifies to make treatment at the right level of difficulty. The first four boxes in the *Clinical Decisions* column are important for *planning treatment*: determining the current level; stating the treatment goal; planning therapy contexts; and specifying therapy stimuli, cues, reinforcement, and responses. Roth and Worthington (2005) are helpful on the topic of therapy conditions, such as contexts and stimuli, cues, and reinforcement. The remaining two boxes in this column are important for *planning measurement*: measuring treatment progress and measuring generalisation, both of which are typically done using non-standardised probes (see Mowrer 1985 for a review of basic data collection and measurement issues). Note that, by reading down the column under any of the levels (1–4), you can see the clinical decisions for that level. By reading across a row, you can see how a particular clinical decision changes as the level changes.

Case examples

Two case examples serve to clarify the chart's sections and demonstrate its clinical application. The children described received individual treatment at the *University of Washington Speech and Hearing Clinic* from a graduate student in speech-language pathology, under my supervision. Both children were developing normally in receptive and expressive language, cognition, and social skills, and had normal hearing thresholds, with speech being the only area of concern. For the purpose of clear illustration, I chose to discuss children with a small set of speech errors. This chart can lend guidance when working with children with more errors or with additional language problems, or when using other models of treatment, such as those that incorporate phonological analysis.

Case 1

'Joanna' was a five-year-old monolingual child whose parents were concerned about intelligibility and age-appropriate speech. Phonological assessment revealed errors on all velars

(/k, g, ŋ/) in single words and connected speech. Joanna was not immediately stimulable for velars when given models and simple instructions for making these sounds. All her substitutions and imitated attempts were /t, d, n/ for /k, g, ŋ/, respectively.

Joanna is a good example of a child who needed to begin at Level 1. With the potential therapy targets all absent, treatment was, by necessity, narrow in scope. The goals were to establish the new targets /k/ and /g/ in simple phonetic forms, and the therapy contexts were restricted to highly structured practice (e.g., table drill or finding stimulus items hidden around the room). The clinician provided maximal cues: tactile cues with a tongue depressor, descriptive names for sounds (e.g., calling /k/ a 'back sound' and referring to it as 'kay'), gestures toward the back of the mouth, verbal instructions, and models were used freely to help Joanna learn about and produce the new velar sounds. The same stimuli were repeated many times, and the only expected responses were /k/ and /g/, first in isolation and then in a few syllables. Concerning /k/ and /g/ 'in isolation', it should be noted that stops cannot exist in isolation, so realisations at this level were actually produced with a whispered or minimally articulated schwa ([kə], [gə]). Reinforcement was frequent and enthusiastic.

Measuring treatment progress at this level was limited to the practice attempts, supported by the clinician cues. Given that Joanna had never produced /k/ or /g/, *any* correct productions were a big step. In the same spirit, our expectations for generalisation were modest, limited to explorations of Joanna's readiness to move ahead to different vowels or new syllable/word positions (i.e., dynamic assessment or stimulability; Hasson and Joffe 2007). It was too soon to worry about generalisation to novel words or connected speech. We knew that more functional gains would come later in treatment. We also did not treat /ŋ/, even though it was absent, but held it as a control behaviour. Had this target remained absent or inconsistent after /k/ and /g/ developed, treatment would have been introduced. Hegde (2002) provides a discussion of measuring control behaviours for treatment efficacy.

Once Joanna produced /k/ and /g/ in a variety of syllables and in some carefully selected CVC words, she met the definition of Level 2: the targets were present but limited to certain activities and contexts. Now the goal was for Joanna to produce targets in varied linguistic forms (new word positions and phonological forms), linguistic levels (phrases and sentences), and activities. Level 2 treatment involved a larger set of practice words and game-like activities that incorporated different types of responses (naming, answering questions). The treatment still remained sufficiently structured to maintain focus on the target and to permit the clinician to provide cues and reinforcement. Note that the structure of therapy, for example, drill versus free play, is an important variable in choosing the right level of treatment, and the interested reader is referred to related discussion by Roth and Paul (2002) on the 'Continuum of Naturalness'.

We anticipated staying at Level 2 for a while longer. We expected to work on the targets in sentences and to fade cues before moving to Level 3, at which point we would help Joanna generalise her productions to conversational speech and natural activities. To our surprise, Joanna suddenly moved to Level 3 independently, using the targets spontaneously throughout the entire session. Parent report supported that changes were occurring at home as well. We therefore used measurements associated with Levels 2 and 3 to document these changes and make further decisions about treatment. Probes of the targets in unpractised words and sentences revealed 100% accuracy; even in conversation and narratives, correct production had risen to slightly above 50%. A probe of /ŋ/ (never treated or practiced) showed 90% correct in words.

Given the speed of these changes, which far outstripped the direct therapy, we concluded that Joanna would likely continue her development independently, especially because her family reinforced her gains and provided a language-rich home. Together with her family, we made the decision to discontinue treatment and follow up as needed at a later time. Subsequently, the family confirmed that Joanna had mastered her sounds and needed no further treatment.

Joanna moved from Level 1 to Level 3 within a 10-week period, which is unusually fast progress, even for a young child. Joanna's strengths were many: she was able to focus and cooperate; she had age-appropriate phonemic awareness and curiosity about what she was learning (e.g., 'why does that word have a 'kay' sound?'); and, despite her initial lack of stimulability, she had a normal motor speech system. These strengths, coupled with a positive therapeutic environment and supportive parents, added up to rapid, well-maintained changes.

Case 2

Let us briefly consider a child who stands in contrast to Joanna. At age 9, 'Robert' was brought to therapy for remediation of /r/. Robert's family had lived in the Middle East for a number of years, and Robert was exposed to several languages. He produced /r/ correctly some of the time in conversational speech. What level of treatment was the correct level for him?

Despite some spontaneous productions in conversational speech (making him appear to be at Level 3), Robert needed treatment at Level 2. He produced some but not all forms of /r/ in words, and he needed to become consistent in phrases and structured sentences. Robert showed excellent progress in sessions as well as generalisation to unpractised words and sentences. However, he still did not produce the targets consistently in conversation; treatment thus moved to Level 3.

The goal for Level 3 was to extend correct productions to more natural communication. The clinician introduced tasks to evoke connected speech (picture description, structured conversations), create practice with new partners, move treatment out of the familiar room to other parts of the clinic, and replace overt cues with subtle, natural reinforcers. By systematically varying the treatment contexts, stimuli, cues, reinforcement, and expected responses, the clinician helped Robert meet Level 3 goals of generalisation. Follow-up after a 3-month break showed that Robert was maintaining his progress and doing well in his daily environment.

Why did Robert begin treatment at Level 2 if he was already producing some correct targets in conversational speech? Robert needed better consistency of his productions, even in simpler tasks. Treatment at Level 3 did not allow sufficient control of therapy conditions to build up that consistency. We did not know if his early multilingual experiences had influenced his articulation development, but the more obvious explanation lay in his speech musculature. Robert had mild low tone in his face and lips, and his speech was sometimes imprecise or weak sounding. He needed to work at a level where he could refine and stabilise his /r/ productions before reinserting them into increasingly complex speech. Though he developed /r/ on his own, he needed treatment to shape his best productions and maintain them under the high processing demands of complex, natural speech.

Conclusion

Working at the right level brings confidence to children and patience to both clinicians and families. By discussing with parents the basics about a child's current level, we can promote realistic expectations and suggest appropriate participation. A simplified chart of levels and corresponding treatment conditions aids the discussion. If more than one target is involved, parents can easily see each target's level on the chart. Even a smart, motivated child can grasp the levels: one nine-year-old girl volunteered that, while she was thrilled to be saying a correct /r/, practising words in the session simply wasn't the same as the way she spoke at home! This led to a discussion of how her treatment would progress in time, and the clinician introduced some functional phrases to support the girl's interest in meaningful communication.

I hope the reader will see that this chart is not meant to impose rules or restrict creativity but to foster logical, careful planning. The concepts it covers are essential to therapy, but the chart is not exhaustive, and a clinician should individualise the activities (even Level 1 activities can be made enjoyable). Although the chart emphasises production practice, other types of learning, such as discrimination exercises or phonemic awareness, can be added. In addition, creative homework assignments can be used at every level, from word awareness or key word assignments at Level 1 to at-home word diaries and creative writing at Levels 3 and 4.

Further, children will vary in how slowly or quickly they progress through the levels. Children may work on different targets at different levels, and some children will need treatment at every level before completing therapy. The guiding principles are to begin at a level that allows a child to be successful, build steadily and systematically toward natural communication, and collect data that support treatment decisions.

Integral stimulation

In the mid-1950s, Robert L. Milisen published an article about a multi-layered program for articulation therapy incorporating imitation and auditory and visual models (Milisen 1954). Milisen's method, called integral stimulation, has shaped the treatment of functional articulation disorders, the dysarthrias, and acquired apraxia of speech. It utilises hierarchical cueing procedures that begin with high levels of support via simultaneous production of slowly spoken simple utterances with visual and tactile cues. The cues are subtly faded and amplified as required until, at the lowest level of support, they fade completely and the client produces delayed repetition of increasingly complex stimulus items. Research by Rosenbeck, Lemme, Ahern, et al. (1973) and Strand and Debertine (2000) shows that integral stimulation intervention in treatment of individuals with apraxia of speech (AOS) is efficacious.

Although they may be unaware of its precise origins, the children's version of integral stimulation is widely used by SLPs/SLTs who treat child speech and language difficulties. It involves a familiar procedure in which the clinician models an utterance and the child *imitates* it, while the clinician ensures that the child's attention is as focused as possible for on *listening to* the model while *looking at* the clinician's face (watching the model, if you like). Integral stimulation proceeds from bottom up, starting with simple phonetic segments and sequences and then short utterances, and building in a hierarchy of difficulty to longer and more phonetically complex stimuli. Integral stimulation can be used on its own when working with children with CAS, but it is more effectively applied in combination with tactile and gesture cues that shape the accuracy of articulatory gestures and prosodic cues (Strand, Stoeckel, and Baas 2006), involving melodic intonation therapy techniques (Helfrich-Miller 1983, 1984, 1994) or contrastive stress (Velleman 2002). A prominent feature of the application of the integral-stimulation-combined-with-prosodic-cues approach with children with CAS is that syllable, word, and sentence stress are emphasised early in therapy, that is, from the outset, and with young children *if possible*.

Dynamic Temporal and Tactile Cueing: DTTC

For non-verbal children with severe CAS, for whom the method described above is too difficult, Strand has developed and tested (Strand, Stoeckel, and Baas 2006; see also Jakielski, Kostner, and Webb 2006) a variation of integral stimulation called *Dynamic Temporal and Tactile Cueing (DTTC) for Speech Motor Learning*. Incorporating principles of motor learning (see above), it can be used with the non-verbal children who struggle unsuccessfully with the task of articulatory imitation and who seem unable to achieve even the remotest approximation for consonants or vowels. DTTC is an explicitly principled, modified version of the *Eight-Step Continuum for Treatment of Acquired Apraxia of Speech* (Rosenbeck, Lemme, Ahern, et al. 1973), originally designed for adult clients with AOS. It allows for what Strand calls 'a continuous shaping of the movement gesture', to (1) improve motor planning and (2) program speech processing as speech and language acquisition progresses. The tiny steps and essential adjustments of the 'therapy dance' within DTTC will have a familiar ring to many clinicians, and are as follows.

1) *Imitation*
   In its implementation, DTTC begins with direct, immediate imitation of natural speech.
2) *Simultaneous production with prolonged vowels (most clinician support)*
   If the child cannot imitate, the task is changed to the simplified, more 'supported' one of *simultaneous production*. At this lower level of difficulty, the SLP/SLT says the utterance at normal volume *with* the child first, very slowly with the addition of touch cues and/or gesture cues as required. Slowing the utterance by sustaining the *vowel* ([si::::] rather than [ssssi]) helps the child, and at the same time lets the SLP/SLT run a 'visual check' to see that the jaw and lip postures are correct (e.g., no jaw slide and acceptable symmetry).
3) *Reduction of vowel length*
   As the simultaneous production phase of therapy advances, the rate of stimuli production is increased (i.e., vowel length is reduced) to sound more natural.
4) *Gradual increase of rate to normal*
   Practice continues at this level to the point where the child synchronises effortlessly with the therapist at normal rate, with normal movement gestures, and without silent posturing.

5) *Reduction of therapist's vocal loudness, eventually miming*

Using delicate timing, the SLP/SLT is then in a position to reduce vocal volume, eventually reaching a point where the clinician is producing a mime (mouthing the utterance) as the child says it aloud. Because of the intellectual closeness within the dyad, this can be a tricky point in therapy, and some children will dutifully follow *exactly* what the adult is doing so that the two are miming at each other! This is obviously not the goal, and children may need explicit instruction to keep their voice 'turned on' even though the adult's is 'off'. The gesture and touch cues may still be needed at this point and will almost certainly be necessary in the next step: the integral stimulation method proper.

6) *Direct imitation*

Ensuring that the child is secure and comfortable with moving to this harder level, the child watches the adult's face while an auditory model is provided. The child attempts to repeat the model and, if successful, does so many times. If unsuccessful, the therapist may backtrack to the simultaneous model or silent mouthing/miming level described above. Eventually all miming is faded, and the child directly imitates and 'repeats' targets numerous times before the final step is introduced.

The key to successful implementation is the therapist's informed observations of and sensitivity to what the child is 'giving' by way of responses. The professional skill and flexibility involved in continually fine-tuning the hierarchy of stimuli and the amount of support provided to enable the child to imitate spontaneously is critical. Auditory (including prosodic), visual, and tactile cues and the level of demand on the child are continually added and faded in each practice trial according to the child's responses. It is especially important with the CAS population, who have good and bad days with their speech-processing capacities, to be prepared to take the therapy 'down a notch' if required, and to explain to parents why this is happening.

7) *Introduction of a one- or two-second s-r delay (least support)*

Once the child is directly imitating the therapist's model with normal rate, prosody he or she can vary, and appropriate articulatory gestures, the therapist inserts a new requirement. This is in the form of a one- to two-second delay before the child imitates, so that the child produces a *very slightly* delayed response. To facilitate this for the children who find the delay difficult and want to 'jump in', miming while the child produces the delayed response can prove helpful.

8) *Spontaneous production*

Finally, the SLP/SLT elicits spontaneous utterances, for example, by asking the child, 'What is this called?, using cloze tasks such as *Twinkle, twinkle __ __*, sentence completion such as *Mother elephant is very big, her baby is __ __*, and the like.

Dr. Edythe Strand, who developed DTTC, is a consultant in the Department of Neurology, Division of Speech Pathology, at the Mayo Clinic in Rochester, Minnesota, and Associate Professor in the Mayo Medical School. Her primary research and clinical interests have been in neurologically mediated communication disorders, especially developmental and acquired AOS, dysarthria, and neurogenic voice disorders. She has published articles and chapters regarding the clinical management of motor speech disorders in children, including treatment efficacy. Responding to Q40, she talks about dynamic assessment (DA) and DTTC.

Q40. Edythe Strand: Child-centred DA

Child-centred DA (Vygotsky 1978; Feuerstein, Rand, Jensen, et al. 1987), DTTC, and integral stimulation are compatible bedfellows, especially early in the sCAS therapeutic encounter, when it is impossible to divorce assessment from therapy. Hasson and Joffe (2007) write that the DA approach sees the positive relationship between therapist and child potentially enhancing the child's performance, feelings of competence, and levels of motivation in both assessment and therapy, cautioning that these benefits must be balanced against the need to obtain reliable and replicable test results. What is the potential contribution of DA to differential diagnosis of SSD; to short-term and longer-term goal-setting, or 'choosing where to start' for children with severe CAS; and how does it interface with DTTC and integral stimulation?

A40. Edythe Strand: DA of motor speech disorders in children

When CAS is suspected, differential diagnosis of a child's SSD is frequently very difficult. One reason for this difficulty is that many children with SSD have co-morbidities such as global developmental delay, structural abnormalities, or hearing loss. As well, their communication impairment frequently involves some combination of language disorder, phonological disorder, pragmatic/communicative intent issues, and perhaps a dysarthria. Clinicians must determine the relative contribution of each to the child's impaired speech production. In doing this, a major challenge for the SLP/SLT is determining whether or not a *motor* speech impairment is a contributory element; difficulties due to planning and programming movement gestures for speech, characteristic of CAS, must be differentiated from phonological or phonetic errors.

The ASHA (2007b) CAS position statement provides a welcome definition of the disorder, listing the behavioural characteristics properly associated with the label. Historically, however, controversy has surrounded the specific speech characteristics associated with CAS (Davis, Jakielski, and Marquardt 1998; Forrest 2003; Caruso and Strand 1999; Mc-Cabe, Rosenthal, and McLeod 1998), imposing difficulties for researchers attempting to develop tests sensitive to and discriminative of children with CAS (McCauley and Strand 2008).

In differential diagnosis of SSD, standardised and non-standardised procedures are typically used. The history, language testing, speech sample, and observations of verbal and nonverbal communication across settings may all contribute to diagnosis. Specific to SSD, the clinician will typically make *independent* observations of the phonetic, phonemic, and phonotactic inventories of younger children. When possible, standardised articulation and phonology tests are also administered in order to complete *relational* analyses, comparing children's performance to that of age-typical peers and adult speakers (Stoel-Gammon, A9). Currently, few standardised measures for speech motor control in children exist, alongside infrequent efforts to examine the psychometric characteristics of them (McCauley 2003). Further, little DA is included within these measures, despite its importance in determining severity and prognosis (Bain 1994).

Dynamic assessment

DAs are employed to evaluate children's performance with support, whereas static assessments evaluate skills without support (Glaspey and Stoel-Gammon 2007). Researchers have investigated DA in language disorders (Bain and Olswang 1995; Olswang and Bain 1996; Hasson and Joffe 2007) and phonological disorders (e.g., Glaspey and Stoel-Gammon 2005, 2007), but its role in childhood motor speech disorders has had little discussion.

By examining a child's responses in varying contexts, DA can facilitate a clinician's ability to differentiate motor impairment in SSD. Observations of spontaneous speech only afford a view of the child's customary production. In most standardised test formats, observations are made of a child attempting an utterance they may be unable to execute correctly, with the child likely producing a habituated response or making a minimal attempt at correct production. Binary scoring then tells us they cannot say the utterance, without suggesting why. But what we see and hear produced spontaneously and in static testing is different from what we perceive when they *try* to correctly produce a specific new word, or one they typically mispronounce. The cueing in DA enables observations of what the child does while really attempting specific movement gestures. In the case of children with suspected CAS, we have the opportunity to evaluate discrete characteristics associated with that label. We may see groping that is unapparent in spontaneous speech, but evident in attempted imitation of specific movement gestures with cueing, inconsistency across trials as cueing occurs, and segmentation of syllables that occurs only when attempting the correct articulatory movement gestures.

Dynamic Evaluation of Motor Speech Skill (DEMSS)

Because DA contributes much to differential diagnosis and treatment planning, I am working with colleagues to develop a dynamic assessment tool, the *Dynamic Evaluation of Motor Speech Skill (DEMSS)*, specifically for younger and/or more severely impaired children, that allows clinicians to judge their responses via multi-dimensional scoring system. The purpose of the *DEMSS* is to differentially diagnose SSD due to difficulty with speech praxis from speech sound errors stemming from other sources. It utilises systematic, progressive cueing to facilitate imitative production of utterances that vary in length and phonetic complexity. Initial data demonstrate the construct validity and reliability of the *DEMSS* (Strand, McCauley and Stoeckel 2006), and we are, at the time of writing, completing an item analysis before revising and re-testing the instrument.

Determining severity and prognosis

In DA, tests need to be sensitive to changes that result from the child's *responses* to cueing; in other words, their *learning*. This is very different from standardised tests, which must show stability over time (Lidz and Pena 1996). Traditional standardised tests allow comparison of a child's performance on a task (e.g., articulation performance) relative to a normative group, at one point in time. Although this may allow some idea of severity, it is quite conceivable that two children may exhibit the same standard score on a measure, but have very different levels of severity and different prognoses for change. This is because most standardised tests do not provide clinicians with the opportunity to observe children's responses to different types of cueing, or their potential to learn via such cueing. DA can facilitate estimates of severity and prognosis because the therapist engages the child across contexts, providing different levels of support, such as tactile cueing, visual attention to the clinician's face, having the child produce the response more slowly, and/or having the child produce the utterance simultaneously with the examiner. Judgments can then be made regarding the child's response to these types and levels of cueing. Such observations facilitate the clinician's judgments regarding how much cueing will be *needed* in early therapy to induce improvement in performance, and how long it may take to achieve initial progress.

Some research in language development has compared static standardised testing to dynamic assessment with respect to predicting whether a child is likely to improve performance quickly with therapy. Olswang and Bain (1996) noted the importance of examining children's capacity to change performance on a difficult task when provided with cueing, demonstrating that DA measures were the best predictors of a child's ability to learn word combinations. Although predictors for change in motor speech performance have not been reported, a good argument can be made for the use of DA procedures for making predictions regarding prognosis.

Prognostic decisions lead clinicians to short-term and long-term goal setting. Non-verbal children's parents often ask, 'Will my child ever talk?' If their child's responses to cueing and facilitation during DA indicate potential as a verbal communicator, then the long-term goal for their child is to establish functional verbal communication. Short-term goals are also facilitated by the DA approach being closely tied to decisions about where to start. Rather than examining at what level (V vs. CV and VC vs. CVC, etc.) the child is successful using binary pass-fail scoring, DA allows observations of the *practice* and the *level of cueing* needed to improve production at varying of levels of phonetic complexity. For example, a non-verbal child exhibiting numerous vowel distortions in isolation, syllables, and words may improve production in all contexts when the clinician helps him/her achieve the initial articulatory position and stay in the steady state of (sustaining) the vowel longer. This would lead to the decision to work at and beyond the CV, VC, and CVC levels. On the other hand, if children cannot improve vowel production, even with maximum cueing and slowed rate, the clinician would choose a smaller stimulus set, fewer vowel targets, and CV and VC syllable shapes at first.

The interface between DTTC and integral stimulation

'Integral stimulation' (Milisen 1954) denotes a therapy approach focused on imitation of auditory and visual models. *DTTC* (Strand, Stoeckel, and Baas 2006) is just one type of integral stimulation, which uses auditory, visual, and tactile cueing. *DTTC*, however, emphasises varying the *temporal* relationship between stimulus and response, maximising cueing at first, and then fading cues over continued practice. This variation in levels of cueing characterises the similarity between *DTTC* and DA. In DA, however, cues are progressively added to determine how *much* help the child needs to improve accuracy of movement gestures. In *DTTC*, cues are maximised at first for utterances the child cannot produce, and then gradually faded as improvement occurs in order to help the child take increasing responsibility for the planning/programming and execution of the movement gestures for the target utterance.

Case example

'Peter', 4;2, attended for comprehensive speech and language evaluation due to concerns regarding his delayed speech acquisition. Since 2;6 he had received individual speech therapy, once weekly at first, building to thrice weekly for the last 14 months, but traditional articulation therapy approaches had evoked little speech progress. His parents' chief concern was whether he would *ever* talk, and they were considering abandoning speech therapy and focusing only on augmentative communication. Peter's receptive language was within the normal range with standard scores between 94 and 101. He initiated communication readily, using sign, gestures, a few intelligible words, and many word approximations understood only by his mother. His Goldman-Fristoe (Goldman and Fristoe 2000) standard score was <40. A dynamic assessment of motor speech skill (*DEMSS*) showed numerous CAS characteristics, including difficulty achieving initial articulatory configurations, with instances of groping and trial-and-error behaviour; numerous vowel distortions which varied with co-articulatory context; prosodic errors; and inconsistency across trials. He was able to produce only 6 of the 68 items correctly in direct imitation without cues (*do, up, mama, papa, booboo,* and *mom*). These results were consistent with his Goldman-Fristoe scores. His *DEMSS* scores, however, also reflected improvement with visual attention to the clinician's face, tactile cueing, slowing, and simultaneous production of the movement gesture with the clinician. His performance improved with progressive cueing on over 65% of utterances and correct production after cues on 28% of incorrect items, although it usually took the maximum cues to achieve correct production. Because of his ability to benefit from cues focused on movement accuracy, a favourable prognosis for functional communication was determined. Considering the severity of his CAS, and his minimal therapy progress to date, intensive therapy was recommended.

Peter was seen for two daily 30-minute therapy sessions over 6 weeks. *DTTC* was used to help Peter take increasing responsibility for planning/programming and executing movement gestures for the selected stimuli. Initial goals focused on producing correct movement gestures for speech; improving his ability to produce CVC, VC, and CV CVC shapes; and improving productive accuracy for the vowels /i/ and /æ/ and the diphthong /aɪ/. Six functional words/phrases were chosen as the initial stimulus set to allow enough mass practice for attaining movement accuracy, yet some distributed practice to facilitate motor learning. The six were: *me, bye, dad, eat, home, hi mom* and *mine*. Within six weeks, he had mastered 5/6 of his original training items and they had generalised to spontaneous speech. He had improved his ability to produce 5 new items (added one at a time as original items were mastered) as well as several additional phrases outside the stimulus set that had been modelled for him at other times throughout the day and through play including, *I win, I won, me too, I'm home,* and *I want*.

This fairly rapid, encouraging improvement likely resulted from more frequent therapy *and* therapy that focused on the principles of motor learning. We maximised the number of practice trials within sessions, using reinforcers that were quick and given only after several responses. Early in treatment, feedback was frequent, immediate, and contained specific information regarding movement performance in order to maximise movement accuracy.

As therapy progressed, feedback became less frequent, with slightly longer delays, and less specificity (knowledge of results) in order to maximise motor learning. We varied rate of movement, starting with slow movement to achieve accuracy, gradually increasing rate to normal. We worked to vary prosody to improve correct lexical stress and avoid habituation of rote prosodic contours. As therapy continued, progress toward correct production of words and phrases became faster. Peter now has many functional words and phrases and continues in therapy.

The Nuffield Centre Dyspraxia Programme Third Edition (NDP3)

Well known in the UK, Australia, and New Zealand, the 1985 and 1992 versions of the Nuffield Programme consisted of many photocopy-free stimulus pictures on loose-bound, A4-sized paper, 'therapy ideas', and NS-OMEs and informational handouts. In 1985, the authors viewed 'articulatory dyspraxia' as a neuromotor disorder. By 1992, linguistic deficits were recognised as part of the condition that was now referred to as Developmental Verbal Dyspraxia (DVD), the preferred UK term for CAS. In this terminology, 'developmental' in the name implies a condition present before birth, 'verbal' means that the disorder has both speech and language aspects, and 'dyspraxia' is defined as a difficulty in achieving purposeful sequential movements in the absence of muscular paresis (Morgan Barry 1995a, b). Joy Stackhouse, who assisted with the NDP3 assessment chapter (pp. 43–72), commented explicitly on 'the unfolding and changing nature of DVD as a condition' and the problems (symptoms) that emerge as the child: progresses across domains; has to deal with increased demands; grows older; and enters each developmental stage (Stackhouse 1992). She saw the speech-processing deficits in DVD as being due to some combination of: (1) phonological misrepresentations in lexicon; (2) inability to plan the speech output; and (3) vocal tract incoordination.

Like previous editions, the NDP3 (Williams and Stephens 2004) has not been scrutinised for its effects, efficacy, and efficiency, and no case studies are available in the peer-reviewed literature, so it enjoys a low level of support. Theoretically, the impact of the psycholinguistic framework (Stackhouse and Wells 1997; Stackhouse, Wells, Pascoe, et al. 2002) is evident, and Williams and Corrin (2004) say, 'A broader based theoretical understanding recognising both motoric and linguistic deficits was adopted, and this continues to be our viewpoint.' The NDP3 Assessment is a static rather than a dynamic assessment (Strand, A40), unaccompanied by reliability, validity, or other statistical data. The sample gathered for analysis may include: segments, CV/VC words, CVC words, CVCV words, multisyllabic words, consonant cluster words, phrases, and sentences. There is provision for evaluating oral-motor skills, including diadochokinesis, prosody, and connected speech. The manual states that the assessment affords 'a sensitive measure of progress', but this is unspecified.

DVD is conceptualised as a difficulty with 'motor programming', requiring therapy that focuses on speech output and 'input skills' such as auditory discrimination. The authors say that they see 'oro-motor skills as valuable pre-speech skills that support the development of accurate speech sounds. Although oro-motor skills may be introduced in isolation, they are soon linked to speech sound production and therefore the NDP is different to oro-motor approaches which are purely designed to develop oro-motor skills' (Williams and Corrin 2004, p. 15). In response to Bowen (2005), Williams, Stephens, and Connery (2006, p. 89) have said, 'We wish to stress that NDP3 is not an oral motor therapy. Although oro-motor therapy may be included at the early stages (as required by the individual child), NDP3 offers a complete remediation program for children with verbal dyspraxia (apraxia of speech) right up to connected speech level. As an illustration, only 35 of the 565 therapy worksheets are concerned with oro-motor aspects.'

The therapy is described as a bottom-up, motor skills learning approach, focusing on motor programming skills, and in its implementation requires from the client frequent (again unspecified), repetitive practice to learn and establish new speech production skills. 'New motor programs for single phonemes and words of different levels of phonotactic structures are created and perfected using cues and feedback. They are established as stored representations by associating them with pictorial images and through frequent practice and repetitive sequencing exercises. As speech is not only a motor skill, but also a linguistic medium, phonological skills are incorporated into the worksheets organised as minimal pairs of words' (Williams 2005, unpublished workshop handout).

Co-author of the NDP3, Pam Williams is a consultant SLT and team manager (developmental disorders) at the Nuffield Hearing and Speech Centre. She has conducted research into the rate, accuracy, and consistency of the diadochokinetic performance of young children with typical speech development (Williams and Stackhouse 1998) and is currently pursuing doctoral studies in speech and language therapy. She is widely known in the UK and Ireland for her workshop presentations on the Nuffield Programme (Williams and Stephens 2004). In her response to Q41, she discusses the unique features of the NDP3 and the relationship between assessment and goal setting.

Q41.   Pam Williams: The Nuffield Programme

The skills children with CAS need to acquire are conceptualised metaphorically in the NDP3 as a 'brick wall', with pre-speech oro-motor skills and single C and V sounds seen as the foundations and word level skills built up in layers of bricks on top of the foundations. Simple CV and VC syllables comprise the first layer, moving up in layers through CVCV, CVC, CVCVC, and multi-syllabic words, clusters, word combinations of phrases and sentences, finally reaching the top layer of connected speech. Can you describe for clinicians interested in using the approach the steps used in this 'multi-layered, multi-target treatment', and how you determine and work from a child's strengths? In what sense is the program 'cumulative', and what has been the impact on it of the psycholinguistic framework?

A41.   Pam Williams: The Nuffield approach to CAS and other severe speech disorders

Treatment planning using the NDP3 (Williams and Stephens 2004), is based on NDP3 Assessment data, which enable the SLP/SLT to establish a baseline for a child's speech production capabilities. In practice, most children start therapy at a single-sound and CV level, with the following two aims. First, to extend the child's phonetic repertoire to include:

/p b t d k g m n h f s w j/ and possibly /ʃ/ and /l/; long vowels and if possible, some short vowels and diphthongs. And second, to increase the number of real words with CV structure the child can produce. In pursuing these aims, therapy target words are carefully selected so as to include as many sounds as possible from the child's phonetic repertoire.

In the NDP3 approach to facilitating the development of intelligible speech in children with CAS and other severe SSDs, therapy proceeds in a hierarchy, with the ability to produce complex phonotactic words or word combinations being dependent on mastery of single phones and simple phonotactic structures. Tasks aimed at expanding the child's phonotactic repertoire are introduced gradually, but only once reasonable competency is evident at single-sound and CV levels. As the child's speech production abilities develop, treatment generally involves working concurrently on several targets at a particular level and also targets at different levels (Stone-Goldman, A39). For example, a child might be working on producing / l/, /f/, /ɔ/, and /ɛ/ at single sound level, voicing contrasts for plosives at CV level, and CVCV words with /m b d n/ in a variety of contexts.

The NDP3 uses sound-cue pictures representing consonants, vowels, and diphthongs (e.g., /b/ is represented by a picture of a ball; /aɪ/ is represented by a picture of an eye), and it is therefore necessary, early in therapy, to teach the child to associate the sound-cue pictures with the sounds they represent. These sound–picture associations are used to help the child build new or modified motor programs (Stackhouse and Wells 1997) for sounds that they cannot say or that they say incorrectly. Typically, the use of the sound-cue pictures is augmented by a range of other facilitators such as: verbal cues, e.g., 'open your mouth wide for this one'; manual cues, such as *Cued Articulation* (Passy 1990); tactile cues, e.g., the therapist gently pushing the child's lips together for bilabial placement; diagrammatic cues, e.g., articulograms (Stephens and Elton 1986) to represent features of a particular sound; and/or orthographic prompts (graphemes).

Oro-motor activities (NS-OME)

For children with the most severe of speech production difficulties who are essentially non-verbal or even non-vocal, it is not possible to work on sounds and words as described below. In such cases, oro-motor activities (NS-OME) are used in an attempt to lay down some basic foundations, from which it may be possible to facilitate speech production (Williams, Stephens, and Connery 2006) These activities might include blowing activities to develop an oral air stream, licking activities to develop tongue movement, lip shape exercises (open, close, round, spread), along with activities to promote discrimination, vocal play, and general sound stimulation.

Getting started: single sounds and CV words

To begin, the clinician introduces four to six sound-cue pictures of consonants and vowels that the child can already produce spontaneously or imitate. Preferably, these should include sounds from different sound classes, maximally opposed (Barlow and Gierut 2002) if possible. The tasks, games, and activities that are provided in the NDP3 reinforce auditory and visual discrimination and production, thereby consolidating the ability to associate the sounds with the related pictures and produce the sounds. Additional sound–picture associations are gradually introduced for sounds the child can already say, while continuing to reinforce those introduced at the beginning, so that they are not 'lost'. Cues and feedback are provided, as required, to ensure articulatory accuracy and consistency of best production. At this point, it is important to ensure that schwa insertion does not creep in, especially after voiceless consonants, as this can become problematic when attempting to promote easy co-articulation between consonants and vowels later in intervention. The child also practices vocal control and prosody; for example, by imitating intonation patterns (rising and falling pitch). As well as working on isolated phones, pictures of CV words are introduced, again building on the child's strengths by starting with words the child can already say, and of course, the particular words will be individual for each client.

Moving on: Teaching sounds

Once the child has some familiarity with a number of consonant and vowel sound-cue pictures and is able to produce the corresponding sounds accurately and consistently, the clinician teaches one or more sounds that the child cannot currently produce spontaneously or imitate. Again, it is not possible or desirable to be prescriptive about the choice of target, because individual children vary so much. Therapists should therefore consider such factors as stimulability and typical developmental acquisition order, but often a trial-and-error approach is necessary. When imitation is not possible, various strategies are utilised, including phonetic placement techniques; visual, verbal, tactile, and kinaesthetic cues; and facilitative contexts, described in the NDP3. While teaching new sounds, interim 'approximations' or 'best productions', such as interdental or dental placements for alveolars, may be accepted at first and later refined.

Individual children learn at different rates, depending on such factors as their age, the severity of their speech difficulty, cognitive capacity, any comorbidities, motivation, and the amount of practice within therapy sessions and elsewhere. In general, with children in the 3- to 7-year age range, we aim for the child to recognise and associate consistently 10 to 15 single sound-cue pictures, and produce or approximate those same 10 to 15 sounds in the first few weeks of therapy. Ideally, these will include a combination of some well-established sounds and some recently learned sounds.

Introducing sequencing

For each new sound that is elicited, frequent repetitive practice is required in order to establish the new motor program. Daily home practice, of 15–20 minutes duration, utilising the materials provided in the NDP3 is recommended to achieve consistent and accurate production. A routine of two or three short practice sessions each lasting 5–10 minutes is suggested, rather than one longer session daily.

Once new motor programs (Stackhouse and Wells 1997) have been established and the child has practised producing sequences involving up to 8 repetitions of the same sound (e.g., /b b b b b b b b/), contrastive sequencing (e.g., /b d b d b d b d/) can be introduced, using the NDP3 worksheets. This challenges the child to retrieve two different motor programs and to utilise motor planning skills to maintain accurate production of the individual sounds throughout the sequence. Some children find this activity very difficult, and for this reason, the starting point should involve two or more distinctive feature contrasts

(Barlow and Gierut 2002) and a slow production rate. Closer feature contrasts should be controlled carefully by SLP/SLT and introduced gradually, with each step challenging the child only slightly. For example, for a child with a /t/ for /k/ replacement, contrastive sequencing might start with /m-k/, then /b-k/, /p-k/, and finally /t-k/. Speed of production can be gradually increased and rhythmic and stress patterning incorporated (Strand and Skinder 1999).

Teaching new CV words

If a child is unable to imitate the clinician's spoken model, new CV words have to be developed by combining two existing established motor programs (C + V = CV). This presents a major challenge for many children, since the process of motor programming is one of the core deficits in CAS (ASHA 2007a). The child needs to learn how to modify the two existing motor programs so that they join smoothly, without the 'gap' in production left earlier in sequencing tasks. Transition worksheets have been specifically designed for this purpose and present the sequence of a consonant and a vowel, followed by the CV word created as they join (e.g., /m/ + /u/ = *moo*; /p/ + /aɪ/ = *pie*). The process of 'sound joining' (co-articulation) is supported by careful modelling and by making explicit the articulatory changes the child needs to achieve (e.g., the inclusion of /h/ or a 'puff of air' between the consonant and vowel) to produce a CV word with a voiceless plosive. The same 'blending' worksheets can be used for 'segmenting' and therefore also help the child develop metalinguistic awareness of the component sounds of words (e.g., *pie* begins with /p/).

Incorporating new CV words into the child's current CV repertoire

As at single-sound level, each newly created CV word has to be practised and consolidated by frequent repetitive practice to establish the new motor program, utilising the NDP3 pictorial materials; for example, the child could post a set of CV cards, with each word occurring four times. Once established, newly created CV words need to be incorporated into the set of CV words the child can already produce, thereby allowing the development of a system of contrasts at the CV level. This aim may be achieved through minimal pair activities (Bowen and Cupples 2006, pp. 287–288), incorporating discrimination and production, and using the therapy cards. In addition, the many prepared minimal pair worksheets in NDP3 may be used. The SLP/SLT needs to select suitable worksheets carefully to ensure the child achieves success but is increasingly challenged, in small graded steps, by the phonetic demands of the individual words in the sequence. For example, for a child who has recently learned to produce *car* accurately, having previously produced it as *tar*, staged sequencing practice might move from a vowel change (e.g., *car, core, car, core*) to an easy placement change (e.g., *car, baa, car, baa*) to a harder placement change (e.g., *tar, car, tar, car*). Verbal cues (e.g., 'remember this one starts with a /k/') and visual cues using the picture symbols (e.g., a small picture of a camera to represent /k/ placed next to the *car* picture) make the phonetic composition of words explicit, helping to clarify phonological representations, as well as establishing the motor program.

Moving beyond CV words

CVCV words with the same phone duplicated (e.g., *mummy, daddy, baby, nanny*) and simple CV + CV 'phrases' (e.g., *no bee, bye boy*) can be introduced, using the NDP3 pictures and worksheets, as soon as the child has established CV syllables involving /b d m n/. Such activities enable children with restricted phonetic repertoires to experience accurate production of two-word utterances, and this can be highly motivating for both the child and parents.

Once the child can produce a range of consonants, vowels, and CV syllables and words, he/she has the building blocks to create words of increasing phonotactic complexity, such as CVCV, CVC, CCV, CVCVC, and multisyllabic words. Once again, the child is required to modify two or more existing motor programs, so that they join together smoothly. Strategies for supporting each level of difficulty, in terms of maintaining accuracy, avoiding sound additions, such as schwa, syllable, or glottal insertion, and ensuring appropriate placement of stress, are provided in the manual. The NDP3 provides transition, blending worksheets for CV + CV = CVCV (e.g., toe + bee = Toby), CV + C = CVC (e.g., boo + t = boot), and C + CV(C) = CCV(C) (e.g., s + tar = star) levels; contrastive sequencing worksheets for CVC and CCV(C) levels (e.g., Lee-leaf, Kate-cake, bed-bread, tar-star); and sets of pictures and cards for all levels. As at single-sound and CV levels, the aim when working at each phonotactic level is to develop accurate motor programs for as wide a range of words as possible and to develop a contrastive system. At the same time, other psycholinguistic processes should be facilitated, including accuracy of phonological representations and phonological awareness skills, as described at CV level.

Word combinations

Once speech production skills have been established in single words, more word combinations (like the *no bee, bye boy* examples referred to above), phrases, and clauses can be introduced. A step-by-step approach is described in the manual and is supported by the pictorial materials, starting with simple and then more complex phrases and clauses, moving on to sentences, and ultimately to connected speech. At each of these levels, the child is challenged to maintain accurate and consistent production as utterances increase in length and complexity, but also to incorporate prosodic features (stress, intonation, rate, rhythm) and word-joining strategies.

Conclusion

The NDP3 is a theoretically grounded treatment package that incorporates a combination of motor, linguistic, and psycholinguistic approaches. The motor aspect is evident in the building of intelligible speech, step by step, from single sounds and simple syllable structures to connected speech. The approach is cumulative, with new phonotactic structures added successively by utilising skills established earlier in treatment. The linguistic aspect is evident in the use of contrastive materials at each level, the introduction of meaningful vocabulary from the earliest stages of therapy, and the inclusion of phrases and sentences in addition to single-sound and single-word levels.

By setting the NDP3 within the context of the psycholinguistic framework (Stackhouse and Wells 1997), it has been possible to explain the rationale for our treatment approach. In particular, we have used the speech-processing box and arrow model (Gardner, A21) to describe the underlying components and processes required at each stage of therapy, such as motor programs, motor programming, motor planning, phonological recognition, and phonological representations. This framework reminds the SLT/SLP that the child with a severe speech disorder has a unique pattern of speech-processing breakdown, which will require a tailor-made therapy program. The NDP3 provides a flexible resource of pictorial materials, as well as a set of therapy procedures and techniques, from which the SLT/SLP can select appropriate components for individual clients.

Early days

In the initial stages of assessment and therapy for children with CAS or suspected CAS (sCAS), parents embark on a huge learning trajectory and may feel swamped with information. It is also a time for hard work for parents as they adjust to the situation and keep the child busy with fun, focused, relevant activities that stem from the child's strengths and interests (Hammer and Stoeckel 2001). According to Hammer and Stoeckel, at this early stage it is important to help parents to:

- Work with the therapist or team, particularly in terms of encouraging the child's motivation, participation, and cooperation in therapy sessions and homework;
- Learn about CAS and relevant techniques to employ at home;
- Question anything not understood, or anything worrying, straight away;
- Be available at key times for participation in sessions, observations, or video viewing;
- Report openly about home practice frequency and the child's responses;
- Work within realistic parameters,
- Understand treatment limitations and prognostic indicators; and
- Have high and reasonable expectations of the child.

Parents, according to Hammer and Stoeckel, will do best if they are shown how to:

- Organise the environment to facilitate communication;
- Make some homework 'invisible' or 'indirect';
- Provide input without always insisting on a response;
- Make some of the homework visible and direct;
- Identify nursery rhymes, songs, and stories that can be used relative to particular targets;
- Use communicative temptations/'desired objects' that are visible but not accessible;
- Employ modelling and recasting techniques optimally;
- Choose targets that will be functional and powerful to motivate the child to *try*; and
- Use fun games and drill-play with frequent 'communication temptations'.

Potential pitfalls parents may be alerted to include:

- Over cueing; for example, providing exaggerated, distorted models;
- Introducing many new targets quickly: new content is best balanced with older content;

- Tackling targets that are too difficult for the child;
- Avoiding practising things the child is 'good at': this is not a waste of time!
- Burnout of child, parents, and other helpers. This is an issue that needs to be considered in relation to homework. Sometimes parents are so eager to do as much as they can that they quickly kill off any good will on the part of the child, exhaust themselves, and face thorny cooperation issues. In the early months, it may be helpful to limit the duration of speech focus at home, and then to expand it gradually if need be so parents are not overwhelmed and the child is not put off.

Within intervention, the clinician's overriding goal is for the child to become as fully functional a communicator as possible by teaching needed skills based on individual and ongoing assessment. Parents need to know that the clinician sees them as the most important members of the treatment team, and integral to any progress, and that he/she will:

- Educate them about CAS and its management;
- Provide information about networking opportunities and available support;
- Teach them specific strategies relative to their child's intervention needs;
- Be flexible with targets and strategies and program implementation;
- Maximise production practice;
- Maximise functional communication goals;
- Maintain high and reasonable expectations of the child within his/her capabilities; and
- Maintain high and reasonable expectations of *them*, within *their* capabilities.

In order to accomplish these objectives, the therapist must be able to:

- Explain goals in clear language and explain changes in treatment strategies, particularly as changes may be misinterpreted as a sign of failure on the part of child, parent, or clinician;
- Genuinely welcome parents' 'why' questions;
- Ensure opportunities for participation, observation, and discussion; and
- Work with parents to motivate and reinforce child's learning.

The child has responsibilities, too. He/she must accept help from the parents and SLP/SLT in the process of learning to communicate more effectively; and ultimately, as an older child or adult, with ongoing professional or non-professional support if wanted, they need to start taking responsibility for maintaining skills, using adaptive strategies and accepting that there will be communicative consequences when they do not.

Homework and the homework habit

No matter how 'in tune', creative, flexible, encouraging, and motivating we, as clinicians, are in therapy sessions, the necessary carryover is unlikely without solid family support. This means that homework has to be understood and implemented properly, one-to-one in good listening and learning conditions, and often. It is essential to impress upon parents that we see this is a collaborative process, that they are not expected to do all the work or to perform miracles, and that their suggestions and feedback are welcome. As the people who know their child best, it is often the parents who can tell us how to get things done without a battle: which rewards will be effective, which activities will be appealing, and the signs we should look for that tell us that the child wants or needs us to 'back off' a little.

If parents can be encouraged to regard 'speech homework' as part of the family's normal routine, it can help enormously. If brief, regular 5- to 7-minute bursts of home-work are as routine as mealtimes and bathing, and as non-negotiable as wearing a car seatbelt or looking both ways before crossing the road (and hopefully not just a job for *one* parent to do with the child), explicitly principled homework is not so difficult for most families to accomplish. Distributed, random bursts of practice with appropriate reinforcement, taken cumulatively, can contribute to significant change. Rehearsal of homework tasks during therapy sessions is valuable as it helps parents build confidence in their skills, and it lets their child know that *their* parents really are part of *their* treatment team. Parents can be engaged early as 'the homework experts' for their own child, compiling power word and phrase lists (words and phrases that are important to the child), collecting speech samples, and making a 'brag book'.

Brag book

A brag book is a small, durable album or picture book, owned by the child and devoted to what the child *can* do, even if it only contains a couple of signs and a few sound effects. It is not a collection of words the adults in the child's life would *like* him/her to say! There is no 'right way' to compile one of these books, but it is quite popular (with children) to start with a few pictures of the child, so that when asked 'Who's this?' they can point to indicate 'me' even if they cannot say it yet; or simply nod when asked 'Is this you?' if they are not yet able to respond with 'Mmm' or 'Yes'. If the child has a few signed or spoken verbs (e.g., *go, stop, eat*) or verbal approximations, these could follow, with photographs of the child engaged in the actions. Favourite toys or foods that they have a sign, sound, or word for might come next, followed by important people (parents, siblings, and grandparents, perhaps), pets, and possessions. Next come all the words and approximations the child can say (including *pooh, wee, bum*, etc. if they are in the repertoire) and the child's sound effects for vehicles, machines, animals, and appliances. For all of these images, it is important to print, in lower case, the intended word or sound effect (e.g., *ee-ee* for mouse) and instructions for executing any signs or gestures, so that anyone who picks up the book knows how to enjoy it with the child. If touch cues, prompts, and imagery are being used, include appropriate graphics and instructions. 'Favourite words' (e.g., *Bob*) or 'good words' (words or phrases that the child says well or is proud of) can go in several times, making sure that there are some easy, fun words at the beginning of the book and again at the end. Songs, rhymes, rebus, and cloze where the child *can* provide the punch line can be included. As the book grows, the pictures can be rearranged so that they are loosely organised by theme and initial sound, encouraging everyone to think in terms of patterns and prosody from early on.

The brag book can include a note or letter from the therapist in accessible, jargon-free language to let the family and significant others know that:

- The emphasis should be on *meaningful* word production and syllable production (e.g., *bee, boo, moo, neigh, go, me too, no way, bye-bye*) and that isolated sounds are really only a goal if they carry meaning (e.g., *sh* for be-quiet, *ss* as a snake sound, *ee-ee* for a mouse sound-effect, etc.), and as a means to an end in stimulability therapy.
- Isolated sound production *may* be used briefly as a means to an end, but that *ba-ba-ba*, *bee-bee-bee*, *ta-ta-ta*, etc. are more desirable than practice drills for [b-b-b-b-b-], [t-t-t-t-], [p-t-p-t-p-t-p-t-p-t-], etc.
- Suprasegmentals (rhythm, melody, stress, loudness, pitch, rate, resonance, and intonation) should be emphasised from the start. This may promote more natural-sounding speech earlier, as opposed to the 'programmed' sound with odd prosody, and the excessive and equal stress (EES) characteristic of many children who have been treated for CAS.
- The desired goal is *many* 'repeats' of therapy targets, whether they are syllables, syllable sequences, single words, or word sequences. The 'repeats' are needed to facilitate optimal, 'automatic' speech production.
- Parents' ingenuity and input, particularly in the initial stages, are necessary to get therapy off to a good start, and we rely on them to help find activities and rewards that are beneficial and also motivating and fun for toddlers and preschoolers.
- They can be reassured that, with appropriate support, most children will start to 'bring the homework to parents', understand what the therapy is for, and take some responsibility for their own practice needs.

Ten tips for intervention for young children with severe CAS

With children who are non-verbal or who have few word approximations, early goals are to:

1) Establish a 'core vocabulary' (a selection of 'power words' like *no, more, go* and *me too*);
2) Select phonetic stimuli, favouring ones that are already spontaneously produced;
3) Start with CV and VC and CVC combinations, *definitely* including isolated vowels, but avoiding isolated consonants unless they carry meaning;
4) Establish the most beneficial facilitators for the child (ask the parents, or *tell* them!);
5) Establish an appropriate stimulus/response relationship;
6) Set criteria for subsequent changes in stimuli (How many correct trials?);
7) Choose reinforcers carefully, knowing that achieving the necessary intensity of drill is difficult, and that it is often hard to maintain the child's attention and cooperation. The aim here is to ensure a sufficient number of responses within a practice session.
8) Watch linguistic load. Keep it simple. Don't use complex carrier phrases or cloze, or awkward prosody.
9) Use alternative and augmentative communication (AAC), including sign and picture exchange to augment verbal attempts, to enhance language development and to

reduce the child's frustration. Reassure parents that AAC will not stifle verbal communication.

10) Keep therapy fresh—sameness and boredom kill *everyone's* motivation.

Which method do you use?

In Chapter 2, there is a section that covers the questions parents of children with SSD ask about severity, prevalence, aetiology, prognosis, therapy, target selection, and goal setting. One question that was not covered was 'Which method do you use?', specifically in relation to children with severe SSD. When parents ask this question, it may be an indication that they believe a 'best method' exists, a favoured 'therapy package' can be accessed, or that there is a certain 'therapy kit' or intervention tool that they should be seeking out. For example, they may ask, 'Are you a PROMPT therapist? (mentioning a widely practiced technique whose effects remain equivocal), or 'Do you do TalkTools?' (naming a popularly applied non-evidence based Oral Motor Therapy product range), or 'Do you do Auditory Integration Training?' [referring to a range of controversial therapies such as *Tomatis*, *Samonas Sound Therapy*, and *The Listening Program*, that have no scientific basis, and about which ASHA (2004c) declared, in a Technical Report, 'AIT has not met scientific standards for efficacy that would justify its practice by audiologists and speech-language pathologists']. The motivation of parents who ask about 'best therapy' and 'miracle cures' is to obtain the best possible services for their children, and many have been advised in good faith to explore options that are supported by neither theory nor evidence (Clark, 2003) and which may appeal to them because they sound more exotic, interesting, and exciting, and even more 'scientific' than mainstream speech and language therapy. Even some clinicians seem to think that a therapy that comes in a box has more appeal than one that comes in the form of a journal article. Some families want to know about complementary, homeopathic, herbal, dietary, astrological, or alternative medicine solutions, needing to ascertain whether the clinician will cooperate with, or at least not actively oppose, their 'alternative practitioners'.

It is important for families to know that there is a range options that includes many commercially available materials and programs, and to appreciate that not all treatments will be suitable for every child, and all treatments have to be individually tailored in response to the child's needs, strengths, challenges, co-morbidities, ongoing assessment outcomes, and response to intervention. In that sense, there is no 'best method', and a 'good method' is one that is adaptable to changes in the child and flexible over time and across settings and conditions. It can be helpful to share with parents that what *we* look for in a therapy is a scientific foundation and its applicability specifically to their child. That is, a therapy that is practicable, based in good theory (Table 1.3, p. 31) and, *ideally* supported by empirical evidence, published in the refereed literature.

Chapter 8

Targets, tips, tricks, and insights

Hollywood cameraman John Alton wrote the first book on cinematography in 1949, calling it *Painting with Light*. This title may have been the inspiration for *The Publicity Photograph* (Galton and Simpson 1958), a radio sketch for *Hancock's Half Hour*. Persuaded by Miss Pugh (Hattie Jacques), Bill (Bill Kerr), and Sid (Sid James) that he needs to update his image, Hancock (Tony Hancock) and Sid consult flamboyant theatrical photographer Hilary St. Clair (Kenneth Williams, he of the soaring triphthongs). When Sid tells St. Clair, 'I want you to take some snaps', he is outraged! '*Snaps*, Sidney? I don't take *snaps*; I *paint* with *light!*'

The topic of 'therapy tips' often arises in Internet discussions and at professional development events. When it does, there can be an urge to mount one's high horse and emulate St. Clair's retort. '*Tips? Tips?* I don't do *tips!* I put solid theory and evidence into practice!' or whatever the SLP/SLT equivalent of painting with light might be. But as seasoned interventionists know, therapy breakthroughs often come when, without abandoning evidence-based practice, we play educated clinical hunches, apply inspired brainwaves shared by mentors and colleagues, simply try something different, or implement a tip or trick from our repertoire that has worked for us before in making our jobs as scientific clinicians easier, especially with more complex clients. This short chapter comprises a compilation of such tips, tricks, and insights, and pointers for where to find meore.

DPD signs

As shown in Boxes 6.1 (p. 206) and 6.4 (p. 239), points 7, 8, 9, and 19, there are four signs that may help us determine whether a child's speech difficulties, or at least *some* of them, are phonological in nature. We should consider the possibility of DPD and a phonological intervention approach if the puzzle phenomenon is evident, if there is a pattern of unusual errors, if the child is marking contrasts 'oddly', and if error sounds are readily stimulable. Two of these giveaway signs, the puzzle phenomenon and marking, can be difficult to 'pick' unless the clinician is actively looking for them, so examples are provided below.

Puzzle phenomenon

The puzzle phenomenon occurs when a child consistently mispronounces sounds where they should occur, but uses them as substitutes where they should not! A 'demonstration' by Dane, father of Quentin, 6;1, exemplifies this.

> Dane: Show her how you say *thumb*.
> Quentin: *Fum*.
> Dane: Now say *sum*.
> Quentin: *Thum*.
> Dane: If he can say *thumb* when he means *sum*, how come he says *fum* when he means *thumb*? I think he's just lazy.

A second example of the puzzle phenomenon comes from the speech data of, Andrew, 4;6.

yellow	/lɛlʊo/	brother	/bwʌzə/
then	/dɛn/	globe	/bloʊb/
those	/douz/	rabbit	/bɹæbɪt/
glove	/gwʌb/	some	/θʌm/
breathe	/bwiv/	thumb	/sʌm/
snooze	/ðuð/	Zoo	/ðu/

Marking

Some of the errors children make deceive our trained ears; when we listen closely, we may find that the errors provide hints that a child knows more than he/she is able to produce, and that their difficulties are phonological and not phonetic. They do so by 'marking' the presence of the correct sound.

Marking with nasality

Uzzia, 5;1, with extensive final consonant deletion, talked about going to [bɛ] (*bed*) and referred to her brother as [bɛ̃]. Although it was easy to hear these as homonyms, it was apparent that Uzzia was *marking* the presence of the /n/ in *Ben* by nasalising the preceding vowel. This hint of a nasal final consonant was consistent with what happens normally, in that vowels preceding nasal consonants are usually nasalised.

Marking with vowel length

Owen, 4;3, also exhibited final consonant deletion, producing bus as [bʌ] and Buzz Lightyear's name as [bʌː], and again these two productions, [bʌ] and [bʌː], were readily mistaken for homonyms. But when we recall that vowels are typically longer before voiced consonants, we would be on safe ground to assume that Owen's lengthening of the short vowel /ʌ/ to [ʌː] meant that he 'knew' the difference between /s/ and /z/ but was not yet able to produce them SFWF.

Table 8.1 Traditional and newer criteria for treatment target selection

Traditional selection criteria	Newer selection criteria
1. Developmental sequence	9. Later developing sounds and structures first
2. Socially important	10. Marked consonants first
3. Stimulable phonemes	11. Non-stimulable phonemes first
4. Minimal meaningful feature contrasts	12. Maximal meaningful feature contrasts
5. Unfamiliar words	13. Systemic function of phonemes
6. Inconsistently erred sounds	14. Sonority sequencing principle
7. Most destructive of intelligibility	15. Least phonological knowledge
8. Most deviant from typical development	16. Lexical properties

Target selection

In the left column of Table 8.1 is a list of eight familiar, traditional target selection criteria that are not strongly based, if at all, in Linguistic theory. In the right column are eight newer criteria with Linguistic underpinnings and empirical support. All sixteen of these are summarised below, and depending on an individual child's intervention needs, any or all may be considered in deciding what to target, and when. The implication here should *not* be taken to read 'out with the old criteria, and in with the new'!

Traditional target selection criteria

1.   Developmental sequence

Working on sound targets in the typical sequence of acquisition is done on the logical assumption that earlier developing sounds are easier for a child to learn first, less frustrating for them to tackle, or easier for the clinician to teach (Hodson 2007; Van Riper and Irwin 1958). A clinician using this strategy might prioritise intervention targets following Shriberg's (1993) early, middle, and late eight acquired sounds, proceeding from the early eight: /m n j b w d p h/ to the middle eight: /t ŋ k g f v ʧ ʤ/ to the late eight: /ʃ ʒ l r s z θ ð/, or they might refer to any number of 'age of acquisition tables' (McLeod 2007a) or 'phonetic mastery tables' (Kilminster and Laird 1978 in Table 1.2, p. 11), or Hodson's (2007) target selection guidelines.

2.   Socially important

The notion of 'social importance' usually implies a significant target for the child or parents in terms of how the child is perceived, and may relate to avoiding embarrassment, as in the following examples. Stoel-Gammon (A9, p. 60) describes Brett, 4;9, who was teased for saying *Bwett*. Tired of the hilarity it generated, the Ayres family were anxious for Gerri, 5;3, to stop calling herself /dɛɹi/ (example used by permission); and Shaun, 4;9, was eager to work on /ʃ/ because he was taunted for saying his name /dɔn/. Many SLPs/SLTs have been asked by parents if the word *truck* might be considered as a target in children who pronounce /tr/ as in *tree* as /f/.

3. Stimulable phonemes

Prioritising for intervention-stimulable phonemes for which a child has most knowledge is based on the interwoven ideas of developmental readiness, ease of learning, and early success as a motivator (Hodson 2007) for the child, and ease of teaching (for the clinician). Traditionally, 'stimulable' has meant that a consonant or vowel can be produced in isolation by the child, in direct imitation of an auditory and visual model with or without instructions, cues, imagery, feedback, and encouragement. For example, a clinician might elicit /f/ simply by providing placement cues and modelling it.

4. *Minimal* meaningful contrasts

Minimal word pairs can be maximally opposed, like *sick-wick*, which differs in place, voice, manner, markedness, and major class; 'nearly maximally opposed', like *big-jig*, which cuts across many featural dimensions but shares the voicing feature; or minimally opposed, like *pat-bat* differing in voice only, *tip-sip* differing in manner only, and *cap-tap* differing in place of articulation only. Targeting error phonemes, or error patterns, using *minimally* opposed words is done on the understanding that it is the most direct way of demonstrating (his/her own) homophony to a child (Dean, Howell, Waters, et al. 1995; Grunwell 1989). So in choosing treatment words for a child exhibiting voiced velar fronting SFWF, word contrasts such as *bug-bud, cog-cod, beg-bed*, and *mug-mud* would be selected, with just one feature difference (in place) between error and target. In the process of constructing minimal pair sets, the clinician would attempt to find phonetically appropriate picturable words representing age-appropriate vocabulary that lend themselves to activities for pre-readers, and in most instances would include printed captions, in lower case, on picture cards and worksheets. For example, *peel* would be printed 'peel', not 'PEEL' or 'Peel', and *Paul* would be printed 'Paul' not 'PAUL' or 'paul' to be consistent with the way early literacy instruction is commonly delivered.

5. Unfamiliar words

Choosing unfamiliar words or low frequency words (in terms of their usage) for treatment stimuli is based on the premise that a child's error production of seldom-spoken or novel words (like *yowie, yabby, Uriah*, and *yen*) will not be as habituated as familiar words (such as *yes, yell, you*, and *yet*), or frozen (fossilised) forms like /lɛlou/ for *yellow*.

6. Inconsistently erred sounds

The principle governing the selection of sounds that are sometimes pronounced correctly is that, because the child demonstrates some knowledge of an inconsistently erred target, it will be easier to learn and teach than a sound for which a child has less (or no) knowledge. For example, following the developmental trend, a child receiving intervention might have acquired velar stops word finally in words like *take* and *big*, but not in other syllable contexts, encouraging the clinician to target /k/ and /g/ pre-vocalically, inter-vocalically, and in clusters, perhaps using facilitative contexts containing final velars (see *Backward chaining* in Chapter 6). Similarly, a child might be producing the /k/ and /g/ in /kl/ and /gl/ clusters but not in other positions, as can happen in typical acquisition, prompting the construction of near minimal pairs, such as *clap-cap, clean-keen;*

glow-go, glad-lad, to facilitate velar stops SIWI. Again, a child may be able to produce the voiceless affricate only in words ending with /ntʃ/, suggesting that practising words such as those found here: http://www.speech-language-therapy.com/nchSFWF-7b.pdf, might be facilitative.

7.   Most destructive of intelligibility

Sometimes an error has such a pervasive, negative impact on intelligibility that it compels consideration as a high treatment priority (Grunwell 1989). A recent example on the author's caseload was Yoshi, 4;2, with English as his first language and a PCC below 30% in both Japanese and English. His mother's second language was Japanese, English was his monolingual father's only language, and his Japanese au pair communicated with him in Japanese and German. In English, Yoshi had widespread glottal insertion before and after utterances and pre- and post-vocalically (as in Japanese). This, coupled with a complete absence of voiced stops had a devastating effect on his intelligibility. Early treatment goals included achieving stimulability of /b d g/ to two syllable positions and elimination of glottal insertion. Yoshi's phonology was unusual in there being no glottal *replacement* evident, only glottal insertion.

8.   Most deviant from typical development (non-developmental errors)

A consensus view of which are the common developmental and non-developmental error patterns, drawn from three sources (Dodd and Iacono 1989; Edwards and Shriberg 1983; Khan and Lewis 1983), is reported by Flipsen Jr. and Parker (2008). Non-developmental patterns include: initial consonant deletion (SIWI); within word consonant deletion (SIWW and SFWW); deletion of unmarked elements of clusters; within word consonant replacement (SIWW and SFWW); errors of insertion and addition (e.g., schwa insertion or addition; vowel addition word finally) and intrusive consonants; backing of stops, fricatives, and affricates; denasalisation; devoicing of stops; idiosyncratic systematic sound preferences; and glottal replacement, unless it is dialectal. Developmental patterns include final consonant deletion; reduplication; weak syllable deletion; cluster reduction; context-sensitive voicing; depalatalisation; fronting of fricatives, affricates, and velars; alveolarisation of stops and fricatives; labialisation of stops; stopping of fricatives and affricates; gliding of fricatives and liquids; deaffrication; epenthesis; metathesis; migration; and vocalisation. Following the recommendation of Grunwell (1989), non-developmental patterns are often given priority, particularly initial consonant deletion, which is only attested in normal development in Finnish, French and possibly Hebrew, and glottal replacement where it is not dialectal. Non-developmental patterns often beg to be eliminated because they can sound 'odd' even to the untrained ear, and they can disrupt prosody.

Newer target selection criteria

9.   Later developing sounds and structures first

Some research suggests selecting later developing sounds (e.g., the late eight acquired consonants: /ʃ ʒ l r s z θ ð/), complex targets (e.g., the marked consonants from a choice of /p t k f v θ ð s z ʃ ʒ tʃ ʤ/ that are missing from the child's inventory), and clusters (but not the adjuncts /st/, /sp/, and /sk/) as early treatment targets because training them will result in greater system-wide change (Gierut, Morrisette, Hughes, et al. 1996). Gierut and colleagues furnish persuasive arguments in favour of devising complex targets that are marked, non-stimulable, late acquired, consistently erred, and presented to the child in high frequency words representing maximally distinct feature oppositions (Baker, A11).

10.   Marked consonants first

Targeting marked properties (features) of phonemes may well facilitate acquisition of unmarked aspects of the system. Markedness is a concept from the study of the sound systems of all natural languages. A marked feature in a language *implies* the necessary presence of another feature, hence the term '*implicational* relationship'. There are languages, like English, that have stops *and* fricatives. There are languages that have stops, but *no* fricatives. But no language has fricatives and no stops. This means that fricatives are a marked class of sounds because the presence of fricatives necessarily implies the presence of stops in a particular language. Thus, it is said that there is an implicational relationship between the fricatives /f v θ ð s z ʃ ʒ/ and stops (Elbert, Dinnsen, and Powell 1984). Another way of putting this is to say that the fricatives, /f v θ ð s z ʃ ʒ/, are marked because they imply stops. Similarly, voiceless sounds, /p t k f θ s ʃ tʃ/, are marked because they imply voiced sounds. Furthermore, consonants imply vowels (Robb, Bleile, and Yee 1999); affricates /tʃ dʒ/ imply fricatives (Schmidt and Meyers 1995); clusters (except for /sp, st, sk/) imply affricates (Gierut and O'Connor 2002); and true clusters with small sonority differences imply true clusters with larger sonority differences (Gierut 1999). Some research suggests we should target the *marked* consonants /p t k f v θ ð s z ʃ ʒ tʃ dʒ/ and clusters, particularly those with small sonority differences, in order to facilitate the acquisition of unmarked ones.

11.   Non-stimulable phonemes first

For well over a decade, sections of the research world have encouraged clinicians to target non-stimulable sounds because if a sound *is* stimulable, it is likely to be added to a child's inventory without direct treatment (Miccio, A15; Miccio, Elbert, and Forrest 1999). As sounds that are *not* stimulable have poorer short-term prognosis than those that are, treatment outcomes are likely to be enhanced when SLPs/SLTs use their skills to address the production of those non-stimulable sounds. Once the sounds are stimulable, in two syllable positions (e.g., /f/ SI and SF in *fie* and *off*, respectively), they are likely to improve even if not targeted directly for treatment beyond that level. Targeting stimulable sounds yields short-term but limited gains, in terms of generalisation (Powell and Miccio 1996), whereas targeting *non-stimulable* sounds via stimulability therapy (Miccio, A15), exploratory sound play, and phonetic placement techniques increases the probability of generalisation, once stimulability has been achieved (Rvachew, Rafaat, and Martin 1999).

12.   Maximal meaningful feature contrasts

The rationale for using maximally opposed, non-proportional contrasts (Gierut 1992) is that the heightened perceptual saliency of the contrasts so formed increases learnability, facilitating phonemic change. This is discussed under *Maximal Oppositions and Empty*

Set in Chapter 4 with examples of treatment targets for Xing-Fu, 4;5, and Vaughan, 5;8, and elaborated by Baker (A11, p. 73).

13.   Systemic function of phonemes

Williams (19A; 2002b, 2003b) describes a non-traditional approach to target selection based on the function of the sound in the child's own system having maximal impact on phonological restructuring. This is explained with examples in Chapter 4 under the heading *Minimal Pair Approaches: Multiple Oppositions*, and by Williams herself in 19A.

14.   Sonority sequencing principle

Sonority is the amount of 'sound' in a consonant or vowel, and it has been represented numerically in a 'sonority hierarchy' (Steriade 1990). Steriade's proposed hierarchy was from most to least sonorous: vowels (=0), glides (=1), liquids (=2), nasals (=3), voiced fricatives (=4), voiceless fricatives (=5), voiced stops (=6), and voiceless stops (=7). Markedness data tell us that consonant clusters are more marked than singletons. Sonority theory adds to the picture by ranking two-element consonant clusters (note: just the two-element ones) in terms of markedness according to their sonority difference scores (Ohala 1999). For example, /kl/ (7 minus 1) has a sonority difference score of 6, whereas /fr/ (5 minus 2) scores 3. As Baker (A11) discusses in more depth, *small* sonority differences of 3 (like /sl/, /ʃr/) or 4 (like /gl/) may promote generalised change to singletons *and* clusters (Gierut 1999; Gierut and Champion 2001; Morrisette, Farris, and Gierut 2006) than other two-element clusters. It should be noted again here that Morrisette, Farris, and Gierut (2006) count initial /s/+ stop 'clusters' as adjuncts and not 'true clusters'.

15.   Least phonological knowledge

Research suggests selecting sounds for which the child has least knowledge because they will be easier to learn (Williams 1991; Barlow and Gierut 2002; Gierut 2001). Applying learnability theory, Gierut (2007) provides support for the position that, in order for efficient learning to occur, we should teach phonologically impaired children complex aspects of the target system, outside of what they have learned already.

16.   Lexical properties

High-frequency words are those words that occur often in the language, like *come, go, good, look, me, now*, and *one*. They are recognised faster by children than low-frequency words. High neighbourhood density words are phonetically similar to many other words. Children recognise and repeat high-density words slower and with less accuracy than low-density words. As well, children name high-density words more accurately than low-density words, suggesting that lexical processing in children entails a high-density disadvantage in recognition and a high-density advantage in production (Storkel, Armbruster, and Hogan 2006). In view of this, in choosing stimulus words, the clinician might consider those that are either high frequency or have low neighbourhood density (Storkel and Morrissette 2002).

Targeting speech perception

There is ample evidence to show that a large component of the SSD population has more difficulty with speech perception than their peers with age-typical speech (Munson, Baylis, Krause, et al. 2006; Munson, Edwards, and Beckman 2005; Rvachew 2007b; Sutherland and Gillon 2007). In an individual client, it is possible that one or more errors are due to the child's inability to hear the difference between his/her customary production and the target correctly produced, but this difficulty may not be readily apparent. Locke's (1980) procedure takes the guesswork out of trying to decide whether a child actually can hear the difference between error and target, at word level, when these are spoken by an adult in word contexts. The form displayed in Table 8.2a allows testing for two different discrimination errors, and instructions for the task

Table 8.2a Locke's Speech Perception–Production Task

Speaker's Name _____	Sex _____	Age _____			

Date: **Date:**

Production Task			**Production Task**		
/	/ → /	/	/	/ → /	/
Target / /	Error / /	Control / /	Target / /	Error / /	Control / /

Stimulus - Class	Response	Stimulus - Class	Response
1. // - Control	yes - NO	1. // - Target	YES - no
2. // - Error	yes - NO	2. // - Control	yes - NO
3. // - Target	YES - no	3. // - Target	YES - no
4. // - Target	YES - no	4. // - Control	yes - NO
5. // - Error	yes - NO	5. // - Error	yes - NO
6. // - Control	yes - NO	6. // - Error	yes - NO
7. // - Control	yes - NO	7. // - Target	YES - no
8. // - Target	YES - no	8. // - Error	yes - NO
9. // - Error	yes - NO	9. // - Target	YES - no
10. // - Target	YES - no	10. // - Control	yes - NO
11. // - Error	yes - NO	11. // - Control	yes - NO
12. // - Control	yes - NO	12. // - Error	yes - NO
13. // - Error	yes - NO	13. // - Target	YES - no
14. // - Target	YES - no	14. // - Control	yes - NO
15. // - Control	yes - NO	15. // - Error	yes - NO
16. // - Error	yes - NO	16. // - Target	YES - no
17. // - Target	YES - no	17. // - Error	yes - NO
18. // - Control	yes - NO	18. // - Control	yes - NO

Mistakes: Error _____ Control _____ Target _____   Mistakes: Error _____ Control _____ Target _____

Table 8.2b Instructions for Locke's Speech Perception–Production Task

1. Under 'production task', enter the target word and the substitution. For example, if the child said 'fumb' for 'thumb', enter thumb → /fʌm/ or /θʌm/ → /fʌm/.
2. Indicate the target sound in the space marked Target (/θ/ in the above example), the substituted sound in the space marked Error (/f/ in the above example), and a related sound as a control in the space marked Control (/s/ might be chosen for this example).
3. In each of the 18 spots under 'Stimulus - Class', fill in the appropriate sounds from #2 above, depending on which item is listed. For example, if the item says Target, write /θ/, if it says Error write /f/, and if it says Control write /s/. This creates the stimuli for the test.
4. Using the target picture as a visual cue, ask the speaker to judge whether or not you said the right word. For example:
   1) Is this 'some'?
   2) Is this 'fumb'?
   3) Is this 'thumb'?
   4) Is this 'thumb'?
   5) Is this 'fumb'? etc.

   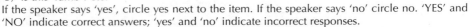

   If the speaker says 'yes', circle yes next to the item. If the speaker says 'no' circle no. 'YES' and 'NO' indicate correct answers; 'yes' and 'no' indicate incorrect responses.
5. Count the mistakes ('yes' and 'no') in each category (Target, Error, Control).
6. The speaker is said to have a problem with perception if 3 or more mistakes in perception are noted in response to the <u>Error</u> stimuli (out of 6 Error stimuli); 3/6 indicates that at least half the child's responses are incorrect, indicating that the child may have trouble distinguishing their customary production from the adult target.
7. Repeat the process for each erred sound suspected to have a perceptual basis.

are in Table 8.2b. For a discussion of perceptually based interventions, see Rvachew (A24, p. 152).

Targeting compensatory errors in the cleft palate population

Velopharyngeal dysfunction is most commonly associated with cleft palate or submucous cleft, but there are other causes, including a short soft palate, adenoidectomy, any neuromotor disorder that causes velopharyngeal insufficiency, craniofacial anomalies, enlarged tonsils, or irregular adenoids. In Q13 (p. 85), Golding-Kushner discusses issues in speech development, assessment, and intervention for children with craniofacial disorders, cleft palate, and velopharyngeal dysfunction; and in this chapter, Dennis Ruscello describes intervention techniques to use (and *not* to use) with this population.

Dr. Dennis Ruscello is a practitioner with an interest in the assessment and treatment of children with SSD, particularly those with structurally based deficits. His research and teaching have focused primarily on this population. Dennis is a member of the West Virginia University Cleft Palate Team and West Virginia University Center for Excellence in Disabilities Pediatric Feeding Team. He holds the Certificate of Clinical Competence in Speech-Language Pathology and is an ASHA Fellow. Dr. Ruscello is the author of a comprehensive book on therapy for child speech impairment (Ruscello 2008a) that includes step-by-step treatment strategies for SSDs with functional, structural, sensory, or neurological bases. What better person to ask in Q42 about the tricks-of-the-trade in the evaluation and treatment of resonance disorders and nasal emission, including context specific nasality, using low tech and 'no tech' procedures?

Q42.   Dennis M. Ruscello: Compensatory errors and cleft lip and palate

Many generalist paediatric SLPs/SLTs rarely encounter children with speech and resonance disorders secondary to cleft palate, craniofacial anomalies, and velopharyngeal
dysfunction (VPD). Terms like pressure-sensitive consonants, nasal rustle (turbulence),
compensatory articulations, prosthetic management, phoneme-specific hypernasality,
glottal substitutions, and the like may be only dimly understood. Karen Golding-Kushner
addresses some of the 'big picture' issues in assessment and treatment in A13. Can you
share with the non-specialist reader the practical strategies and techniques they should
know about when approaching this population, and the therapy tools they should have
to hand, and dispel some of the myths surrounding VPD and its management?

A42.   Dennis M. Ruscello: Treating compensatory errors in the cleft palate population: Some treatment techniques

Before discussing treatment techniques for children with VPD, it is important to emphasise
several points. First, these patients have a structurally based problem that can manifest
in different resonance and speech disorders. Second, many SLPs/SLTs see such clients
infrequently, so have limited relevant content knowledge and clinical skills. Third, these
children have heterogeneous speech production characteristics that may include developmental variation, obligatory errors, and compensatory errors.

Developmental variation occurs in the speech of children acquiring the sound system(s)
of their language(s) (Bernthal and Bankson 2004). These may be outgrown or persist,
requiring treatment, and are unrelated to structural problems. Obligatory errors result from
structural differences, which influence negatively the physiologic movement(s) requisite
to correct sound production (Golding-Kushner 2001; Ruscello, Tekieli, and Van Sickels
1985). Generally, obligatory errors are distortions of the intended sound and typically
resolve spontaneously once structural defects are corrected (Kummer, Strife, Grau, et al.
1989; Moller 1994). Finally, compensatory errors involve substitutions for individual sounds
or sound classes and are typical in children with VPD (Golding-Kushner 2001; Kummer
2001a). They include glottal stops, nasal snorts, velar fricatives, pharyngeal fricatives,
pharyngeal stops, and mid-dorsum palatal stops.

A study conducted by Hardin-Jones and Jones (2005) gives the reader an impression
of the incidence of resonance and speech production errors in children with repaired cleft
palate. Of 212 preschool children, 78 subjects (approximately 37%) had moderate to severe
hypernasality, while 53 (25% of the group) had compensatory errors. The most frequent
compensatory errors, in order, were glottal stops, glottal fricative /h/, nasal substitutions,
mid-dorsum palatal stops, pharyngeal fricatives, and posterior nasal fricatives.

Treatment techniques for compensatory errors

The treatment of hypernasality is generally accomplished through surgery or the fabrication
of a speech appliance; treatment of compensatory errors, however, is the responsibility of
the SLP/SLT. Such treatment is important because research demonstrates that elimination of compensatory errors positively influences velopharyngeal movement (Henningsson

and Isberg 1986). Treatment techniques for compensatory errors have been described in several study reports, treatment reviews, and texts (Golding-Kushner 1995, 2001, 2004; Kummer 2001b; McWilliams, Morris, and Shelton 1984; Peterson-Falzone, Hardin-Jones, and Karnell 2001; Peterson-Falzone, Trost-Cardamone, Karnell, et al. 2006; Ruscello 2008a; Trost-Cardamone and Bernthal 1993). The techniques are based primarily on judicious clinical decision-making and a modicum of treatment efficacy research, as the evidence base (Baker and McLeod 2004) is quite limited. I use the following treatment techniques differentially with children with cleft palate who have compensatory errors. Each has a specific purpose and rationale, tied to the research literature. They are divided into techniques used during acquisition (while a child is acquiring correct conscious production of a target sound) and during automatisation (when *automatic* spontaneous correct production is becoming established) or techniques that may be used in both phases of target sound practice (Ruscello 1993). The acquisition techniques are suitable for preschoolers as young as 3;0, with stimuli presented in a picture-reading format. The automatisation tasks are appropriate for school-aged children from 6;0 and beyond. Self-monitoring techniques incorporate acquisition and automatisation activities for children aged 3;0 upwards.

Acquisition

Imitative modelling

Imitative modelling is important in early treatment. The practitioner should ensure that stimuli are spoken with normal loudness, because excessive loudness or overstimulation may cause children to produce practice stimuli similarly. This is best avoided, since children with cleft palate are at risk for hyperfunctional voice disorders (Peterson-Falzone, Trost-Cardamone, Karnell, et al. 2006), and undue loudness may mask the SLP/SLT's perception and accurate assessment of imitative productions.

Non-speech sound stimulation and nonce words

Eliciting a target 'pressure sound' (obstruent) can be very difficult with some children, because they revert to their customary substitution during sound stimulation trials or, if they are backing, produce another posterior-based articulation (i.e., a non-target glottal or velar production). Accordingly, it is helpful to begin with the sound in *isolation* for target fricatives. Stops and affricates are elicited in CV contexts, since they are produced with obstruction of the vocal tract prior to release to an adjacent vowel. I have also found it useful to incorporate nonspeech sounds, in order to reduce error sound interference (Ruscello 2008a). For example, I may ask a child to whistle with their tongue for /s/, which of course they all say they cannot do! I then furnish instructions regarding tongue placement and lip position. I follow this with a whistle sound made with the tongue tip. Sometimes, the child's imitative token is judged to be /s/ in isolation. The child receives positive verbal feedback, continuing to practice until the target is elicited with the verbal cue alone ('Make the whistle sound.'). After /s/ production is stabilised through practice, I inform the child that the 'whistle sound' is really /s/.

Another approach to reducing contextual interference is the use of nonce words. A nonce item is a sound combination that is not a free morpheme, and may or may not have a permissible phonological structure. It is generally paired with a picture or line drawing, for example ⊕, to assign meaning to it. 'Billy, this is a sud.' (The clinician proffers ⊕.) 'Say sud.' In this way, the child rehearses a 'word unit,' absent from his/her lexicon in order to reduce interference from the error response.

Nasal occlusion

During practice trials at the isolation, nonce, and word levels, I have children gently pinch their nostrils with their thumb and forefinger (Golding-Kushner 2001). I emulate this while producing the stimuli, to cue them. Because the children have obligatory VPD, nasal occlusion helps them generate and sustain adequate air pressure for plosive, fricative, and affricate target production. It also provides auditory and tactile feedback for the child as targets are uttered (Kummer 2001b).

Imagery

For some children, using imagery helps them distinguish between target sound(s) and their substitution error(s). Because many compensatory errors preserve manner of articulation, but change place to a more posterior point of articulation (Trost-Cardamone and Bernthal 1993), a place distinction can be made. For example, if a child substituted /ʔ/ for /t/ and /d/, a place-based distinction between 'throaties' and 'tippies', respectively, can be made (Klein 1996b; and see Chapter 4 for a discussion of Imagery Therapy, and Table 6.5 for imagery names and verbal and gesture cues and reminders). Introductory identification trials are used to contrast glottal error productions and the alveolar target(s), enabling the child to make the appropriate auditory distinction with the associated image. Once able to make the distinction, children are queried periodically during practice trials. 'Billy, did you make the tippy sound or the throaty sound? Yes, you did make the tippy sound. Good job!'

Automatisation

Speed drills

Speed drills can assist in the automatisation of a target sound (Ruscello 1993). The child practises the target in context, while the SLP/SLT manipulates speaking rate. The goal is to increase rate of production, maintaining high levels of response accuracy. Speed drills consist of speech output by the client in practice sets, across training trials, with a gradual reduction in the time necessary to produce it. For instance, the clinician may present 20 phrases, to be read or 'picture-read' citation-naming style. The client has to read (or 'read') aloud the phrases using the target sound correctly. The time needed to produce the phrases and the accuracy rate for the practice set are recorded and shared with the child, providing feedback. The client is then instructed to read the 20 phrases taking less time, while maintaining the accuracy rate. Time and accuracy rate are again taken, and the results are discussed with the client. Additional practice sets can be completed, aiming to reduce time and sustain accuracy. Speed drills may also be performed with words or sentences, at the therapist's discretion. Speed drills can be interspersed throughout treatments as a supplementary activity. If the child's performance deteriorates during speed drills, the clinician should withdraw them, re-introducing them when the child appears ready (applying clinical judgement).

Auditory masking

Also designed to automate targets, auditory masking was developed by Manning, Keappock, and Stick (1976) to *assess* the automatic use of a target sound. The authors hypothesised that a client relies on auditory information during the automatisation phase of treatment, and interfering with auditory information provides an indication of the extent to which an individual is using a target sound automatically. The following is a description of a potentially effective treatment variation that I employ. The client reads or picture-reads a list of words, phrases, or sentences containing the target, and an accuracy rate is established. The client is then instructed that he/she will read the material again, wearing a headset through which noise will be played. Masking noise from an audiometer is audio recorded and the audiotape played through a headset, while the client produces the stimuli. Comparative accuracy rates between the masking and non-masking conditions are then discussed with the client.

Acquisition/Automatisation

Self-monitoring

Self-monitoring tasks are included in a number of treatments (Bernthal and Bankson 2004; Shriberg and Kwiatkowski 1987), and the author has found that self-monitoring can be useful with this client population. They include the client: (1) monitoring correct and incorrect productions of targets in production practice; (2) identifying, discriminating, and/or monitoring the production of another speaker, such as the clinician or caregiver; and (3) assessing the accuracy of his/her productions in more spontaneous treatment activities, such as conversational exchanges (Koegel, Koegel, and Ingham 1986). My preference is to employ self-monitoring in conversation or during automatisation tasks. Initially, a topic is introduced and the child is instructed that 'one idea at a time' will be discussed and to be sure to make the 'new sound' correctly. The use of limited spontaneous speech reduces any possible frustration for the child without destroying spontaneity. When the conversation ends, the child is queried regarding a word or words containing the target sound. The child identifies words containing the target sound, indicating the accuracy of those productions. As the child's self-monitoring skills improve, conversations increase in length.

Caregiver involvement

Ideally, caregivers are involved in their children's treatment, but the type of involvement varies (Ruscello 2008a). I meet with the caregiver, discuss the child's SSD and any co-existing communication disorders, and the proposed treatment, answering their questions. Stressing the importance of careful monitoring of hearing acuity, in light of the high incidence of conductive hearing loss in this population (Peterson-Falzone, Hardin-Jones, and Karnell 2001), I ask caregivers to provide verbal feedback to the child regarding speech progress, and to project a positive attitude to treatment. If a caregiver is willing to take a more active role, I involve the person in the treatment process, encouraging home activities that provide additional opportunities for practice. Crucially, the actively involved caregiver must first be trained to discriminate between correct and incorrect responses, because the child must receive reliable response information from both caregiver and SLP/SLT. I recommend that the caregiver carry out short practice sessions of approximately 8–10 minutes daily, recording the accuracy of the child's responses. These data are discussed each week with the caregiver, and modifications to practice material or sessions are made as needed.

Non-speech oral motor treatment (NS-OMT)

One treatment technique that I do not recommend is NS-OMT. The overwhelming majority of children with cleft palate do not have muscle weakness or muscle tone problems, and even if they did, NS-OMT divorced from speech production activities would not be indicated (Ruscello 2004, 2008b). NS-OMT techniques, such as blowing, sucking, or specific resistance exercises to 'improve' lip, tongue, or palate strength are not indicated. Moreover, efficacy studies of intervention designed to improve velopharyngeal function for speech through NS-OMT have largely been unsuccessful (Ruscello 2004, 2008b; Tomes, Kuehn, and Peterson-Falzone 2004). The clinician (and caregiver) should avoid NS-OMT activities and treat compensatory speech errors by using task-specific speech therapy.

Summary

The techniques described herein are used by the author in the treatment of children with cleft palate who present with compensatory errors. Most are based on research, but the reader must be mindful that large-scale treatment studies have not been undertaken to validate the treatment efficacy of each. Consequently, it is important for the SLP/SLT to measure the client's performance, so that the efficacy of the techniques can be assessed empirically and necessary changes made.

Words and pictures

The quest for suitable picture pairs representing age-appropriate vocabulary can be disappointing. Many of the published cards and worksheets intended for child speech intervention include words selected because they can be represented pictorially by an artist. It is rare to find materials that take account of the necessary linguistic and developmental criteria. As a consequence, clinicians often find that words need to be discarded because they are too challenging for a child with a particular speech error. For example, words pairs like *kite-tight, coat-tote, cart-tart, can-tan, Ken-ten, corn-torn, code-toad* are unsuitable in the early stages of working on voiceless velar fronting because the assimilatory effects of the alveolars /t/, /d/, and /n/ likely promote productions like /taɪt/ for *kite* and /tɛn/ for *Ken*.

On the topic of velars, there are few picturable English CVCs for the voiced velar–alveolar opposition SFWF to choose from without resorting to proper nouns (*Doug-Dud*) and fictional words, such as the names of 'aliens', monsters, and creatures (*Zig-Zid*). The picturable real words are *big-bid, bag-bad, bug-bud, cog-cod, beg-bed, mug-mud, leg-lead, hag-had, rig-rid, dig-did, rogue-road, sag-sad*, available at http://www.speech-language-therapy.com/tx-/d-vs-g-SFWF.pdf and not many more. Of these, *dig-did* probably needs to be rejected because *did* may feed the tendency for *dig* to be pronounced /dɪd/; *bag-bad, hag-had*, and *rogue-road* will not be suitable if clinicians or parents regard *bad, hag*, and *rogue* as scary, pejorative, or politically incorrect. Some children don't like pictures of 'sad' because it makes them sad, so *sag-sad* may be unacceptable; and *big-bid, cog-cod, beg-bed, leg-lead, hag-had, rig-rid, dig-did, rogue-road*, and *sag-sad* are likely to be problematic because *bid, did*, and *rid* are difficult conceptually, and *cod, cog, lead* (the metal or in a pencil), *hag*, and *rogue* may be unfamiliar to the child. That leaves three potential pairs, which may actually be enough to work with: *bug-bud, beg-bed*, and *mug-mud*. One could go through a similar process of elimination with the minimal word pairs for the voiced velar–alveolar contrast SIWI (http://www.speech-language-therapy.com/tx-/g-vs-d-SIWI.pdf). The word pairs are: *go-dough, gown-down, game-dame, got-dot, gull-dull, guy-dye, gear-deer, ghee-D, guide-died*, and *gig-dig*, and *gown-down, got-dot*, and *guide-died* may promote unwanted assimilation effects.

Words that are familiar in one linguistic milieu may be unfamiliar in another. For example, the luggage compartment of a car is called a *trunk* in the US and a *boot* in Australia; a *jersey* in the UK is called a *sweater* in the US and a *jumper* in Australia and New Zealand; a *pacifier* in the US is a *dummy* in the UK, Australia, and New Zealand. Depending on where you are, a dumpster is a skip, a lorry a truck, an elevator a lift, a queue is a line, and a courgette is a zucchini. Because of these differences, vowel pronunciation differences, and other difficulties associated with commercially available picture resources, clinicians, like the author, often elect to make their own materials that are linguistically, developmentally, and culturally suited to their clients.

Many home-made consonant worksheets including minimal pairs are freely available for colleagues to download from http://www.speech-language-therapy.com/txresources.html, and singleton and contrastive word lists can be found at http://www.speech-language-therapy.com/wordlists.html. Other resources are linked to http://www.speech-language-therapy.com/freebies.htm. The vocabulary used in the resources represents (non-rhotic) Australian English pronunciation, and although most of the words and minimal pairs will 'work' in other dialects of English, users may need to discard some. They were made in Microsoft Word, with copyright-free pictures from Microsoft Clip Art and Media (http://www.office.microsoft.com/clipart) and converted into portable document files (pdf) using Adobe Acrobat (the program, not the free reader). Colleagues are free to save them to their own computers and customise them to suit individual clients and service delivery models. Among the resources are informational slide shows for consumers, consonant worksheets, minimal pairs, listening lists, a description of the 'butterfly procedure' for working on palatalised and lateralised fricatives and affricates, and a page of 'therapy facts and tricks'. The resources in the facts and tricks page include pictures for the Aspiration Trick for Stopping and Prevocalic Voicing, facilitative contexts for affricates, Llama Therapy for /l/, and the Treasure

Technique for /ɹ. As well, there are pictures for backward chaining for /k/, described in Chapter 6.

Inspiration online

A final source of tips, tricks, and insights, not to mention good solid theory and evidence, can be found in the daily discussion among members of the phonologicaltherapy group (Bowen 2001), in the message archive, and in the groups' outstanding collection of links and resource files. People join phonologicaltherapy for a variety of reasons. Some enjoy sharing their knowledge, many love a good exchange of ideas, and lots like to ask questions and have them answered—and they usually *are* answered. Others, especially those in academic settings, are keen to stay in touch with the 'clinical reality' and stay appraised of what clinicians in the field are thinking and doing, whereas people in isolated work settings join for support and contact with peers. Many members appreciate, and constantly access, the extensive collection of child speech-related links and informational files, including important journal articles, available on the group Web site. The primary topic for the group is children's speech sound disorders, including developmental phonological disorders, childhood apraxia of speech, functional articulation disorders, and speech production difficulties associated with craniofacial differences. Discussions also concern 'older' children whose phonological or other speech sound difficulties persist, and who have phonological awareness, literacy, and language-processing problems. Most members of the group are SLPs/SLTs and Linguists, including clinicians, university teachers, and researchers. There are also many undergraduate and graduate students of communication sciences and disorders, and a few consumers.

Chapter 9

Working with PACT

PACT is an acronym for a family-centred phonological assessment and intervention approach to SSD called *Parents and Children Together* (Bowen, in press; Bowen and Cupples 2006). The acronym implies an agreement between parents, child, and clinician that all are actively involved in the therapy process, and the name itself reflects the child and family focus of the approach. Administered in planned blocks and breaks, PACT is 'broad-based' because, while concentrating mostly on the phonemic (phonological or linguistic) level, it *also* takes account of phonetic and auditory perceptual factors, because the difficulties children with phonological disorders experience may not be exclusively 'phonological'. It directly targets speech perception and intelligibility in children with phonological disorder, and it may also indirectly impact morphosyntax and phonological awareness (particularly phonemic awareness) and hence literacy acquisition. This chapter comprises an account of PACT, a case study of 'Josie', and two contributions (Dodd, A43 and James, A44) relating to issues that arose in Josie's management. The story of Josie will be familiar to readers who participated in the *Moderate and Severe Speech Sound Disorders* Master Class around Australia and New Zealand in 2007–2008.

Primary population

PACT was designed for three-to-six year olds and validated as an effective treatment for children in this age range diagnosed with mild, moderate, and severe phonological disorders (Bowen 1996a; Bowen and Cupples 1999a, b). The children in the efficacy study were typical of children with intelligibility difficulties in that they did not necessarily have 'pure' phonological disorder. Whereas children with language impairment were excluded from the study and each of the children's major communication disability was at the phonological level, the major disability was often accompanied by phonetic execution and auditory perceptual difficulties, and some participants were treated for dysfluency during the speech intervention process. The rationale for developing a therapy for preschoolers and younger school children was twofold. First, intelligibility difficulties may be obvious in two and three year olds, but diagnosis of SSD is usually elusive until some time in a child's fourth year; and second, we wanted to develop an intervention that families could access before their children started school, potentially pre-empting or minimising literacy acquisition difficulties.

Secondary population

Clinicians have reported acceptable outcomes with PACT with other populations, but such implementation has not been tested experimentally. The 'other' children have included: 3;0-to-6;0 year olds with language processing and production issues *and* SSD; and children with speech production issues ≤10 years with SLI; ≤10 years with pragmatic issues; growing up bilingual (and multilingual; Ray 2002) and with developmental delay; as well as children with clefts, autism spectrum disorder, Down syndrome, Fragile X syndrome, Williams syndrome, and cochlear implants. Although not designed specifically for children with CAS, it has been incorporated, with integral stimulation therapy (Strand, Stoeckel, and Baas 2006), and compatible techniques that follow the principles of motor learning (Schmidt and Lee 2000), to help treat children diagnosed with CAS.

Theoretical basis

PACT is based on the assumptions that phonemic change is (1) gradual and motivated by homophony; (2) enhanced through metalinguistic awareness of phones and the phonemic system; and (3) facilitated by heightened perceptual saliency of contrasts because it increases their learnability. PACT embraces the foundation of all minimal pair approaches (Fey 1992a) by systematically modifying groups of sounds produced in error; emphasising the establishment of feature contrasts to mark meaning distinctions rather than accurate sound production; and making it explicit to children that the function of phonology is communication. This is achieved in PACT by working at word level and above, using naturalistic parent–child communicative contexts, increasing the child's (and parents') metaphonological awareness, and targeting phonological, phonetic, and perceptual levels as required.

Empirical support

In the efficacy study, a longitudinal matched groups design was employed, with assessment, treatment, and re-assessment (probe) phases. Fourteen children were treated under typical clinical conditions, and treatment was withheld from eight matched children on waiting lists. At probe, the treated children showed accelerated and highly selective improvement in their productive phonology [$F(1,20) = 19.36$, $P < 0.01$], whereas the untreated eight did not. No such selective improvement was observed in the treated children in either receptive vocabulary or Mean Length of Utterance in Morphemes, attesting to the specific effect of the therapy. PACT is practicable (Robey and Schultz 1998) under conditions of everyday practice in terms of the in-clinic component (Bowen and Cupples 1998, 1999a), and it is feasible and often enjoyable for interested families implementing homework and follow-up away from the clinic (Bowen and Cupples 2004).

Assessment

A 200-utterance CS or 200-word CS and *Quick Screener* (Bowen 1996b, after Dean, Howell, Hill, et al. 1990) SW sample usually provide sufficient data to allow independent and relational analyses (Stoel-Gammon, A9) and diagnosis, or provisional diagnosis, of phonological impairment. Additional testing is sometimes necessary, and this might entail administration of the DEAP (Dodd, Crosbie, Zhu, et al. 2002) or the HAPP-3 (Hodson 2004), the Locke Speech Perception–Production Task (Locke 1980; see Tables 8.2a and 8.2b, p. 287–288), and an imitative PCC (Johnson, Weston, and Bain 2004). Speech assessment within the PACT approach, whether initial or ongoing, is integral to intervention. As parents play a central role in management, it is highly desirable for them to be aware—through observation, participation, and explanation—of the speech-language assessment process. Essential components of data gathering are the case history interview; an audiological evaluation by an Audiologist; pragmatics, voice and fluency screening; an oral musculature examination; and a CS sample of 200 utterances, if possible, noting that, for some children, single word tokens may predominate. Within the case history interview, parents are asked to provide an intelligibility rating using a scale of 1 to 5: (1) completely intelligible; (2) mostly intelligible; (3) somewhat intelligible; (4) mostly unintelligible; and (5) completely unintelligible. This is recorded on the *Quick Screener* data collection form displayed in Figure 9.1.

If the child's output is so unintelligible that the clinician cannot even guess the content, or if time is short or the child's cooperation difficult to establish, an imitative PCC procedure is used rather than the conversational PCC procedure (Flipsen Jr., A10). Johnson, Weston, and Bain (2004) found that PCCs derived from conversational samples did not differ significantly from PCCs drawn from sentence imitation, using age-appropriate vocabulary, syntax, and representative distribution of speech sounds in children aged 4 to 6. They concluded that 'the sentence imitation procedure offers a valid and efficient alternative to conversational sampling'. In their experiment, a wordless picture book, *Carl Goes to Daycare* (Day 1993), provided visual stimuli for the repetition task, and the short sentences the children repeated after the examiner included, 'Watch them dance', 'He got cold', and 'Time to go home'.

Quick Screener

Speech assessment begins with the administration of the *Quick Screener*, while parents observe, using the data collection form displayed in Figure 9.1. The SLP/SLT phonetically transcribes in full, with necessary diacritics, the child's production of the first word 'cup' and immediately assigns a score which goes in the 'CC' (consonants correct) column. For example, if the child says [kʌp] the score is 2; if he/she says [kʌ], [ʌp], [tʌp], or [gʌp] the score is 1; and if he/she says [ʌ] or [tʌ] the score is zero. Each word is scored for consonant production in this way. There are approximately 100 consonants in the sample, depending on the dialect of English, so a tentative single-word PCC can be estimated quickly, with parents watching, by adding the figures in the CC columns and calling the sum a percentage. For example, if the child scores 55 consonants correct, his/her tentative PCC, or screening PCC, is 55%. There is also provision on the form to record vowel errors. The vowel and diphthong targets on the data collection form reflect non-rhotic Australian English, and these can be changed by the therapist for other

Quick Screener

SINGLE-WORD SCREENING SAMPLE USING THE METAPHON STIMULUS VOCABULARY

Dean, E., Howell, J., Hill, A., & Waters, D. (1990). Metaphon Resource Pack. Windsor, Berks: NFER Nelson

Date of Birth	Observer(s)
Today's date	Examiner

① completely intelligible ② mostly intelligible ③ somewhat intelligible ④ mostly unintelligible ⑤ completely unintelligible

#	TARGET	TRANSCRIPTION	CC	#	TARGET	TRANSCRIPTION	CC
1	cup	ʌ		23	jam	æ	
2	gone	ɒ		24	house	aʊ	
3	knife	aɪ		25	path	a	
4	sharp	a		26	door	ɔ	
5	fish	ɪ		27	smoke	oʊ	
6	kiss	ɪ		28	bridge	ɪ	
7	sock	ɒ		29	train	eɪ	
8	glass	a		30	chair	ɛə	
9	watch	ɒ		31	red	ɛ	
10	nose	oʊ		32	spoon	u	
11	mouth	aʊ		33	plane	eɪ	
12	yawn	ɔ		34	fly	aɪ	
13	leaf	i		35	sky	aɪ	
14	thumb	ʌ		36	sun	ʌ	
15	foot	ʊ		37	wing	ɪ	
16	toe	oʊ		38	splash	æ	
17	snake	eɪ		39	tent	ɛ	
18	van	æ		40	salt	ɒ	
19	fast	a		41	crab	æ	
20	girl	ɜ		42	sweet	i	
21	stairs	ɛə		43	sleeve	i	
22	big	ɪ		44	zipper	ɪ ə	

Check ɔɪ boy ɪə ear　　　**SUBTOTAL CC:**　　　　　　　　　　　　　　**TOTAL CC:**

TENTATIVE single word phonetic inventory (≈100 consonants in sample) and PVC (47 vowels/diphthongs in sample)

Vowels	i	ɪ	ɛ	æ	a	ʌ	ə	ɜ	ɒ	ɔ	ʊ	u	Vowels correct (47)　　　%
Obstruents	p	b	t	d	k	g	f	v					Consonants correct (≈ 100)　　%
Obstruents	θ	ð	s	z	ʃ	ʒ	tʃ	dʒ	STIMULABILITY				MARKED p t k f v
Sonorants	m	n	ŋ	l	r	w	j	h					θ ð s z ʃ ʒ tʃ dʒ

List phonological processes/record observations

Figure 9.1 'The Quick Screener Data Collection form (Bowen, 1996b, after Dean, Howell, Hill, et al. 1990).

dialects of English. If the child mispronounces the vowel or diphthong in a word, the vowel or diphthong is circled by the therapist and later tallied to calculate a screening percentage of vowels correct (PVC) using the formula VOWELS CORRECT $\div$ 47 $\times$ 100 = PVC (again, while parents observe). It should be remembered that the PCC and the PVC derived from the screener are *screening* (tentative) measures, although it has been observed clinically that there is little variation in PCC and PVC scores between data gathered via the *Quick Screener* and larger data sets.

Using the *Quick Screener* analysis form displayed in Figure 9.2, the clinician summarises the child's phonological processes as percentages of occurrence, if this is considered useful, and records pertinent observations, including the therapist's own intelligibility rating. These outcomes are discussed in the child's hearing. It is explained to parents that the child's continued presence during discussion demonstrates to the child that his/her parents are important partners in the therapy process. It also helps to acknowledge parents, up front, as the homework experts and experts on their own child.

The word set contained in *Quick Screener* is based on the *Metaphon Resource Pack Screening Test* developed by Dean, Howell, Hill, et al. (1990) with the word 'gun' changed to 'gone', and is freely available at http://www.speech-language-therapy.com/tx-a-quickscreener.html. Word productuctions can be elicited using the *Metaphon Resource Pack Screening Test* easel book, or The *Quick Screener* pictures presented as a slide show, or printed on cards. The author prefers the slide show option, not least because children usually find it interesting and fun, *and*, quite remarkably, frequently ask to do it 'again'! The data collection form has space for recording stimulability data and the child's inventory of marked consonants. In stimulability testing, the child is asked to directly imitate vowels in isolation and CVs, usually [ba bi bu] etc. focusing on vowels and diphthongs already circled on the form; and consonants of interest in CV or VC contexts, or both, but not usually in isolation. Marked consonants in the child's inventory are circled, from a choice of /p t k f v θ ð s z ʃʒ t ʃ dʒ/. The stimulability and markedness data are later used in the decision-making process for treatment target selection.

Assessing progress

It is usual to reassess, using the *Quick Screener*, with parent observation, at the beginning of each block (immediately after a break), allowing parents, who are often particularly interested in the inventories and percentages, to observe any changes. Additional testing may be required; for example, the DEAP, HAPP-3 or the Locke Task might be repeated. Any decision to terminate or continue therapy is made jointly with parents.

Goals and Goal Attack

Table 1.3 (p. 31) provides a schema within which to view three levels of intervention goal. The basic goal of PACT is to work at word level or above to encourage phonological reorganisation, thus facilitating the emergence of clear speech. This basic goal is achieved by increasing a child's consonant, vowel, syllable-shape, syllable-stress, phonotactic, and suprasegmental repertoires and accuracy; and by promoting generalisation of new

Velar fronting

#	Target SI	0 / 1	#	Target SF	0 / 1
1	cup		7	sock	
6	kiss		17	snake	
2	gone		22	big	
20	girl		37	wing	
	TOTAL	/4		TOTAL	/4

Palato-alveolar fronting

#	Target SI	0 / 1	#	Target SF	0 / 1
4	sharp		5	fish	
30	chair		9	watch	
23	jam		28	bridge	
	TOTAL	/3		TOTAL	/3

Word-final devoicing

#	Target	0 / 1	#	Target	0 / 1
41	crab		43	sleeve	
31	red		10	nose	
22	big		28	bridge	
				TOTAL	/6

Backing

#	Target SI	0 / 1	#	Target SF	0 / 1
16	toe		15	foot	
39	tent		42	sweet	
26	door		31	red	
	TOTAL	/3		TOTAL	/3

Stopping of fricatives

#	Target SI	0 / 1	#	Target SF	0 / 1
5	fish		13	leaf	
15	foot		11	mouth	
14	thumb		6	kiss	
7	sock		38	splash	
36	sun		43	sleeve	
4	sharp		10	nose	
18	van				
44	zip(per)				
	TOTAL	/8		TOTAL	/6

Stopping of affricates

#	Target SI	0 / 1	#	Target SF	0 / 1
30	chair		9	watch	
23	jam		28	bridge	
	TOTAL	/2		TOTAL	/2

Pre-vocalic voicing

#	Target	0 / 1	#	Target	0 / 1
25	path		5	fish	
16	toe		14	thumb	
6	kiss		36	sun	
			4	sharp	
				TOTAL	/7

Liquid/glide simplification

#	Target	0 / 1	#	Target	0 / 1
9	watch		12	yawn	
13	leaf		31	red	
				TOTAL	/4

Initial consonant deletion

#	Target	0 / 1	#	Target	0 / 1
3	knife		7	sock	
22	big		30	chair	
18	van		12	yawn	
				TOTAL	/6

Final consonant deletion

#	Target SI	0 / 1	#	Target SF	0 / 1
23	jam		10	nose	
44	zip		5	fish	
31	red		28	bridge	
				TOTAL	/6

Initial cluster reduction

#	Target SI	0 / 1	#	Target SI	0 / 1
33	plane		43	sleeve	
8	glass		27	smoke	
28	bridge		17	snake	
29	train		32	spoon	
41	crab		21	stairs	
34	fly		35	sky	
42	sweet		38	splash	
				TOTAL	/14

Final cluster reduction

#	Target	0 / 1	#	Target	0 / 1
19	fast		40	salt	
39	tent				
				TOTAL	/3

Figure 9.2 Quick Screener Analysis form

segments, structures, and prosodic features to increasingly challenging contexts and situations. The intermediate goal is to target groups of sounds related by an organising principle (processes, rules, or patterns), addressing phonetic and perceptual levels as required. Specific intervention goals are to target a sound, sounds, or syllable structures, using horizontal strategies: targeting several sounds within a sound class or manner of production, or syllable structure category, and/or targeting more than one process or deviation or structure simultaneously.

Goal selection and attack strategies are primarily therapist-driven and explained to parents. Multiple goals are addressed in and across treatment sessions and within homework, sequentially and simultaneously, and rarely cyclically. For example, Emeline, 5;1, in session four of her second therapy block, had three concurrent goals. First, a phonetic goal to produce /dʒ/ and /tʃ/ in onset and coda in six practice words; second, a phonological goal to recognise distinctions in input, and to mark distinctions in output in short phrases between the cognate pairs /p b/, /t d/, and /k g/ (e.g., with Emeline instructing and adult to 'Touch the *pea/bee*', 'Touch the *toe/doe*', 'Touch the *cap/gap*'; and then switching roles); and a generalisation goal to use the voiceless fricatives /f/, /s/, and /ʃ/ in conversational speech in untrained words in the therapy session and during an agreed daily period at home.

Materials and equipment

The materials and equipment required consist of toys, vowel and consonant pictures on cards and worksheets, a 'speech book' (exercise book, ring binder, or scrapbook), drawing and 'making' materials and equipment, rewards such as stamps and stickers, a computer for slideshows and the administration of the *Quick Screener*, and an audio recorder to record therapy snippets. It is helpful but not essential for the family to have a computer and audio recorder. Pictures in speech books and on cards usually include printed captions to clarify what the target words are meant to be. Captions are printed consistent with the way in which early literacy instruction is commonly delivered, with all words printed in lower case, and capital letters used only for the beginnings of proper nouns. Such pictures are available to clinicians and families at http://www.speech-language-therapy.com/freebies.htm.

Intervention

Therapy sessions

The child is seen by the clinician for 50–60 minutes (usually 50 minutes) once per week in therapy blocks. The minimum parent participation involves the parent joining the therapist and child for 20 minutes at the end of a session, or 10 minutes at the beginning and end; and the maximum parent participation sees parents staying 50–60 minutes. The parent assumes the role of a dynamic collaborator in a treatment triad with child and therapist. Segments of parent participation always require the child's continued involvement, to properly demonstrate what should happen at home. The following is an outline of a 50-minute session for Iain, 5;7, with his father Gordon and a therapist, towards the end of his second treatment block (of three) in which one treatment target was addressed.

Iain had a persistent /n/ for /l/ sound replacement SIWI, and over the previous two weeks, had *finally* become stimulable for /l/ in CVs by dint of every phonetic placement technique the therapist knew—or at least it felt that way! Gordon left Iain with the therapist for 15 minutes while he dropped his wife Lucinda at a railway station and took seven-year-old Bruce to school, returning for the final 35 minutes of the session with Iain's brother Fergus, 18 months, who played happily alone while work proceeded. Iain had already engaged in items 1 to 3 with the therapist.

1. Rhyming auditory bombardment using five pictured, captioned (in lowercase printing), minimal pairs: snip-slip, snap-slap, snow-slow, snug-slug, sneak-sleek, was presented. The pairs were spoken to Iain at a comfortable conversational loudness level, and then he played a quick game of 'Point to the one I say', with the therapist saying the words and Iain pointing.
2. Next was auditory input cloze with the same captioned pictures, with Iain saying the sn-words that he was already able to pronounce correctly:
   Adult: Slow rhymes with. . . Iain: snow
   Adult: Slap rhymes with. . . Iain: snap, etc.
3. A minimal pairs 'silent sorting' task followed. Four cards (name, night, knots, and nine) were placed on the table, and Iain was encouraged to 'think the words' as he placed a rhyming word (from a choice of lame, light, lots, and line) beside each (see Figure 9.3).

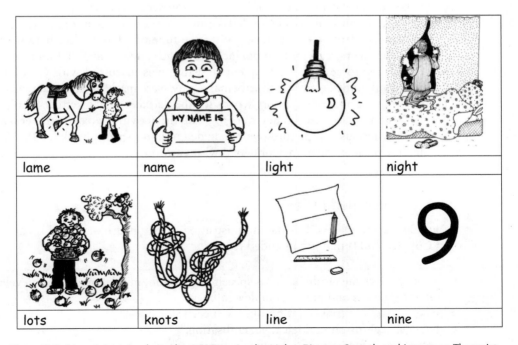

| lame | name | light | night |
| lots | knots | line | nine |

Figure 9.3 /l/ vs. /n/ minimal word pairs. Drawing by Helen Rippon, Speech and Language Therapist www.blacksheeppress.co.uk

4. Gordon began participating in the session at this point. Iain was shown a page of pictures of late, lei, lap, let, light, lock, lick, lame, lead, lit, and lice, and told, 'This time, Iain, you be the teacher and tell me if I say these words the right way or the wrong way.' Taking the role of 'student', Gordon made deliberate random errors, emulating Iain's sound replacement (e.g., 'Nate' for 'late', 'neigh' for 'lei', 'nap for 'lap' as single-word inputs or in short utterances, e.g., 'He is *late* for school' vs. 'He is *Nate* for school'). All Iain had to do was tell the 'student' whether he was right or wrong without modelling correct pronunciation.

5. The therapist, and then Gordon, presented a 'Fixed-up-one Routine' for /n/ vs. /l/.

6. The clinician presented a homophony confrontation task with lei-neigh, lap-nap, lame-name, and low-no, and this was the one task not included in homework.

7. All three rehearsed a Knock-Knock joke (Knock, knock. Who's there? Lettuce. Lettuce who? Lettuce in!). This was then recorded several times on the same tape with Iain saying 'Lettuce' and 'Lettuce in' and his father saying 'Who's there' and 'Lettuce who?'

8. The auditory bombardment was delivered again and recorded on the same tape. It consisted of *snip-slip, snap-slap, snow-slow, snug-slug, sneak-sleek*, as in item one above, followed by fifteen words in sequence: *leaf, lamb, lock, label, lead, lie, lake, lion, lip, letter, lunch, llama, lamp, lettuce.*

9. Homework, comprising activities 2–4 and 6–8, was explained by the clinician, demonstrated by the clinician and Iain, and then rehearsed by Iain and Gordon. Iain tried the Knock-Knock joke out on his father several more times, and the tape with the joke and bombardment sequences, with a running time of 2.5 minutes, was played.

10. In the context of putting 'children' on a toy school bus, Gordon, therapist, and Iain sang 'Lettuce-in, lettuce-in, lettuce-in', 'Lettuce-go, lettuce-go, lettuce-go', and 'Lettuce-out, lettuce-out, lettuce-out' to the tune of 'Here we go, here we go, here we go' on the tape to take home, increasing the running time to 4 minutes.

11. How to reinforce /l/ using frequent recasting was discussed with Gordon (parent education), and suggestions for thematic play were made around the words 'llama' and 'line' and making up more words for the 'lettuce song' ('Lettuce stop', 'Lettuce start', 'Lettuce see', etc.). They were to do all the activities except number 6 at home, and instructions and pictures were included in Iain's speech book for Lucinda, who shared over half the homework-load with Gordon.

Intervention scheduling

A unique feature of PACT is its administration in planned blocks and breaks (Bowen and Cupples 2004) that are intended to:

- accommodate the gradualness of speech acquisition, mimicking typical development;
- allow for spurts and plateaus in development;
- make 'space' for consolidation of new speech skills;
- make 'space' for phonological generalisation;
- make 'space' for untrained spontaneous gains; and
- provide periodic respite, allowing families to refresh and regroup.

Dosage

The initial block and break are usually about 10 weeks each, and then the number of therapy sessions per block tends to reduce while the period between blocks remains more or less constant at 10 weeks. A typical schedule is 10 weeks on, 10 weeks off, 8 weeks on, 10 weeks off, 4–6 weeks on. It is suggested to parents that, during the breaks, they do no formal practice for up to 8 weeks. In the 2 weeks prior to the next block, they are asked to enjoy looking through the speech book with the child a few times and to do any activities the child wants to do. Although they don't do homework or revision in the breaks, the child's parents continue to provide modelling corrections, reinforcement of revisions and repairs, and pursue metalinguistic activities, incidentally, as opportunities arise, using the strategies learned in 'parent education' in the therapy block(s).

Typically those children with phonological disorder *only* have needed a mean of 21 consultations for their output phonology to fall within age-expectations, so many are ready for discharge at the end of their second block (about 30 weeks after initial assessment) or immediately after their second break (about 40 weeks after initial assessment). A small number of children engaged in PACT have required a third block; fewer have needed four; and there is no record of a child needing more than four treatment blocks. Children with phonological disorder as well as mild language or fluency difficulties have required about the same volume of therapy for speech, but most have continued having intervention for longer to address their other, non-speech goals.

Target selection

Like goal selection and attack, target selection (with exceptions like Shaun's wanting to work on /ʃ/ in order to pronounce his own name correctly) is therapist-driven, and the reasons certain targets are given preferential treatment are explained to parents. As part of a stopping pattern, Shaun, 4;9, called himself 'Dawn'. An adult neighbour whose name actually was Dawn, apparently oblivious to the misery it evoked and angry requests from Shaun to 'Stop it', teased him endlessly to the point where *all* he and his mother were interested in doing in therapy was to work on /ʃ/. In selecting treatment targets, the clinician uses linguistic criteria, taking into account motivational factors and attributes of the child and the parents; is flexible in terms of feature contrasts; and applies evidence and clinical judgement. Traditional and newer criteria (see Table 8.1, p. 282) may be applied to isolating optimal targets.

Sometimes it is necessary to fall back on other, more traditional criteria. Take Tessa for example. Superficially, Tessa 5;10, was a perfect candidate for a least knowledge approach using high-frequency lexical targets because she had a phonetic inventory of only 13 consonants, a PCC of 38%, and extensive homophony. Or *was* she? She was a fretful, diffident child with wary, apprehensive parents, ready to abandon therapy if the clinician attempted anything 'too hard'. These three were unsuited to complex maximal oppositions or empty set feature contrasts, for which Tessa had least knowledge. They needed to ease into therapy via a gentler, albeit less potent, approach using unmarked, stimulable, inconsistently erred, early developing sounds; low-frequency words with low neighborhood density; and minimal feature contrasts. Once they were all ready to trust the clinician's target choices and confront more difficult tasks, Tessa took more risks, handling the challenges of multiply opposed word sets within the Multiple Exemplar Training component of PACT.

PACT components

PACT has five dynamic and interacting components: Parent Education (Family Education), Metalinguistic Training, Phonetic Production Training, Multiple Exemplar Training (Auditory Input and Minimal Contrasts Therapy), and Homework. The therapy involves the child, primary caregiver(s), and therapist; and sometimes significant others, including older siblings, grandparents, and teachers, become involved in homework.

1. Parent Education (Family Education)

Rationale

Recognising that PACT will not suit every child or every family, we hypothesised that arming interested parents with techniques (e.g., modelling, recasting, fostering repair strategies, and thematic play) related to their own child's intervention needs, and by working with them collaboratively, we would tap a unique and powerful 'therapeutic resource'. Unique because a child (usually) only has one set of parents, and powerful because (usually) parents likely spend the most time with their child and are most motivated to help. Through supportive Parent Education, they would be guided to use 'speech time' optimally in Homework and incidentally in real (not contrived) communicative contexts as natural opportunities arose. This might lead to the need for less consultation and fewer child–clinician contact hours, and ensure that planned breaks from therapy were used more productively.

Methods

Incorporating simple principles of adult learning (Knowles 1970), parents learn techniques, explained in plain-English (Bowen 1998a, b), including: delivering modelling and recasting, encouraging self-monitoring and self-correction, using labelled praise, and providing focused auditory input. Employing clinical judgement and responding to parent feedback, Parent Education is delivered according to need (Bowen and Cupples 2004). It may happen in the form of modelling, counselling, direct instruction, observation, scripted routines, participation, and discussion in assessment and therapy sessions, as well as role-playing and rehearsal. For some families, this involves independent reading of handouts and publications (Bowen 1998a, b; Flynn and Lancaster 1996) and viewing relevant informational slideshows (http://www.speech-language-therapy.com/shows.html) e-mailed to them or accessed from the Internet and viewed on home computers, and later discussed. Some families need more support than this and are 'talked through' informational handouts and view individualised (for their child) slide shows in-clinic, explained carefully by the therapist.

Written information is provided in a speech book that often becomes a prized possession of the child's, particularly if it features his/her own artwork. It is used to facilitate communication between therapist, family, and others involved (e.g., grandparents or teachers). It includes current targets and goals, a progress record, homework activities, developmental norms, and information about therapy for SSD. Parents and teachers are encouraged to contribute to the book: recording progress, commenting on homework content and performance, noting favourite activities or their own innovations, and often giving important pointers to the therapist that might otherwise be unavailable. For instance, Bowen and Cupples (2004) reported that Sophie, 4;3, with a moderate to severe SSD, talked constantly at home and was animated and chatty in the clinic, but that her teacher surprised (and enlightened) the therapist and her parents when she wrote in the speech book: 'I enjoy working with Sophie and doing the activities in her book. She is very responsive in the one-on-one– loves it – but if I try to involve another child or two she clams up completely. I think you should know that she never speaks to her kindy peers – only to teachers and the aide, and only one-to-one, and in a quiet voice we can hardly hear.' This information led to providing preschool personnel with strategies that increased Sophie's communication with her peers.

Discussion

Parents of the children in the efficacy study were not 'selected' in any sense and were not forewarned prior to initial consultation that they would be asked to participate in the therapy. Nonetheless, all the families rose to the task willingly, becoming actively involved in therapy sessions and in homework which they did in 5- to 7-minute bursts once, twice or three times daily, as recommended. On average, homework was done 24 times per week (4 families), 18 times per week (1 family), 12 times per week (7 families), 8 times per week (1 family), and 6 times per week (1 family) (Bowen, in press; Bowen and Cupples 2004).

Parents vary in the amount and style of information they need, some performing well with little explanation, learning best via observation and rehearsal. Others want a lot of 'training' before being comfortable performing activities at home. Although it is encouraged without insisting, some parents are shy when it comes to rehearsing homework tasks in the clinic with the therapist watching. Educational levels appear to have little bearing on how readily parents comprehend and work with concepts, expressed in plain-English, such as 'sound patterns', 'sound classes', 'reinforcement', 'modelling', 'labelled praise', 'revisions and repairs', 'progressive approximations', 'shaping', and 'gradualness of acquisition'. Subjectively, it seems some parents have an instinct, 'feel', or 'gene' for this sort of thing, and some appear to have missed out! Some are intuitive 'natural teachers', and some are not. Despite this, it is amazing what parents will *learn* to do well with adequate levels of support when they perceive that their child stands to benefit. Parents with personal histories of communication difficulties similar to their child's may be endowed with a special empathy, although some of them may have residual issues affecting their capacity to reflect on language function and to enjoy language play (Crystal 1996, 1998).

In delivering parent education, it is imperative to:

- avoid overwhelming families with information at any point;
- circumvent giving them the impression that they have to become 'mini-therapists';

- provide parents with opportunities to rehearse new skills if appropriate, while being sensitive that some adults find it embarrassing and difficult (or culturally inappropriate) to play;
- create an atmosphere in which parents can feel comfortable in questioning anything not understood, share their perspectives, and exercise choice; and
- listen to their ideas respectfully and incorporate them where possible.

2. Metalinguistic training

Rationale

This component was inspired by a fascinating article by Dean and Howell (1986) that proposed a role for guided discussion and meta-language in helping children reflect on the features or properties of phonemes, and the structure of syllables, with a view to improving their awareness of when and how to apply phonological repair strategies. Dean, Howell, and colleagues went on to develop *Metaphon*, an approach that centres on dialogue between therapist and child with only passing references to parents. We wanted to take these ideas in a new direction, actively engaging parents, still with the aim of increasing children's metaphonological awareness, and their capacity to reflect on their own speech performance.

Excited by the practical connections between Ingram's (1976) schema of underlying representation, surface form and mapping rules, and the Dean and Howell (1986) suggestions for developing linguistic awareness, it struck us that, if they were only implemented for a short period in weekly therapy sessions, their effects might not be optimal. Our plan was to provide parents with training, scripts, and informational handouts (later to become Bowen 1998a, and in French, Bowen 2007). We reasoned that if *child*, and *clinician* and *parents*, and *teachers* where applicable, used a common language around sound and syllable properties, and the reasons for, and the communicative consequences of homophony, it would improve the accuracy of that child's knowledge of the system of phonemic contrasts and increase the likelihood of spontaneous self-corrections. This would be especially the case if *all* the adults involved (not just the SLP/SLT) knew how to reinforce them. Metalinguistic Training fosters 'phonological discoveries' by the child. His/Her capacity to *perceive*, *talk about*, *reflect upon*, and *revise and repair* homophonous productions is enhanced via simple routines and systematic feedback delivered by parents.

Methods

Using guided discussion (Dean and Howell 1986), child, parents, and clinician talk and think about the properties of the speech sound system and how it is organised to convey meaning, incorporating simple metaphonological and phonological awareness (Hesketh, A22) activities. In finding a common language to describe phonemic features and syllable shapes, the clinician can borrow from many sources, including Klein's (1996a, b) 'imagery terms' or 'imagery labels' (e.g., poppy, windy, throatie, and tippy, discussed in Chapter 4); the *Metaphon* (Dean, Howell, Hill, et al. 1990) terms such as long, short, front, back, noisy, growly, whisper, and quiet; and the imagery names and cues in Table 6.5 (p. 242).

Activities, at home and in therapy, involve sound picture associations (e.g., /ɹ/ is a roaring lion sound; /tʃ/ is a choo-choo train; /f/ is a bunny rabbit sound, because it is made with teeth like a bunny); phoneme segmentation for onset matching (e.g., kangaroo starts with /kə/); awareness of rhymes and sound patterns (e.g., games with minimal pairs like *tie-die*; and near minimal pairs like *tie-tight*); rudimentary knowledge of the concept of 'word'; understanding the idea of words and longer utterances 'making sense'; awareness of the use of revision and repair strategies using 'judgement of correctness' games (e.g., *The boy tore his shirt* vs. *The boy tore his cert*) and the 'fixed-up-one routine'; and playing with morphophonological structures to produce lexical and grammatical innovations (e.g., *pick* vs. *picks*).

The use of spontaneous revisions and repairs is fostered, particularly at home, by use of the fixed-up-one routine. The routine is a metalinguistic technique that allows adults to talk simply to children about revisions and repairs. Scripts, such as the one displayed in Figure 9.4, are provided to introduce them to the technique, and various versions of it are available (http://www.speech-language-therapy.com/tx-self-corrections.html) with an instructional slideshow (http://www.speech-language-therapy.com/shows.html). Also with regard to self-monitoring and making revisions and repairs, the child is encouraged to *notice* phoneme collapses or homonymy (e.g., *boo* and *blue* realised homophonously as /bu/).

Discussion

The 1986 suggestions of Dean and Howell were adopted and extended, allowing metalinguistic awareness to be targeted in naturalistic, supportive clinic *and home* settings. Expressions that crop up constantly in the context of PACT being discussed with parents are 'talking task', 'listening task', 'thinking task', 'fixed-up-ones', 'word', 'rhyme', 'making sense', 'two-step word', and 'remember the 50:50 split'. The latter refers to the general recommendation that the 50:50 split between 'talking tasks' vs. 'thinking and listening tasks' that is observed in therapy sessions is also observed at home.

Sometimes a family will generate its own appropriate terminology, and memorable offerings have included 'Bob', 'Bobs', and 'fix-its' in relation to 'fixed-up-ones' (Bob the Builder's motto is 'Can we fix it? Yes we can') and 'Einstein' and 'Einstein Time' in relation to listening and thinking tasks! 'Einstein Time' and 'Nice one, Einstein!' were the brainchild of Sebastian's father, who was intrigued by the author's framed picture of Einstein, adorned with a thinks bubble that read 'THINKING'. The picture is sometimes put on the table during 'thinking tasks', such as judgment of correctness games, silent sorting of word-pairs, 'point to the one I say' activities, and word classification games, to cue everyone that 'thinking' is supposed to be happening!

3. Phonetic production training

Rationale

'Phonological disorders arise more in the mind than in the mouth', according to Grunwell (1987), and phonological therapy is, by definition, linguistic, meaning-based, focussed

The 'fixed-up-one routine' for the velar-alveolar contrast

car	key
1) Say to your child, "Listen to this. If I accidentally said 'tar' when I wanted to say 'car' it wouldn't sound right. I would have to fix it up and say 'car' wouldn't I? Did you hear that fixed-up-one? I said 'tar' then I fixed it up and said 'car'".	**2)** Say to your child, "Listen. If I said 'tee' it wouldn't sound right. I would have to fix it up and say 'key'".
girl	goat
3) "If I said 'dirl' instead of 'girl' I would have to do a fixed-up-one again. I would have to <u>think</u> to myself not 'dirl' its 'girl'. Did you hear that fixed-up-one?"	**4)** "'Hairy doat' isn't right is it? I need to do a fixed-up-one and say 'hairy goat'".
corn	cup
5) "What would I have to do if I accidentally said 'torn' for this one? I would have to do a ..." [fixed-up-one]	**6)** Would I have to do a fixed-up-one if I said 'tup' for this one?"

Self-corrections for the velar stop consonants 'k' and 'g'
Adults continually make little mistakes when they speak. They barely notice these mistakes at a conscious level, and quickly correct themselves, and go on with what they are saying. This process of noticing speech mistakes and correcting them as we go is called making revisions and repairs, or self-corrections. Many children with speech sound difficulties are not good at self-correcting. They find it difficult to monitor their speech (i.e., they find it hard to listen to it critically) and make corrections.

At home this week, introduce the idea of a 'fixed-up-one' (make up your own term for this if you like), or the process of noticing speech mistakes and then saying the word(s) again more clearly, specifically in relation to the stop consonants 'k' and 'g'. Go through the six-step routine shown above two or three times, and talk about fixed-up-ones. Have some fun making up other 'mistakes' with 'k' and 'g' words, that need <u>thinking about</u> and <u>correcting</u>.

Find more speech games and ideas for parents and their children at
www.speech-language-therapy.com/tx-self-corrections.html

Figure 9.4 An example of the Fixed-up-One Routine. Drawing by Helen Rippon, Speech and Language Therapist www.blacksheeppress.co.uk

on activating a child's underlying system for phoneme use, and 'in the mind'. But, having said that, some children with phonological disorder need help at the phonemic level *and* the phonetic level. In other words, they must be taught to make the sounds and structures.

Methods

Phonetic production training is integrated with metalinguistic training and multiple exemplar training. It uses stimulability techniques (Miccio 2005; Bleile 2004, 2006) and sound elicitation and phonemic placement procedures (Secord, Boyce, Donohue, et al. 2007) wherein the therapist teaches a child to generate absent or distorted phones *beyond* isolated sound level, or failing that, to produce approximations of consonants in the same sound class in CV (onset) and VC (coda) combinations. Homework for phonetic targets includes listening and production, observing the 50:50 split.

Discussion

It is rarely necessary to train intervocalic (SIWW or SFWW) stimulability or to train all vowel and diphthong contexts. For instance, having taught /tʃu/ and /utʃ/, one seldom has to teach /tʃu tʃi tʃɔ tʃaɪ tʃoʊ tʃeɪ tʃa/ and /utʃ itʃ ɔtʃ aɪtʃ oʊtʃ eɪtʃ atʃ/, etc. Children usually proceed from syllable to word level, having demonstrated the capacity to produce the phone in CV and/or VC contexts. Introductory stimulability or pre-practice tasks may be at individual sound (segment) and 'nonsense syllable' level, even involving 'syllable drill', but not for long. Once a child is stimulable for a target, or is producing a passable approximation, or a phone in the same sound class, in syllables or words, therapy moves onto the phonemic level and all activities are 'meaning based' at word level and beyond (Bowen and Cupples 2006). The child does production practice of a few target words, usually no more than six. It is important to know that 'phonetic production training' does not imply traditional articulation therapy (Van Riper 1978) or adaptations of it (e.g., Raz, A4).

4. Multiple exemplar training

Rationale

Focused auditory input and the heightened perceptual saliency of phones, structures, and contrasts, provided by the therapy activities, increases the learnability of new sounds, syllable structures, and word contrasts.

Methods

Multiple exemplar training has two overlapping aspects: auditory input and minimal contrasts (minimal pairs) therapy. Auditory input involves listening lists, alliterative input, and thematic play; and minimal contrasts therapy uses minimal, maximal, or multiple oppositions between words. Listening lists comprise word lists of up to 15 words with a common phonetic feature (e.g., *sail, seat, sigh, sew, seed, sum, sack, sun, sand, sea, sock, soup, silly, seal, saw, soap*) or up to seven word pairs (e.g., *sock-shock, sour-shower; sack-shack, sip-ship, sell-shell, Sue-shoe, save-shave*) or triplets (e.g., *seat-sheet-cheat, sigh-shy-chai, sip-ship-chip, sore-shore-chore, Sue-shoe-chew*) or target, error, and 'foil' (e.g., *pie-bye-boo, pig-big-boo, Paul-ball-boo, pin-bin-boo, pug-bug-boo, pat-bat-boo, poi-boy-boo*) to the child. Foils are introduced to make some sequences more rhythmical and fun, and more enticing for the child to dance, jog, march, or bop to. Sometimes the words are pictured and sometimes not (see http://www.speech-language-therapy.com/txresources.html). Alliterative input can be provided via stories, songs, rhymes, games, and worksheets, such as one for /k/ SIWI depicting a *cat*: in a *cupboard*, with a *kite*, in a *coat*, in a *corner*, in a *kennel*, being *carried*, behind a *curtain*, and in a *cap*.

Thematic play or auditory input therapy (Lancaster, A20) involves playing games and reading books to the child that give rise to frequent repetitions of targets. Bowen (in press) describes an activity for 'Bruno', 4;2, who was learning /f/ SFWF. In one therapy session, and for a week in homework, he listened to the story of Jeff and Steph and the scarf (shown in Figure 6.1, p. 248). In related homework, Bruno played minimal contrast games using the work sheet illustrated in Figure 9.5. At intervals, outside of formal homework, Bruno played a game with his father where a superhero jumped off a roof, and he played with Smurf figurines with both parents. In fact, he took the Smurfs almost everywhere, constantly pretending to be a Smurf; and, for a period, Smurfs became his main conversational topic (briefly supplanting Thomas the Tank Engine)—*exactly* what was needed to provide intense and interesting (to him) input for final /f/.

In minimal contrasts therapy, a child sorts, with as much help as is required, words pictured and captioned on cards according to their sound properties, in sessions and for homework, and engages in homophony confrontation tasks (in sessions but not for homework), such as the ones below.

1. **'Point to the one I say.'**
   Child points to pictures of the words, spoken by the adult in random order (e.g., sheet, sip, sell, ship, shell, seat) or rhyming order (e.g.: seat-sheet, sip-ship, sell-shell).
2. **'Put the rhyming words with these words.'**
   Three to nine cards are presented (e.g., pin, pea, pack, pole), and the child puts rhyming cards beside them (bin, bee, back, bowl).
3. **'Say the word that rhymes with the one I say.'**
   Adult says words with the target phoneme; child says rhyming non-target words (adult: 'floor'; child: 'four'; adult: 'flake'; child: 'fake'), with the child saying carefully selected words that he/she can already say.
4. **'Give me the word that rhymes with the one I say.'**
   Adult says the non-target word, and the child selects the rhyming word containing the target sound. For example, in working on velar fronting: Adult says 'tea'; Child selects a picture of 'key'. Adult says 'tool'; Child selects a picture of 'cool'. Adult says 'tape'; Child selects a picture of 'cape'.
5. **'Tell me the one to give you.'**
   This is a homophony confrontation game, and it is the only task that it not included in homework. It needs a skilled, light touch and can easily go wrong, especially if the child is pushed too hard. In a game context, the adult responds to the word

Rhyming Pairs /f/ SFWF

laugh	scarf	off	cough
Jeff	Steph	wife	knife
half	calf	laugh scarf off cough Jeff Steph wife knife calf half	scarf laugh cough off Steph Jeff knife wife half calf

/f/ vs. /p/ SFWF

cough	cop	Steph	step
wife	wipe	cuff	cup
sniff	snip	cough cop Steph step wife wipe cuff cup sniff snip	cop cough step Steph wipe wife cup cuff snip sniff

Final /f/ vs. no final consonant

la	laugh	Y	wife
Lee	leaf	low	loaf
scar	scarf	la laugh Y wife Lee leaf low loaf scar scarf	laugh la wife Y leaf Lee loaf low scarf scar

Figure 9.5 Minimal pair and near minimal pair sets. Drawing by Helen Rippon, Speech and Language Therapist www.backsheeppress.co.uk

actually said (e.g., Child says [tɪn] for 'chin' and is handed 'tin'). The aim is for the child to recognise communicative failure and attempt a revised production.

6. **'You be the teacher: tell me if I say these words the right way or the wrong way.'**
   Adult says individual words or phrases, and the child judges whether they have been said correctly; for example, puddy tat vs. pussy cat. The child judges: right/wrong; yes/no; silly/OK.

7. **'Silly Sentences'**
   The child judges whether or not a sentence is a 'silly one'; for example, One-two buckle my doo vs. One-two buckle my shoe; Mary had a little lamb vs. Mary had a whittle wham.

8. **'Silly Dinners'**
   Adult says what he/she wants for dinner, and the child judges whether it is a 'silly dinner': I want jelly/deli; I want fish and chips/ships; I want green peas/bees; I want a cup of coffee/toffee. With activities 6, 7, and 8, it is important to explain clearly to parents that the child does not have to 'correct you'.

9. **'Shake-ups and Match-ups'**
   The child is shown four pictures, for example, tie-time, two-toot. The pairs are said to the child rhythmically several times. Cards are 'shaken up' in a container and tipped out. The child then arranges them, with help if necessary, 'the same as they were before' (i.e., in near minimal pairs).

10. **'Find the two-step words.'**
    With adult assistance, the child sorts pictured near minimal pair words with consonant clusters SIWI or SFWF from contrasting words with singleton consonants SIWI or SFWF (e.g., feet-fleet, fat-flat, fake-flake).

11. **'Walk when you hear the 2-steps.'**
    Child 'finger-walks' two steps (to a destination) upon hearing a consonant cluster SIWI as opposed to a singleton SIWI (e.g., the child 'walks' for 'true', but not 'two' or 'roo').

Discussion

Suggestions for multiple exemplar activities 1–11 above are provided to parents. It should be noted, however, that, for many families, the suggestions actually trigger their creativity and they come up with innovative and appropriate games, activities, and books that are perfect for their child (and inspiring for the clinician).

5. Homework

Rationale

Homework administered by a parent or parents provides children with practice, reinforcement, opportunities to generalise, and opportunities for discovery. It allows families to hone, generalise, and enjoy the 'teaching skills' learned in therapy sessions. By engaging in activities autonomously, families are free to experiment, creating new opportunities for learning in natural, functional contexts. As their knowledge, skills, and confidence grow, most will innovate, making up new games and fun routines, and some even instigate apposite 'next steps' in therapy. Because homework suggestions are not rigid, homework is conducive to internal development and families can shape it to fit their interests, preferences, and culture. Homework can assume the family 'stamp' as well as the clinician's 'style', influencing the form, content, and conduct of sessions in dynamic and attention-grabbing ways, letting the adults concerned create activities a child genuinely likes and is responsive to.

Methods

Homework comprises short bursts of formal home activities and the use of appropriate speech stimulation techniques (e.g., modelling corrections) when opportune. Homework comprises activities from the most recent session, delivered in 5- to 7-minute bursts once, twice, or three times daily, one-to-one with an adult in good listening conditions. Examples of 'good' and 'poor' listening conditions are discussed. Practices can be as little as 10 minutes apart (e.g., practice-story-practice-story-practice-story; practice-craft-practice-craft-practice-craft, with the 50:50 split observed between listening–thinking tasks vs. talking tasks. Parents are encouraged to make the homework regular, brief, naturalistic, encouraging, and fun. Instructions and activities go in a homework book and are explained as often as required. If, for some reason, homework does not happen for a day or days, parents are asked not to 'compensate' by doing more than three practices subsequently. It is suggested that they combine homework with activities the child likes, such as colouring and cutting, story reading, or going to a park or favourite spot sometimes to do it.

Discussion

If one family member (e.g., the father in Iain's case) usually accompanies the child and participates in therapy sessions, other family members (e.g., mother and grandparents) can learn from their example during homework sessions and by watching their application of modelling, recasting, and other techniques. The system will fall down if one parent does 'the bringing' to therapy and the other parent does *only* the formal homework without good communication between the two, as sometimes happens.

Case study

Background

'Josie' attended a rural New South Wales Community Health Speech Pathology clinic with her mother six times between the ages of 5;2 and 5;5 for an assessment and five 'language stimulation group' sessions conducted by a locum SLP because she was a late talker and her speech was unintelligible. At 5;11, she was referred back to Community Health by a school nurse, attending an intake clinic with her father 'David' for a speech assessment only. In a 20-minute session, an 88-word, 3-position screener called the *Articulation Survey* was administered by a second SLP who diagnosed Developmental Verbal Dyspraxia (DVD) and added Josie to a therapy waiting list. She had normal audiograms at 6;1 and 6;7.

Referral

Six months after diagnosis, Josie was referred to the author by a District School Counsellor (Educational Psychologist). Referral was prompted by Josie's teacher, concerned about her language development, disinterest in and difficulty with pre-reading and phonological awareness activities, and her air of unhappiness at school.

Initial presentation

Bright, bubbly, and co-operative, Josie, 6;5, presented for initial consultation towards the end of her first year of school (Kindergarten in NSW). The first session involved taking a history and administering a CELF-P requested by school personnel. Josie performed in the mid-average range: Receptive Language Score 103, Expressive Language Score 100, and Total Language Score 101. Apart from late language acquisition, poor intelligibility, and a maternal family history of speech and literacy difficulties, Josie's history was unremarkable. The conversational speech sample excerpt and the *Quick Screener* data displayed in Figures 9.6 and 9.7, respectively, were gathered at 6;6 in the second session (4 weeks after the first), and the analysis displayed in Figure 9.8 was done while her parents watched. At 6;6, her mother 'Maureen' and half-sister 'Emma' assigned Josie an intelligibility rating of (2) mostly intelligible. The author gave her (3) somewhat intelligible; and David and her teacher gave her ratings of (4) mostly unintelligible.

Screening Process

Steps 1–4 were performed during the session, and Steps 5–10 were performed after it.

Single-word sample

1. The first step in this quick screening analysis was to examine the single-word sample (Figure 9.7), tally Josie's consonants correct out of approximately 100 (depending on the dialect of English), and calculate a tentative Percentage of Consonants Correct (PCC; tentative because this is a small, slightly inexact, single-word *screening* sample). With scoring erring on the generous side, her single-word PCC was 30%. Later it was found that both her conversational and imitated PCCs were slightly lower than this at 27%, indicating an unusually severe SSD for a child of 6;6.

2. Using the analysis form (Figure 9.8), phonological processes with their percentages of occurrence and other obvious errors were noted as follows: velar fronting 25% SI and SF; prevocalic voicing 57%; gliding of liquids 100%; final consonant deletion 66%; stopping of fricatives 25% SI; stopping of affricates 100% SF; and cluster reduction 100% SI and SF. Gliding of fricatives and affricates SI was prevalent, as was deletion of fricatives WF, glottal replacement, and /n/ dentalised, interdental, or produced /n^d/.

3. Counting each vowel and diphthong as one vowel, her vowels correct out of 47 were tallied and a tentative Percentage of Vowels Correct (PVC) calculated. With vowel errors in twelve words (fish, kiss, bridge, wing, leaf; foot; van, crab, splash;

Josie: eː ə jʌn̪ᵈ ʌn̪ᵈ muːn ɒuːn wʌn̪ᵈ daɪd
There's a sun   and   moon   on   one   side

ʌn̪ᵈ θə daɪ ɔn̪ᵈ θi ʌdə daɪd wɪʔ ə bweɪndoʊ ‖
and   the sky on the other side with a rainbow.

θə hæʊdɔ ɪd bwakʌm ɒʔ
The handle is broken off,

doʊ jʌ ki jɔ pʰʌn̪ᵈ ɪn ɪt dɔn̪ᵈ jʌ ‖
so   you keep your pens in it, don't you?

weː dɪd θʌʔ kʰʌ kʌm θoʊm eːbwə ‖
Where did the cup come from, ever?

Caroline: My friend Anna gave it to me.

Josie: wəd ɪʔ jɔ bɜθdeɪ ‖
Was   it   your   birthday?

Caroline: No, it was just for a present.

Josie: weː ju daʔ wen θə hæju pʰʌw ɒʔ ‖
Were you sad when the handle fell off?

Caroline: Actually, it didn't have a handle when she gave it to me.

Josie: jɔ ban̪ᵈ geɪ ju ə kʰʌ wɪʔ noʊ hæʊdɔ ‖
Your friend   gave you a cup with no handle.

aɪ miːn jaɪ hæjoʊ ‖
I   mean, like hello!

ʃi wədʔ ə bwi gʊᵈ judə ‖
She wasn't a very good chooser.

Caroline: Do you like it?

Josie: jet ɪtᵈ weːdi bwədi ‖
Yes.   It's   really   pretty.

Caroline: I like it too, even though it has no handle.

Josie: bʌʔ ɪʔ wə bi betə wɪʔ ə hæʊdoʊ ‖
But   it   would be better with a handle.

Figure 9.6 An excerpt from Josie's conversational speech sample at 6;6

#	TARGET	TRANSCRIPTION		CC	#	TARGET	TRANSCRIPTION		CC
1	cup	ʌ	kʰʌ	1	23	jam	æ	jiæm	1
2	gone	ɒ	kʰɒn	1	24	house	aʊ	hæʊ	1
3	knife	aɪ	naɪ	1	25	path	a	pʰa	1
4	sharp	a	wja:		26	door	ɔ	dɔ	1
5	fish	ɪ	de		27	smoke	oʊ	moʊ	1
6	kiss	ɪ	de		28	bridge	ɪ	mweʔ	
7	sock	ɒ	wj:ɒk	1	29	train	eɪ	ɹeɪ n	2
8	glass	a	wja		30	chair	ɛə	jɛə	
9	watch	ɒ	bwɒʔ	1	31	red	e	wje:	
10	nose	oʊ	noʊ	1	32	spoon	u	bun	1
11	mouth	au	mau	1	33	plane	eɪ	veɪ	
12	yawn	ɔ	jɔn	2	34	fly	aɪ	fnaɪ	
13	leaf	i	wjəi		35	sky	aɪ	fnaɪ	
14	thumb	ʌ	θʌn̪d	1	36	sun	ʌ	jʌn̪d	1
15	foot	ʊ	bɒʔ		37	wing	ɪ	weɪ n	1
16	toe	oʊ	tʰoʊ	1	38	splash	æ	bwʌʃ	1
17	snake	eɪ	fneɪʔ	1	39	tent	e	denʔt	2
18	van	æ	bweɪn	1	40	salt	ɒ	jɒut	1
19	fast	a	bʰa		41	crab	æ	mbwa	
20	girl	ɜ	gwɜʊ	1	42	sweet	i	bwiʔ	1
21	stairs	eə	dʰe		43	sleeve	i	bwiʔ	
22	big	ɪ	bɪ	1	44	zipper	ɪ	wɪbə	
boy bɔɪ ear ɪə			SUBTOTAL CC:	15				TOTAL CC:	30

Figure 9.7 Josie's initial Quick Screener data at 6;6

house, stairs, and ear), her PVC was about 74% (35/47). Her productions of girl and salt were not factored in because they were dialectal.

Single word *and* conversational speech sample

4. Referring to the single-word (SW) and conversational speech (CS) sample, the vowels and consonants present were listed to record Josie's vowel and consonant inventories.
5. The marked consonants present in her SW and CS samples were circled on the form. Her marked consonants were /p t k f θ/, with /v/ and /ʃ/ considered marginal because they occurred infrequently and neither were present in both samples.
6. Any vowel and/or consonant inventory constraints were noted. Her SW consonant constraints were /ŋ ð s z tʃ dʒ l/, and her CS constraints were /ŋ v ð s z ʒ tʃ dʒ l ɹ/. There were no vowel inventory constraints, and one missing diphthong /ɪə/.

Velar fronting 25% SI 25% SF

#	Target SI	0 / 1	#	Target SF	0 / 1
1	cup	0	7	sock	0
6	kiss	1	17	snake	0
2	gone	0	22	big	0
20	girl	0	37	wing	1
	TOTAL	1/4		TOTAL	1/4

Palato-alveolar fronting

#	Target SI	0 / 1	#	Target SF	0 / 1
4	sharp	0	5	fish	0
30	chair	0	9	watch	0
23	jam	0	28	bridge	0
	TOTAL	/3		TOTAL	/3

Word-final devoicing

#	Target	0 / 1	#	Target	0 / 1
41	crab	0	43	sleeve	0
31	red	0	10	nose	0
22	big	0	28	bridge	0
				TOTAL	/6

Backing

#	Target SI	0 / 1	#	Target SF	0 / 1
16	toe	0	15	foot	0
39	tent	0	42	sweet	0
26	door	0	31	red	0
	TOTAL	/3		TOTAL	/3

Stopping of fricative 25% SI

#	Target SI	0 / 1	#	Target SF	0 / 1
5	fish	0	13	leaf	0
15	foot	1	11	mouth	0
14	thumb	0	6	kiss	0
7	sock	0	38	splash	0
36	sun	0	43	sleeve	0
4	sharp	0	10	nose	0
18	van	1			
44	zip(per)	0			
	TOTAL	2/8		TOTAL	/6

Stopping of affricates   100% SF

#	Target SI	0 / 1	#	Target SF	0 / 1
30	chair	0	9	watch	1
23	jam	0	28	bridge	1
	TOTAL	/2		TOTAL	2/2

Pre-vocalic voicing 57%

#	Target	0 / 1	#	Target	0 / 1
25	path	0	5	fish	1
16	toe	0	14	thumb	0
6	kiss	1	36	sun	1
			4	sharp	1
				TOTAL	4 /7

Liquid/glide simplification gliding 100%

#	Target	0 / 1	#	Target	0 / 1
9	watch	0	12	yawn	0
13	leaf	1	31	red	1
				TOTAL	/4

Initial consonant deletion

#	Target	0 / 1	#	Target	0 / 1
3	knife	0	7	sock	0
22	big	0	30	chair	0
18	van	0	12	yawn	0
				TOTAL	/6

Final consonant deletion 66%

#	Target SI	0 / 1	#	Target SF	0 / 1
23	jam	0	10	nose	1
44	zip	0	5	fish	1
31	red	1	28	bridge	1
				TOTAL	4/6

Initial cluster reduction 100% SI

#	Target SI	0 / 1	#	Target SI	0 / 1
33	plane	1	43	sleeve	1
8	glass	1	27	smoke	1
28	bridge	1	17	snake	1
29	train	1	32	spoon	1
41	crab	1	21	stairs	1
34	fly	1	35	sky	1
42	sweet	1	38	splash	1
				TOTAL	14 /14

Final cluster reduction 100%

#	Target	0 / 1	#	Target	0 / 1
19	fast	1	40	salt	1
39	tent	1			
				TOTAL	3/3

Figure 9.8 Josie's initial Quick Screener analysis at 6;6

7. Phonotactic combinations were recorded to assess Josie's syllable/word shape inventory. She only produced one- and two-syllable combinations, and her inventory was C, V, CV, VC, CVC, CCV, CCVC, CCCV, CVCV, CCVCC, and CCVCVC.

8. Idiosyncratic or unusual features were noted as dentalised alveolars, glottal replacement, gliding of fricatives and affricates, vowel and diphthong errors, schwa

insertion, final consonant deletion, and no words beyond two syllables in the CS sample.

9. The data were perused for chronological mismatch, and one example was found in her correct production of /θ/ as in 'birthday' in all obligatory contexts.

10. The syllable stress inventory (assuming typical stress patterns) was recorded as S = strong and W = weak. The SW words she produced in the CS excerpt were representative of the entire CS sample (zipper, better, other, handle, birthday, rainbow, broken, chooser, really, and pretty). There were no other word stress patterns apart from one WS in 'hello' when mimicking Emma's 'cool' production with strong emphasis on the second syllable.

11. Extensive homonymy was evident (e.g., *where*, *were*, and *red* were produced identically).

12. Her contrastive phones (phonemes) were /n m w j p b t d/, and it was interesting to see that /n m w j p b d/ were in the Early 8 and /t/ was in the Middle 8 with no Late 8 consonants functioning as phonemes. Her non-contrastive phones were /h g k f ɹ ʃ θ/.

13. Subsequent administration of the Locke Task showed that she could not reliably discriminate between the liquid /l/ from the glide /j/ or the liquid /ɹ/.

14. Subsequent administration of the DEAP inconsistency assessment revealed consistent production with only two items, *helicopter* and *vacuum cleaner*, produced inconsistently.

From this screening (1–12 above) and her performance during language testing 1 month before, it was evident that Josie had a severe phonological disorder with phonemic, perceptual, and phonetic issues, and CAS was ruled out. Parental permission was obtained to share these data, including videos of therapy, for teaching purposes. Permission to show the videos was later withdrawn.

Josie's family

The family were eager to be involved in therapy, especially if it meant the number of sessions could be reduced. They were drought affected and on a tight budget, residing 100 km (62 miles) over difficult terrain from the clinician's practice. Josie's household comprised her father (David, 52); mother (Maureen, 38); half sister (Emma 15), who was home-schooled by Maureen and David and who was Maureen's child; and her twin brother and sister ('Jasper' and 'Ruby', 4;2). David had two sons ('Ben', 16, and 'Aaron', 14) living overseas with their mother ('Rebekah', 54). Maureen was not in paid employment, and David sent regular child support payments and school fees to Rebekah. The family was cheerful and close-knit, spending much time together and with a wide circle of friends, especially around sport, local government, community, and outdoor activities. Emma assumed a 'mothering' role with Josie, Jasper, and Ruby. David volunteered that he was 'Type A', 'a news junkie', and 'obsessed with finances and the price of petrol'. No one disagreed.

There was a maternal family history of speech and literacy issues, and Maureen and Emma (described as 'learning disabled' by the school psychologist who referred Josie) were poor readers and spellers. Ruby was a late talker and unintelligible and waiting for

SLP assessment at Community Health. Ben, Aaron, and Jasper were reported to have 'excellent communication skills' (like David). Maureen was a calm, competent person who had completed 4 years of high school, 2 years of a hairdressing apprenticeship, and a Child Care Certificate at an Institute of Technical and Further Education (TAFE). She was employed as a preschool assistant prior to Josie's birth. She did not drive a car due to epilepsy. David had a law degree and a master's degree in business administration and was engaged in a new venture as proprietor of a specialist book publishing company, working from home on the family farm.

Therapy planning for Josie

Although (marked) /ʃ/ appeared in Josie's CS output, she was not stimulable for it in the true sense. The (marked) affricates /tʃ/ and /dʒ/ and the (marked) fricatives /s/ and /z/ were never present in output and were also non-stimulable; so consonant inventory expansion was a priority. First, /tʃ/ was selected for stimulability training. The reasoning behind this was that there is evidence to suggest that targeting the marked voiceless affricate consonant might: (1) evoke the emergence of *unmarked* consonants, and (2) promote generalisation to /dʒ/. A second marked consonant, /s/, was selected for stimulability training because it might help promote cluster development and generalise to /z/ and other fricatives and unmarked features. Consideration was given to targeting the later developing and marked /ð/, but this idea was rejected. Because Josie already had the voiceless cognate /θ/ in her repertoire, it was felt that working on /ð/ might not have as much impact on her overall system as /s/. On the other hand, late-developing, non-stimulable, unmarked /l/ looked like a good candidate for therapy, especially since the Locke Task revealed that Josie could not reliably discriminate the liquid /l/ from the glide /j/. In hindsight, it *might* have been more fruitful to target /ɹ/ early on. Thinking about /l/ led naturally to deciding about her clusters. Clearly, with 100% cluster reduction in her SW sample, and only /bw/ SIWI in her CS sample, clusters were a high priority. It was decided that targeting /l/ clusters was not the best option for her. Rather, targeting the adjuncts /st/, /sp/, and /sk/, although it might not stimulate generalisation to other clusters, might give her the 'idea' of producing clusters and help in adding the singletons /s/ and subsequently /z/ to her repertoire (via generalisation) and possibly even the voiced dental fricative /ð/. In hindsight, this was *not* the smartest move, and /l/ clusters might have been the better targets. Because of family finances and the high cost of petrol, it was decided to spread the therapy as much as was practical, with David eagerly committing to being 'very hands on'.

Agent, scheduling, and dosage

David and Maureen were 'stuck' when it came to choosing an SLP for their daughter. They had virtually no choice with the closest SLP almost 2 hours' drive away over unsealed and mountain roads, entailing heavy petrol consumption over the round trip. They certainly did not have the luxury of questioning whether the author would be the 'best' therapist for them, whether they wanted to 'go privately', or whether the assessment administered would lead to service delivery that would fit easily with their busy family life. They did, however, consider whether the intervention offered was 'scientific' and whether the therapist was properly credentialed and experienced, with David asking searching questions.

Their main consideration in proceeding was to minimise and 'budget' the number of appointments. In the event, Josie was seen 15 times over 12.5 face-to-face hours, spread over almost 12 months, with the support of a homework program conscientiously administered by her parents and teenage sister. The dosage and scheduling described for Josie was mainly the result of the parents' wishes, influenced by the therapist's suggestions on how appointments could be best deployed. Aware of this, and powerless to do anything about it, they would ask periodically whether the spread-out appointment schedule might adversely affect Josie's progress, thereby pinpointing a knowledge gap. Little is known about the effects of service delivery: in terms of the primary *agent* of therapy, appropriate *dosage*, and optimal *scheduling*, and how they relate to outcomes. This is a knowledge gap that concerns Barbara Dodd, and she discusses it in A43.

The question itself came from Australian SLP Lauren Osborne who graduated from the University of Sydney, and began working in a community setting with paediatric clients in 2006. Her clinical interests include working with culturally and linguistically diverse populations, children with phonological impairment, and preschool-aged children with language impairment. The major challenge she faced in her first year in the workforce was the lengthy waiting list at her workplace, and trying to make the most of the limited number of therapy sessions available to each client. For her, the most rewarding aspects of being an SLP are seeing parents and teachers understand that they have an important role in helping children with speech and language impairments and seeing children's speech and language skills improve.

Dr. Barbara Dodd is a research professor at the Perinatal Research Centre, University of Queensland, Australia, and in the Department of Language and Communication Sciences, City University, London, UK. Her research interests include children's changing speech and language abilities in the areas of listening, speaking, and thinking; the need for differential diagnosis of different types of SSD and the links between diagnosis and intervention approach; the evaluation of the types of research evidence available on intervention approaches; and issues in SLP/SLT service delivery. The author of a key reference book (Dodd 2005) and the classification system for phonological disorder and CAS discussed in Chapter 2, she is widely published in the peer reviewed literature and is lead author of the *Diagnostic Evaluation of Articulation and Phonology (DEAP)* (Dodd, Crosbie, Holm, et al. 2002).

Q43. Barbara Dodd: Determining duration and frequency of therapy

There was silence from several thousand participants when Lauren Osborne posted a message (http://health.groups.yahoo.com/group/phonologicaltherapy/message/12449) to the phonologicaltherapy list in 2007:

I'm doing a Quality Improvement Project at work at the moment, based around how we are managing waiting list times. One of the questions which came up (from a non-SLP colleague) was, 'Do you know how much therapy these children need?' I honestly didn't know, but promised to look it up! I've managed to find a few articles, but I'm not finding it easy! At this stage I'm wondering if there is a lack of research into the area, or if it's that my searching strategy is lacking something. I was hoping someone out there would be able to help! I'm basically interested in how much therapy is needed to successfully treat/manage communication difficulties/disorders (speech-based, and others) in children. When I say how much - I'm thinking both in number/length of sessions, and length of time (weeks/months/years etc). If anyone can point me in the right direction, I'd appreciate it!

How would you tackle this important and frequently asked question?

A43.   Barbara Dodd: Finding the correct dose of intervention for developmental speech impairment

The effect of service delivery on intervention outcome has recently been recognised as a huge gap in the knowledge base of SLP (Kamhi 2006b). For example, Alex Johnson, the 2006 president of ASHA, identified the dearth of information on service delivery as a challenge for professional practice (Uffen 2006). One reason why lack of knowledge about service delivery has become an issue is the current emphasis on evidence-based practice. Evidence-based practice requires in-depth understanding of the effects of a range of service delivery factors: dosage; scheduling (e.g., weekly vs. twice weekly); agent of therapy; group vs. individual vs. consultative models; age at which specific types of intervention will be most cost-effective for specific impairments; and where intervention should best occur (e.g., classroom or clinic). As illustrated by Josie's case, there is also the problem of what type of service delivery is most appropriate when SLP services are difficult to access.

In response to the question posed, a brief summary of the available research literature on dosage and scheduling is presented. There are, however, three major problems.

Effect of type of speech impairment and population

Studies usually focus on specific client groups. The findings made for that client group may not hold for other types of communication impairments or for children from different language learning contexts (e.g., bilingual or socially disadvantaged backgrounds).

Effect of type of intervention content

Studies do not always specify the type of intervention approach used. Different intervention approaches may give rise to different outcomes when service delivery remains constant, and different service delivery may affect the outcome of a specific intervention approach.

Effect of the interaction between aspects of service delivery

Little is known about how service delivery factors interact. For example, dosage and scheduling used in successful group intervention may not result in cost-effective intervention if a child is seen individually or by an agent of therapy. Further, carers' involvement in therapy is likely to affect outcome (Bowen and Cupples 2004).

It seems likely, then, that client group, intervention approach, and type of service delivery interact to affect outcome. Perhaps that is why so few research studies focus on service delivery in SLP. Scheduling service provision that is long-term, occurring over months or years, is more complex than the brief interventions typical of most publicly funded health or education settings. Therapy cannot be measured in the same way, for example, as a pharmaceutical, so dosage cannot necessarily be predetermined. Policy designed to reduce the cost of speech-language intervention by rationing the amount of therapy and encouraging the use of non-professional agents of intervention is likely to have hidden consequences (e.g., children failing to achieve at school). Until the effect on outcome of different types of service delivery is known, however, the profession lacks the evidence to argue the case for more resources for people with communication impairments.

Dosage and scheduling

The amount of intervention provided varies in research reports of therapy efficacy. The six studies included in Law, Garrett, and Nye's (2004) meta-analysis of 'phonological intervention studies' included dosages of 23 hours (Almost and Rosenbaum 1998), 7.5 hours (Lancaster 1991; Shelton, Johnson, Ruscello, et al. 1978), and 6 hours (Glogowska, Roulstone, Enderby, et al. 2000; Munro 1999). One study did not provide information about dosage. The studies used a range of therapeutic approaches (auditory discrimination, minimal pairs, 'table-top activities') and scheduling. They had very different outcomes. Glogowska et al. (2000) reported no benefit of therapy, whereas Lancaster (1991) reported a 45% reduction in error pattern occurrence.

The amount of therapy given in selected research reports in SLP journals (2004–2008) that described studies of intervention for speech difficulties is shown in Table A43.1. Surprisingly few studies were found. The range of dosage was enormous, many studies far exceeding what is typical for many if not most SLP/SLT services. Table A43.1 also gives information about scheduling (i.e., intervals between sessions and length of sessions). Again, there is considerable variation.

It is difficult to compare these studies' outcomes because of differences in the ways in which they are reported. Nevertheless, detail about outcomes for studies using a specific service delivery approach is important for clinicians seeking information about cost-effective intervention. Gierut (2004b) reported an increase of between 28% and 88% in phoneme accuracy that was calculated from children's productions of non-word therapy targets, rather than a standardised test of untreated, real word production. She also reported a mean increase of three phonemes as a measure of generalisation from the same data. In contrast, Broomfield and Dodd (2005) reported an increase of 16% in PCC on a standardised assessment, with a mean increase of four phonemes and seven clusters and suppression of a mean of two error patterns per child. Baker and McLeod's (2004) measure related to suppression of one error pattern. These differences in outcome are striking, particularly given variation in dosage.

A recent paper by Warren, Fey, and Yoder (2007) argued the need for research on effectiveness to specify the intensity of intervention: the *dose* (number of target trials properly given in a session); *dose frequency* (number of sessions per week); and *total duration* (number of weeks) of therapy received. They proposed a cumulative intervention intensity, which is a product of dose × frequency × total duration. The examples given from their current research on language disorder for low-intensity therapy was 60 targets in a 60-minute session once per week for 40 weeks, whereas high-intensity treatment was

Table A43.1 Reports of intervention studies 2004–2008

Article	Population, Age, Intervention	Dosage (hours)	Scheduling
Advances in Speech-Language Pathology/International Journal of Speech-Language Pathology			
Dodd, et al. (2008)	N = 19, 3-6 years, PC	6	1 × wk, 30 m
Crosbie, et al. (2006)	N = 1, 7;0, CV	8	2 × wk, 30 m
American Journal of Speech Language Pathology			
Adler-Brock, et al. (2007)	N = 2; 12/14, ultrasound for /r/	14	? × wk, 60 m
Rvachew (2004)	N = 34, 3;5–4;11, PA + LK + clinician chosen therapy	4 + 10	? × wk, 15+ m 1–2 × wk, 50 m
International Journal of Language and Communication Disorders			
Bernhardt & Major (2005)	N = 19, 6;1–8;5, PA, non-linear	36	3 × wk, 45 m
Pascoe, et al. (2005)	N = 1, 6;5, CVC words	30	2 × wk, 60 m
Crosbie, et al. (2005)	N = 18 4;8–6;5 years, PC, CV	8	2 × wk, 30 m
Denne, et al. (2005)	N = 20 5;0–7;0, group PA	12	1 × wk, 90 m
Moriaty & Gillon (2006)	N = 3, 6;3–7;3, PA, LK	7	3 × wk, 45 m
Hesketh, et al. (2007)	N = 42, 4;0–4;6, group PA	30	2/3 × wk, 30 m
Child Language Teaching and Therapy			
Baker & McLeod (2004)	N = 2, 4 years, PC	10–31	2 × wk, 45 m
Other Journals			
Gierut (2004b)	Overview treatment studies	19	3 × wk, 60 m

Abbreviations: PC, phonological contrast; CV, core vocabulary; PA, phonological awareness; LK, letter knowledge; CVC, consonant-vowel-consonant; wk, week; m, minutes; N, number children; ?, not reported.

60 targets in a 60-minute session 5 times per week for 40 weeks. The total amount of therapy given seems huge in comparison to the dose of therapy generally reported by clinicians in Australia, New Zealand, or the UK.

A randomised control trial of intervention for speech impairment

One example of the dosage typically available in UK speech and language therapy services was provided by Broomfield and Dodd (2004a). They reported a randomised control trial of 320 children with speech impairment who were referred to a Paediatric Speech and Language Therapy Service in the United Kingdom. This study differentially diagnosed subtypes of speech impairment, specified the content of the therapeutic approaches implemented, and described the clinical pathway (including service delivery). Statistical analyses investigated treatment vs. no treatment outcome. In addition, the effect of a number of factors on outcome was reported: dosage, age for cost-effective intervention for specific impairments, case history factors, and co-morbidity with other language disorders.

The study had three groups (see Table A43.2), evaluating the effect of treatment vs. no-treatment and dosage. The type and duration of the intervention offered was determined by the nature and severity of each child's speech disorder. The available intervention programs were: traditional articulation therapy (Van Riper 1963), phonological contrast therapy (Dean, Howell, Waters, et al. 1995), and core vocabulary therapy (Dodd and Bradford 2000). The clinical pathway is shown in Table A43.3. Each intervention program

Table A43.2 Randomised control trial: study design

Treatment Group (TG)	TG1	TG2	TG3
Initial assessment	month 0	month 0	month 0
Phase 1 (1–6 months)	intervention	NO intervention	intervention
Midpoint assessment	month 6	month 6	month 6
Phase 2 (6–12 months)	NO intervention	intervention	intervention
Final assessment	12 months	12 months	12 months

was planned to run for six sessions, usually weekly for 30–45 minutes. Some programs were applicable in both group and individual settings. Groups of up to six children usually attended weekly for 60 minutes, with two staff, one of whom may have been an SLT assistant. The direct therapy time then was 4.5 hours in addition to assessment and diagnostic therapy (usually about 4 hours), as shown in the clinical pathway in Table A43.3.

The major finding was that the mean increase in PCC for all children receiving treatment was 23% ($N = 212$) as compared with 2% ($N = 101$) for children receiving no treatment. Findings for subgroups of speech impairment indicated that the therapy and service delivery approaches chosen were all associated with positive change. The group of children in TG3, who received double the amount of intervention, made significant additional progress but not to the same extent as they had during the first episode of intervention. That is, most progress in speech accuracy was achieved during the first six sessions.

Age of intervention

The data were further analysed to identify the age at which the specific intervention received had the best outcome given the service delivery model chosen. Children with articulation

Table A43.3 Clinical pathway for randomised control trial of speech disorder

Clinical Pathway	Data	Action
Speech assessment	Within normal range 6–12 months delay >12-month delay/disorder	Discharge Put on review Go to next step
Diagnostic therapy and therapy selection	Observation in group sessions focusing on listening, attention, discrimination, concepts	Progress monitored for 2–10 sessions; no progress, go to next step
Differential diagnosis	Articulation disorder Phonological delay Consistent phonological disorder Inconsistent phonological disorder	Articulation disorder Phonological contrast Phonological contrast Core vocabulary
Future therapy	Repeat initial steps, break if therapy focus changes.	
Articulation therapy	If 6+ and targets mastered but not generalised, intensive group.	

disorder did best when treatment was given once they reached seven years. Poorer outcomes were noted for children five years and younger. Children with phonological delay did best when receiving treatment at five years and older. In contrast, the outcome of treatment for consistent phonological disorder was better for children up to four years of age. If treatment was not provided in the preschool years, the severity of their impairment increased. Children with inconsistent phonological disorder made most progress when they were three years of age. The data suggested that the earlier intervention is provided for phonological disorder, the better the outcome, indicating that it may be easier to shape a developing system than one that is well established.

Effect of other factors

Case history factors affecting outcome of intervention included socio-economic status, family history of speech and language disorders, reported behavioural difficulties, and co-morbidity of other language problems. One surprising finding was that children with reported behavioural difficulties had a positive response to intervention. Perhaps their difficult behaviour reflected their frustration with their impaired ability to communicate, motivating their positive response to therapy. Greater severity at referral was related to slower response to intervention, particularly for children with delayed phonological acquisition. Further studies are needed to untangle how population and case history information should influence service delivery, particularly prioritisation for intervention.

Three aspects need to be considered in research to build knowledge of best practice. Accurate and specific differential diagnosis underpins advances in appropriate intervention, which must be delivered using appropriate dosage and scheduling by an appropriately qualified professional agent of intervention. If knowledge about one of these components is deficient, the outcome for the client is likely to be diminished.

Josie's therapy

Intervention commenced in November, and the content of her 15 (out of a possible 17) therapy sessions and brief details are listed in the next section. The reader may download from http://www.speech-language-therapy.com/04mc-therapy-for-josie.htm many of the specific materials used in Josie's intervention.

November to December Age 6;6–6;7: 4 sessions over 4 weeks
Session 1: 40 Minutes
Present: Josie, Maureen, and Emma

1) Stimulability Training (Phonetic Production Training) for /tʃ/ and /s/.
2) Sound-Picture-Symbol associations for all fricatives and affricates.
3) Auditory Discrimination Training for liquid /l/ vs. the glide /j/ in CV words.
4) Auditory Discrimination Training for all fricatives and affricates in CV words.
5) Auditory Bombardment (Focused Auditory Input): /tʃ/ words SIWI (*hat shop chop*, etc).
6) Near Minimal Pairs Games for /st/, /sp/, and /sk/ SIWI vs. /t/, /p/, and /k/ SIWI.

7) Homework: 2–6 above, and Thematic Play for the voiceless affricate /tʃ/ SIWI. Thematic play was around Chinese cooking (with vocabulary like Chinese, China, chopsticks, chicken chow mein, and choy sum), taking advantage of David's being an adventurous cook and the family's interest in Chinese culture and cuisine.

Session 2: 40 Minutes
Present: Josie, Maureen, and Emma

Josie was now stimulable for /tʃ/ SIWI in syllables and CV words *chew, chore, cha-cha-cha*, and with intense concentration could imitate /s/ in isolation.

1) Verbal and visual imagery were introduced for /tʃ/ (the train sound), /dʒ/ (the tired train sound), and /s/ and the glides (/j/ or [ja ta] – the yes sound, and /w/ or [wa wa] – the cry-baby sound). Imagery was emphasised in sound-sorting games in which Josie had to select between glides and affricates (to target her idiosyncratic gliding of affricates and fricatives).
2) Judgement of correctness game chew, chore, cha-cha-cha vs. Sue, saw, sah-sah-sah.
3) Judgement of correctness game chew, chore, cha-cha-cha vs. ewe, your, ya-ya-ya.
4) Auditory Discrimination Training for all fricatives, affricates, and glides. Josie quickly learned to discriminate these, although she still had difficulty discriminating liquids from glides at word level. Emma enjoyed playing these games frequently with Josie.
5) Auditory Bombardment (Focused Auditory Input): /tʃ/ words SIWI and /s/ words SIWI
6) Production practice of 10 /tʃ/ SIWI CV and CVC words.
7) Near minimal pairs games for Final Consonant Deletion.
8) Homework: 4–7 above and practising producing /s/ in isolation.

Session 3: 40 Minutes
Present: Josie and David (40 minutes)

1) Minimal Triplets game with: chew, shoe, sue; chip, ship, sip; chore, shore, sore.
2) Rhyming cloze task: shoe rhymes with ch. . . , Sue rhymes with ch. . . , etc. for /tʃ/ SIWI.
3) Rhyming cloze task: ewe rhymes with ch. . . , woo rhymes with ch. . . , etc. for /tʃ/ SIWI.
4) Increased use of /ʃ/ was noted in conversation. Stimulability for /ʃ/ SI and SF was now present, so 8 production practice words for /ʃ/ WF were provided.
5) Production practice words for /tʃ/ WI were also provided.
6) 'Itchy Archie' was elicited, and Josie was promised a special sticker if she could still say it after the school holidays.
7) Games 4 and 5 from Session 2 were continued, using different words and syllables.
8) Near minimal pairs games for FCD (bee beach, cow couch, A aitch, sir search, pea peach)
9) Homework: 1–3 above.

Session 4: 1 hour, 50 minutes
Present: David, Maureen, and Emma

This was a parent education session without Josie. It included PowerPoint shows on modelling, recasting, and revisions and repairs. Detailed homework instructions for working with Josie in 5- to 7-minute 'bursts', once, twice, or three times daily in the summer holidays were given. David kept in touch by e-mail, even attaching Josie's drawing of Itchy Archie as a Christmas card! The family's tasks were to model and reinforce /st/, /sp/, and /sk/, final consonant inclusion, and to do activities around /tʃ/, /dʒ/, and /s/, talking about the imagery and sound-letter-symbol associations, and to maintain stimulability. In this session, the difficulties both Maureen and Emma had with language processing and production, particularly the production of consonant clusters and polysyllabic words, contrasted markedly with David's verbal abilities and quick grasp of what was needed.

Consonant clusters and polysyllabic words

During Josie's initial consultation, it emerged that there was a maternal family history of speech and literacy issues. Maureen and Emma were poor readers and spellers, and Ruby was a late talker with unintelligible speech. Maureen's conversation was characterised by many mispronunciations. For example, each time she attended with Josie, she mentioned that they would go to the village afterwards for an *advocargo sandwich*. She referred several times to a NSW state politician (The Hon Danna Vale MP) as *dallavale*, and frequently substituted *weave* for *we* (*If weave get there early. . .*), and referred repeatedly to the *ditstrict slimming carnival* (district swimming carnival), apparently without noticing. In addition, there were examples of subtle schwa insertion, especially with /pl/ and /bl/ in onset, in words like *platter*, *place*, *blister*, and *blame* (/pəlætə/, /pəleɪs/, /bəlɪstə/, /bəleɪm/) and schwa deletion in words like *Malouf* and *believe* (/mluf/, /bliv/). From this speech behaviour in her mother, and the many citation-naming and spontaneous-speech consonant deletions Josie made at the outset—with words that included: *binoculars, butterfly, Beijing, carnival, computer, Dolly Magazine, Dumbledore, florist, mistake, octopus, play station, rain forest, Slim Dusty* (the family dog), *spaghetti*, and *triangle*—Josie might have been expected to have particular difficulty conquering clusters and polysyllables, but she did not.

Dr. Debbie James is an academic and speech pathologist, conducting research at the University of South Australia. Her expertise and research interests involve children with oral and written speech and language problems; children's ability with polysyllabic word production; language and literacy; speech improvement; and children's development of speech and language. Both Josie and Maureen were interesting relative to research by Dr. James into the possible clinical significance of consonant cluster errors, mispronunciation of polysyllabic words, and consonant deletion errors, and she explores this possibility in A44.

Q44.   Deborah G. H. James: Underlying representations and surface forms

An interesting feature of Josie's intelligibility rating at 6; 6 by her parents was that, even though both spent an equivalent amount of time with her, her mother who may have had 'fuzzy' underlying representations and who had many speech errors in output found her to be 'mostly intelligible', whereas her father, who was highly competent verbally, found her 'mostly unintelligible'. Can you comment on the probable relationship in individuals with persistent errors with polysyllabic words and words containing clusters, between underlying representation and surface form? In working with children who appear to have persistent errors with clusters and polysyllables, what testing would you suggest, and what are the clinical implications and the directions therapy might take?

A44.   Deborah G. H. James: The relationship between the underlying representation and surface form of long words

The term 'long words' refers here to words of three or more syllables and 'short words' to words of one or two syllables. When more specificity is required, 'multisyllabic words' refers to words of two or more syllables, monosyllabic words to one-syllable words, and disyllabic words to two-syllable words. However, in the literature, 'polysyllabic' and 'multisyllabic' words are used variously. For Davis (1998), polysyllabic words have four or more syllables, whereas other scholars have applied 'polysyllabic words' and 'multisyllabic words' to words of two or more syllables. Clusters are contiguous consonant sequences occurring at the edges of syllables, abiding by the phonotactic, or sequencing constraints, of the ambient language.

Underlying phonological representations and long words and cluster errors

The notion that erroneous surface forms of long words and words containing clusters re-flect weak underlying phonological representations (UR) of them is fascinating. If the idea holds, it may also have intriguing clinical implications for assessment *and* intervention. UR is the term used to describe the storage of the word's phonological information in long-term memory (Stackhouse and Wells 1997). I think the genesis of this relationship is in the broader positive relationship between the quality of someone's speech output and their corresponding UR. Accumulating evidence that accurate speech output depends on a robust UR indicates that the more accurate a person's output, the more accurate and fine-grained is the corresponding UR (Hesketh, Dima, and Nelson 2007; Sutherland and Gillon 2005, 2007). This, in turn, suggests that output status may be an indicator of the UR quality. It also implies dependency between the two, namely, improvement in one pre-supposes improvement in the other. Indeed, intervention studies show that interven-tion designed to enhance the quality of the UR, through phonological processing tasks (including phonological awareness tasks), *and* output resulted in changes in output (Baker 2000; Bowen and Cupples 1999a; Habers, Paden, and Halle 1999). Further, programs that focussed on UR only resulted in changes in output (Moriarty and Gillon 2006; Weiner 1981a), whereas simultaneously treating UR *and* output proved more effective than only treating output (Gillon 2000; Hesketh, Dima, and Nelson 2007).

An asymmetrical relationship

This UR-to-output relationship, however, appears asymmetrical, and clinicians, especially those working with children's literacy, regularly face the conundrum of a child with typical speech output alongside poor phonological processing (Scarborough and Brady 2002).

The asymmetry recedes when the number of syllables in words used for testing speech is manipulated, as evidenced by studies where test stimuli included words of differing syllable numbers. Where speech testing relied on short words, the relationship between speech and phonological processing was either absent or weak (Bishop and Adams 1990; Catts 1993). By contrast, a relationship *was* present when speech testing included nine or more long words (Elbro, Borstrøm, and Petersen 1998; Larrivee and Catts 1999; Leitão, Hogben, and Fletcher 1997; Lewis and Freebairn 1992; Lewis, Freebairn, and Taylor 2000b, 2002; Stothard, Snowling, Bishop, et al. 1998). These findings suggest that long words, which have *more syllables* and *more stress variations*, provide unique information; the question is, why? We can start answering this question by exploring the structure of syllables via the rubric of non-linear phonology.

The internal structure of syllables

Syllable constituents include onsets, rimes, nuclei (vowels), and codas (the final consonant or consonant cluster, if any). These constituents are modelled hierarchically, as displayed in the onset-rime tree in Figure A44.1. The rime is the obligatory syllable head and its partner, the onset, is optional, allowing for words without onsets, such as *eye* and *egg*. In English, the consonants in the onset vary in number from zero to three. The rime contains the obligatory nucleus and its partner, the offset, or coda and, like the onset, is optional; in English, the coda can have zero to four consonants. Consequently, syllables shapes vary from one-sound words like *owe* /oʊ/ to eight-sound words like *strengths* /strɛŋkθs/.

The nucleus is the most prominent syllable constituent because it is the most sonorous (Baker, A11), consequent to vocal tract openness. Conversely, the constituents at the syllable edges, the onsets and codas, are the least prominent, consequent to a less open vocal tract. The onsets and codas comprise either singleton consonants or clusters. Different syllables have different sonority profiles because of the different syllable shapes and the sonority characteristics of the sounds that fill the syllable constituents. Some syllables have a greater and sharper change in sonority from the edge to the nucleus than others, so are more salient than syllables with less distinct contrasts in sonority between their edges and the nucleus. These different sonority profiles have implications for speech acquisition because children tend to say words and/or syllables with more distinct contrasts

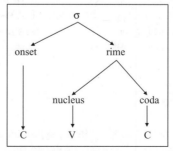

Key: σ = syllable

Figure A44.1 The structure of a syllable

more accurately than those with less distinct contrasts (Kehoe 2001). For example, *bat* is a more salient syllable and word than *man* because a greater sonority differential exists between its edges and nucleus than that of *man*. This is so because voiceless stops are less sonorous than nasals, giving rise to greater contrast. Similarly, syllables beginning or ending with consonant clusters are also less salient than their near minimal pair counterparts with singleton consonants in these slots because the change in sonority from the syllable edge to the nucleus is more gradual. For example, the change in sonority from the onset to the nucleus in *black* is more gradual than in *back*. This theory predicts that it is easier for children to extract sufficient details from *bat* and *back* than *man* and *black* to yield adult-like renditions, so adult-like renditions of *bat* and *back* will probably emerge before those of *man* and *black*. For all four words, the UR in young children is likely to be holistic but, possibly, the UR of *man* and *black* has to be more fine-grained than that of *bat* and *back* to yield an output of equivalent accuracy. This same logic applies to long words, that is, the UR of long words may need to be even more fine-grained to yield an output of equivalent accuracy to short words so that the additional phonological constituents are present in the output. Further, some of the unique features of long words may strain extraction abilities more than short words.

Another difference between multisyllabic words and monosyllabic words is in the types of consonant sequences they can contain. The consonant sequences that can occur in multisyllabic words are consonant clusters and coda-onset sequences whereas the only consonant sequences that can occur in monosyllabic words are consonant clusters. Coda–onset sequences occur when codas and onsets abut at syllable edges, consequent to the linking of syllables in them. This generates sequences such as k.t/, /m.b/, /dʒ.t and /m.bj/ at the junction between the first and second syllable in: o*c*t*opus, ham*burger, veg*etables*, and am*bulance*, respectively, and /p.t/ at the junction of the third and fourth syllables in *helicopter*. As none of these sequences are legal onset clusters and only some are legal coda clusters (Clark and Yallop 1995), this underscores the need to employ multisyllabic words in testing so these aspects of phonology are sampled.

Stress

Short and long words differ in the levels of stress therein. Monosyllabic words have one level of stress, disyllabic words have two, and long words may have as many levels as they have syllables. For example, *catamaran* with four syllables has four levels of stress, as displayed in Figure A44.2, as does, *hippopotamus* with five syllables. Your first reaction may be 'Sorry? There are only three levels of stress, primary, secondary, and weak, that can apply to words, and for *hippopotamus*, there are only strong and weak syllables'. This is true (Roca and Johnson 1999). However, more levels can occur because of the metrical structure of words.

Metrical structure

Within metrical phonology (Selkirk 1984), syllables gather to form feet, and feet gather into prosodic words. Speakers of English prefer to arrange syllables within prosodic words so strong and weak ones alternate (Roca and Johnson 1999). A foot typically consists of two syllables; a head one which is strong, and second one which is marked for secondary or

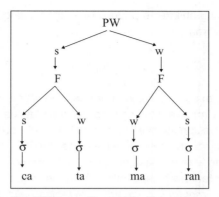

Key: PW = prosodic world F = foot;
S = strong; W= weak σ = syllable

Figure A44.2 The metrical structure of catamaran

weak stress. Prosodic words contain one or more feet. In prosodic words of more than one foot, one foot is more prominent than the other, which implies different levels of stress in a word. *Catamaran* has two feet. The first two syllables form the first and head foot, which is more prominent than the second foot that comprises the third, weak syllable and the fourth, strong syllable. Because the first foot is more prominent than the second foot, so too is its strong syllable more prominent than its counterpart in the second foot, and the same holds for the two weak syllables in both feet, resulting is four different levels of stress.

Another important feature of stress specific to long words is within-word *weak* syllables, such as the two in ca*ta.ma*ran. In short words, weak syllables can form either the whole word, such as *the* in a phrase like *the cat*, or they can occur first or last in DSWs (e.g., *giraffe* or *cola*), but they cannot occur within words in these contexts. The importance of checking children's ability to realise within-word weak syllables, or non-final weak syllables, is underscored by the findings of Aguilar-Mediavilla, Sanz-Torrent, and Serra-Raventos (2002), who reported that language-impaired children, aged 3;10 to 4;10, had more difficulty with them than their typically developing peers.

Assessment implications

Based on the above information and my own research findings (James 2006), I echo Stackhouse (1985), Watts (2004), and Young (1991, 1995), who recommended that long words be included routinely in child speech assessment. Importantly, their inclusion enhances *content validity* of testing because a wider array of phonological variables is sampled, including stress, non-final weak syllables, and coda–onset consonant sequences. It also enhances *construct validity* because they reveal age-related differences between groups of typically developing children that are not evident in short words (James 2006; James, van Doorn, McLeod, et al. 2008). For example, metathesis occurred in disyllabic and polysyllabic words but not in monosyllabic words. Also, age differences for metathesis only occurred in polysyllabic words and not in the disyllabic words. They also reveal disorder-related differences, as for some children, their impairments are only apparent in polysyllabic words and not in short words (see James 2006, for a literature review). Their exclusion risks not identifying children's phonological processing and speech output difficulties only evident in long words.

Caveat

For the reasons expounded above, some long words are easier for children to say than others. Thus, it is important to use those long words that are clinically useful. James (2006) showed that the uniting features for clinically useful words were (a) non-final weak syllables with sonorant onsets or codas, especially the liquid /l/; (b) consonant sequences, especially those requiring an anterior/posterior articulatory movement; and (c) consonants that shared place or manner features, especially sonorants. The following 10 long words: *ambulance, hippopotamus, computer, spaghetti, vegetables helicopter, animals, caravan, caterpillar,* and *butterfly*, proved to be the most clinically useful of the 39 long words used in the study.

Therapy

Given the evidence that working with phonological awareness brings about positive changes in the output, coupled with the assumption that accurate PSW production requires a more fine grained UR than short words, I recommend including long words among the usual therapy targets and techniques. One example is to incorporate long words into *focused auditory input* (Hodson 2007) and *Auditory Input Therapy* Lancaster, Keusch, Levin, Pring, and Martin (in press) *, perceptually based interventions* (Rvachew, A24), and *minimal pair therapy* (Barlow and Gierut 2002). Alternatively, one could work with families of long words, such as those displayed in Table A44.1, exploring their similarities and differences.

In conclusion, by using long words in the management of paediatric speech impairment, several clinical efficiencies can be achieved. Clinicians can sample and expose children to a greater array of phonological variables than short words permit. This is especially relevant for clinicians working with school-aged children because developmental changes occur more frequently in long words with few, if any, in short words. It also seems that working with these variables is simultaneously enhancing the UR, thereby working on phonological awareness (for literacy) as well as speech output.

Table A44.1 Quasi minimal pairs and word families in long words

Root word; *ward*	Words with C+/jul/*	Words with initial weak syllable	Some quasi minimal pairs
ward	binoculars	spaghetti	*reminder,*
award/ing	ridiculous	zucchini	*remember*
reward/ing	funicular	tomato	*remainder*
toward	meticulous	potato	*veranda*
forward	folliculous	banana	*Miranda*
backward	fasciculus	pyjamas	Kur*anda*
			su*rrender*

* These words were listed by Gilbert and Johnson (1978).

Josie 6;9 PCC SW 65% CS 50%

#	TARGET	TRANSCRIPTION		CC	#	TARGET	TRANSCRIPTION		CC
1	cup	ʌ	kʌp	2	23	jam	æ	tʃæm	1
2	gone	ɒ	gɒn	2	24	house	aʊ	hæʊ	1
3	knife	aɪ	naɪp	1	25	path	a	pas	1
4	sharp	a	ʃap	2	26	door	ɔ	dɔ	1
5	fish	ɪ	bɪʃ	1	27	smoke	oʊ	smoʊk	3
6	kiss	ɪ	kɪt	1	28	bridge	ɪ	wɪtʃ	0
7	sock	ɒ	ʃɒk	1	29	train	eɪ	tɹeɪn	3
8	glass	a	gwatʃ	1	30	chair	ɛə	tʃɛə	0
9	watch	ɒ	wɒtʃ	2	31	red	e	wed	1
10	nose	oʊ	noʊdᶻ	1	32	spoon	u	sbun	2
11	mouth	aʊ	maʊp	1	33	plane	eɪ	pweɪn	2
12	yawn	ɔ	jɔn	2	34	fly	aɪ	jaɪ	0
13	leaf*	i	jəip	0	35	sky	aɪ	skaɪ	2
14	thumb	ʌ	θʌm	2	36	sun	ʌ	sdʌn	2
15	foot*	ʊ	bʊt	1	37	wing	ɪ	wɪn	1
16	toe	oʊ	toʊ	1	38	splash	æ	pwæʃ	2
17	snake	eɪ	sneɪk	3	39	tent	e	tent	3
18	van	æ	bwæn	1	40	salt	ɒ	sdɒt	2
19	fast	a	bast	2	41	crab*	æ	wab	1
20	girl	ɜ	gɜʊ	1	42	sweet	i	swit	3
21	stairs*	eə	sdez	2	43	sleeve	i	swid	1
22	big	ɪ	bɪg	2	44	zipper	ɪ	sɪp	1
boy bɔɪ ear e ə		SUBTOTAL CC:		32		* VowelReplacement		TOTAL CC:	65

Figure 9.9 Josie's second Quick Screener record form at 6;9

Session 5: 1 Hour, 10 Minutes
Present: Josie, Maureen, and David

The Quick Screener was administered again (Figure 9.9) with parents observing, and discussed. Josie was now stimulable for all consonants to two syllable positions except /l/ and /f/. Her SW PCC was 65% and her CS PCC 50% in the clinic. There had been improvement in syllable structure with a significant reduction in final consonant deletion from 66% to zero, glottal replacement was almost eliminated, and she was tackling longer words, but with pervasive weak syllable deletion. Velar fronting was now confined to the velar nasal only. The occurrence of prevocalic voicing, which had not been directly targeted, had dropped to 14% (previously 57%). Similarly, cluster reduction had dropped from 100% to 50% SI and 83% SF. Gliding of liquids had not changed and still stood at 100%, and stopping of fricatives (bearing in mind that she had been *gliding* fricatives) had risen to 50% SI and 83% SF. There were vowel replacements in words 13, 14, 21, and 41, and it appeared that the minimal pair work for consonants, and possibly the increased attention to speech generally at home, was having a beneficial effect on vowel production also.

1) The adjuncts /st/, /sp/, and /sk/ needed more work. This was tackled by using a multiple oppositions approach, using imagery cues, and the fixed-up-one routine for *all* s-clusters (not just the three s + voiceless stop adjuncts).

2) Polysyllabic words for production practice, focusing on weak syllable inclusion, were provided.

3) /s/ vs. /ʃ/ minimal pair activities were done in the session and given for homework, along with /st/, /sp/, and /sk/ SIWI for production practice. The family were instructed to model /s/ constantly in all contexts, including polysyllables.

4) Homework: 3 and 4 above, with Josie being rewarded strongly for performing self-corrections.

February to April, age 6;9–6; 11 – 5 sessions over 8 weeks (2 cancellations)
Session 6
Present: Josie, Maureen, Emma, and Maureen's sister

Maureen's sister, who normally minded the twins while Josie came to therapy, drove Josie, Emma, and Maureen to the appointment because David was working. Josie was not well and they only stayed briefly. No homework was provided and, Josie was unable to attend her appointment the following week because she was still unwell.

Session 7: 60 Minutes
Present: Josie and David

1) The whole session was devoted to clusters ,'two step words' (cluster words), 'three-part words', and 'four part words' (polysyllables), with 'finger walking' and silent tapping of syllables.

2) Using pictures from her 'speech book', Josie took great pleasure in making up her own (rather bizarre) fixed-up-one routine for clusters.

3) Homework: Reinforcement of self-corrections by David, Maureen, and Emma, and Josie was to take the speech book to school for a pat on the back from her teacher, who rose to the occasion!

Session 8: 40 Minutes
Present: Josie and David

1) The velar nasal was introduced in minimal pairs (win wing, pin ping, bun bung, etc.), with multiple exemplar games and thematic play. At home, they modelled the velar nasal, modelled polysyllables (to target weak syllable deletion), and did daily production practice of polysyllables.

2) Josie was still unable to produce /f/ in CVs, but she could in VCs provided they were not real words that she knew (e.g., she could produce *uff* and *eef*, but not *if*, *off*, and *eff*).

3) Homework: She was given a challenge to 'perfect' -iff, -off, -aff, and -uff over the next week.

Session 9: 40 Minutes
Present: Josie and David

1) Although clusters continued to be problematic, the velar nasal generalised within a week!

2) Playing a hunch that we could capitalise on her recent success with nasals, nasal clusters SF were emphasised for a week, particularly /-ŋk/ (sink, pink, wink, drink, link, etc.), but also /-nt/ and /-nd/.

3) Building on '–iff, -off, -aff, and uff', 'iffy offy, affy, and uffy' were established in the session and sent home to 'perfect'.
4) A judgement of correctness task and a fixed-up-one routine for homework, and a list of final /-ŋk/, /-nt/, and /-nd/ words for production practice were provided (three of each).
5) Homework: 3 and 4 above.

Session 10: 40 Minutes
Present: Josie, Maureen, and David

The Quick Screener (Figure 9.10) was administered and discussed, with David doing most of the scoring! The final cluster strategy worked, and by the next session, Josie was using them inconsistently in *careful* conversational speech.

1) Minimal pair games for stopping of fricatives were introduced.
2) Using a backward chaining technique, Josie managed at long last to produce /f/ SIWI, so: iffy-fee, offee-fee, affy-fee.

#	TARGET	TRANSCRIPTION		CC	#	TARGET	TRANSCRIPTION		CC
1	cup	ʌ	kʌ p	2	23	jam	æ	dʒ æ m	2
2	gone	ɒ	g ɒ n	2	24	house	aʊ	h æʊ s	2
3	knife	aɪ	n aɪ s	1	25	path	a	pas	1
4	sharp	a	ʃ a p	2	26	door	ɔ	d ɔ	1
5	fish	ɪ	ʃ ɪ ʃ	1	27	smoke	oʊ	s m oʊ k	3
6	kiss	ɪ	k ɪ s	2	28	bridge	ɪ	ɹ ɪ dʒ	2
7	sock	ɒ	s ɒ k	2	29	train	eɪ	t ɹ eɪ n	3
8	glass	a	g w a s	2	30	chair	ɛə	tʃ ɛə	1
9	watch	ɒ	w ɒ tʃ	2	31	red	e	ɹ e d	2
10	nose	oʊ	n oʊ z	2	32	spoon	u	s p u n	3
11	mouth	au	m au θ	2	33	plane	eɪ	p w eɪ n	2
12	yawn	ɔ	j ɔ n	2	34	fly	aɪ	s w aɪ	0
13	leaf	i	j i s	0	35	sky	aɪ	s k aɪ	2
14	thumb	ʌ	θ ʌ m	2	36	sun	ʌ	s ʌ n	2
15	foot	ʊ	s ʊ t	1	37	wing	ɪ	w ɪ ŋ	2
16	toe	oʊ	t oʊ	1	38	splash	æ	s p ɹ æ ʃ	3
17	snake	eɪ	s n eɪ k	3	39	tent	e	te n t	3
18	van	æ	b æ n	1	40	salt	ɒ	s ɒ t	2
19	fast	a	s a s t	2	41	crab*	æ	ɹ a b	2
20	girl	ɜ	g ɜ ʊ	1	42	sweet	i	s w i t	3
21	stairs*	eə	s t e z	3	43	sleeve	i	s w i z	1
22	big	ɪ	b ɪ g	2	44	zipper	ɪ	z ɪ p	2
		SUBTOTAL CC	38					TOTAL CC	82

Figure 9.10 Josie's third Quick Screener record form at 7;1

3) Homework: The family was to maintain Josie's ability to produce /f/ SIWI and model in general. No specific homework was given, and Josie was asked to put her speech book and other materials away in a safe place and have a break. This was presented as a reward for a terrific effort on her part.

June: 3 sessions over 4 weeks, age 7;1
Session 11: 1 Hour, 10 Minutes
Present: Josie, Maureen, and David

Josie's single word and conversational PCCs were now around about the same. Disappointingly for her, she was barely stimulable for /f/ SIWI and SFWF, and there had been no functional generalisation. She was still not stimulable for /l/, but she was now usually replacing /l/ with liquid /ɹ/ and not a glide /j/, and this replacement of a liquid with a liquid was interpreted as progress.

1) We decided to focus on /f/ and /v/ concurrently, using a combination of traditional phonetic production training and multiple exemplar activities and the aspiration trick (the f-hat, f-heat strategy; see http://www.speech-language-therapy.com/tx-facts-and-tricks.html).
2) Homework: /f/, /f/, and more /f/! And /v/!

Session 12: 40 Minutes
Present: Josie, Maureen, and David

1) Production practice of /f/ SI and /fr/ SI words.
2) Production of /ft/ using lexical innovation (laugh/laughed, cough/coughed, etc.).
3) Auditory bombardment using /f/ vs. /v/ minimal pairs (fat-vat, fine-vine, fail-veil, etc.).
4) Auditory discrimination games for /r/ and /l/ (lung-rung, lead-read, list-wrist, etc.).
5) Homework: 1–4 above and modelling and frequent recasting for /f/ and /v/.

Session 13: 40 Minutes
Present: Josie, David, Maureen, and Emma

This was an interesting session in which the family reviewed progress and future plans. Josie's name had come up on the Community Health waiting list, and they had been informed, to their surprise, that she had already been seen once at school by a newly appointed SLP. They were torn between staying with someone they knew and accessing a local service minutes by car from their home, commencing in late January. They decided to proceed with three scheduled appointments in September (2 sessions) and November (1 session) before changing to the new clinician. Therapy and homework were the same as for Session 12, with different vocabulary and games, plus auditory bombardment for /l/ SIWI.

September: 2 sessions over 4 weeks, age 7;3–7;4
Session 14: 40 Minutes
Present: Josie and David

1) More work on /f/ and /v/ in story retelling and narrative tasks. Both targets were beginning to show functional generalisation. This was *so* exciting for Josie, who commented, 'Ept, uh eff is my hard one, isn't it? But I can do it when I think!'

2) Homework: none, other than praising Josie, who was self-monitoring constantly.

Session 15: 40 Minutes
Present: Josie and David

1) In the session, /l/ was elicited in 'la' for the first time!
2) Homework: production practice: la-la-laugh, la-la-laugh, la-la-last, etc. and auditory bombardment for /l/ SIWI and SIWW.

November: 1 Session Age 7;6
Session 16: 40 Minutes
Present: Josie, David, Maureen, and Emma

The Screener was administered for the final time at the parent's request while the family observed (Figure 9.11). Her PCC in SW and CS was 93% or thereabouts. Josie was able to produce laugh, last, llama, latte, Lana, etc. perfectly, but was unable to produce /l/ preceding vowels other than /a/. Her speech was fully intelligible, and the only outstanding difficulties were with /l/ and a tendency to replace /eə/ with /e/ or /ɛ/. Josie was looking forward to seeing the Community Health SLP in the New Year. The case notes and a brief report were provided to David and Maureen for them to share with the SLP. Attempting to execute a smooth changeover, the author left two telephone

#	TARGET	TRANSCRIPTION		CC	#	TARGET	TRANSCRIPTION		CC
1	cup	ʌ	k ʌ p	2	23	jam	æ	dʒ æ m	2
2	gone	ɒ	g ɒ n	2	24	house	aʊ	h æʊ s	2
3	knife	aɪ	n aɪ f	2	25	path	a	p a θ	2
4	sharp	a	ʃ a p	2	26	door	ɔ	d ɔ	1
5	fish	ɪ	f ɪ ʃ	2	27	smoke	oʊ	s m oʊ k	3
6	kiss	ɪ	k ɪ s	2	28	bridge	ɪ	b ɹ ɪ dʒ	3
7	sock	ɒ	s ɒ k	2	29	train	eɪ	t ɹ eɪ n	3
8	glass	a	g w a s	2	30	chair	eə	tʃ eə	1
9	watch	ɒ	w ɒ tʃ	2	31	red	e	ɹ e d	2
10	nose	oʊ	n oʊ z	2	32	spoon	u	s p u n	3
11	mouth	aʊ	m aʊ θ	2	33	plane	eɪ	p w eɪ n	2
12	yawn	ɔ	j ɔ n	2	34	fly	aɪ	f w aɪ	1
13	leaf	i	ɹ i f	1	35	sky	aɪ	s k aɪ	2
14	thumb	ʌ	θ ʌ m	2	36	sun	ʌ	s ʌ n	2
15	foot	ʊ	f ʊ t	2	37	wing	ɪ	w ɪ ŋ	2
16	toe	oʊ	t oʊ	1	38	splash	æ	s p ɹ æ ʃ	3
17	snake	eɪ	s n eɪ k	3	39	tent	e	t e n t	3
18	van	æ	v æ n	2	40	salt	ɒ	s ɒ t	2
19	fast	a	f a s t	3	41	crab*	æ	k ɹ a b	3
20	girl	ɜ	g ɜ ʊ	1	42	sweet	i	s w i t	3
21	stairs*	eə	s t e z	3	43	sleeve	i	s w i v	2
22	big	ɪ	b ɪ g	2	44	zipper	ɪ	z ɪ p	2
		SUBTOTAL CC		44			TOTAL CC		93

Figure 9.11 Josie's fourth and final Quick Screener record form at 7;6

messages at the SLPs workplace and e-mailed her, but received no response. David also requested that the SLP speak to the author and was told that Josie's speech difficulties were so mild that case discussion was unnecessary.

Epilogue

The following May, Maureen visited unexpectedly with her sister, but not Josie, to report progress. Josie, now 8;0, had been seen by her new therapist for a language assessment over two sessions. She had a Composite Language Score of 100 on the CELF-4 Australian. She was grouped with two boys for weekly 30-minute sessions to work on a common target, /l/, in the lunch period at school, and a Reading Recovery teacher did individual 'l-homework' (but not Reading Recovery) with Josie and each of the boys twice weekly. No speech (or other) homework was sent home for any of the children. She had 8 group therapy sessions over 8 weeks with the SLP and 12 individual sessions with the Reading Recovery teacher, and was dismissed from therapy because she had reached the maximum allocation. Maureen was unsure, but she thought /l/ had not improved. She had not spoken to the SLP since the CELF-4 assessment. Maureen happily reported that Josie had maintained her other progress and was doing quite well academically in Year 2 (the third year of formal schooling in NSW). Plans to home-school her had been suspended for the time being because Josie was now enjoying school. Maureen said she and David might re-contact 'if the ells don't come good'.

Josie made remarkable progress with comparatively little SLP intervention in terms of therapist hours, and one has to wonder whether the outcome would have been so positive if her intervention had happened in the hands of a non-SLP within a typical (and increasingly prevalent) consultative framework or through an aide (McCartney, Boyle, Bannatyne, et al. 2005). She was on the author's caseload from 6;5 to 7;6. In that time, she had a language assessment (one session), an initial speech assessment (1 session), and 15 intervention sessions, some of which incorporated ongoing assessment as required. She had 2 missed appointments due to illness. In all, she had 12.5 hours of in-clinic face-to-face intervention, requiring 3 to 4 hours of preparation for sessions by the clinician, plus the therapist's Einstein Time! Her family's dedication to keeping scheduled appointments, participating in sessions, learning relevant skills, helping Josie to maintain a positive attitude, implementing homework meticulously, and making it fun provides a wonderful example of what can be achieved even with tight limitations on the amount of intervention that can be administered. It also exemplifies the value of the SLP/SLT taking the time to plan explicitly principled therapy; the advantages of careful target selection with an eye to generalisation across a child's phonological system; the benefits of painstaking stimulability training; and the profound changes that can occur when the clinician manages every aspect of intervention him/herself, in person, in a team effort with child and family.

Acknowledgment

Thanks are extended to Josie and her family for sharing their story; and to two of her SLPs for their willing participation in providing assessment data and other information.

Chapter 10

Directions and reflections

In this closing chapter, Benjamin Munson, John Bernthal and Megan Overby, Suzanne Purdy, Suze Leitão, and Joan Rosenthal traverse a breadth of topics, including a rarely considered one in the context of child speech. It concerns sociophonetics, gender stereotyping, and social indexing, and Munson (A45) approaches it with enthusiasm and empathy. By contrast, Bernthal and Overby (A46) address a prominent hot topic: the escalating and worrying teacher–researcher and doctoral shortages in our profession. Then, Purdy (A47) provides an account of the important links between hearing and SSD, providing expert guidance from an Audiology perspective. Next, Leitão (A48) reflects on the art and science of clinical thinking in everyday practice and the knotty issues that can arise. Finally, and inspirationally, Rosenthal (A49) presents her key components of a practitioners' survival kit.

Sociophonetics

In the world of phoneticians, the burgeoning field of sociophonetics resides at the intersection of sociolinguistics and phonetics. Most of its work has involved descriptive accounts of phonetic and phonological variation within regional dialects, speech styles, or (social) speech groups, and attempts to explore the relationship between phonetics and phonology (Ohala 1990). By comparison, there has been scant exploration of the relationship between phonetic and phonological variation and how speech is perceived. Roberts (2002) provides a summary of available data which suggest that children acquire knowledge of sociolinguistic variation from the earliest stages, although little is known about *how* variation comes to be learned in the course of language acquisition. Many social factors systematically shape variation in speech production, including individual differences such as age, gender, ethnicity, and socio-economic status (Labov 1994–2001), and the influence of social groups and networks with which speakers are associated (Eckert 2000a; Milroy 1987). Sociophonetics has applications in pedagogy, foreign language teaching, forensic phonetics, and multi-layered transcription (Müller 2006). In SLP/SLT, it has undeniable implications for understanding of child-directed speech ('parentese'), therapy discourse, style-shifting, speaker- and listener-oriented articulatory control, register, code switching, and for deepening cultural and linguistic sensitivity.

Dr. Benjamin Munson is as Associate Professor in Speech Language Hearing Sciences at the University of Minnesota, Minneapolis. His many research interests include relationships among phonology, metaphonology, and the lexicon; speech production in phonological impairment; the cognitive and linguistic bases of phonological development and disorders in children; gender typicality in children's speech, including when and how children learn to express gender through speech, with a particular focus on how this learning interacts with more general aspects of language learning; and sociophonetics.

Q45. Benjamin Munson: Sociophonetics and child speech practice

Quite inadvertently, Van Borsel, Van Rentergem, and Verhaeghe (2007) pointed to the importance of SLPs/SLTs having informed views of linguistic variation, enabling them to distinguish genuine pathology from natural non-standard variation, and this is clearly an area where sociophonetics can help. What are the methods of enquiry in this non-traditional area of study? Can you explore for the interested clinician or clinical researcher the likely impact of, and clinically relevant research areas in children's SSDs for, sociophonetics as its literature base mushrooms and interfaces with clinical phonology?

A45. Benjamin Munson: Pathology or social indexing?

As practicing SLPs/SLTs know, the articulatory and perceptual characteristics of speech sounds vary from talker to talker, and within talkers, from utterance to utterance. For instance, phonetic detail can vary across talkers due to anatomic and dialectal differences; and within talkers, as a function of ambient noise (Lane and Tranel 1971) or the presumed language abilities of the person being addressed (Bradlow 2002). Determining whether a variation reflects pathology, warranting treatment, or whether it is normal is a challenge faced whenever we differentiate between language impairment and first-language interference in children from culturally and linguistically diverse backgrounds. Understanding of, and sensitivity to, the sources of variation simplify the task of forming these judgments.

Imagine two girls growing up in North America who demonstrate *superficially* equivalent pronunciation patterns, apparently omitting within word /r/ as in *every*, substituting /f/ for /θ/ word finally as in *bath*, and omitting final /t/ and /d/ as in *hat* and *bad*, respectively. One girl has these errors because of a problem in phonological acquisition and requires intervention. The other does not have errors per se, but rather, sound patterns that indicate successful acquisition of a variant of English, African American English, in which these are the speech community's pronunciations (for a review, see Thomas 2007). The second girl requires no intervention, except perhaps to say that, if she were to interact with people in dialectally diverse speech communities, she might benefit from explicit instruction in appropriate code-switching.

Assessing whether variation is pathological or not can be complex, and certainly not always as straightforward, for US clinicians at least, as the comparison above suggests.

Take for example the labiodental variants of /r/, transcribed as [ʋ], in some dialects of English in the UK. Superficially, they sound like /r/ misarticulations that occur in typical acquisition. An improbable interpretation of this variant is that it represents a widespread, persistent speech error, but as Foulkes and Docherty (2000) show, rates of use of [ʋ] are highly linked to social stratification. Indeed, its use might signal, intentionally or unintentionally, membership of different social groups, rather than social-group differences in the incidence of misarticulation.

Sociophonetics

Sociophonetics melds methodologies and theoretical constructs from several disciplines, including experimental phonetics, psycholinguistics, and sociolinguistics. Foulkes (2005) summarises how sociophoneticians catalogue variation in the sound structure of language echoing social-group membership, in production and perception, and how this interacts with other linguistically based phonetic variation: segmental and prosodic. Perceptual studies in this sub-field reveal that listeners readily associate different pronunciation variants with social categories, often in ways contrary to the actual use of these variants in a population. Niedzielski (1999) illustrates this in an influential study of vowel perception by people in Detroit, Michigan. Participants were presented with synthesised vowels in a speaker identification task, and told that the vowels were modelled on the productions of either Detroiters, or residents of nearby Windsor, Ontario, who speak a different English dialect. Labelling of the Windsor vowels, by the Detroit participants, showed tactic knowledge of the ways that people within that dialect region speak. Interestingly, the labels listeners gave for vowels presumed to be produced by Detroiters exposed social stereotypes of the speech of Detroiters that did not match their actual vowel productions.

A qualitatively similar case comes from Munson and Zimmerman (2006). They examined listeners' perception of men's sexual orientation according to how /s/-initial words were produced. A popular-culture stereotype in North America and in much of the Commonwealth of Nations holds that gay men lisp. Although the term 'lisp' has fallen out of scientific use among SLPs/SLTs, it clearly connotes a misarticulation. Published studies on /s/ variation and sexual orientation in men show that individuals' production of /s/ is associated with both actual and perceived sexual orientation (Linville 1998; Munson, McDonald, DeBoe, et al. 2006). The distinctive /s/ associated with gay- and gay-sounding men's speech, however, is arguably a hyper-correct /s/, and not a lisp, as its acoustic characteristics serve to better differentiate it from the acoustically similar sounds /ʃ/ and /θ/ than the heterosexual and heterosexual-sounding men's /s/ (Jongman, Wayland, and Wong 2000). Munson and Zimmerman found that listeners label a talker as gayer-sounding when presented with stimuli containing a hyper-correct /s/ than when presented with stimuli containing /s/ with average acoustic characteristics. Nearly identical scores were elicited when listeners rated tokens containing a frontally misarticulated /s/, even though its acoustic characteristics differed markedly from those of hyper-correct /s/.

Other research demonstrating that listeners' expectations affect speech perception complements these findings. For example, expectations about talker gender and social class affect the categorisation of speech sounds (Hay, Warren, and Drager 2006; Strand and Johnson 1996). Strand and Johnson showed that acoustically equivalent American-English lingual fricatives are labelled differently depending whether listeners believed they are listening to a man (favouring a /s/ response) or to a woman (favouring a /ʃ/ response), perhaps signifying tacit knowledge of sex differences in production of these sounds. Hay, Warren, and Drager showed that listeners in New Zealand label the acoustically ambiguous diphthongs in *hair* and *here* differently depending on whether they are led to believe they are produced by a woman or a man and by a working-class or a middle-class person.

The cases of sexual orientation and /s/, and /r/ variation in the UK, are particularly interesting, illustrating that considerable variation in pronunciation can occur *within* a speech community, without appearing to be due to obvious anatomic or physiologic differences. Moreover, their origins appear to be different from those for regional dialects, the formation of which may be related to factors such as migration and language contact (Trudgill 2004). But surely labiodental /r/ ([ʋ]), hyper-articulated /s/, and very local phonetic variants within high school cliques (Eckert 2000b; Mendoza-Denton 2007) cannot result from such factors. Rather, they appear to be instances of groups of individuals exploiting permissible variation in speech to convey social categories, *alongside* propositional linguistic information.

Consequences of variation

In addition to understanding the *causes* of variation, SLPs/SLTs must understand its *consequences*. Consider the fairly robust finding that English-speaking women are more articulate than men (Bradlow, Toretta, and Pisoni 1996). Perceptual studies reviewed in Munson and Babel (2007) show that many listeners make tacit associations between hyperarticulation and sex typicality of speech. What if children held these stereotypes, too? If they did, they might judge less-articulate male peers as more masculine sounding, and more-articulate female peers as more feminine sounding. This in turn might promote a powerful social motivation for some children, particularly young boys, to resist speech and language therapy aimed at improving intelligibility, because 'success' might manifest as a boy sounding less boy-like! Then again, imagine a child with a [t] for /s/ substitution being taught /s/ in therapy. One likely and reasonable instructional strategy would be for the clinician to model a hyper-articulate /s/. The social meaning associated with that phonetic variant in some English-speaking contexts might make boys in particular averse to learning it.

A child who is taught only one variant of /s/ in therapy is ill-equipped to manipulate its characteristics to convey different social registers, unless therapy promotes spontaneous learning of the full range of /s/ variants through encoding and emulation of different models in the population. To this end, peer-modelling might be incorporated into therapy.

Implications for practice

When clinical SLPs/SLTs are proactive in incorporating ethnographic analysis into their practice, especially with culturally and linguistically diverse populations, they examine the range of phonetic variation throughout the communities in which a child communicates. They develop both taxonomies of phonetic variants and observations of the communicative functions of these variants, much as Eckert (2000b) and Mendoza-Denton (2007) did when researching sociophonetic variation in high school students' speech. Ethnographic analysis holds promise for a rich and detailed picture, more complex, more informative, and more culturally apt than traditional descriptive approaches to child speech, a suggestion that is consistent with many of the works assembled by Müller (2006).

Ethnographic analysis was not employed when Van Borsel, Van Rentergem, and Verhaeghe (2007) examined an almost 23% incidence of what they characterised as dentally misarticulated /s/ in Belgian university students aged 18 to 22, reported to be 'native speakers of Dutch'. Their incidence fluctuated as a function of some variables rarely cited as being associated with misarticulation rates, such as university field of study. The lowest rates of interdental /s/ were among humanities students, with higher values for natural sciences and social sciences students, and a significant majority of those identified as lisping were unaware that they were assessed as such. Carefully indicating that their finding might not be new, they cite a palatographic study (Dart 1991) that revealed dental articulation of /s/ and /z/ by French-speaking (42.1%, p. 48) and English-speaking (22.8%, p. 50) adults with no obvious speech, language, or hearing impairments. Moreover, Van Borsel and colleagues concede that no definitive interpretation of their findings exists. They speculate, however, that they might reflect increased social tolerance to imprecision in articulation, or to the influence, on Dutch pronunciation, of English in which /θ/ and /s/ and their voiced cognates are phonemic.

How might these authors have incorporated insights from sociophonetics into their study? First, by examining more incisively the distribution of variants relative to actual or perceived social categories, especially in view of their intriguing finding that these categories differed as a function of university course. Were the students marking their affiliation to humanities or the sciences with distinctive patterns of phonetic variation? Then, analysis of listener perceptions of the participants' /s/ production might have yielded surprising insights. For example, the dental sound might have been associated more strongly with affiliation with a particular social group than with a judgment that the person produced speech less accurately. It is interesting to reflect on how such a finding might help explain why the variant is present. Consider, for example, that this research took place in Belgium, where many languages, including Belgian French and Flemish (the Belgian variant of Dutch), are spoken. As shown by Dart, French has a higher rate of dental fricative productions than English. Perhaps the higher use of dental fricative in certain groups relates to their exposure to or social identification with the French-speaking population in that country. That, of course, is mere speculation on this author's part, but it shows how sociophonetic methods could have been used to flesh out Van Borstel and colleague's findings. If, in the analysis, these variants actually indicated pathology, then it might be reasonable to suggest that Belgian logopedistes consider treating them more aggressively in children and adolescents.

But, if these are indeed normal sociophonetic variants, then they do not warrant treatment in the traditional sense, although they might legitimately be the subject of a regimen to increase talkers' linguistic flexibility. That is, SLPs/SLTs should not be blind to the fact that non-pathological variation may be associated with negative judgments by some listeners, especially where they index membership in a group that is itself stigmatised. In this regard, Van Borstel and colleagues cite references in support of their argument that frontal lisping can be associated with negative evaluative judgments.

An individual's communicative effectiveness, broadly speaking, resides in part on their ability to fluently switch among different phonetic variants in socially appropriate contexts, and SLPs/SLTs are best positioned, in terms of their knowledge and skill bases, to help people who find this problematic. But it must be emphasised that a population that speaks a non-standard variant is *not* a disordered population, and their presenting 'condition' is not a disorder. By carefully assessing whether productions are deviant, as opposed to normal, socially stratified variants, SLPs/SLTs can ensure that they do not improperly treat normal variation as pathology.

SLPs/SLTs should also be aware that a variant perceived negatively in one context or by one group may be perceived positively in another context or by another group. The association between /s/ and men's sexuality in the many English-speaking countries is a case in point. Whereas this variant is associated with both actual and perceived sexual orientation, it is also associated with hyper-articulate speech. A man whose habitual /s/ demonstrates these characteristics would be ill-advised to change his /s/ characteristics in all communicative contexts, as doing so would prevent him from projecting the positive characteristics that are associated with clear-sounding speech.

The doctoral shortage in higher education

It seems that clinicians who do research, or 'hands on scientists', are an endangered species. ASHA has identified both a critical shortage and a continuing attrition of PhD and other doctoral level faculty in the US whose magnitude will affect the professional preparation of SLPs and the conduct of research in communication sciences and disorders. In a highly publicised focused initiative, ASHA is working to increase the number of doctoral teacher–scholars and students who choose higher education as a career option. The aim is to fill academic faculty/researcher vacancies in human communication sciences and disorders over the next decade at least, to achieve a balance between supply and demand. Part of this initiative manifests as Web content specifically promoting PhD education and teacher–researcher careers. The advertising highlights the lack of overt encouragement for clinicians, including experienced ones, to step outside traditional roles and pursue doctoral studies.

Chapter 1 includes discussion of the research–practice gap and the culture of separation that can exist between theorists, researchers, and practitioners. But heartening signs of constructive alliances between lab and clinic, within the higher degree process, are also revealed. It was with this in mind that Q46 was put to Dr. John Bernthal, an ASHA past president, professor and chair of the Department of Special Education and Communication Disorders, and director in the Barkley Memorial Center at the University of Nebraska-Lincoln. Famously and indispensably for the readers of and contributors to this book, he is co-author with Dr. Nicholas Bankson of five editions of *Articulation and Phonological Disorders*, and with Bankson and Peter Flipsen, Jr. of the sixth edition (Bernthal, Bankson, and Flipsen 2009). Bernthal's co-author here is Dr. Megan Overby, an Assistant Professor at The College of St. Rose in Albany, NY. After working as a public school SLP for nearly two decades, she returned to academia, receiving her PhD from the University of Nebraska-Lincoln in 2007. Her teaching and research interests include phonology, language, and literacy. She is assisting The College of St. Rose to prepare to launch a PhD program in Communication Sciences and Disorders.

Q46. John E. Bernthal and Megan S. Overby: The teacher–researcher supply in communication sciences and disorders

It is tempting to suppose that the theory-therapy-research-practice gap closes a fraction each time a clinical SLP/SLT enrolls in a doctoral program with a view to conducting clinical research in communication sciences and disorders. How would you set about encouraging clinicians to take this path; what is the process; does it differ from place to place; and what, for you, are the burning research questions in child speech?

A46. John E. Bernthal and Megan S. Overby: The teacher–researcher shortage: Possible future directions

In this contribution, we discuss the shortages of teacher–researchers in SLP/SLT. The current shortages and those projected in the next decade require implementing multiple, diverse recruitment strategies of PhD candidates. One recruitment strategy is to target practicing clinicians with applied research interests. We review some of the reasons this strategy may be viable relative to PhD preparation in English-speaking countries and identify a few of the potential applied research questions which may be of interest to practicing clinicians.

The shortage of PhD scholars in SLP academic programs in North America has been recognised for some time, and we hear similar reports from around the world. For example, in 2002, ASHA identified an emerging shortage of teacher–researchers. Approximately 7% of doctoral faculty positions were unfilled in 2001 with the gap anticipated to widen over time (ASHA 2002a). Because the shortage was expected to adversely affect the preparation of future professionals and researchers, increasing the number of PhD scholars, teachers, and researchers became a priority for ASHA. Since 2004, ASHA has adopted focused initiatives to increase the number of students recruited into the profession (ASHA 2004–2007).

The largest pool of potential future researchers–teachers consists of practicing clinicians. Some practitioners have the skills, knowledge, and potential to make major contributions as future teacher–researchers. If the shortage of SLP/SLT doctoral candidates is to be addressed, fostering interest among current practitioners to pursue doctoral study and employment at colleges and universities is urgently needed. One way to encourage clinicians to pursue doctoral study is to help them recognise the similarities between clinical practice and applied research. Each clinical case is, in effect, a research study, and competent clinicians treat their clinical cases in such a manner. Clinicians routinely develop hypotheses about a problem, collect baseline data, provide a treatment, analyse the results, and then adjust the treatment if merited. These experiences and the resulting clinical skills that practitioners acquire can provide a transition to more formal research activities.

Clinical experiences can dictate the focus of the research program of an individual who decides to seek a career in research. The second author of this contribution came to a doctoral program with specific research interests generated from her years of practice as an SLP in the US public schools. During her practice, literacy (reading and spelling) became a major focus of educational instruction and she developed an interest in the area. Dr. Overby noticed an apparent connection between SSD and literacy skills, but her review of the literature revealed limited research findings to illuminate her clinical practice. What she detected as a clinician, coupled with an insufficient theoretical explanation and limited evidence for the hypothesised connection, motivated her to pursue a PhD. Megan's interest developed into a nascent research agenda, became the focus of her PhD program, and remains a priority for her continued research. This is just one example of an applied research interest that emerged from a clinician's day-to-day practice.

In order to recruit clinicians into PhD programs, it may be beneficial for current researchers to share the rewards that can be found in a career in teaching and research. For many researchers, these include the extension and expression of scholarship, expanding personal discovery of thought, theory, and application of ideas. It can be gratifying for a university faculty member to assist in the development of research and clinical skills of practitioners and researchers, knowing that graduates will improve the quality of life for individuals with communication disorders.

Research preparation

The clinician who is interested in doctoral study may not be acquainted with the process. In general, the overall format for doctoral study does not differ from place to place, although the specific requirements differ across programs. The focus of PhD programs across the world is to prepare an individual to conduct research. This means that the student will take coursework and complete independent study that provides theory and information related to the student's research interests. Doctoral programs typically require learning of research tools, such as research methods and statistics, and participation in research projects leading to a dissertation. The specific requirements across universities may vary quite widely in terms of expectations for statistics courses, preparation for college/university teaching, major and minor area requirements, qualifying exams, and research requirements. All programs require a major research project (a dissertation or thesis) followed by an examination and defence of the research project.

Unfortunately, many clinicians wish or need to pursue PhD education on a part-time basis, but, although some individuals have had success on a part-time basis, the best model appears to be a full-time period of concentrated study. Full-time study is more efficacious than part-time study because it allows the individual to focus single-mindedly on the goal of developing and addressing research questions and provides continuous access to resources. It engages the student in the depth and breadth of academic pursuit, which is difficult on a part-time basis.

There are programs in the US that consist of collaborative or joint PhD programs across different institutions. Although all PhD programs require a full-time period of concentrated study (i.e., full-time study on site), joint programs may allow students to reduce their usual 3–5 years of residence at the lead institution. In addition, these programs may offer distance classes and provide a critical mass of faculty mentors when such a critical mass is not available at a single institution.

A doctoral degree with a focus on child SSD and/or language disorders is typically not obtained solely within an SLP/SLT program, but includes coursework in related areas, such as Education, Psychology, Linguistics, or Neurosciences. Frequently, study and/or research in a particular speciality area associated with SSD, such as children with autism spectrum disorders, CAS, language impairment, and/or literacy problems is also a part of a degree program. One of the advantages of a doctoral degree that includes study in a related area is the different perspective such study can bring to the speech and language issues being researched.

Research needs

Many clinicians develop applied research questions that can have a major impact on the field of SSD. SLPs/SLTs can bring clinical interests and questions to the table that are critical to the advancement of the profession. This book includes discussion of many topics which have direct application to the field of child SSD—stimulability, target selection, cycles therapy, multiple opposition therapy, etc. Examination of the effectiveness of these, and other instructional issues, is important to the field of child SSD.

Some of the most pressing research questions for child SSD are related to treatment efficacy. SLPs/SLTs can successfully treat many children with SSD, but we do not have the data to determine which treatment strategies or approaches are most efficient. Nor do we have good dismissal criteria. We also need to identify subgroups of children with SSD and find the most effective and efficient treatment programs across and within subgroups. Another area where we need information is in predicting which children with SSD will self-correct and which require early remediation and intervention. Little is known about the optimum frequency of therapy or the most effective delivery models of therapy (e.g., use of speech aides/assistants and parents). Finally, more information is needed about the role of genetics in speech and language delays and disorders and whether different treatment approaches work better for children with a specific genetic predisposition. Most of these research needs listed above are issues with direct clinical application and of interest to practising clinicians.

In addition to research questions, a major concern in the field is the research-to-practice gap. How do we get the evidence available into common practice? For example, Kamhi (2006) reported that research findings support the idea that complex phonological targets are useful in clinical practice (Baker, A11), yet SLPs/SLTs do not commonly consider phonological complexity when selecting targets. In contrast, the use of non-speech oral motor practice, discussed by Lof (A30), continues to be used in the field although the evidence available suggests that this is not an effective practice to change speech production (Lof 2007). These are but two examples of practice lagging behind research findings. Perhaps if more clinicians pursued PhD degrees, conducted applied research, and presented it in clinical forums, this gap between research and practice could be reduced.

The shortage of PhD students is real, and the need for applied research is greater than ever. Addressing these issues necessitates using multiple, diverse recruitment strategies. A quick review of pressing research questions leads to the conclusion that most of the questions are applied issues. It becomes clear, then, that encouraging practicing clinicians to pursue doctoral programs is a practical and promising means to help fill the gap in educating the next generation of clinicians and researchers.

A view from audiology

In the industrialised world at least, almost every child with SSD who is assessed by an SLP/SLT is also assessed by an Audiologist. But apart from the resultant audiogram and tympanogram carefully filed with the child's other details, there is often little overt appreciation of this essential input. Furthermore SLP/SLT clinicians who are not dually qualified in Audiology may have a poor grasp of hearing issues relative to this population. For one significant example, the high incidence of conductive hearing loss in children with cleft palate (Peterson-Falzone, Hardin-Jones, and Karnell 2001) is well known, but the generalist SLP/SLT may not know how and with what frequency hearing acuity should be monitored.

Dr. Suzanne Purdy is Associate Professor and Head of Speech Science at the University of Auckland. She began her career as a clinical audiologist in 1981 and, after completing her PhD at the University of Iowa in 1990, worked as a lecturer and researcher in the Audiology and Speech Science programs at the University of Auckland in New Zealand and at National Acoustic Laboratories in Australia. Her research interests are wide-ranging but have focussed on auditory processing, auditory evoked potentials, auditory plasticity, and outcomes for profoundly deaf children and adults using cochlear implants.

Q47. Suzanne Purdy: Audiology and speech pathology

What would an Audiologist like to be able to tell an SLP/SLT working with child speech in terms of the normal speech spectrum and audibility of speech sounds with different types of hearing loss? Are there particular screening, referral, and management consideration to be taken into account with indigenous, low SES, CALD, and other special populations; what are the research needs and directions; what communication and collaboration would you like to see between SLPs/SLTs and Audiologists; and are there any good news stories?

A47.   Suzanne C. Purdy: Hearing and children's speech sound disorders

Kent's (2000) model of spoken language production emphasises the acoustic analysis of speech as the basis for successful phonetic and prosodic processing. Because hearing loss degrades the perceived acoustic characteristics of the speech signal, there is a strong link between impaired speech perception and impaired speech production. Evidence for these links comes from preschoolers and infants. In preschoolers, greater degrees of hearing loss are associated with more severe SSD (Schonweiler, Ptok, and Radu 1998); and infants with hearing loss have delayed onset of consistent canonical babbling and delayed consonant development (Moeller, Hoover, Putman, et al. 2007). Moeller and co-workers assessed infants with hearing loss, aged 10–24 months, over a 14-month period, finding that they produced significantly fewer fricatives and affricates [f, v, θ, ð, s, z, ʃ, ʒ, tʃ, dʒ] than otologically typical controls. They also found considerable individual variability in speech development for children with the same degree of hearing loss, so the link between perception and production is not completely straightforward.

Relating the acoustics of the speech signal to the audiogram

The audiogram such as the one displayed in Figure A47.1 (mild high frequency hearing loss), is a graph of hearing thresholds measured in *decibels hearing level* (dB HL) as a function of *speech frequency* measured in Hertz (Hz). The 0 dB HL level on the audiogram represents the softest sound heard, on average, at each frequency by young, otologically

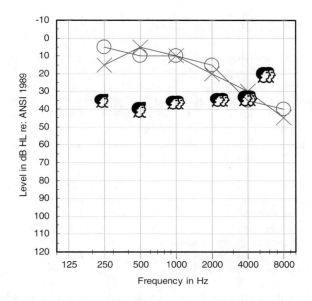

Figure A47.1 Pure tone audiogram showing mild bilateral, high-frequency hearing loss. Circles indicate right ear and crosses indicate left ear hearing thresholds. Hearing thresholds are considered normal if they are in the range −10 to +15 dB HL (Clark 1981). The dB HL scale represents hearing levels relative to the hearing of young 'otologically normal' 18–30 year olds. The face symbols on the graph represent the average speech level in each frequency region for conversational speech (59 dB SPL at 1 m) spoken by an adult female (Cox and Moore 1988). Even with this mild hearing loss, the highest frequency speech sounds (fricatives such as /s/) are close to the threshold of hearing, and speech energy above 4000 Hz is not audible. At greater distances, more of the speech signal will be inaudible. The term 'speech banana' is a term used to refer to the speech spectrum since speech is softest in both the very low and high frequencies and loudest at low-mid frequencies, producing a banana shape when plotted on the audiogram. Hearing thresholds of 16–25 dB HL are classified as slight hearing loss, 26–40 dB as mild, 41–55 dB as moderate, 56–70 dB as moderate-severe, 71–90 dB as severe, and >90 dB as profound (Clark 1981).

normal adults. Some people with normal hearing can hear at even softer levels than the average, so people *can* have hearing thresholds of −5 dB HL or −10 dB HL. Although human hearing spans the frequency range from 20 Hz to 20,000 Hz in young people, audiologists routinely test hearing from 250 to 8000 Hz because this frequency region encompasses most of the speech signal (see Box 10.1). If time is short when testing young children, the frequencies tested may only include 500, 1000, 2000, and 4000 Hz. The softest and highest pitched sounds in English are /s/ and /ʃ/ (Pittman, Stelmachowicz, Lewis, et al. 2003). Although these phonemes have frequency spectra that contain significant energy at frequencies above 4000 Hz, audiologists do not routinely test frequencies above 4000 Hz in young children. This is partly because modern hearing aids have a limited frequency 'bandwidth' so that aided frequencies above 4000 Hz are generally not audible for a person with hearing loss. Because the high-frequency English consonants are very quiet, even a mild high-frequency hearing loss will make these sounds inaudible, unless the speaker is very close to the listener (Pittman, Stelmachowicz, Lewis, et al. 2003). When filtered by a hearing aid, /s/ and /ʃ/ are very similar. It is not surprising, therefore, that children with mild or greater hearing losses commonly misarticulate fricatives (Elfenbein, Hardin-Jones, and Davis 1994; Moeller, Hoover, Putman, et al. 2007).

Box 10.1 Pure tone audiometry and tympanometry

Pure tone audiometry (PTA): PTA is the technique used to measure hearing thresholds. Tones are usually presented via earphones, but sometimes a loudspeaker is used with young children (this tests the 'better' ear only). The softest level at which tones are detected is the hearing threshold (measured in dB HL; the average normal hearing threshold of 0 dB HL). In preschoolers, PTA is performed using a conditioned play response. PTA is usually performed in children aged 6–24 months using Visual Reinforcement Audiometry (VRA), with infants making a head turn response to the tones, reinforced by presentation of an illuminated, moving mechanical puppet (Northern and Downs 2002).

Tympanometry: Tympanometry is the technique used to objectively measure middle ear function (Ramakrishnan, Sparks, and Berryhill 2007). The tympanometer probe, which is inserted into the ear, contains a pressure pump, a tone generator, and a microphone to measure the sound in the ear. As the pressure in the ear canal changes from positive to negative (relative to external air pressure), a normal eardrum will first be 'clamped' by the pressure, then released, then clamped again. This results in a peak in the measured tympanogram at or near normal air pressure, as shown in Figure A47.2. The peak indicates the maximum admittance of the middle ear (energy flow through the system) and should occur at close to 0 decaPascals (daPa) pressure, if the middle ear is normally aerated via the Eustachian tube.

When considering the effects of hearing loss on speech perception and production, key aspects of the speech signal are its intensity, frequency content, and timing. The intensity of the speech signal decreases with distance; for example, the speech level reduces by 6 dB when distance doubles. Typically, speakers automatically adjust their vocal effort to compensate for increased listener distance, but increased effort cannot *fully*

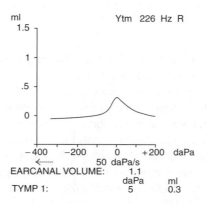

Figure A47.2 This is a normal 'Type A' tympanogram recorded with an air pressure pump speed of 50 daPa/s (decaPascals per second). The ear canal volume of 1.1 mL is estimated based on the admittance at +200 daPa pressure, when the eardrum is clamped with a positive pressure and there is reduced energy flow through the middle ear. In this example, the peak occurs close to zero pressure, at 5 daPa, with a normal peak admittance value of 0.3 mL. The term 'admittance' refers to the flow of energy through a mechanical system (in this case, the eardrum, middle ear space, and middle ear ossicles). Peaks that occur below −100 daPa ('Type C' tympanograms) indicate that there is negative pressure behind the eardrum. Flat 'Type B' tympanograms indicate either a perforation in the eardrum (if volume is high) or a blocked middle ear (if volume is low), usually due to OME (ASHA 1990).

compensate (Michael, Siegel, and Pick 1995). The important temporal (timing) aspects include suprasegmental factors, such as rate, pauses between words and sentences and variations in pitch across utterances, and segmental factors, such as voice onset time (VOT) and timing of vowel formant frequency transitions. Listeners with sensorineural hearing loss (SNHL) have impaired temporal processing, making it difficult for them to detect short gaps in sound or rapid sound transitions (Lister and Roberts 2005), which may impact on speech production. Lane and Perkell (2005) review the literature on the VOT (the interval from plosive release to the onset of voicing of a vowel) in pre- and postlingually deafened speakers and conclude that 'there is a tendency for the difference between voiced and voiceless VOT to be reduced, to the point for many speakers that there is in effect a substitution of the voiced for the voiceless cognate' (e.g., 'toe' realised as [dou]).

Does otitis media cause SSD?

Otitis media with effusion (OME), widely referred to as 'glue ear', is common amongst preschool children (Simpson, Thomas, van der Linden, et al. 2007). OME is generally associated with hearing levels of about 25 dB HL on average and is typically worse in the low frequencies. Some children with persistent OME have mild to moderate hearing loss (Fria, Cantekin, and Eichler 1985). The treatment of OME remains controversial, with a recent *Cochrane Review* concluding that 'grommets only offer a short-term hearing improvement in children with simple glue ear' (Lous, Burton, Felding, et al. 2005, p. 2). Many studies have explored the relationship between OME and a range of outcomes, including speech, language, learning, and auditory processing (Lous, Burton, Felding, et al. 2005; Roberts, Rosenfeld, and Zeisel 2004), with poor consensus. Shriberg and his colleagues reviewed 27 early studies published between 1969 and 1996 that examined whether OME is a risk factor for SSD. They concluded that '(a) there is limited evidence for a strong correlative association between early OME and concurrent or later speech disorder, and (b) there is no evidence for a direct causal association between OME and speech disorder' (Shriberg, Flipsen, Thielke, et al. 2000, p. 80). Roberts and colleagues (2004) determined that severity of hearing loss, rather than the number of OME episodes, is a key predictor of speech and language outcomes. OME presence is commonly monitored via tympanometry (see Box 10.1 and Figure A47.2), which measures energy transmission through the middle ear. Research in this area is hampered by poor subject specificity in many studies, particularly the lack of information on severity of hearing loss.

The impact of OME and poor hearing on early speech development is reflected in restricted phonetic inventories, a preference for bilabial stops, word initial glottal replace- ment, nasal deviations, and limited production of velars, liquids and obstruents (Petinou, Schwartz, Mody, et al. 1999; Rvachew, Slawinski, Williams, et al. 1999). Shriberg, Flipsen, and Thielke (2000) reported a retrospective study of Native American children, finding that OME-positive participants had an almost fivefold increase in risk for SSD. In general, it seems that a positive history of middle ear disease may increase risk for SSD, but the average effect size may be relatively small compared with other risk factors, such as family history (Lewis, Freebairn, Hansen, et al. 2007), prematurity (Salt and Redshaw 2006), or low birthweight (Rvachew, Creighton, Feldman, et al. 2005). OME is likely to have greater impact when several risk factors co-occur, when hearing loss is more severe, or when onset is earlier. OME risk factors are summarised in Table A47.1.

Table A47.1 Influence of socioeconomic status and other demographic factors on otitis media (OM) risk

Studies	Study design	Outcomes
Jacoby, Coates, Arumugaswamy, et al. (2008)	Prospective cohort study of children undergoing routine clinical examinations by an ear, nose, and throat specialist up to age of 2 years ($N = 82$ Aboriginal and $N = 157$ non-Aboriginal children).	OM diagnosed at least once in 74% of Aboriginal children and 45% of non-Aboriginal children. Passive smoking increased risk of OM in Aboriginal children, and in non-Aboriginal children not attending childcare.
Lubianca Neto, Hemb, and Brunelli (2006)	Systematic review of literature (1966–2005) on modifiable risk factors for recurrent acute OM.	Established risk factors are use of pacifiers and care in daycare centres. Probable risk factors are lack of breastfeeding, presence of siblings, craniofacial abnormalities, passive smoking, and presence of adenoids.
Paterson, Carter, Wallace, et al. (2006, 2007)	Prospective study of Pacific children residing in New Zealand (NZ), $N = 656$, screened for middle ear disease at age 2 years of age.	Population prevalence 27% for OME or acute otitis OM. Middle ear disease in Pacific children more severe than in NZ children of European descent. Ear discharge, frequent coughs and colds, snoring, breathing problems, and being exposed to a large number of other children (through daycare or church) increases risk of OME.
Pugh, Burke, and Brown (2004)	Cross-sectional study of $N = 359$ children in preschool to third grade (182 native Hawaiian; 177 non-native Hawaiian).	Group differences in tympanometry findings indicate ethnic differences in middle ear function.
Overturf (2000)	American Academy of Pediatrics Committee on Infectious Diseases review of literature (technical report).	Streptococcus pneumoniae most common cause of a range of illness, including acute OM, in children. Children at increased risk of pneumococcal infections include healthy Native American (American Indian and Alaska Native) and African American children.
Bluestone (1998)	Review of literature.	Chronic suppurative otitis media (CSOM) is a problem in developing nations and in certain populations. Highest rates of CSOM found in Inuits of Alaska, Canada and Greenland, Australian Aboriginals, and certain Native American tribes.
Paradise, Rockette, Colborn, et al. (1997)	Large ($N = 2253$) prospective study of Western Pennsylvania children aged 2 months to 2 years.	Low socioeconomic status (SES) (estimated from the type of health insurance and maternal education) most important demographic factor associated with occurrence of OME.

Intervention

Children with moderate to profound SNHL are likely to be fitted with hearing aids and receive interventions such as SLT once hearing loss is identified (ASHA 2002b). Comparatively recent studies of profoundly deaf children with cochlear implants (CI) indicate significant improvements in pre-first-word vocalisations (Kishon-Rabin, Taitelbaum-Swead, Ezrati-Vinacour, et al. 2004), phonetic inventory (Blamey, Barry, and Jacq 2001), phoneme accuracy (Connor, Craig, Raudenbush, et al. 2006), phonological development (Doble 2006; Kim and Chin 2008), and speech intelligibility (Calmels, Saliba, Wanna, et al. 2004; Lejeune and Demanez 2006). Speech is, however, typically delayed by the period without sound, and speech errors persist in some children even when hearing loss is identified early and intervention occurs before 6–12 months of age. Peng, Weiss, Cheung, et al. (2004) reported that 6- to 12-year-old Mandarin-speaking CI users with approximately 2–6 years implant experience had fewest speech errors for plosives and most errors for nasals, affricates, fricatives, and the lateral approximant /l/. Blamey, Barry, and Jacq (2001) found a plateau in performance 5–6 years after implantation, with eight phones failing to attain a 50% criterion in five or more out of a group of nine children (/ɔɪ, ʊə, ʒ, t, s, z, tʃ, θ/).

Policies on intervention for mild hearing loss are less consistent than for more severe losses. In many countries, children with mild hearing loss may not receive any assistance, despite evidence for school difficulties in this population (Bess, Dodd-Murphy, and Parker 1998; Yoshinaga-Itano, Johnson, Carpenter, et al. 2008). Classroom amplification systems have been shown to improve learning outcomes in indigenous Australian children who are at high risk for OME and consequent hearing loss (Massie and Dillon 2006). The impact of these systems on speech has not been reported.

There are few published studies of SLP/SLT outcomes for children with hearing loss. One of the basic tenets of Auditory Verbal Therapy (AVT), a widely adopted therapy approach for children with SNHL which emphasises listening over looking, is that hearing loss should be identified early and optimal amplification should be provided to enhance access to the speech signal (Lim and Simser 2005). Optimising access to the speech signal is a key requirement for AVT. Hence, the distance between the child and the speaker is an important consideration (Lim and Simser 2005). Although AVT is widely promoted as a therapy approach for children with SNHL (Caleffe-Schenck 1992), Rhoades (2006) reviewed the outcomes of AVT research and concluded that there is little high-level evidence supporting AVT.

Paatsch, Blamey, Sarant, et al. (2006) demonstrated improvements in PCC, speech perception, and reading aloud after speech production training delivered by a teacher of the deaf to children with mild to profound hearing loss. Children were trained individually or in groups of two or three for 20 minutes each school day. This study also showed improvements in knowledge of word meanings, speech perception, and reading aloud after vocabulary training. For the reading aloud task, children read words presented randomly on a computer screen and were scored on the accuracy of their whole-word productions. Visual feedback has been a useful component of speech therapy with individuals with hearing loss. For example, Parsloe (1998) and Pantelemidou, Herman, and Thomas (2003) reported speech improvements in individual case studies of hearing-impaired children using electropalatography (EPG) therapy. Massaro and Light (2004) reported improved speech production that generalised to non-trained items after using a computer-animated talking head to train correct articulation in seven hearing-impaired children aged 8–13 years.

Ultrasound and EPG have also been used successfully in hearing-impaired adolescents and adults (Bernhardt, Gick, Bacsfalvi, et al. 2003; Bernhardt, Gick, Bacsfalvi, et al. 2005).

Communication and collaboration between SLPs/SLTs and audiologists

Although the role of the SLP/SLT has changed with improvements in both early identification and hearing technology, the need remains for ongoing speech therapy for many children with hearing loss. Although the relative risk of SSD across populations is unknown, differences in the incidence of otitis media (see Table A47.1) and SNHL indicate that there will be population differences affecting the need for SLP/SLT in children with hearing loss. In New Zealand, SNHL is more common in Pacific and Māori children than in children of European or Asian descent (Giles and O'Brien 1991; Greville 2007). Variations in infant and maternal health and vaccination programs, consanguinity, and other genetic factors contribute to population differences in SNHL (Bener, Eihakeem, and Abdulhadi 2005; Smith, Bale, and White 2005; Attias, Al-Masri, Abukader, et al. 2006).

Audiological assessment is always recommended for children with SSD, but it is particularly important for children with OME histories. Children with earlier onset of OME, more OME episodes, and poorer hearing thresholds are at greater risk for SSD. Timely referral to an otolaryngologist is recommended because more aggressive medical management may occur if there is speech delay or disorder combined with poor audiology results (Lous, Burton, Felding, et al. 2005). If a child has craniofacial abnormalities and/or a syndromal condition commonly associated with OME and/or SNHL (Golding-Kushner, A13; Ruscello, A42), management of the speech and hearing difficulties and ear health will require a close and ongoing partnership between professionals and families (Greig, Papesch, and Rowsell 1999; Shott, Joseph, and Heithaus 2001).

Research needs

Large-scale, prospective longitudinal studies are needed to determine the impact of OME on speech, using speech measures that are associated with longer term outcomes (Lewis, Shriberg, Freebairn, et al. 2006). Key variables that need to be considered in such studies include hearing thresholds, persistence of OME, treatment, risk factors (SES, ethnicity, language environment, etc.), and factors that predict the persistence of SSD, such as family history (Bishop, Price, Dale, et al. 2003). Little is known about the efficacy of different speech therapy approaches for children with moderate to profound hearing loss, and hence there is considerable need for large-scale, well-controlled studies in this area. There are no well-controlled studies of the effectiveness of AVT for SSD in hearing-impaired children. Given the widespread use of the AVT approach, there is a great need for further research to determine whether the listening focus of AVT is optimal, whether visual feedback alone or a combined approach might be better, or whether there are characteristics of individual children, such as differences in hearing loss and speech perception, that make them better suited for one therapy approach over another. With the advent of universal newborn hearing screening, most permanent SNHL should be identified early; however, some children with hearing loss who receive appropriate amplification from an early age have speech errors that persist. Further research is needed to determine reasons for this individual variability and optimal therapy approaches for these children.

Case illustration

Huia, 18;0, was born with bilateral profound deafness, diagnosed at 14 months, presumed due to recessive inheritance. She was fitted with high-powered hearing aids, which she ceased wearing after receiving a right-sided CI at 5;2. Her CI file indicates that, at implantation, she could sign 3- to 4-element phrases, finger spell place names and family names, and with prompts could produce a low-frequency long vowel, /b/, and /m/. Huia attended both a mainstream preschool and a preschool at a local school for deaf children. She continued at the school for deaf until 7;0, with 2 hours per week at a mainstream primary school, after which she was in a 'deaf unit' in a mainstream school from age 8–11 years, and in mainstream classrooms from 12-18 years, with weekly assistance from a Resource Teacher of the Deaf and a note-taker in high school for some academic subjects.

Huia used New Zealand Sign Language until she received her CI, and was introduced to spoken English only after implantation, starting to speak at 7;0. She received weekly habilitation with an SLT trained in AVT for 5 years after the CI, which focused on making a transition from full signing to becoming as oral as possible. The aim was to develop her auditory skills and her receptive and expressive language. When habilitation ceased, her file indicates that she could speak clearly and sign to her deaf peers, use lip reading, and utilise both syntactic and semantic information to identify or establish the meaning of unknown words.

Huia came to our clinic at 17;7, after 7 years with no direct SLT input. Pre-therapy standard scores for the *Comprehensive Assessment of Spoken Language* (Carrow-Woolfolk 1999) ranged from 67 to 101 (Total Score 80). Her scores for Synonyms, Inference, and Pragmatic Judgement subtests were below 80. Formal testing showed that she had speech recognition scores of 33% for words presented in noise at 5 decibels signal-to-noise ratio (a noise level that would be better than some classrooms). Huia described her difficulties as follows: 'Although I have pretty good results with my exams I find that going to school is hard because it is very noisy. It is hard for some of my friends to understand what I am saying and I sometimes don't know what they are talking about. The really embarrassing moments happen when I think I have understood somebody and then I realise by the look on their faces that I missed the point.'

Huia was assessed before and after 5 months of weekly therapy using an AVT approach. Post-therapy, CASL scores improved and ranged from 86 to 108. The biggest gain was in understanding 'inference', where her standard score improved from 67 to 87. Presumably this increase reflected a focus in therapy on word meanings, multiple meanings for a given word, and non-literal figurative language. Speech therapy focused on improving her ability to hear the different voice quality yielded by nasal versus oral voice projection. Her HAPP-3 (Hodson 2004) scores improved from 74.1% errors pre-therapy to 10.3% errors post-therapy, with significant reductions in speech errors involving nasalisation and cluster reduction. Huia improved her ability to listen, perceive errors in her own speech, listen to adult target models and then imitate them, but with limited generalisation to spontaneous conversation.

This enthusiastic, competent young woman received her CI at a later-than-optimum age. Despite this, she has developed intelligible speech and is now engaged in tertiary study with note-taker support. Huia has a supportive family and is highly motivated to improve her speech and listening skills. No doubt she would have benefited from ongoing habilitation after her CI, if this had been available to her. Unfortunately, because of limited availability of SLT resource to support children with hearing loss, Huia was discharged from therapy at a time when she would have benefited from ongoing input.

Acknowledgement

Thank you to Liz Fairgray and 'Huia' for their assistance with the case illustration.

Choices

The term 'best available evidence' is frequently taken to mean research-based knowledge, but as a process guiding intervention, EBP integrates a variety of data sources, including case studies by clinicians. The process also incorporates systematic ongoing education of professionals and informed involvement of clients, while taking account of systemic policies and procedures, and challenges in application, such as unduly large caseloads, personnel shortfalls, scarcity of material resources, and time constraints, necessitating many choices. In the hurly burly of practice, most choices in speech assessment and intervention incorporate elements of clinical thinking and clinical judgement, often involving that highly prized ingredient: clinical intuition. We know these phenomena, recognising that they occur somewhere between clinical observations and clinical decision-making, but they elude precise definition and are difficult, if not impossible, to teach. As clinicians making decisions, we rely on the evidence base, sound theory, and as much of 'the literature' as we can tackle in our full schedules, as well as client perspectives and our own insights and experiences. This is often in situations where time is limited, access is poor, data are missing or ambiguous, and there are competing long- and short-term trade-offs to contend with.

A Fellow of Speech Pathology Australia, Dr. Suze Leitão has a long-standing clinical and research interest in children with speech and literacy difficulties. She is a senior lecturer on the speech pathology course in the School of Psychology at Curtin University of Technology in Western Australia, and runs a small private practice specializing in children with spelling and reading difficulties. Her current research includes a longitudinal study of the development of phonological representations and literacy outcomes for a cohort of children with speech and language impairment. In recent years, her teaching in the areas of professional issues and clinical science have caused her to reflect on the mix of art and science involved in clinical decision-making in this age of EBP.

Q48. Suze Leitão: Clinical thinking

In the messy real world, manualised procedures and the science of therapy often have to give way to the art of therapy. But here's the rub: the so-called art has to be consistent with our moral frameworks, ethical codes, and 'the science'. Can you reflect on these issues in relation to children's speech and literacy difficulties?

A48.   Suze Leitão: Clinical decision-making: Art and science

Over the years of clinical practice, I have often had to reach out for help from mentors and peers when faced with a situation where I felt doing things 'by the book' was not the right thing to do. I have strong memories of a letter a mother sent me where she berated me at length for talking to her about her son's severe speech difficulties while he was in the room. As a young clinician, I had felt that describing the extent of his difficulties to him (aged 12) and his mother was the accurate and truthful way to give feedback and explain why I thought he needed therapy urgently at his age. Looking back, I now see that, whereas the objective data may have led me to a clinical decision regarding therapy based on evidence, which I explained as clearly as I could, there were a number of other issues I needed to consider. Consultation with professionals from other walks of life, such as psychology and family therapy, may have benefited my approach with this client, for example. Understanding the family dynamics and relationships may have influenced the way I approached the feedback session. And not only 'looking back at', but also 'reflecting on' the episode in order to make sense of it and try to understand it, allowed me to learn from it and incorporate this knowledge into my own developing clinical decision-making skills. Needless to say, I never saw the family again and do not know if he received treatment!

In my current role teaching clinical science to speech pathology students, I have even more cause to reflect on my own frameworks for decision-making. There is nothing better for sharpening the mind than teaching others! Unpacking the process and content of clinical decision-making in my role as a clinical educator and lecturer has opened my eyes to the complexity of what students often think we do seamlessly.

So what factors do we consider when we approach the task of making clinical decisions? Our own framework of morals and values is one place to start. For example, most, if not all, cultures place value on telling the truth. Our professional codes of ethics are another very useful guide. For example, the Speech Pathology Australia code of ethics, an aspirational framework, places strong emphasis on truth, balancing doing good with not causing harm, fairness, and autonomy. The law and our legal responsibilities to our clients and our profession provide us with another key set of principles. And this is all before we get to the evidence base for our profession, our theoretical underpinnings, and the data we collect! So clinical decision-making should really be quite easy then? Giving advice to families and clients a piece of cake? Just a matter of creating some decision-making trees with yes/no junctions and procedural manuals, and always sticking to the 'truth'?

Well, no, not really.

Unfortunately the world is a messy place. To a large extent, clinical decision-making in its moral, ethical, and legal frameworks is about relationships and context. Clinical decision-making requires us to analyse and interpret—to combine science with art, yet still maintain our professional integrity and do the right thing by our clients.

In one place where I used to work, children were not considered eligible for services if they were considered to have 'dyspraxia' (CAS), as the educational policy of the time was that this somewhat controversial condition did not affect language development. The term 'phonological disorder', on the other hand, or 'speech and language disorder', was acceptable! So how would a diagnostic decision tree help me decide what was the 'truth' to put in my reports?

What about the times I have made a decision not to put a particular finding or test result in a report? Sometimes a decontextualised test result may show strengths not reflected in real-life performance or vice versa. What about the times when I have had a diagnosis or 'label' in my head, collected enough data to confirm this, yet did not use the label? Would putting these in writing just muddy the waters when read by another professional, who may have decision-making powers? Does leaving it out represent the truth?

'David', 6;6, came to see me on the recommendation of his teacher. He presented with severe and complex speech difficulties. His parents felt treatment would be a waste of time because he would grow out of it, eventually achieving intelligible speech under his own steam. Based on my assessment, the evidence directed me to choose non-stimulable, later developing more complex targets. However, I felt I needed to demonstrate that my treatment could produce change quickly so I selected a stimulable, earlier developing sound that was not really impacting on his intelligibility. Although this didn't draw on the evidence base for effective and efficient therapy, David learned this quickly and his parents decided that they would keep coming (for a while anyway)!

Parents of children with severe and persistent speech and literacy difficulties often contact me for advice regarding 'cures' they have read about in the papers or seen on the television or Internet. Many of these programs are expensive and involve signing a contract for a substantial fee and time frame. Some of these push a scientific or pseudoscientific approach, whereas others rely heavily on testimonials. I was recently contacted by a family who had embarked on such a program and rang me after 6 weeks to tell me that they had seen some progress but were finding the payments difficult and couldn't decide whether to continue or try and get their money back. What to say? There was little solid research behind the program, but the family had not seen much progress with more traditional therapy. As Powell (A34, p. 199) puts it: the use of controversial treatments is not prohibited by most codes of professional ethics, but to be ethical in our practice we need to balance beneficence with non-maleficence (do good and not do harm). Like Stoeckel (A35, p. 215), I wondered how I could provide them with a variety of resources and help them evaluate the program yet remain supportive and respectful of their choices. I had to acknowledge that they had already spent a large sum of money that they wouldn't get back and that they might be up for more payments whatever their choice, to continue or withdraw. This kind of investment does tend to bias one's evaluation of progress!

The evidence base for our profession is lacking, there is no doubt (Rosenthal, A49). But we do have a growing basis to support our clinical practice and our clinical decision-making. We must treat every client in a scientific manner: gather our data and analyse them carefully. I recommend that SLPs/SLTs carefully consider the evidence you do have, but interpret it within the wider context that includes client-, family-, clinician- and even wider, maybe agency- or service-related factors and frameworks. Set up hypotheses that match your clinical evidence, but don't ignore those intuitive hunches! Reflect on, and learn from, those messy real-life clinical contexts that we work in. The outcomes of our decisions may not be what we expect and this may, or may not, be a bad thing. What is important, is that we learn from them and continue to develop our clinical decision-making skills whether we are student, novice, or experienced.

To re-iterate, our clinical decision-making may well involve a mix of scientific objective facts and artistic subjective interpretations. That is the real world of decision-making.

However, every decision we make will be framed by our own personal and professional moral and ethical codes and life experience and must be consistent with that.

Electronic communication with each other

Clinical thinking, decision-making, and access to the evidence base have been enhanced by the development of e-mail, the Internet, and the availability of discussion groups, listservs, and other electronic mailing lists (Bowen 2003). Even so, nowhere is the complexity of keeping up with the child speech field more evident than in the extensive discussion that takes place on the phonologicaltherapy list (Bowen 2001). There, some of the frequently asked questions expose the confusion, concern, and even embarrassment of highly trained professionals from around the world who do not feel they have a working grasp of recent applications of research to assessment and therapy. Encouragingly, however, the list's posts *also* tell a lot about the eagerness of the participating academics to appreciate the workaday reality of clinicians, and vice versa. Professional Internet discussions around the management of SSD also tend to showcase a lack of information literacy among participants (Bowen 2003), with practitioners preferring the best available (anecdotal) advice of colleagues and mentors over current, published, best available evidence. They reveal the tendency to habitually turn to old favourite, well-thumbed texts, handouts from continuing professional development (CPD) or continuing education unit (CEU) events, and Google or other search-engine and Internet 'finds' for elucidation.

The Association of Speech and Language Therapists in Independent Practice (ASLTIP) provides information on independent SLT throughout the UK and supports members of the RCSLT who are in independent practice. The majority of its members work with children and child speech and language issues. ASLIP has a members-only discussion group of approximately 350 members and 3 list moderators. Observation of 8,000 of the group's messages from June 2004 to June 2008, with an eye to the styles of online peer support provided relative to child speech topics, was made possible by the ASLTIP executive and members agreeing, by popular vote, to this surveillance. Approximately 20% of all posts related to SSD. An exhaustive list of the SSD-related topics raised over the 4 years comprises: auditory discrimination, backing, blocks and breaks attendance schedules, Bowen (1998a, b, 2001), case discussion, cleft lip and palate, Colour Coding; Core Vocabulary Therapy, cued articulation, DEAP, education and videoconferencing, glottal insertion, glue ear, horns and straws therapy, hyponasality, intelligibility, Johansen Sound Therapy, lateral-s, Makaton, materials and book recommendations, Metaphon, minimal pairs word lists, mouth gym exercises, NDP3, older dyspraxic children, oral motor muscle-based therapy, oro-motor work, PACT, PROMPT, palatal-s, pictures, phonetic placement and stimulability, phonological awareness, phonology work, psychological effects of phonological delay, 'recipe' speech therapy (cookbook therapy), reducing speech rate, SATPAC, STAP assessment, self-monitoring, suck-swallow-breathe, TalkTools, TalkTools support group, The Listening Programme, the phonologicaltherapy group, the role of SENCOs, the role of Speech Therapy aides, SpeechLink, TinyEYE, tongue tie, tongue exercises, VPD and nasal emission, velar fronting, video-teleconferencing, voicing errors, vowel therapy, word lists, worksheets, and verbal dyspraxia. The most frequent SSD topics were around Bowen (1998a), Cued Articulation, Johansen Sound Therapy [one of the Auditory Integration Therapies that ASHA (2004d) has cautioned against], phonetic placement and stimulability techniques, oromotor work, and Talk-Tools. Many therapy approaches (e.g., the Psycholinguistic framework and Phoneme Awareness Therapy) and EBP were not mentioned; bibliographic citations were infrequent and uniformly incomplete. Except for condemnation of the SpeechLink methodology and concerns over the adequacy of the STAP articulation test (see Table 2.6, p. 59) being administered by aides, all suggestions to employ untested approaches, such as Sound Therapy and NS-OMT, and to attend related training events were accepted uncritically. Questions and advice tended to focus on intervention, particularly in the form of 'therapy tips', with little discussion devoted to assessment, target selection, therapy approach selection, or goal setting. Advice was often given based on minimal client information. As with most professional electronic mailing lists, only a small proportion of subscribers actually posted, with about 12 individuals providing answers to SSD questions on a regular basis. Overall, the 'tone' of the ASLTIP discussion group was supportive, friendly, informal, and 'safe'. As a discussion group not specifically set up to focus on SSD, the ASLTIP mailing list appears to be quite representative. Levels of discussion are similar on Desiree Rusch-Winterbottom's Yahoo group (http://www.health.groups.yahoo.com/group/SLPtalk/) with a lot of peer support, and much enthusiasm for non-evidence-based approaches such as NS-OMT. There is emphasis on EBP on the ASHA SID1 listserv, but very little discussion of SSD, and to date never in-depth. There is probably more SSD-related support for SLPs/SLTs seeking help on the consumer-oriented Apraxia-KIDS listserv and message boards (Gretz, A7) than there is on any of the 'professional' forums mentioned in this paragraph.

By contrast, the phonologicaltherapy group (Bowen 2001) is devoted to professional discussion of child speech development and disorders and related issues, such as literacy acquisition. Established by the author in December 2001, its international membership of speech-language professionals, linguists, students, and consumers (who mainly observe discussions) exceeds 5,000 at the time of writing, increasing at the current rate of approximately 500 every 6 months. Participants are from 74 countries: including the Arab Emirates, Argentina, Australia, Bahrain, Bangladesh, Belgium, Bosnia and Herzegovina, Brazil, Brunei Darussalam, Cameroon, Canada, Chile, Colombia, Croatia, Cyprus, Denmark, Egypt, Estonia the Falkland Islands, Finland, France, Germany, Ghana, Gibraltar, Greece, Hong Kong, Hungary, Iceland, India, Indonesia, Iran, Iraq, Ireland, Israel, Italy, Japan, Jordan, the Republic of Korea, Kyrgyzstan, Lebanon, Malaysia, Malta, Mexico, the Netherlands, New Zealand, Niue, Norway, Pakistan, Palestine, the People's Republic of China, the Philippines, Poland, Portugal, Qatar, the Republic of China (Taiwan), Romania, the Russian Federation, Saudi Arabia, Singapore, South Africa, Spain, Sri Lanka, Sweden, Switzerland, Syria, Tanzania, Turkey, Tuvalu, the UK, the United Arab Emirates, the USA, Yemen, Yugoslavia and Zimbabwe. Over half the membership of phonologicaltherapy (58.74%) comprises SLPs from the US.

In the last 4 years, the volume of posts per month has ranged from 56 to 410 with a mean of a little over 200 per month. Discussions tend to be focused on SSD, covering a broad range of clinical, theoretical, and empirical topics across the areas of phonetic, phonemic, structural, and motor speech disorders. Although the list maintains a clinical focus, addressing topics of current interest in clinical phonology, it also addresses controversial topics. For the most part, an evidence-based perspective is maintained, and at the same time, clinicians are encouraged by the list-owner and other members (including fellow clinicians) to establish practice-based evidence for accountability and quality assurance.

In general, the mood is collegial and supportive, but debate can be fiery at times, and there is the odd post in which someone begs forgiveness for stating their case undiplomatically! Exchanges between academics, between clinicians, and between academics and clinicians are especially interesting and helpful, and in general, the group provides a useful resource, peer support, and opportunities for learning. By fostering communication between clinicians, student clinicians, and researchers, the reach of information is expanded not only to 'places' outside the classroom, but also across linguistic and cultural boundaries. The list is a powerful resource for educators and students as well as clinicians. In fact, several university faculty members from at least 13 countries (e.g., Australia, Canada, Egypt, Eire, India, Israel, Korea, Malaysia, New Zealand, South Africa, Taiwan, the UK, and the USA) include the phonologicaltherapy list in their course syllabi and require students to audit and critically appraise list interchanges and resources when discussing them in class. Information obtained from the lists is cited in lectures, workshops, and books. It has proven to be an innovative instructional tool that reaches a far wider audience than any other professional medium.

Web site

In the early stages of establishing *speech-language-therapy dot com* (Bowen 1998b), there was huge and problematic variation in the standards of content of the Web sites purporting to represent our profession on the international stage (Bowen 2003). Of particular concern was the quality of information for consumers, students, and professionals about children's SSDs. Although there was some information of an exceptionally high standard, much was inaccurate, simplistic, badly written, difficult to locate, and rarely adequately referenced. As well, controversial practices (Duchan, Calculator, Sonnenmeier, et al. 2001) were often presented misleadingly, and dubious treatments were prominently represented, with slick Web sites touting untested cures and products. Unfortunately, little has changed.

Here was an irresistible challenge, begging a problem-based learning approach. Instead of starting with a particular aspect of information and communication technology (ICT), such as building a Web site, and then designing content to fit it, the site started with goals that allowed for a variety of technology uses throughout its implementation. The overriding goal was to get key information from the research evidence base 'out there'. In the process, challenges were met, new friendships forged, research networks expanded, and novel and useful skills gained.

Our professional knowledge base and skills in oral and written communication, coupled with a little study, hands-on practice and peer support mean that motivated SLPs/SLTs are perfectly poised to play their part in harnessing the Net for our profession. Using problem-based strategies, and understanding that we are tackling an international medium, we can critically and systematically evaluate Web resources, improve what is there, and fill the gaps we find. The effects of doing so are potentially far-reaching in terms of improving heath information delivery. The essence of the task is to think in terms of creating an exemplary, global, SLP/SLT 'Web presence' that the profession can celebrate.

No one need 'own' such a project. Just as the Internet has no central headquarters, no regulatory body overseeing its content, no ethics committee, and no censor, once an agreed blueprint based on existing codes of ethics and standards of practice was set up, self-assessed contributions could come from the pooled resources of national associations, educational institutions (faculty and students), practitioners working singly or in groups, consumer advocates, and experts in a variety of communication disorders and ICT-related fields (Bowen 2003). The Internet influences our world-view and the way we practice. It changes the way we communicate and alters our language irretrievably, inspiring new words, and new meanings for old words. One of the new words, 'networking', is used popularly to refer to the establishing of communication links with other people as a means of exchanging ideas and information. The challenge for our profession in harnessing the Net is to become international networkers, focused on quality of client care, in the common goal of creating a Web presence worthy of personal and professional pride, and universal recognition.

Survival and progress

In 2007, when the author's contemporary B. May Bernhardt received Q32 and an early draft of Chapter 5, she was on sabbatical leave, far from her office in Vancouver. Although not in work mode, she responded almost immediately by e-mail: 'Caroline – Thanks for trying with this book. I don't expect it will change the world like most books don't, but it at least gets at the knowledge translation issue . . . which is key if we are to advance the field a tiny centimetre before we retire.' The word 'retire' prompted a 2002 memory of lively dinner conversation at Lassaters Casino, Alice Springs, central Australia, when she told of relishing the prospect of retirement. Among others at the table were Sharynne McLeod (A1), Peter Flipsen, Jr. (A10), Roslyn Neilson (A17), Nicole Watts Pappas (A25), Tom Powell (A34), Deb James (A44), and John Bernthal (A46). Perhaps each person thought fleetingly about retirement before the conversation changed direction, and maybe there were others at the table who thought for a moment of Joan Rosenthal and other colleagues who *had* retired.

Already a highly regarded authority in SLP/SLT clinical and academic circles when the author began practice in Sydney, Australia in 1971, Joan Rosenthal was *the* person to ask for help with knotty child speech cases. She was variously referred to as a role model, an expert, the oracle, and a guru—but always unassuming, she never behaved like a celebrity SLP! Theory-related and steeped in years of practical experience, her therapy approach to CAS and other developmental speech sound problems was always 'find what works with the individual child'. That was the evidence base that she trusted, stressing that 'what works' of course could change for an individual over time. It seems a satisfactory and rather neat way to round off this work that the first person the author ever consulted for a second opinion, with dozens of questions, should be the person to answer the last question here so many years later.

Q49. Joan Rosenthal: Resiliance in the workplace

Change and progress are frequent words for clinical SLPs/SLTs in their pursuit of effective, efficient, and efficacious management for each child with an SSD. All too frequently the quest takes place in work environments that are impacted by political apathy, misguided public policy, funding shortfalls, unstable levels of staffing, unmanageable waiting lists, and too little time. And as you have pointed out, another sort of change that clinicians have to deal with is that children with the more severe speech problems have long-term support and intervention needs that alter as they grow older and their conditions unfold. All this is set against the background of an information explosion in the peer-reviewed print and electronic media that leaves most of us reeling and unable to keep apace. And yet there is something that drives us to persevere: the intellectual and practical challenge, or the perceived needs of the client that require our special expertise, or the wish to help, or our compulsion to play out the professional role. Or maybe it is to do with our personal perspective and the sheer fascination with the task at hand. As the American author Henry Miller (1891–1980) said, 'The moment one gives close attention to anything, even a blade of grass, it becomes a mysterious, awesome, indescribably magnificent world in itself.' What do you think, and what would be in your survival kit for clinicians and clinical educators as they tackle the complex working world of children's SSDs?

A49. Joan Rosenthal: Key components of a survival kit: Theory, evidence, and experience

Caroline, and readers,

The first point I'd like to make is that our professional evidence base is sketchy, although it's constantly developing. Still, there's not yet enough science in our knowledge of SSDs, our understanding of what is behind them, and our certainty about how we can effectively and efficaciously help children and their families through them, to rely on the published evidence base for our therapy. The same applies to knowing how and what to assess. But the limitations in our published evidence base don't mean that, as clinicians, we work in the dark in intervention. Every piece of intervention we apply is an experiment and needs to be treated as such. Do we continue? Is it working? Can we build on it? Do we need to look at the presenting problem from another angle entirely? The client's response provides the evidence. So my survival kit would contain my theoretical knowledge (continually built on by what you dramatically and accurately describe as the information explosion) hitched to my senses: what I see, hear, and intuit from my client. This indeed provides fascination with the clinical task at hand: selecting from choices about what to do, interpreting what we observe by way of response from our clients, and making further choices about what to do next.

My second point is that, not uniquely among the health professions, SLP/SLT can be beset by fads. The longer you are in this profession and working with SSD, the more you'll be exposed to our fads. They are part and parcel of the information explosion, and they are also a response to our lack of evidence-based knowledge. They come; they sweep away what has gone before; they are adopted with enthusiasm and often with expense. They spawn workshops, continuing education, even certification, sometimes research. And after a while, the next fad arrives. Experience of a succession of fads can give rise to some cynicism, but in a survival kit, I would prefer to find some healthy skepticism.

What relates these two topics: the limited evidence base and the succession of fads in intervention? There in the middle is the here-and-now: the client's behaviour and our response to it, and our behaviour and the client's response to it. Our here-and-now observation provides evidence (that can be linked to the published evidence base and that can inform our reaction to the current fad).

The third item in my survival kit would be a reminder message that flashes on an internal screen: value experience. One's individual and growing experience is a further source of evidence. I remember after my first year of practice as a speech therapist (as it was then in Australia) thinking: 'I've learned more in this year than I did in all the years of my training'. That was not an indictment of my course of study. Indeed, my course of study prepared me to be an independent learner, to be a perceptive and critical observer of my own therapy. The result was that my clinical experience provided me with a stream of evidence and a concomitant stream of questions. Look how this works! Why didn't that work? What if. . .? Experience hones one's skills as a clinician, develops wisdom as well as knowledge.

The final item in my survival kit is an understanding that the development of expertise is a two-way street. There is an obligation to share such wisdom as we have acquired, and to learn from what others can contribute. Consider how you can do this. It may be by mentorship, by sharing with colleagues, by brainstorming over clinical problems, by writing, by teaching. It may also be by asking questions, by expressing ignorance, by acknowledging feelings of uncertainty and need for support. I'll confess that it was a weakness of mine, especially as a fairly recent graduate, to try to give the impression that I knew everything—doubtless from fear that someone would discover how little I did know! But it helps to realise that we have a community of wisdom. Value it and be part of it.

Conclusion

As students, clinicians, clinical educators, academics and researchers in our funny, quirky, specialised world of children with SSD, and their families, we are all workers, thinkers, and life-long learners. Our work, thinking and learning with this fascinating, rewarding, challenging, engaging, and sometimes frustrating population often meets the four critical criteria of all problem-based learning tasks. The problems we face are open-ended with no 'right' answers and no single route to solutions. The problems are authentic, related to real life. They are complex, involving a variety of skills, a breadth of content, and depth of thought. And they are open to self-assessment, so that we learners can determine for ourselves what work we must do in order to advance to more expert levels of performance. I hope this book will help.

References

ASHA (1990). *Guidelines for screening for hearing impairment and middle ear disorders. ASHA,* 32 (Supp1 2), 17–24.

ASHA (1994). *Continuing Education Board Manual.* Rockville, MD: ASHA.

ASHA (2001). *Scope of Practice in Speech-Language Pathology.* Retrieved December 29, 2007 from http://www.asha.org/NR/rdonlyres/4FDEE27B-BAF5-4D06-AC4D-8D1F311C1B06/0/19446_1.pdf.

ASHA (2002a). *Ph.D. Program Survey Report.* Retrieved December 19, 2007 from: http://www.asha.org/members/phd-faculty-research/reports/phd_survey_sum.html.

ASHA (2002b). *Guidelines for audiology service provision in and for schools* [Guidelines]. Available from: http://www.asha.org/policy

ASHA (2004a). *American Speech-Language-Hearing Association 2004 Schools survey report: Caseload characteristics.* Rockville, MD: ASHA.

ASHA (2004b). *Preferred Practice Patterns for the Profession of Speech-Language Pathology.* Retrieved July 31, 2007 from: http://www.asha.org/docs/html/PP2004-00191.html.

ASHA (2004c). *Evidence-based practice in communication disorders* (Position Statement). Retrieved February 1, 2008 from: http://www.asha.org/NR/rdonlyres/B1DF75A7-83A0-4F78-8A09-4113139CE5CE/0/JCCEBPReport04.pdf.

ASHA (2004d). *Auditory Integration Training* [Technical Report]. Retrieved March 5, 2009 from: http://www.asha.org/policy.

ASHA (2004–2007). *Focused Initiatives.* Retrieved January 2, 2008 from: http://www.asha.org/about/leadership-projects/national-office/focused-initiatives.html.

ASHA (2005). *Evidence-based practice in communication disorders* [Position Statement]. Retrieved March 5, 2009 from: http://www.asha.org/members/deskref-journals.

ASHA (2006a). *Focused initiative: evidence-based practice.* Retrieved July 13, 2007 from: http://www.asha.org/members/ebp/.

ASHA (2006b). *2006 Schools Survey Report: Caseload Characteristics.* Rockville, MD: ASHA.

ASHA (2007a). *Childhood Apraxia of Speech* [Position Statement]. Retrieved February 25, 2008 from: http://www.asha.org/policy.

ASHA (2007b). *Childhood Apraxia of Speech* [Technical Report]. Retrieved February 25, 2008 from: http://www.asha.org/docs/html/TR2007-00278.html.

ASHA (n.d.). *Questions for consumers to ask about products or procedures for hearing, balance, speech, language, swallowing, and related disorders.* Retrieved December 29, 2007 from: http://asha.org/public/speech/consumerqa.htm.

Abrahamsen, E., & Flack, L. (2002, November). Do sensory and motor techniques improve accurate phoneme production? Paper presented at the *American Speech-Language-Hearing Association Annual Convention*, Atlanta, GA.

Adams, M. J., Treiman, R., & Pressley, M. (1996). Reading, writing and literacy. In I. Sigel and A. Renninger (Eds). *Handbook of Child Psychology, Volume 4: Child Psychology in Practice.* New York, NY: Wiley.

...ck, M., Bernhardt, B., Gick, B., & Bacsfalvi, P. (2007). The use of ultrasound in remedi-
...of North American English /r/ in 2 adolescents. *American Journal of Speech – Language
...ology*, *16*, 128–140.

...-Mediavilla, E. M., Sanz-Torrent, M., & Serra-Raventos, M. (2002). A comparative study
...the phonology of pre-school children with specific language impairment (SLI), language
...ay (LD) and normal acquisition. *Clinical Linguistics & Phonetics*, *16*(8), 573–596.

Air, D. H., Wood, A. S., & Neils, J. R. (1989). Considerations for organic disorders. In N. A. Creaghead, P. W. Newman, and W. A. Secord (Eds). *Assessment and Remediation of Articulatory and Phonological Disorders* (2nd Edition). Columbus, OH: Merrill Publishing Company, pp. 265–301.

Allport, G. (1924). *Social Psychology*. Boston, MA: Houghton-Mifflin Co.

Almost, D., & Rosenbaum, P. (1998). Effectiveness of speech intervention for phonological disorders: A randomized control trial. *Developmental Medicine & Child Neurology*, *40*(5), 319–325.

Alton, J. (1949, republished 1995). *Painting with Light*. Berkeley, CA: University of California Press.

American Psychiatric Association. (1994). *Diagnostic and Statistical Manual of Mental Disorders* (4th Edition). Washington, DC: APA.

Andrews, N., & Fey, M. E. (1986). Analysis of the speech of phonologically impaired children in two sampling conditions. *Language, Speech, and Hearing Services in Schools*, *17*, 187–198.

Anthony, A., Bogle, D., Ingram, T. T. S., & McIsaac, M. W. (1971). *Edinburgh Articulation Test*. Edinburgh: Churchill Livingstone.

Anthony, J. L., & Lonigan, C. J. (2004). The nature of phonological awareness: Converging evidence from four studies of preschool and early grade school children. *Journal of Educational Psychology*, *96*, 43–55.

Apel, K. (1999). Checks and balances: Keeping the science in our profession. *American Journal of Speech-Language Pathology*, *30*, 98–107.

Apel, K., & Self, T. (2003). Evidence-based practice: The marriage of research and clinical service. *The ASHA Leader*, *8*(16), 6–7.

Apraxia-kids.org (2004). A Comparison of Childhood Apraxia of Speech, Dysarthria, and Severe Phonological Disorder. Retrieved March 20, 2008 from: http://www.apraxia-kids.org/site/c.chKMI0PIIsE/b.980831/apps/s/content.asp?ct=464135.

Aram, D. M., & Hall, N. E. (1989). Longitudinal follow-up of children with preschool communication disorders: Treatment implications. *School Psychology Review*, *18*, 487–501.

Arlt, P. B., & Goodban, M. J. (1976). A comparative study of articulation acquisition as based on a study of 240 normals, aged three to six. *Language, Speech, and Hearing Services in Schools*, *7*, 173–180.

Armstrong, S., & Ainley, M. (1988). *The South Tyneside Assessment of Phonology*. Northumberland: Stass Publications.

Armstrong, S., & Ainley, M. (1992). *The South Tyneside Assessment of Phonology* (2nd Edition). Northumberland: Stass Publications.

Arvedson, J., Clark, H., Frymark, T., et al. (2007, November). The effectiveness of oral-motor exercises: An evidence-based systematic review. *Paper presented at the American Speech-Language-Hearing Association Annual Convention*, Boston, MA.

Attias, J., Al-Masri, M., Abukader, L., et al. (2006). The prevalence of congenital and early-onset hearing loss in Jordanian and Israeli infants. *International Journal of Audiology*, *45*(9), 528–536.

Austin, D., & Shriberg, L. D. (1996). *Lifespan reference data for ten measures of articulation competence using the Speech Disorders Classification System (SDCS)* (Tech. Rep. No. 3). Phonology Project, Waisman Center, University of Wisconsin-Madison.

Norms

Bahr, D. C. (2001). *Oral Motor Assessment and Treatment: Ages and Stages*. Boston, MA: Allyn and Bacon.

Bailey, D. B., McWilliam, P., & Winton, P. J. (1992). Building family-centred practices in early intervention: A team-based model for change. *Infants and Young Children, 5*(1), 73–82.

Bain, B. (1994). A framework for dynamic assessment in phonology: Stimulability revisited. *Clinics in Communication Disorders, 4*(1), 12–22.

Bain, B. A., & Dollaghan, C. A. (1991). The notion of clinically significant change. *Language, Speech, and Hearing Services in Schools, 22,* 264–270.

Bain, B. A., & Olswang, L. B. (1995). Examining Readiness for Learning two-word utterances by children with specific expressive language impairment: Dynamic assessment validation. *American Journal of Speech-Language Pathology, 4*(1), 81–91.

Baker, E. (2000). *Changing nail to snail: A treatment efficacy study of phonological impairment in children*. Unpublished PhD thesis, University of Sydney, Sydney.

Baker, E. (2004). Phonological analysis, summary and management plan. *ACQuiring Knowledge in Speech, Language and Hearing, 6*(1), 14–21.

Baker, E. (2006). Management of speech impairment in children: The journey so far and the road ahead. *Advances in Speech-Language Pathology, 8*(3), 156–163.

Baker, E. (2007). Using sonority to explore patterns of generalisation in children with phonological impairment. Paper presented at the *Speech Pathology Australia National Conference*, Sydney, Australia.

Baker, E., & Bernhardt, B. (2004). From hindsight to foresight: working around barriers to success in phonological intervention. *Child Language Teaching and Therapy, 20*(3), 287–318.

Baker, E., Carrigg, B., & Linich, A. (2007). What's the evidence for... the cycles approach to phonological intervention? *ACQuiring Knowledge in Speech, Language and Hearing, 9*(1), 29–31.

Baker, E., Croot, K., McLeod, S., & Paul, R. (2001). Tutorial paper: Psycholinguistic models of speech development and their application to clinical practice. *Journal of Speech, Language, and Hearing Research, 44,* 685–702.

Baker, E., & McLeod, S. (2004). Evidence-based management of phonological impairment in children. *Child Language Teaching and Therapy, 20*(3), 265–285.

Baldwin, D. A., & Markham, E. M. (1989). Establishing word-object relations: A first step. *Child Development, 60,* 381–398.

Ball, L., Beukelman, D., & Bernthal, J. (November, 1999). Communication Characteristics of Children with DAS. Poster presented to the *American Speech-Language-Hearing Association Convention*, San Francisco, CA.

Ball, M. J. (2007). Articulatory foundations of speech acquisition. In S. McLeod (Ed). *The International Guide to Speech Acquisition*. Clifton Park, NY: Thomson Delmar Learning.

Ball, M. J., & Gibbon, F. E. (2002). *Vowel Disorders*. Woburn, MA: Butterworth-Heinemann.

Ball, M. J., & Kent, R. D. (Eds). (1997). *The New Phonologies: Developments in Clinical Linguistics*. San Diego, CA: Singular.

Bandura, A. (1994). Self-efficacy. In V. S. Ramachaudran (Ed). *Encyclopedia of Human Behavior, Vol. 4)*. New York: Academic Press, pp. 71–81. [Reprinted in H. Friedman (Ed). *Encyclopedia of Mental Health*. San Diego, CA: Academic Press, 1998.]

Bankson, N. W., & Bernthal, J. E. (2004). Treatment approaches. In J. E. Bernthal and N. W. Bankson (Eds). *Articulation and Phonological Disorders* (5th Edition). Boston, MA: Allyn and Bacon, pp. 292–347.

Barlow J. A. (2001) Recent advances in phonological theory and treatment [Special Issue]. *Language, Speech, and Hearing Services in Schools, 32,* 225–298.

Barlow, J. A. (2002) Recent advances in phonological theory and treatment, Part II [Special issue]. *Language, Speech, and Hearing Services in Schools, 33,* 4–69.

Barlow, J. A., & Gierut, J. A. (2002). Minimal pair approaches to phonological remediation. *Seminars in Speech and Language*, 2(1), 57–67.

Barr, J., McLeod, S., & Daniel, G. (2008). Siblings of children with communication impairments: Cavalry on the hill. *Language, Speech, and Hearing Services in Schools*, 39(1), 21–32.

Bashir, A., Grahamjones, F., & Bostwick, R. (1984). A touch-cue method of therapy for developmental verbal apraxia. *Seminars in Speech and Language*, 5(2), 127–128.

Bates, S. A. R., Watson, J. M. M., & Scobbie, J. M. (2002). Context-conditioned error patterns in disordered systems. In M. J. Ball & F. E. Gibbon (Eds). *Vowel Disorders* Woburn, MA: Butterworth-Heinemann, pp. 145–185.

Bauman-Waengler, J. (2004). *Articulatory and Phonological Impairments: a Clinical Focus* (2nd Edition). Boston, MA: Allyn and Bacon.

Bazyk, S. (1989). Changes in attitudes and beliefs regarding parent participation and home programs: An update. *The American Journal of Occupational Therapy*, 43(11), 723–728.

Beckman, D. A., Neal, C. D., Phirsichbaum, J. L., Stratton, L. J., Taylor, V. D., & Ratusnik, D. (2004). Range of movement and strength in oral motor therapy: A retrospective study. *Florida Journal of Communication Disorders*, 21, 7–14.

Bell, A. M. (1849). *A new elucidation of the principles of speech and elocution.* Published by the author.

Bell, A. M. (1886). *Essays and Postscripts on Elocution.* New York, NY: E. S. Werner.

Bener, A., Eihakeem, A. A., & Abdulhadi, K. (2005). Is there any association between consanguinity and hearing loss. *International Journal of Pediatric Otorhinolaryngology*, 69(3), 327–333.

Bennet, T., Zhang, C., & Hojnar, L. (1998). Facilitating the full participation of culturally diverse families in the IFSP/IEP process. *Infant-Toddler Intervention. The Transdisciplinary Journal*, 8(3), 227–249.

Benson, D. F., Dobkin, B. H., & Gonzalez, L. J. (1994). Assessment: Melodic intonation therapy. Report of the therapeutics and technology assessment subcommittee of the American Academy of Neurology. *Neurology*, 44, 566–568.

Berners-Lee, T. (2002). The World Wide Web - Past Present and Future: Exploring universality. *Japan Prize Commemorative Lecture.* Retrieved July 12, 2007 from: http://www.w3.org/2002/04/Japan/Lecture.html.

Bernhardt, B. (1990). *Application of nonlinear phonological theory to intervention with six phonologically disordered children.* Unpublished doctoral dissertation, University of British Columbia.

Bernhardt, B. (1992). The application of nonlinear phonological theory to intervention. *Clinical Linguistics & Phonetics*, 6, 283–316.

Bernhardt, B. (2004). Introduction to the Issue: Maximizing success in phonological intervention. *Child Language Teaching and Therapy*, 20, 195–198.

Bernhardt, B. (2005). Selection of phonological goals and targets: Not just an exercise in phonological analysis. In A. Kamhi and K. Pollock (Eds). *Phonological Disorders in Children: Clinical Decision-Making in Assessment and Intervention.* Baltimore, MD: Paul H. Brookes, pp. 109–120.

Bernhardt, B., Brooke, M., & Major, E. (2003). Acquisition of structure versus features in nonlinear phonological intervention. Poster presented at the Child Phonology Conference, UBC, July 2003, Vancouver, BC, Canada.

Bernhardt, B., Gick, B., Bacsfalvi, P., & Adler-Bock, M. (2005). Ultrasound in speech therapy with adolescents and adults. *Clinical Linguistics & Phonetics*, 19(6–7), 605–617.

Bernhardt, B., Gick, B., Bacsfalvi, P., & Ashdown, J. (2003). Speech habilitation of hard of hearing adolescents using electropalatography and ultrasound as evaluated by trained listeners. *Clinical Linguistics & Phonetics*, 17(3), 199–216.

Bernhardt, B., & Gilbert, J. (1992). Applying linguistic theory to speech-language pathology: The case for nonlinear phonology. *Clinical Linguistics & Phonetics*, 6, 123–145.

Bernhardt, B., Gilbert, J., & Ingram, D. (Eds). (1996). *Proceedings of the UBC International Conference on Phonological Acquisition.* Somerville, MA: Cascadilla Press.

Bernhardt, B., & Holdgrafer, G. (2001a). Beyond the Basics I: The need for strategic sampling for in-depth phonological analysis. *Language, Speech, and Hearing Services in Schools, 32,* 18–27.

Bernhardt, B., & Holdgrafer, G. (2001b). Beyond the Basics II: Supplemental sampling for in-depth phonological analysis. *Language, Speech, and Hearing Services in Schools, 32,* 28–37.

Bernhardt, B. & Major, E. (2005). Speech, language and literacy skills 3 years later: a follow-up study of early phonological and metaphonological intervention. *International Journal of Language & Communication Disorders, 40*(1), 1–27.

Bernhardt, B., & Stemberger, J. P. (1998). *Handbook of Phonological Development from the Perspective of Constraint-based Nonlinear Phonology.* San Diego, CA: Academic Press.

Bernhardt, B., & Stemberger, J. P. (2000). *Workbook in Nonlinear Phonology for Clinical Application.* Austin, TX: Pro-Ed.

Bernhardt, B. H., & Stemberger, J. P. (2007). Phonological impairment. In P. Lacy (Ed). *Handbook of Phonology.* Cambridge, UK: Cambridge University Press, pp. 573–593.

Bernhardt, B., Stemberger, J., & Major, E. (2006). General and nonlinear phonological intervention perspectives for a child with a resistant phonological impairment. *Advances in Speech-Language Pathology, 8,* 190–206.

Bernhardt, B., & Stoel-Gammon, C. (1994). Nonlinear phonology: Introduction and clinical application, *Journal of Speech and Hearing Research, 37,* 123–143.

Bernstein Ratner, N. (2006). Evidence-based practice: An examination of its ramifications for the practice of speech-language pathology. *Language, Speech, and Hearing Services in Schools, 37,* 257–267.

Bernthal, J. E., & Bankson, N. W. (Eds) (1994). *Child Phonology: Characteristics, Assessment, and Intervention with Special Populations.* New York, NY: Thieme Medical, pp. 110–139.

Bernthal, J. E., & Bankson, N. W. (2004). *Articulation and Phonological Disorders* (5th Edition). Boston, MA: Allyn & Bacon.

Bernthal, J. E., Bankson, N. W., & Flipsen, P., Jr. (2009). *Articulation and Phonological Disorders* (6th Edition). Boston, MA: Pearson Education.

Berry, M. D., & Eisenson, J. (1942). *The Defective in Speech.* New York: Appleton-Century-Crofts.

Berry, M. D., & Eisenson, J. (1956). *Speech Disorders: Principals and Practices of Therapy.* New York, NY: Appleton Century Crofts.

Bess, F. H., Dodd-Murphy, J., & Parker, R. A. (1998). Children with minimal sensorineural hearing loss: prevalence, educational performance, and functional status. *Ear & Hearing, 19*(5), 339–354.

Betz, S. K., & Stoel-Gammon, C. (2005). Measuring articulatory inconsistency in children with developmental apraxia. *Clinical Linguistics & Phonetics, 19,* 53–66.

Bird, J., Bishop, D. V. M., & Freeman, N. H. (1995). Phonological awareness and literacy development in children with expressive phonological impairments. *Journal of Speech and Hearing Research, 38,* 446–462.

Bishop, D. V. M., & Adams, C. (1990). A prospective study of the relationship between specific language impairment, phonological disorders and reading retardation. *The Journal of Child Psychology and Psychiatry, 31*(7), 1027–1050.

Bishop, D. V. M., Price, T. S., Dale, P. S., & Robert, P. (2003). Outcomes of early language delay: II. Etiology of transient and persistent language difficulties. *Journal of Speech Language and Hearing Research, 46*(3), 561–575.

Blache, S. E. (1982). Minimal word pairs and distinctive feature training. In M. Crary (Ed). *Phonological Intervention: Concepts and Procedures.* San Diego, CA: College-Hill Press Inc.

Blamey, P. J., Barry, J. G., & Jacq, P. (2001). Phonetic inventory development in young cochlear implant users 6 years postoperation. *Journal of Speech, Language, and Hearing Research, 44,* 73–79.

Bleile, K. M. (1995). *Manual of Articulation and Phonological Disorders: Infancy Through Adulthood*. San Diego, CA: Singular.

Bleile, K. M. (2002). Evaluating articulation and phonological disorders when the clock is running. *American Journal of Speech-Language Pathology, 11*, 243–249.

Bleile, K. M. (2004). *Manual of Articulation and Phonological Disorders: Infancy Through Adulthood* (2nd Edition). Clifton Park, NY: Thomson Delmar Learning.

Bleile, K. M. (2006). *The Late Eight*. San Diego, CA: Plural Publishing.

Bluestone, C. D. (1998). Epidemiology and pathogenesis of chronic suppurative otitis media: Implications for prevention and treatment. *International Journal of Pediatric Otorhinolaryngology, 42*(3), 207–223.

Boh, A., Csiacsek, E., Duginske, R., Meath, T., & Carpenter, L. J. (2006). Counseling parents of children with CAS. Annual Convention of the American Speech-Language-Hearing Association, Miami, FL, November 2006.

Boone, D. R., & McFarlane, S. C. (2000). *The Voice and Voice Therapy*. Needham Heights, MA: Allyn & Bacon.

Bonilha, L, Moser, D., Rorden, C., Bylis, G., & Fridriksson, J. (2006). Speech apraxia without oral apraxia: Can normal brain function explain the physiopathology? *Brain Imaging, 17*(10), 1027–1031.

Boshart, C. (1998). *Oral Motor Analysis and Remediation Techniques*. Temecula, CA: Speech Dynamics.

Bowen, C. (1996a). *Evaluation of a phonological therapy with treated and untreated groups of young children*. Unpublished doctoral dissertation. Macquarie University.

Bowen, C. (1996b). *The Quick Screener*. Retrieved November 21, 2007 from http://www.speech-language-therapy.com/tx-a-quickscreener.html.

Bowen, C. (1998a). *Developmental Phonological Disorders: A Practical Guide for Families and Teachers*. Melbourne: The Australian Council for Educational Research.

Bowen, C. (1998b). *Speech-language-therapy dot com*. Retrieved October 17, 2007 from www.speech-language-therapy.com/.

Bowen, C. (2001). *Phonologicaltherapy: phonological therapy discussion group*. Retrieved September 24, 2008 from: http://health.groups.yahoo.com/group/phonologicaltherapy.

Bowen, C. (2003). Harnessing the Net: A challenge for Speech Language Pathologists. The 2003 Elizabeth Usher Memorial Lecture. In C. Williams and S. Leitão (Eds). *Nature, Nurture, Knowledge, Proceedings of the Speech Pathology Australia National Conference*, Hobart, 9–20.

Bowen, C. (2005). What is the evidence for·... ? Oral motor therapy. *ACQuiring Knowledge in Speech, Language, and Hearing, 7*, 144–147.

Bowen, C. (2007). *Les difficultés phonologiques chez l'enfant: guide à l'intention des familles, des enseignants et des intervenants en petite enfance*. Caroline Bowen, Rachel Fortin, traductrice et adaptatrice. Montréal: Chenelière-éducation.

Bowen, C. (in press). Parents and children together (PACT) intervention for children with speech sound disorders. In A. L. Williams, S. McLeod, and R. McCauley. (Eds). *Interventions for Speech Sound Disorders in Children*. Baltimore, MD: Paul Brookes.

Bowen, C., & Cupples, L. (1998). A tested phonological therapy in practice. *Child Language Teaching and Therapy, 14*(1), 29–50.

Bowen, C., & Cupples, L. (1999a). Parents and children together (PACT): A collaborative approach to phonological therapy. *International Journal of Language & Communication Disorders, 34*(1), 35–55.

Bowen, C., & Cupples, L. (1999b). A phonological therapy in depth: a reply to commentaries. *International Journal of Language & Communication Disorders, 34*(1), 65–83.

Bowen, C., & Cupples, L. (2004). The role of families in optimizing phonological therapy outcomes. *Child Language Teaching and Therapy, 20*, 245–260.

Bowen, C., & Cupples, L. (2006). PACT: Parents and children together in phonological therapy. *Advances in Speech-Language Pathology, 8*(3), 282–292.

Bradlow, A. (2002). Confluent talker- and listener-oriented forces in clear speech production. In C. Gussenhoven, T. Rietveld, and N. Warner (Eds). *Papers in Laboratory Phonology VII.* Cambridge: Cambridge University Press, pp. 241–273.

Bradlow, A., Torretta, G., & Pisoni, D. (1996). Intelligibility of normal speech I: Global and fine-grained acoustic-phonetic talker characteristics. *Speech Communication, 20*, 255–272.

Braine, M. D. S. (1974). On what might constitute a learnable phonology. *Language, 50,* 270–299.

Bridgeman, E., & Snowling, M. (1988). The perception of phoneme sequence: A comparison of dyspraxic and normal children. *British Journal of Disorders of Communication, 23,* 245–252.

Bronfenbrenner, U., & Morris, P. A. (1998). The ecology of developmental processes. In R. M. Lerner (Ed). *Handbook of Child Psychology: Volume 1: Theoretical Models of Human Development.* New York, NY: John Wiley and Sons, pp. 993–1027.

Broomfield, J., & Dodd, B. (2004a). The nature of referred subtypes of primary speech disability. *Child Language Teaching and Therapy, 20,* 135–151.

Broomfield, J., & Dodd, B. (2004b). Children with speech and language disability: Caseload characteristics. *International Journal of Language and Communication Disability, 39,* 303–324.

Broomfield, J. & Dodd, B. (2005). Clinical effectiveness. B. Dodd (Ed). *Differential diagnosis and treatment of children with speech disorder,* 2nd Ed. London: Whurr, pp. 211–229.

Brown, C. (2007). Identifying a standard assessment and of speech sound disorders (SSD) in children: Comments on Prezas and Hodson, Rvachew and Lewis. *Encyclopedia of Language and Literacy Development.* London, ON: Canadian Language and Literacy Research Network, pp. 1–5. Retrieved December 3, 2007 from: http://www.literacyencyclopedia.ca/pdfs/topic.php?topld=38.

Bruce, B., Letourneau, N., Ritchie, J., Larocque, S., Dennis, C., & Elliott, M. R. (2002). A multisite study of health professionals' perceptions and practices of family-centred care. *Journal of Family Nursing, 8,* 408–429.

Bunton, K., & Weismer, G. (1994). Evaluation of a reiterant force-impulse task in the tongue. *Journal of Speech and Hearing Research, 37,* 1020–1031.

Byrd, K., & Cooper, E. (1989). Apraxic speech characteristics in stuttering, developmentally apraxic, and normal speaking children. *Journal of Fluency Disorders, 14,* 215–229.

Caleffe-Schenck, N. (1992). The auditory-verbal method: description of a training program for audiologists, speech language pathologists, and teachers of children with hearing loss. *Volta Review, 94,* 65–68.

Calmels, M. N., Saliba, I., Wanna, G., et al. (2004). Speech perception and speech intelligibility in children after cochlear implantation. *International Journal of Pediatric Otorhinolaryngology, 68*(3), 347–351.

Camarata, S. M. (1993). The application of naturalistic conversation training to speech production in children with speech disabilities. *Journal of Applied Behavior Analysis, 26,* 173–182.

Camarata, S. M. (1995). A rationale for naturalistic speech intelligibility intervention. In M. E. Fey, J. Windson, and S. F. Warren (Eds). *Language Intervention: Preschool Through the Elementary Years.* Baltimore, MD: Paul H. Brookes Publishing Co., pp. 63–84.

Cameron, J., Banko, K. M., & Pierce, W. D. (2001). Pervasive negative effects of rewards on intrinsic motivation: The myth continues. *The Behavior Analyst, 24,* 1–44.

Campbell, T. F. (2003). Childhood apraxia of speech: Clinical symptoms and speech characteristics. In L. D. Shriberg and T. F. Campbell (Eds). *Proceedings of the 2002 Childhood Apraxia of Speech Research Symposium.* Carlsbad, CA: Hendrix Foundation, pp. 37–47.

Campbell, T. F., & Bain, B. A. (1991). How long to treat: A multiple outcome approach. *Language, Speech, and Hearing Services in Schools, 22,* 271–276.

Campbell, T. F., Dollaghan, C. A., Janosky, J. E., & Adelson, P. D. (2007). A performance curve for assessing change in Percentage of Consonants Correct- Revised. *Journal of Speech, Language, and Hearing Research, 50*, 1110–1119.

Campbell, T. F., Dollaghan, C. A., Rockette, H. E., et al. (2003). Risk factors for speech delay in three-year-old children. *Child Development, 74*, 346–357.

Cantwell, D. P., & Baker, L. (1987). Clinical significance of childhood communication disorders: Perspectives from a longitudinal study. *Journal of Child Neurology, 2*, 257–264.

Carrow-Woolfolk, E. (1999). *Comprehensive Assessment of Spoken Language (CASL)*. Bloomington, MN: Pearson Assessments.

Carter, B., & McGoldrick, M. (1999). *The Expanded Family Life Cycle: Individual, Family and Social Perspectives* (3rd Edition). Needham Heights: Allyn & Bacon Publishers.

Carter, E. T., & Buck, M. W. (1958). Prognostic testing for functional articulation disorders among children in the first grade. *Journal of Speech and Hearing Disorders, 23*, 124–133.

Carter, J. A., Lees, J. A., Murira, G. M., Gona, J., Neville, G. B. R., & Newton, C. R. J. C. (2005). Issues in the development of cross-cultural assessments of speech and language for children. *International Journal of Language & Communication Disorders, 40*(4), 385–401.

Caruso, A. J., Ludo, M., & McClowry, M. T. (1999). Perspectives on stuttering as a motor speech disorder. In A. Caruso and E. Strand (Eds). *Clinical Management of Motor Speech Disorders in Children*. New York, NY: Thieme-Stratton, pp. 319–344.

Caruso, A. J., & Strand, E. A. (1999). *Clinical Management of Motor Speech Disorders in Children*. New York, NY: Thieme Publishing Co.

Carroll, J. M., Snowling, M. J., Hulme, C., & Stevenson, J. (2003). The development of phonological awareness in preschool children. *Developmental Psychology, 39*, 913–923.

Casby, M. W. (2001). Otitis media and language development: A meta-analysis. *American Journal of Speech-Language Pathology, 10*, 65–80.

Caspari, S. (2007). Working guidelines for the assessment and treatment of childhood apraxia of speech: A review of ASHA's 2007 position statement and technical report [Electronic Version]. Retrieved March 5, 2009 from: http://www.speechpathology.com/articles.

Catts, H. W. (1993). The relationship between speech-language disabilities and reading disabilities. *Journal of Speech and Hearing Research, 36*, 948–958.

Chapman Bahr, D. (2001). *Oral Motor Assessment and Treatment: Ages and Stages*. Boston, MA: Allyn & Bacon.

Chappell, G. E. (1973). Childhood verbal apraxia and its treatment. *Journal of Speech and Hearing Disorders, 38*, 362–368.

Chegar, B. E., Tatum, S. A., Marrinan, E., & Shprintzen, R. J. (2006). Upper airway asymmetry in velo-cardio-facial syndrome. *International Journal of Pediatric Otorhinolaryngology, 70*, 1375–1381.

Childhood Apraxia of Speech Association of North America (CASANA). (1997).Retrieved March 5, 2009 from http://www.apraxia-kids.org.

Chin, S. B. (1996). The role of the sonority hierarchy in delayed phonological systems. In T. W. Powell (Ed). *Pathologies of Speech and Language: Contributions of Clinical Phonetics and Linguistics*. International Clinical Phonetics and Linguistics Association, pp. 109–117.

Chin, S. B. (2006). Realization of complex onsets by pediatric users of cochlear implants. *Clinical Linguistics & Phonetics, 20*(7), 501–508.

Chomsky, N. (1959). A review of B. F. Skinner's *Verbal Behavior. Language, 35*, 26–58.

Chomsky, N. (1965). *Aspects of the Theory of Syntax*. Cambridge, MA: MIT Press.

Chomsky, N. (1995). *The Minimalist Program*. Cambridge, MA: MIT Press.

Chomsky, N., & Halle, M. (1968). *The Sound Pattern of English*. New York: Harper and Row.

Chumpelik, D. (1984). The PROMPT system of therapy: Theoretical framework and applications for developmental apraxia of speech. *Seminars in Speech and Language, 5*, 139–156.

Clark, H. M. (2003). Neuromuscular treatments for speech and swallowing: A tutorial. *American Journal of Speech-Language Pathology, 12*(4), 400–415.

Clark, H. M. (2005). Clinical decision making and oral motor treatments. *The ASHA Leader*, *10*(8), 8–9.

Clark, H., Hensen, P., Barber, W., Stierwalt, J., & Sherrill, M. (2003). Relationships among subjective and objective measures of tongue strength and oral phase swallowing impairments. *American Journal of Speech-Language Pathology, 12*, 40–50.

Clark, J., & Yallop, C. (1995). *An Introduction to Phonetics and Phonology* (2nd Edition). Oxford: Basil Blackwell.

Clark, J. G. (1981). Uses and abuses of hearing loss classification. *ASHA, 23*(7), 493–500.

Clarke-Klein, S., & Hodson, B. (1995). A phonologically based analysis of misspellings by third graders withdisordered-phonology histories. *Journal of Speech and Hearing Research, 38*, 839–849.

Cohen, J. H., & Diehl, C. F. (1963). Relation of speech sound discrimination ability to articulation-type speech defects. *Journal of Speech and Hearing Disorders, 28*, 187–190.

Cole, K., Maddox, M., & Lim, Y. (2006). Language is the key: Constructive interactions around books and play. In R. McCauley and M. Fey (Eds). *Treatment of Language Disorders in Children*. Baltimore, MD: Paul Brookes, pp. 149–174.

Colone, E., & Forrest, K. (2000, November). Comparison of treatment efficacy for persistent speech sound disorders. Poster presented at the annual convention of the American *Speech-Language-Hearing Association Convention*, Washington, D.C.

College of Speech Therapists (1959). *Terminology for Speech Pathology*. London: College of Speech Therapists.

Comenius, J. A. (1659). *Orbis Sensualium Pictus* (Facsimile of first English edition of 1659). Adelaide: Sydney University Press.

Connor, C. M., Craig, H. K., Raudenbush, S. W., Heavner, K., & Zwolan, T. A. (2006). The age at which young deaf children receive cochlear implants and their vocabulary and speech-production growth: Is there an added value for early implantation? *Ear and Hearing, 27*(6), 628–644.

Costello, J., & Onstine, J. (1976). The modification of multiple articulation errors based on distinctive feature theory. *Journal of Speech and Hearing Disorders, 41*, 199–215.

Cox, R. M., & Moore, J. N. (1988). Composite speech spectrum for hearing and gain prescriptions. *Journal of Speech & Hearing Research, 31*(1), 102–107.

Crais, E. (1991). Moving from "parent involvement" to family-centred services. *American Journal of Speech-Language Pathology*, September, 5–8.

Crais, E. (1992). 'Best practices' with preschoolers: Assessing and intervening within the context of a family-centered approach. In J. Damico (Ed). *Best Practices in School Speech-Language Pathology, 2*, 33–43.

Crais, E., Poston Roy, V., & Free, K. (2006). Parents' and professionals' perceptions of family-centered practices: What are actual practices vs. what are ideal practices? *American Journal of Speech-Language Pathology, 15*, 365–377.

Crary, M. A. (1984). Phonological characteristics of developmental verbal dyspraxia. *Seminars in Speech and Language, 5*, 71–83.

Crary, M. A. (1993). *Developmental Motor Speech Disorders*. San Diego, CA: Singular Publishing Group.

Crary, M. A., Landess, S., & Towne, R. (1984). Phonological error patterns in developmental verbal dyspraxia. *Journal of Clinical Neuropsychology, 6*(2), 157–170.

Creaghead, N. A., Newman, P. W., & Secord, W. A. (1989). *Assessment and Remediation of Articulatory and Phonological Disorders* (2nd Edition). Columbus, OH: Merrill.

Crosbie, S., Holm, A., & Dodd, B. (2005). Intervention for children with severe speech disorder: A comparison of two approaches. *International Journal of Language & Communication Disorders, 40*, 467–491.

Crosbie, S., Pine, C., Holm, A., & Dodd, B. (2006). Treating Jarrod: A core vocabulary approach. *Advances in Speech-Language Pathology, 8*(3), 316–321.

Crystal, D. (1972). The case of linguistics: a prognosis. *British Journal of Disorders of Communication*, 7, 3–16.

Crystal, D. (1991). *A Dictionary of Linguistics and Phonetics*. Oxford: Basil Blackwell.

Crystal, D. (1996). Language play and linguistic intervention. *Child Language Teaching and Therapy*, 12, 328–344.

Crystal, D. (1998). *Language Play*. London: Penguin Books.

Cummings, E. E., & Firmage, J. G. (1994). *E. E. Cummings: Complete Poems 1904–1962*. New York: Vintage.

D'Antonio, L. L., Muntz, H. R., Marsh, J. L., Marty-Grames, L., & Backensto-Marsh, R. (1988). Practical application of flexible fiberoptic nasopharyngoscopy for evaluating velopharyngeal function. *Plastic and Reconstructive Surgery*, 82, 611–618.

Daniel, B., & Wassel, S. (2002). *The Early Years. Assessing and Promoting Resilience in Vulnerable Children 1*. London: Jessica Kingsley Publishers.

Dart, S. N. (1991). *Articulatory and Acoustic Properties of Apical and Laminal Articulations*. Ph.D. Dissertation, Department of Linguistics, University of California, Los Angeles. Reprinted as UCLA Working Papers in Phonetics, 79, 1–155.

Davis, B. L. (1998). Consistency of consonant patterns by word position. *Clinical Linguistics & Phonetics*, 12(4), 329–348.

Davis, B., Jacks, A., & Marquardt, T. P. (2005). Vowel patterns in developmental apraxia of speech: three longitudinal case studies. *Clinical Linguistics & Phonetics*, 19, 249–274.

Davis, B., Jakielski, K., & Marquardt, T. (1998). Developmental apraxia of speech: Determiners of differential diagnosis. *Clinical Linguistics & Phonetics*, 12(1), 25–45.

Davis, B. L., & MacNeilage, P. F. (1990). The acquisition of vowels: A case study. *Journal of Speech and Hearing Research*, 33, 16–27.

Davis, B. L., & MacNeilage, P. F. (1995). The articulatory basis of babbling. *Journal of Speech and Hearing Research*, 38, 1199–1211.

Davis, B. L., & Velleman, S. L. (2000). Differential diagnosis and treatment of developmental apraxia of speech in infants and toddlers. *Infant-Toddler Intervention*, 10(3), 177–192.

Dawes M., Summerskill, W., Glasziou P., et al. (2005). Second International Conference of Evidence-Based Health Care Teachers and Developers. Sicily statement on evidence-based practice. *BMC Medical Educaton*, 5(1), 1.

Day, A. (1993). *Carl Goes to Daycare*. New York, NY: Farrar, Straus, & Giroux.

Dean, E., & Howell, J. (1986). Developing linguistic awareness: A theoretically based approach to phonological disorders. *British Journal of Disorders of Communication*, 21, 223–238.

Dean, E., Howell, J., Hill, A., & Waters, D. (1990). *Metaphon Resource Pack*. Windsor, Berks: NFER Nelson.

Dean, E. C., Howell, J., Waters, D., & Reid, J. (1995). Metaphon: A metalinguistic approach to the treatment of phonological disorder in children. *Clinical Linguistics & Phonetics*, 9, 1–19.

Deem, R., & Brehony, K. J. (2000). Doctoral students' access to research Cultures – are some more equal than others? *Studies in Higher Education*, 25, 149–165.

Denne, M., Langdowne, N., Pring, T., & Roy, P. (2005). Treating children with expressive phonological disorders: does phonological awareness therapy work in the clinic? *International Journal of Language & Communication Disorders*, 40(4), 493–504.

Dhooge, I. J. (2003,). Risk factors for the development of otitis media. *Current Allergy and Asthma Reports*, 3(4), 321–325.

Dinnsen, D. A., & Elbert, M. A. (1984). On the relationship between phonology and learning. In D. A. Dinnsen, M. A. Elbert, and G. Weismer (Eds). *Phonological Theory and the Misarticulating Child*. Rockville, MD: ASHA, pp. 59–68.

Dinnsen, D. A., & Gierut, J. A. (2008). Optimality theory: A clinical perspective. In M. J. Ball, M. Perkins, N. Muller, et al. (Eds). *Handbook of Clinical Linguistics*. Malden, MA: Blackwell, pp. 439–451.

Doble, M. (2006). *Development of oral communication in infants with a profound hearing loss: pre- and post-cochlear implantation.* Unpublished PhD thesis, The University of Sydney.

Dodd, B. (1995). *Differential Diagnosis and Treatment of Children with Speech Disorder.* London: Whurr Publishers.

Dodd, B. (2005). *Differential Diagnosis and Treatment of Children with Speech Disorder* (2nd Edition). London: Whurr.

Dodd, B. (2007). Evidence-based practice and speech-language pathology: Strengths, weaknesses, opportunities and threats. *Folia Phoniatrica et Logopaedica, 59,* 118–129.

Dodd, B. J., & Bradford, A. (2000). A comparison of three therapy methods for children with different types of developmental phonological disorder. *International Journal of Language & Communication Disorders, 35,* 189–209.

Dodd, B., Crosbie, S., McIntosh, B., et al. (2008). The impact of selecting different contrasts in phonological therapy. *International Journal of Speech-Language Pathology, 10*(5), 334–345.

Dodd, B., Crosbie, S., MacIntosh, B., Teitzel, T., & Ozanne, A. (2000). *Pre-School and Primary Inventory of Phonological Awareness.* London: The Psychological Corporation.

Dodd, B., Crosbie, S., Zhu, H., Holm, A., & Ozanne, A. (2002). *Diagnostic Evaluation of Articulation and Phonology (DEAP).* London: Psychological Corporation.

Dodd, B., & Gillon, G. (2001). Exploring the relationship between phonological awareness, speech impairment and literacy. *Advances in Speech-Language Pathology, 3*(2), 139–147.

Dodd, B., Holm, A., Crosbie, S., & McIntosh, B. (2006). A core vocabulary approach for management of inconsistent speech disorder. *Advances in Speech-Language Pathology, 8*(3), 220–230.

Dodd, B., Holm, A., Hua, Z., and Crosbie, S. (2003). Phonological development, a normative study of British-English speaking children. *Clinical Linguistics & Phonetics, 17,* 617–643.

Dodd, B., Hua, Z., Crosbie, S., Holm, A., & Ozanne, A. (2003). *Diagnostic Evaluation of Articulation and Phonology (DEAP).* London: Psychological Corporation.

Dollaghan, C. A. (2004). Evidence-based practice in communication disorders: what do we know, and when do we know it? *Journal of Communication Disorders, 37,* 391–400.

Dollaghan, C. A. (2007). *The Handbook for Evidence-Based Practice in Communication Disorders.* Baltimore: Paul H. Brookes.

Dollaghan, C., & Campbell, T. (1992). A procedure for classifying disruptions in spontaneous language samples. *Topics in Language Disorders, 12,* 56–68.

Drummond, S., & Asher, J. (2005). Developmental Verbal Apraxia and Phonological Disorders: Speech and Non-Speech Performances. Presented at the *American Speech-Language-Hearing Association Convention,* November.

DuBois, E., & Bernthal, J. E. (1978). A comparison of three methods of obtaining articulatory responses. *Journal of Speech and Hearing Disorders, 43,* 295–305.

Duchan, J. F. (2001). *History of Speech-Language Pathology in America.* Retrieved February 22, 2008 from: http://www.acsu.buffalo.edu/~duchan/history.html.

Duchan, J. F. (2006). How conceptual frameworks influence clinical practice: evidence from the writings of John Thelwall, a 19th-century speech therapist. *International Journal of Language & Communication Disorders, 41*(6), 735–744.

Duchan, J., Calculator, S., Sonnenmeier, R., Diehl, S., & Cumley, G. (2001). A framework for managing controversial practices. *Language, Speech, and Hearing Services in Schools, 32,* 133–141.

Dunn, L. M., & Dunn, L. M. (1997). *Peabody Picture Vocabulary Test-III.* Circle Pines, MN: American Guidance Service.

Dunn, L. M., Dunn, L. M., & Williams, K. T. (1997). *Peabody Picture Vocabulary Test, 3rd.* Circle Pines, MN: AGS.

Ebersöhn, L., & Eloff, I. (2006). Identifying asset-based trends in sustainable programmes which support vulnerable children. *South African Journal of Education, 26*(3), 457–472.

Eckert, P. (2000a). *Linguistic Variation as Social Practice*. Oxford: Blackwell.

Eckert, P. (2000b). *Linguistic Variation as Social Practice: The Construction of Identity in Belten High*. New York, NY: Wiley.

Edwards, J., Fox, R. A., & Rogers, C. L. (2002). Final consonant discrimination in children: Effects of phonological disorder, vocabulary size, and articulatory accuracy. *Journal of Speech, Language, and Hearing Research*, 45, 231–242.

Edwards, M. L. (1983). Selection criteria for developing therapy goals. *Journal of Childhood Communication Disorders*, 7, 36–45.

Edwards, M. L. (1992). In support of phonological processes. *Language, Speech, and Hearing Services in Schools*, 23, 233–240.

Edwards, S. M. (1995). Optimizing outcomes of nonlinear phonological intervention. Unpublished Master's thesis, University of British Columbia.

Ehri, L. C. (1989). The development of spelling knowledge and its role in reading acquisition and reading disability. *Journal of Learning Disabilities*, 22, 356–365.

Eisenson, J. (1968). Developmental aphasia: A speculative view with therapeutic implications. *Journal of Speech and Hearing Disorders*, 33, 3–13.

Eisenson, J., & Ogilvie, M. (1963). *Speech Correction in the Schools*. New York: Macmillan.

Ekelman, B. L., & Aram, D. M. (1983). Syntactic findings in developmental verbal apraxia. *Journal of Communication Disorders*, 16(4), 237–250.

Elbert, M. (1989). Generalisation in treatment of phonological disorders. In L. McReynolds and J. Spradlin (Eds). *Generalisation Strategies in the Treatment of Communication Disorders*. Toronto: B. C. Decker, Inc, pp. 31–43.

Elbert, M. (1992). Consideration of error types: A response to Fey's 'Articulation and phonology: Inextricable constructs in speech pathology.' *Language, Speech, and Hearing Services in Schools*, 23, 241–246.

Elbert, M., Dinnsen, D., & Powell, T. (1984). On the prediction of phonological generalisation learning pattern. *Journal of Speech and Hearing Disorders*, 49, 309–317.

Elbert, M., Dinnsen, D., & Weismer, C. (Eds) (1984). *Phonological Theory and the Misarticulating Child* (ASHA Monographs No. 22). Rockville, MD: ASHA.

Elbert, M., & Gierut, J. (1986). *Handbook of Clinical Phonology: Approaches to Assessment and Treatment*. San Diego, CA: College-Hill Press.

Elbro, C., Borstrøm, I., & Petersen, D. K. (1998). Predicting dyslexia from kindergarten: The importance of distinctness of phonological representations of lexical items. *Reading Research Quarterly*, 33, 36–60.

Eldridge, M. (1965). *A History of the Australian College of Speech Therapists*. Melbourne, Melbourne University Press.

Eldridge, M. (1968a). *A History of the Treatment of Speech Disorders*. Edinburgh & London: E. & S. Livingstone.

Eldridge, M. (1968b). *A History of the Treatment of Speech Disorders*. Melbourne: F.W. Cheshire.

Elfenbein, J. L., Hardin-Jones, M. A., & Davis, J. M. (1994). Oral communication skills of children who are hard of hearing. *Journal of Speech & Hearing Research*, 37(1), 216–226.

Ellis Weismer, S., & Robertson, S. (2006). Focused stimulation: Approach to language intervention. In R. McCauley and M. Fey (Eds). *Treatment of Language Disorders in Children*. Baltimore, MD: Paul Brookes, pp. 175–202.

Erickson, K. (2007). Children with atypical phonological development: Assessment profiles and rates of change. Unpublished Master's thesis, University of British Columbia.

Fairbanks, G. (1940). *Voice and Articulation Drillbook*. New York: Harper.

Fazio, B. B. (1997). Learning a new poem: Memory for connected speech and phonological awareness in low-income children with and without specific language impairment. *Journal of Speech, Language, and Hearing Research*, 40, 1285–1297.

Felsenfeld, S., Broen, P. A., & McCue, M. (1992). A 28-year follow-up of adults with a history of moderate phonological disorder: Linguistic and personality results. *Journal of Speech and Hearing Research*, *35*, 1114–1125.

Felsenfeld, S., Broen, P. A., & McGue, M. (1994). A 28-year follow-up of adults with a history of moderate phonological disorder: Educational and occupational results. *Journal of Speech and Hearing Research*, *37*(6), 1341–1353.

Fenson, L., Dale, P. S., Reznik, J. S., Thal, D., Bates, E. Hartung, J., et al. (1993). *MacArthur Communicative Development Inventories*. San Diego, CA: Singular.

Ferguson, C. A. (1968). Contrastive analysis and language development. *Monograph Series on Language and Linguistics*, *21*, 101–112, Georgetown University.

Ferguson, C. A. (1978). Learning to pronounce: The earliest stages of phonological development in the child. In F. D. Minifie and L. L. Lloyd (Eds). *Communicative and Cognitive Abilities: Early Behavioural Assessment*. Baltimore, MD: University Park Press, pp. 273–297.

Ferguson, C., & Farwell, C. (1975). Words and sounds in early language acquisition. *Language*, *51*, 419–439.

Ferguson, C. A., & Macken, M. (1980). Phonological development in children: Play and cognition. *Papers and Reports on Child Language Development*, *18*, 138–177.

Ferguson, C. A., Peizer, D. B., & Weeks, T. A. (1973). Model-and-replica phonological grammar of a child's first words. *Lingua*, *3*, 35–65.

Feuerstein, R., Rand, Y., Jensen, M. R., Kaniel, S., & Tzuriel, D. (1987). 'Prerequisites for assessment of learning potential: the LPAD model'. In C. S. Lidz (Ed). *Dynamic Assessment: An Interactional Approach to Evaluating Learning Potential*. New York, NY: The Guilford Press.

Fey, M. E. (1985). Clinical forum: Phonological assessment and treatment. Articulation and phonology: Inextricable constructs in speech pathology. *Human Communication Canada*. Reprinted (1992) *Language, Speech, and Hearing Services in Schools*, *23*, 225–232.

Fey, M. E. (1992a). Phonological assessment and treatment. Articulation and phonology: An introduction. *Language, Speech, and Hearing Services in Schools*, *23*, 224.

Fey, M. E. (1992b). Phonological assessment and treatment. Articulation and phonology: An addendum. *Language, Speech, and Hearing Services in Schools*, *23*, 277–282.

Fey, M. E., & Stalker, C. (1986). A hypothesis testing approach to treatment of a child with an idiosyncratic (morpho)phonological system. *Journal of Speech and Hearing Disorders*, *41*, 324–336.

Fielding-Barnsley, R., & Purdie, N. (2005). Teachers' attitude to and knowledge of metalinguistics in the process of learning to read. *Asia-Pacific Journal of Teacher Education*, *33*(1), 65–76.

Fields, D., & Polmanteer, K. (2002, November). Effectiveness of oral motor techniques in articulation and phonology treatment. Poster presented at the *American Speech-Language-Hearing Association Convention*, Atlanta, GA.

Fisher, S. E., Vargha-Khadem, F., Watkins, K. E., Monaco, A. P., & Pembrey, M. E. (1998). Localisation of a gene implicated in a severe speech and language disorder. *Nature*, *18*, 168–170.

Flahive, L., Hodson, B., & Velleman, S. (2005, November). Apraxia AND phonology. Seminar at the annual meeting of the American Speech-Language-Hearing Association, San Diego, CA.

Fletcher, S. G. (1972). Time-by-count measurement of diadochokinetic syllable rate. *Journal of Speech and Hearing Research*, *15*, 757–762.

Flipsen, P., Jr. (2002, May). Causes and speech sound disorders. Why worry? Presentation at the *Speech Pathology Australia National Conference*, Alice Springs, Northern Territory, Australia.

Flipsen, P., Jr. (2006). Measuring the intelligibility of conversational speech in children. *Clinical Linguistics & Phonetics*, *20*(4), 303–312.

Flipsen, P., Jr., Hammer, J. B., & Yost, K. M. (2005). Measuring severity of involvement in speech delay: Segmental and whole-word measures. *American Journal of Speech-Language Pathology*, *14*, 298–312.

Flipsen, P., Jr., & Parker, R. G. (2008). Phonological patterns in the speech of children with cochlear implants. *Journal of Communication Disorders*, *41*(4), 337–357.

Flynn, L., & Lancaster, G. (1996). *Children's Phonology Sourcebook*. Oxford: Winslow Press.

Forrest, K. (2002). Are oral-motor exercises useful in the treatment of phonological/articulatory disorders? *Seminars in Speech and Language*, *23*, 15–25.

Forrest, K. (2003). Diagnostic criteria of developmental apraxia of speech used by clinical speech-language pathologists. *American Journal of Speech-Language Pathology*, *12*(3), 376–380.

Foulkes, P. (2005). Sociophonetics. In K. Brown (Ed). *Encyclopedia of Language and Linguistics* (2nd Edition). Amsterdam: Elsevier, pp. 495–500.

Foulkes, P., & Docherty, G. (2000). Another chapter in the story of /r/: 'labiodental' variants in British English. *Journal of Sociolinguistics*, *4*, 30–59.

Fowler, C. A. (1995). Speech production. In J. L. Miller and P. D. Eimas (Eds). *Handbook of Perception and Cognition: Speech, Language and Communication*. San Diego, CA: Academic Press, pp. 29–61.

Fox, A. V., Dodd, B., & Howard, D. (2002). Risk factors for speech disorders in children. *International Journal of Language & Communication Disorders*, *37*(2), 117–131.

Fox, M. (2001). *Reading Magic*. New York, NY: Harcourt, Inc.

Fria, T. J., Cantekin, E. I., & Eichler, J. A. (1985). Hearing acuity of children with otitis media with effusion. *Archives of Otolaryngology*, *111*(1), 10–16.

Giles, M., & O'Brien, P. (1991). The prevalence of hearing impairment amongst Maori schoolchildren. *Clinical Otolaryngology & Allied Sciences*, *16*(2), 174–178.

Greig, A. V., Papesch, M. E., & Rowsell, A. R. (1999). Parental perceptions of grommet insertion in children with cleft palate. *Journal of Laryngology & Otology*, *113*(12), 1068–1071.

Greville, A. (2007). *New Zealand Deafness Notification Data January–December 2005*. Report prepared for National Audiology Centre, Auckland District Health Board.

Guralnick, M. J. (2001). A developmental systems model for early intervention. *Infants and Young Children*, *1*(2), 1–18.

Galton, R., & Simpson, A. (1958). *The Publicity Photograph*, BBC Radio. Retrieved September 17, 2008 from http://www.archive.org/details/Hancocks_Half_Hour.

García Col, C., & Magnuson, K. (2000). Cultural differences as sources of developmental vulnerabilities and resources. In J. P. Shonkoff and S. J. Meisels (Eds). *Handbook of Early Childhood Intervention* (2nd Edition). Cambridge: Cambridge University Press, pp. 94–114.

Gardner, H. (1997). Assessment of developmental language disorders. In C. Adams, M. Edwards, and B. Byers Brown (Eds). *Developmental Disorders of Language* (2nd Edition). London: Whurr, pp. 135–160.

Gardner, H. (2006). Assessing speech and language skills in the school-age child. In J. Stackhouse and M. Snowling (Eds). *Dyslexia, Speech and Language* (2nd Edition). London: Whurr, pp. 74–97.

Gardner, H., Froud, K., McClelland, A., & van der Lely, H. K. J. (2006). Development of the Grammar and Phonology Screening (GAPS) test to assess key markers of specific language and literacy difficulties in young children. *International Journal of Language & Communication Disorders*, *41*(5), 513–540.

Gascoigne, M. (2006). Supporting children with speech language and communication needs within integrated children's services. *RCSLT Position paper*. London: RCSLT.

Gerber, S. E. (1998). *Etiology and Prevention of Communicative Disorders* (2nd Edition). San Diego, CA: Singular Publishing Group, Inc.

Gereau, S. A., Steven, D., Bassila, M., Sher, A. E., Sidoti, E. J., Jr., & Morgan, M. (1988). Endoscopic observations of Eustachian tube abnormalities in children with palatal clefts. In

D. J. Lim, C. D. Bluestone, J. O. Klein, et al. (Eds). *Symposium on Otitis Media*. Toronto: B. C. Decker, pp. 60–63.

Geren, J., Snedeker, J., & Ax, L. (2005). Starting over: A preliminary study of early lexical and syntactic development in internationally adopted preschoolers. *Seminars in Speech and Language*, 26, 44–53.

Gibbon, F. E., & Mackenzie Beck, J. (2002). Therapy for abnormal vowels in children with phonological impairment. In M. J. Ball and F. E. Gibbon (Eds). *Vowel Disorders*. Woburn, MA: Butterworth-Heinemann, pp. 217–248.

Gibbon F., Shockey, L., & Reid, J. (1992). Description and treatment of abnormal vowels in a phonologically disordered child. *Child Language Teaching and Therapy*, 8, 30–59.

Gierut, J. (1989). Maximal opposition approach to phonological treatment. *Journal of Speech and Hearing Disorders*, 54, 9–19.

Gierut, J. (1992). The conditions and course of clinically induced phonological change. *Journal of Speech and Hearing Research*, 35, 1049–1063.

Gierut, J. A. (1998). Treatment efficacy: Functional phonological disorders in children. *Journal of Speech, Language, and Hearing Research*, 41, S85–S100.

Gierut, J. A. (1999). Syllable onsets: Clusters and adjuncts in acquisition. *Journal of Speech, Language, and Hearing Research*, 42, 708–726.

Gierut, J. (2001). Complexity in phonological treatment: Clinical factors. *Language, Speech, and Hearing in Schools*, 32, 229–241.

Gierut, J. A. (2004a, Summer). Clinical application of phonological complexity. *CSHA Magazine*, 6-7, 16.

Gierut, J. A. (2004b). Enhancement of learning for children with phonological disorders. *Sound to Sense June 11–13*, MIT, B164–B172.

Gierut, J. (2007). Phonological complexity and language learnability. *American Journal of Speech-Language Pathology*, 16(1), 6–17.

Gierut, J. A., & Champion, A. H. (2001). Syllable onsets II: Three-element clusters in phonological treatment. *Journal of Speech, Language, and Hearing Research*, 44, 886–904.

Gierut, J., Elbert, M., & Dinnsen, D. (1987). A functional analysis of phonological knowledge and generalisation learning in misarticulating children. *Journal of Speech and Hearing Research*, 30, 462–479.

Gierut, J. A., Morrisette, M. L., Hughes, M. T., & Rowland, S. (1996). Phonological treatment efficacy and developmental norms. *Language, Speech, and Hearing Services in Schools*, 27, 215–230.

Gierut, J. A., & O'Connor, K. M. (2002). Precursors to onset clusters in acquisition. *Journal of Child Language*, 29, 495–517.

Gilbert, J. H. V., & Johnson, C. E. (1978). Temporal and sequential constraints on six-year-olds' phonological productions: Some observations on the ambliance phenomenon. *Journal of Child Language*, 5, 101–112.

Gillon, G. (1998). The speech-literacy link: Perspectives from children with phonological speech disorders. *New Zealand Speech-Language Therapists Association Biennial Conference Proceedings*, Dunedin 14–17 April, 1998. Supplementary (1), pp. 1–6.

Gillon, G. T. (2000). The efficacy of phonological awareness intervention for children with spoken language impairment. *Language, Speech, and Hearing Services in Schools*, 31(2), 126–141.

Gillon, G. (2002). Follow-up study investigating benefits of phonological awareness intervention for children with spoken language impairment. *International Journal of Language & Communication Disorders*, 37(4), 381–400.

Gillon, G. T. (2004). *Phonological Awareness: From Research to Practice*. New York: Guilford Press.

Gillon, G. T. (2005). Facilitating phoneme awareness development in 3- and 4-year-old children with speech impairment. *Language, Speech, and Hearing Services in Schools*, 36, 308–324.

Gillon, G. T. (2006). Phonological awareness: A preventative framework for preschool children with spoken language impairment. In R. McCauley and M. Fey (Eds). *Treatment of Language Disorders in Children: Conventional and Controversial Approaches*. Baltimore, MD: Paul H. Brookes, pp. 279–307.

Gillon, G., Moriarty, B., & Schwarz, I. (2006). *Evidence Based Practice: An Update of Best Practices in Speech-Language Therapy*. Wellington: Ministry of Education.

Gillon, G. T., & Schwarz, I. E. (1998). *An International Literature Review of Best Practices in Speech and Language Therapy for Preschool and School Aged Children*. Wellington: Ministry of Education.

Gillon, G. T., & Schwarz, I. E. (2001a). *An International Literature Review of Best Practices in Speech and Language Therapy: 2001 Update*. Wellington: Ministry of Education.

Gillon, G., & Schwarz, I. (2001b). Screening spoken language skills for academic success. *Proceedings of the 2001 Speech Pathology Australia National Conference: Evidence and Innovation*, Melbourne.

Girolametto, L., & Weitzman, E. (2006). It Takes Two to Talk -The Hanen Program for Parents - Early language intervention through caregiver training. In R. McCauley and M. Fey (Eds). *Treatment of Language Disorders in Children*. Baltimore, MD: Paul Brookes, pp. 77–104.

Glaspey, A. M., & Stoel-Gammon, C. (2005). Dynamic assessment in phonological disorders: The scaffolding scale of stimulability. *Topics in Language Disorders: Clinical Perspectives on Speech Sound Disorders*, 25(3), 220–230.

Glaspey, A., & Stoel-Gammon, C. (2007). A dynamic approach to phonological assessment. *Advances in Speech-Language Pathology*, 9(4), 286–296.

Glennen, S. (2002). Pre-adoption questions for parents. Retrieved February 19, 2008 from: http://pages.towson.edu/sglennen/PreAdoptionQuestions.htm.

Glennen, S. (2005). New arrivals: Speech and language assessment for internationally adopted infants and toddlers within the first months home. *Seminars in Speech and Language*, 26, 10–21.

Glennen, S. (2007a). Predicting language outcomes for internationally adopted children. *Journal of Speech, Language, and Hearing research 50*, 529–548.

Glennen, S. (2007b). International adoption speech and language mythbusters. *Perspectives on Communication Disorders and Sciences in Culturally and Linguistically Diverse Populations*, 14(3), 3–8.

Glennen, S. (2007c). Speech and language in children adopted internationally at older ages. *Perspectives on Communication Disorders and Sciences in Culturally and Linguistically Diverse Populations*, 14(3), 17–20.

Glennen, S., & Bright, B. (2005). Five years later: Language in school-age internationally adopted children. *Seminars in Speech and Language*, 26, 86–101.

Glennen, S., & Masters, G. (2002). Typical and atypical language development in infants and toddlers adopted from Eastern Europe. *American Journal of Speech-Language Pathology*, 11, 417–433.

Glogowska, M., & Campbell, R. (2000). Investigating parental views of involvement in pre-school speech and language therapy. *International Journal of Language & Communication Disorders*, 35(3), 391–405.

Glogowska, M., Roulstone, S., Enderby, P., & Peters, T. (2000). Randomised controlled trial of community based speech and language therapy in preschool children. *British Medical Journal*, 321, 923–926.

Golding-Kushner, K. J. (1995). Treatment of articulation and resonance disorders associated with cleft palate and VPI. In R. J. Shprintzen and J. Bardach (Eds). *Cleft Palate Speech Management: A Multidisciplinary Approach*. St. Louis, MO: Mosby, pp. 327–351.

Golding-Kushner, K. J. (2001). *Therapy Techniques for Cleft Palate Speech and Related Disorders*. San Diego, CA: Singular.

Golding-Kushner, K. J. (2002). Velopharyngeal insufficiency (VPI) and apraxia. Retrieved April 10, 2008 from http://www.apraxia-kids.org/site/c.chKMI0PIIsE/b.980831/apps/s/content.asp?ct=464507.

Golding-Kushner, K. J. (2004). Treatment of sound system disorders associated with cleft palate speech. *SID 5 Newsletter*, 14, 16–19.

Golding-Kushner, K. J. (2005). Speech and language disorders in velo-cardiofacial syndrome. In K. Murphy and P. Scambler (Eds). *Velo-Cardio-Facial Syndrome: A Model for Understanding Microdeletion Disorders*. Cambridge: Cambridge University Press, pp. 181–199.

Golding-Kushner, K. J. (2007a). Speech and language therapy. In D. Landsman (Ed). *A Practical Handbook for Educating Children with Velo-cardio-facial Syndrome and Other Developmental Disabilities*. San Diego, CA: Plural Publishing.

Golding-Kushner, K. J. (2007b). Teletherapy: using technology to solve the problem. *Fourteenth International Scientific Meeting of the Velo-Cardio-Facial Syndrome Educational Foundation, Inc.*, Plano, TX.

Goldman, R., & Fristoe, M. (2000). *Goldman-Fristoe Test of Articulation* (2nd Edition). Circle Pines, MN: American Guidance Service.

Goldsmith, J. A. (1972). *Autosegmental Phonology*. MIT doctoral dissertation.

Goldstein, B. (1996). Error groups in Spanish speaking children. In T. W. Powell (Ed). *Pathologies of Speech and Language: Contributions of Clinical Phonetics and Linguistics*. New Orleans: International Clinical Phonetics and Linguistics Association.

Goldstein, K. (1948). *Language and Language Disturbances*. New York: Grune and Stratton.

Goodman, K. (1976). Reading: a psycholinguistic guessing game. In H. Singer and R. B. Ruddell (Eds). *Theoretical Models and Processes of Reading*. Newark, DE: IRA.

Goozee, N., Purcell, A., & Baker, E. (2001). Sonority and the acquisition of consonant clusters in a child with cleft-lip and palate. *Proceedings of the Speech Pathology Australia National Conference*, Melbourne.

Gordon-Brannan, M., & Hodson, B. (2000). Severity/intelligibility measures of prekindergartners' speech. *American Journal of Speech-Language Pathology*, 9, 141–150.

Gosling, A. S., and Westbrook, J. I. (2004). Allied health professionals' use of online evidence: a survey of 790 staff working in the Australian public hospital system. *International Journal of Medical Informatics*, 73(4), 391–401.

Granger, R. (2005). *Word Flips*. Greenville, SC: Super Duper Publications.

Gray, S. I., & Shelton, R.I. (1992). Self-monitoring effects on articulation carryover in school-age children. *Language, Speech, and Hearing Services in Schools*, 23, 334–342.

Gretz, S. (1997). *Apraxia-KIDS: A program of the Childhood Apraxia of Speech Association*. Retrieved August 1, 2007 from: http://www.apraxia-kids.org.

Gross, G. H., St. Louis, K. O., Ruscello, D. M., & Hull, F. M. (1985). Language abilities of articulatory-disordered school children with multiple or residual errors. *Language, Speech, and Hearing Services in Schools*, 16, 171–186.

Gruber, F. A. (1999). Probability estimates and paths to consonant normalization in children with speech delay. *Journal of Speech, Language, and Hearing Research*, 42, 448–459.

Gruber, F. A., Lowery, S. D., Seung, H.-K., & Deal, R. (2003). Approaches to speech/language intervention and the true believer. *Journal of Medical Speech-Language Pathology*, 11(2), 95–104.

Grunwell, P. (1975). The phonological analysis of articulation disorders. *British Journal of Disorders of Communication*, 10, 31–42.

Grunwell, P. (1981). *The Nature of Phonological Disability in Children*. New York: Academic.

Grunwell, P. (1983). Phonological development in phonological disability. *Topics in Language Disorders, 3*, 62–76.

Grunwell, P. (1985a). *Phonological Assessment of Child Speech (PACS)*. Windsor: NFER-Nelson.

Grunwell, P. (1985b). Developing phonological skills. *Child Language Teaching and Therapy, 1*, 65–72.

Grunwell, P. (1987). *Clinical Phonology* (2nd Edition). Baltimore, MD: Williams & Wilkins.

Grunwell, P. (1989). Developmental phonological disorders and normal speech development: A review and illustration. *Child Language Teaching and Therapy, 5*, 304–319.

Grunwell, P. (1992). Process of phonological change in developmental speech disorders. *Clinical Linguistics & Phonetics, 6*, 101–122.

Grunwell, P. (1997). Developmental phonological disability: Order in disorder. In B. W. Hodson and M. L. Edwards (Eds). *Perspectives in Applied Phonology*. Gaithersburg, MD: Aspen Publications.

Guralnick, M. J. (2001). A developmental systems model for early intervention. *Infants and Young Children, 14*(2), 1–18.

Guralnick, M. J. (2005). An overview of the developmental systems model for early intervention. In M. J. Guralnick (Ed). *The Developmental Approach to Early Intervention*. Baltimore, MD: Paul H. Brookes, pp. 3–28.

HPC (2007). *Standards of proficiency: Speech and language therapists. Health Professions Council*. Retrieved on November 3, 2007 from http://www.hpc-uk.org/assets/documents/ 10000529Standards_of_Proficiency_SLTs.pdf.

Habers, H. M., Paden, E. P., & Halle, J. W. (1999). Phonological awareness and production: Changes during intervention. *Language, Speech, and Hearing Services in Schools, 30*, 50–60.

Hahn, E. (1960). Communication in the therapy session: A point of view. *Journal of Speech and Hearing Disorders, 25*(1), 18–23.

Hall, C., & Golding-Kushner, K. J. (1989). Long-term follow-up of 500 patients after palate repair performed prior to 18 months of age. *Sixth International Congress on Cleft Palate and Related Craniofacial Anomalies*. Jerusalem, Israel.

Hall, D. M. B., & Elliman, D. (Eds) (2003). *Health for All Children*, 4th Edition. Oxford: Oxford University Press.

Hall, P. K. (1989). The occurrence of developmental apraxia of speech in a mild articulation disorder: A case study. *Journal of Communication Disorders, 22*, 265–276.

Hall, P. K. (2000a). A letter to the parents of a child with developmental apraxia of speech. Part I. Speech characteristics of the disorder. *Language, Speech, and Hearing Services in Schools, 31*, 169–172.

Hall, P. K. (2000b). A letter to the parents of a child with developmental apraxia of speech. Part II. The nature and causes of DAS. *Language, Speech, and Hearing Services in Schools, 31*, 173–175.

Hall, P. K. (2000c). A letter to the parents of a child with developmental apraxia of speech. Part III. Other problems often associated with the disorder. *Language, Speech, and Hearing Services in Schools, 31*, 176–178.

Hall, P. K. (2000d). A letter to the parent(s) of a child with developmental apraxia of speech. Part IV: Treatment of DAS. *Language, Speech, and Hearing Services in Schools, 31*, 179–181.

Hall, P. K., Hardy, J. C., & La Velle, W. E. (1990). A child with signs of developmental apraxia of speech with whom a palatal lift prosthesis was used to manage palatal dysfunction. *Journal of Speech and Hearing Disorders, 55*(3), 454–460.

Hall, P. K., Jordan, L. S., & Robin, D. A. (1993). *Developmental Apraxia of Speech: Theory and Clinical Practice*. Austin, TX: Pro-Ed.

Halle, J., Ostrosky, M., & Hemmeter, M. L. (2006). Functional communication training: A strategy for ameliorating challenging behavior. In R. McCauley and M. Fey (Eds). *Treatment of Language Disorders in Children*. Baltimore, MD: Paul Brookes, pp. 509–546.

Hallett, T. L. (2002). The impact of technology on teaching, clinical practice and research. *The ASHA Leader*, 7(11), 4–5, 13. Retrieved on July 12, 2007 from: http://www.asha.org/about/publications/leader-online/archives/2002/q2/f020611.htm.

Hammer, D., & Stoeckel, R. (2001). Teaching and Talking Together: Building a Treatment Team. Presentation at the annual convention of the American Speech-Language-Hearing Association, New Orleans, Louisiana.

Hammer, C. S., & Weiss, A. L. (2000). "African American" mothers' view of their infants' language development and learning environment. *American Journal of Speech-Language Pathology*, 9(2), 126–140.

Hanson, M. L. (1983). *Articulation*. Philadelphia, PA: W.B. Saunders Co.

Hardin-Jones, M. A., & Jones, D. L. (2005). Speech production of preschoolers with cleft palate. *Cleft Palate-Craniofacial Journal*, 42, 7–13.

Hartley, L. P. (1953). *The Go-Between*. New York, NY: Alfred A. Knopf.

Harris, Z. (1951). *Methods in Structural Linguistics*. Chicago, IL: Chicago University Press.

Hasson, N., & Joffe, V. (2007). The case for dynamic assessment in speech and language therapy. *Child Language Teaching and Therapy*, 23(1), 9–25.

Hatcher, P. J., Hulme, C., & Ellis, A. W. (1994). Ameliorating early reading failure by integrating the teaching of reading and phonological skills: The phonological linkage hypothesis. *Child Development*, 65, 41–57.

Hawk, S. S. (1933). *Speech Disorders*. New York, NY: Harcourt Brace & Co.

Hay, J., Warren, P., & Drager, K. (2006). Factors influencing speech perception in the context of merger-in-progress. *Journal of Phonetics*, 34(4), 58–84.

Hayden, D. (2006). The PROMPT model: Use and application for children with mixed phonological-motor impairment. *Advances in Speech-Language Pathology*, 8(3), 265–281.

Hayden, D., & Square, P. (1994). Motor speech treatment hierarchy: A systems approach. *Clinics in Communication Disorders*, 4, 162–174.

Hayden, D., & Square, P. (1999). *Verbal Motor Production Assessment for Children (VMPAC)*. USA: Psych Corp.

Healy, T. J., & Madison, C. L. (1987). Articulation error migration: a comparison of single word and connected speech samples. *Journal of Communication Disorders*, 20, 129–136.

Hegde, M. N. (2002). *Treatment Procedures in Speech-Language Pathology* (3rd Edition). Austin, TX: Pro-Ed.

Hegde, M. N., & Pena-Brooks, A. (2007). *Treatment Protocols for Articulation Disorders*. San Diego, CA: Plural Publishing.

Helfrich-Miller, K. R. (1983). The use of melodic intonation therapy with developmentally apractic children: A clinical perspective. *Journal of the Pennsylvania Speech-Language-Hearing Association*, 11–15.

Helfrich-Miller, K. R. (1984). Melodic intonation therapy with developmentally apraxic children. *Seminars in Speech and Language*, 5, 119–125.

Helfrich-Miller, K. R. (1994). Clinical perspective: Melodic intonation therapy for developmental apraxia. *Clinics in Communication Disorders*, 4(3), 175–182.

Henderlong, J., & Lepper, M. R. (2002). The effects of praise on children's intrinsic motivation: A review and synthesis. *Psychological Bulletin*, 128(5), 774–795.

Henningsson, G. E., & Isberg, A. M. (1986). Velopharyngeal movements in patients alternating between oral and glottal articulation: A clinical and cineradiographical study. *Cleft Palate Journal*, 23, 1–9.

Hesketh, A. (2004). Early literacy achievement of children with a history of speech problems. *International Journal of Language & Communication Disorders*, title~t713393930~all~issueslist~39 (4), 453–468.

Hesketh, A., Adams, C., & Nightingale, C. (2000). Metaphonological abilities of phonologically disordered children. *Educational Psychology*, 20, 484–498.

Hesketh, A., Adams, C., Nightingale, C., & Hall, R. (2000). Phonological awareness therapy and articulatory training for children with phonological disorders: a comparative outcome study. *International Journal of Language & Communication Disorders*, 35, 337–354.

Hesketh, A., Dima, E., & Nelson, V. (2007). Teaching phoneme awareness to pre-literate children with speech disorder: a randomized controlled trial. *International Journal of Language & Communication Disorders,title~t713393930~all~issueslist~42(3)*, 251–271.

Hewitt, T. W. (2006). *Understanding and Shaping Curriculum: What We Teach and Why*. Thousand Oaks, CA: Sage Publications.

Hewlett, N. (1990). Processes of development and production. In P. Grunwell (Ed). *Developmental Speech Disorders*. Edinburgh: Churchill Livingstone.

Hixon, T., Hawley, J., & Wilson, K. (1982). The around-the-house device for the clinical determination of respiratory driving pressure: A note on making the simple even simpler. *Journal of Speech and Hearing Disorders*, 47, 413.

Hoch, L., Golding-Kushner, K. J., Sadewitz, V., & Shprintzen R. J. (1986). Speech therapy. *Seminars in Speech and Language: Current Methods of Assessing and Treating Children with Cleft Palates*, 7(3), 313–326.

Hodge, M. (2002). Nonspeech oral motor treatment approaches for dysarthria: Perspectives on a controversial clinical practice. *Perspectives on Neurophysiology and Neurogenic Speech and Language Disorders*, 12(4), 22–28.

Hodge, M., Salonka, R., & Kollias, S. (2005, November). Use of nonspeech oral-motor exercises in children's speech therapy. Poster presented at the *American Speech-Language-Hearing Association Convention*, San Diego, CA.

Hodge, M., & Wellman, L. (1999). Management of children with dysarthria. In A. Caruso & E. Strand (Eds). *Clinical Management of Motor Speech Disorders in Children*. New York, NY: Thieme, pp. 209–280.

Hodson, B. (1980). *The Assessment of Phonological Processes*. Danville, IL: Interstate.

Hodson, B. (1982). Remediation of speech patterns associated with low levels of phonological performance. In M. Crary (Ed). *Phonological Intervention, Concepts and Procedures*. San Diego, CA: College-Hill Press Inc.

Hodson, B. (1992). Clinical forum: Phonological assessment and treatment. Applied phonology: Constructs, contributions and issues. *Language, Speech, and Hearing Services in Schools*, 23, 247–253.

Hodson, B. (1994). Determining phonological intervention priorities: Expediting intelligibility gains. In E. J. Williams and J. Langsam (Eds). *Children's Phonology Disorders: Pathways and Patterns*. Rockville, MD: American Speech-Language-Hearing Association.

Hodson, B. (1997). Disordered phonologies: What have we learned about assessment and treatment? In B. Hodson and M. Edwards (Eds). *Perspectives in Applied Phonology*. Gaithersburg, MD: Aspen, pp. 197–224.

Hodson, B. (2003). Hodson Computerized Analysis of Phonological Patterns. Wichita, KS: PhonoComp Software.

Hodson, B. (2004). *Hodson Assessment of Phonological Patterns* (3rd Edition). Austin, TX: Pro-Ed.

Hodson, B. (2005). *Enhancing Phonological and Metaphonological Skills of Children with Highly Unintelligible Speech*. Rockville, MD: ASHA.

Hodson, B. (2006). Identifying phonological patterns and projecting remediation cycles: Expediting intelligibility gains of a 7 year old Australian child. *Advances in Speech-Language Pathology*, 8(3), 257–264.

Hodson, B. (2007). *Evaluating and Enhancing Children's Phonological Systems: Research and Theory to Practice*. Greenville, SC: Thinking Publications/Super Duper.

Hodson, B. W., Chin, L., Redmond, B., & Simpson, R. (1983). Phonological evaluation and remediation of speech deviations of a child with a repaired cleft palate: A case study. *Journal of Speech and Hearing Disorders, 48,* 93–98.

Hodson, B. W., & Paden, E. P. (1981). Phonological processes which characterize unintelligible and intelligible speech in early childhood. *Journal of Speech and Hearing Disorders, 46,* 369–373.

Hodson, B. W., & Paden, E. (1983). *Targeting Intelligible Speech: A Phonological Approach to Remediation.* San Diego, CA: College-Hill Press.

Hodson, B. W., & Paden, E. P. (1991). *Targeting Intelligible Speech: A Phonological Approach to Remediation* (2nd Edition). Austin, TX: Pro-Ed.

Hodson, B. W., Scherz, J. A., & Strattman, K. H. (2002). Evaluating communicative abilities of a highly unintelligible child. *American Journal of Speech-Language Pathology, 11,* 236–242.

Hoffman, P. R. (1983). Interallophonic generalization of /r/ training. *Journal of Speech and Hearing Disorders, 48,* 215–221.

Hoffman, P.R. (1990). Spelling, phonology, and the speech-language pathologist: A whole language perspective. *Language, Speech, and Hearing Services in Schools, 21,* 238–243.

Hoffman, P. R. (1992). Synergistic development of phonetic skill. *Language, Speech, and Hearing Services in Schools, 23,* 254–260.

Hoffman, P. R. (1993). A whole-language treatment perspective for phonological disorder. *Seminars in Speech and Language, 14,* 142–151.

Hoffman, P. R., Daniloff, R. G., Bengoa, D., & Schuckers, G. (1985). Misarticulating and normally articulating children's identification and discrimination of synthetic [r] and [w]. *Journal of Speech and Hearing Disorders, 50,* 46–53.

Hoffman, P. R., & Daniloff, R. G. (1990). Evolving views of children's disordered speech sound production from motoric to phonological. Special Series: Speech-language pathology and audiology: Looking back on the past 25 years. *Journal of Speech-Language Pathology and Audiology, 14,* 13–22.

Hoffman, P. R., & Norris, J. A. (1989). On the nature of phonological development: Evidence from normal children's spelling errors. *Journal of Speech and Hearing Research, 32,* 787–794.

Hoffmann, P. R., Norris, J. A., & Monjure, J. (1990). Comparison of process targeting and whole language treatments for phonologically delayed preschool children. *Language, Speech, and Hearing Services in Schools, 21,* 102–109.

Hoffman, P. R., Schuckers, C. H., & Daniloff, R. G. (1980). Developmental trends in correct /r/ articulation as a function of allophone type. *Journal of Speech and Hearing Research, 23,* 746–756.

Holder, W. D. D. (1669). *Elements of Speech*: an essay of inquiry into the natural production of letters: with an appendix concerning persons deaf and dumb. London: Royal Society.

Holm, A., Crosbie, S., & Dodd, B. (2007). Differentiating normal variability from inconsistency in children's speech: normative data. *International Journal of Language & Communication Disorders, 42*(4), 467–486.

Howard, S., & Heselwood, B. (2002). The contribution of phonetics to the study of vowel development and disorders. In M. J. Ball and F. E. Gibbon (Eds). *Vowel Disorders.* Woburn, MA: Butterworth-Heinemann, pp. 37–82.

Howell, J., & Dean. E. (1994). *Treating Phonological Disorders in Children: Metaphon Theory to Practice.* London: Whurr.

Hughes, S. (1992). Serving cultural diverse families of infants and toddlers with disabilities. *Infant Toddler Intervention. The Transdisciplinary Journal, 2*(3), 169–177.

Hulme, C., Hatcher, P., Nation, K., Brown, A., Adams, J., & Stuart, G. (2002). Phoneme awareness is a better predictor of early reading skill than onset-rime awareness. *Journal of Experimental Child Psychology, 82,* 2–28.

Iglesias, A., & Quinn, R. (1997). Culture as context for early intervention. In S. K. Thurman, J. R. Cornwell, and S. R. Gottwald (Eds). *Contexts of Early Intervention: Systems and Settings.* Baltimore, MD: Paul H. Brookes, pp. 55–71.

Individuals with Disabilities Education Improvement Act [IDEA] (2004). Public Law 108–446. 20 USC 1400, 108th Congress.

Ingram, D. (1974). Phonological rules in young children. *Journal of Child Language, 1,* 49–64.

Ingram, D. (1976). *Phonological Disability in Children.* London: Edward Arnold.

Ingram, D. (1981). *Procedures for the Phonological Analysis of Children's Language.* Baltimore, MD: University Park Press.

Ingram, D. (Ed). (1983). Case studies of phonological disorders. Special issue of *Topics in Language Disorders, 2*(3), vii–ix

Ingram, D. (1986). Explanation and phonological remediation. *Child Language Teaching and Therapy, 2,* 1–9.

Ingram, D. (1989a). *Phonological Disability in Children* (2nd Edition). London: Cole & Whurr.

Ingram, D. (1989b). *First Language Acquisition: Method, Description and Explanation.* Cambridge: Cambridge University Press.

Ingram, D. (1997). Generative phonology. In R. D. Kent and M. J. Ball (Eds). *The New Phonologies: Developments in Clinical Linguistics.* San Diego, CA: Singular Press, pp. 7–33.

Ingram, D. (1998). Research-practice relationships in speech-language pathology. *Topics in Language Disorders, 18*(2), 1–9.

Ingram, D., & Ingram, K. (2001). A whole word approach to phonological intervention. *Language, Speech, and Hearing Services in Schools, 32,* 271–283.

Ingram, K., & Ingram, D. (2002). Commentary on 'Evaluating articulation and phonological disorders when the clock is running.' *American Journal of Speech-Language Pathology, 11,* 257–258.

Irvin, R., West, J., & Trombetta, M. (1966). Effectiveness of speech therapy for second grade children with misarticulations predictive factors. *Exceptional Children, 32,* 471–479.

Irwin, L. (1993). *Partnerships in Early Intervention. A Training Guide on Family-Centered Care, Team Building and Service Coordination.* Waisman Centre: University of Wisconsin, Module 1, pp. 19–21.

Irwin, D., Pannbacker, M., Powell, T. W., & Vekovius, G. T. (2007). *Ethics for Speech-Language Pathologists and Audiologists: An illustrative Casebook.* Clifton Park, NY: Thomson Delmar Learning.

Isberg, A., & Henningsson, G. (1987). Influence of palatal fistulas on velopharyngeal movements: A cineradiographic study. *Plastic and Reconstructive Surgery, 79,* 525–530.

Jacobson, J. W., Foxx, R. M., & Mulick, J. A. (2005). *Controversial Therapies for Developmental Disabilities: Fad, Fashion, and Science in Professional Practice.* Mahwah, NJ: Lawrence Erlbaum Associates.

Jacoby, P. A., Coates, H. L., Arumugaswamy, A., et al. (2008). The effect of passive smoking on the risk of otitis media in Aboriginal and non-Aboriginal children in the Kalgoorlie-Boulder region of Western Australia. *Medical Journal of Australia, 188*(10), 599–603.

Jakielski, K. J., Kostner, T. L., & Webb, C. E. (2006, June). Results of integral stimulation intervention in three children. Paper presented at the *5th International Conference on Speech Motor Control.* Nijmegen: The Netherlands.

Jakobson, R. (1941/1968). *Child Language, Aphasia and Phonological Universals.* The Hague: Mouton.

James, D. G. H. (1997). The need to use polysyllabic words in the assessment and analysis of speech. *The Australian Communication Quarterly, Autumn,* 6–8.

James, D. G. H. (2001a). An item analysis of words for an articulation and phonological test for children aged 2 to 7 years. *Clinical Linguistics & Phonetics, 15*(6), 457–485.

James, D. G. H. (2001b). Use of phonological processes in Australian children aged 2 to 7;11 years. *Advances in Speech-Language Pathology, 3*(2), 109–127.

James, D. G. H. (2006). *Hippopotamus is so hard to say: Children's acquisition of polysyllabic words.* Unpublished PhD thesis, University of Sydney, Sydney.

James, D. G. H., van Doorn, J., & McLeod, S. (1998). Children's acquisition of polysyllabic words in the age range of 5 to 7 years: The use of epenthesis. In K. Hird (Ed). *Speech Pathology Australia National Conference 1998 Proceedings.* Fremantle, WA: Curtin Printing Services and Curtin University of Technology, pp. 163–174.

James, D. G. H., van Doorn, J., McLeod, S., & Esterman, A. (2008). Patterns of consonant deletion in typically developing children aged 3 to 7 years. *International Journal of Speech-Language Pathology, 10*(3), 179–192.

Jamieson, D. G., & Rvachew, S. (1992). Remediation of speech production errors with sound identification training. *Journal of Speech-Language Pathology and Audiology, 16,* 201–210.

Jewett, J. (2003). A labor of love in Bosnia. *The ASHA Leader, 11*(7), 20–21, 27.

Joffe, B., & Reilly, S. (2004). The evidence base of the evaluation and management of motor speech disorders in children. In S. Reilly, J. Douglas, and J. Oates (Eds). *Evidence Based Practice in Speech Pathology.* London: Whurr Publishing.

Joffe, B., & Serry, T. (2004). The evidence base for the treatment of articulation and phonological disorders in children. In S. Reilly, J. Douglas, and J. Oates (Eds). *Evidence Based Practice in Speech Pathology.* London: Whurr.

Joffe, V. L. (2008). Minding the gap in research and practice in developmental language disorders. In V. L. Joffe, M. Cruice, and S. Chiat (Eds). *Language Disorders in Children and Adults: New Issues in Research and Practice.* Chichester: John Wiley Publishers.

Joffe, V. L., & Pring, T. (2003, September). Phonological therapy in clinical settings: What do we do and how effective is it? *Paper presented at the CPLOL 5th European congress*, Edinburgh.

Joffe, V. L., & Pring, T. (2008). Children with phonological problems: A survey of clinical practice. *International Journal of Language & Communication Disorders, 43*(2), 154–164.

Johnson, C. A., Weston, A. D., & Bain, B. A. (2004). An objective and time-efficient method for determining severity of childhood speech delay. *American Journal of Speech-Language Pathology, 13,* 55–65.

Johnson, C. J. (2006). Getting started in evidence-based practice for childhood speech-language disorders. *American Journal of Speech-Language Pathology, 15*(1), 20–35.

Johnson, D. E. (2000). Medical and developmental sequelae of early childhood institutionalization in Eastern European adoptees. In C. A. Nelson (Ed). The Minnesota Symposia on Child Psychology: The Effects of Early Adversity on Neurobehavioral Development. *Minnesota Symposium on Child Psychology, 31,* 113–162.

Johnston, P. (2004). *Choice Words: How Our Language Affects Children's Learning.* Portland, ME: Stenhouse.

Jones, D. (1967). *An Outline of English Phonetics* (9th Edition). Cambridge: Heffer.

Jongman, A., Wayland, R., & Wong, S. (2000). Acoustic characteristics of English fricatives. *Journal of the Acoustical Society of America, 108,* 1252–1263.

Kamhi, A. G. (1992). The need for a broad-based model of phonological disorders. *Language, Speech, and Hearing Services in Schools, 23,* 261–268.

Kamhi, A. G. (2004). A meme's eye view of speech-language pathology. *Language, Speech, and Hearing in Schools, 35,* 105–111.

Kahmi, A. G. (2006a). Prologue: Combining research and reason to make treatment decisions. *Language, Speech, and Hearing Services in Schools, 37*(4), 255–257.

Kamhi, A. G. (2006b). Treatment decisions for children with speech-sound disorders. *Language, Speech, and Hearing Services in Schools, 37*(4), 271–279.

Kamhi, A. G., & Pollock, K. E. (Eds). (2005). *Phonological Disorders in Children: Clinical Decision Making in Assessment and Intervention*. Baltimore: Paul H Brookes.

Karlin, I., & Strazzula, M. (1952). Speech and language problems of mentally deficient children. *Journal of Speech and Hearing Disorders*, 7, 286.

Karlsson, H. B., Shriberg, L. D., Flipsen, P., Jr., & McSweeny, J. L. (2002). Acoustic phenotypes for speech-genetics studies: Toward an acoustic marker for residual /s/ distortions. *Clinical Linguistics & Phonetics*, 16, 403–424.

Kathard, H., Naude, E., Pillay, M., & Ross, E. (2007). Improving the relevance of speech-language pathology & audiology research and practice. *South African Journal of Communication Disorders*, 54, 3–7.

Kaufman, N. (1995). *Kaufman Speech Praxis Test*. Detroit, MI: Wayne State University Press.

Kaufman, N. (2005). *Kaufman Speech Praxis Workout Book*. Gaylord, MI: Northern Speech Services.

Kearns, K. P. (1986). Flexibility of single-subject experimental designs. Part II: Design selection and arrangement of experimental phases. *Journal of Speech and Hearing Disorders*, 51, 204–213.

Kehoe, M. (2001). Prosodic patterns in children's multisyllabic word patterns. *Language, Speech, and Hearing Services in Schools*, 32, 284–294.

Kent, R. (1982). Contextual facilitation of correct sound production. *Language, Speech, and Hearing Services in Schools*, 13, 66–76.

Kent, R. D. (2000). Research on speech motor control and its disorders: a review and prospective. *Journal of Communication Disorders*, 33(5), 391–427; quiz 428.

Kent, R. (2004). Normal aspects of articulation. In J. E. Bernthal and N. W. Bankson (Eds). *Articulation and Phonological Disorders*. Boston, MA: Allyn & Bacon, pp. 1–62.

Kerridge, I., Lowe, M., & Henry, D. A. (1998). Ethics and evidence-based medicine. *British Medical Journal*, 316, 1151–1153.

Kewley-Port, D., Watson, C. S., Elbert, M., Maki, K., & Reed, D. (1991). The Indiana Speech Training Aid (ISTPA) II: Training curriculum and selected case studies. *Clinical Linguistics & Phonetics*, 5, 13–38.

Khan, L. M., & Lewis, N. P. (1990). Phonological process therapy in school settings: The bare essentials to meeting the ultimate challenge. *National Student Speech Language Hearing Association Journal*, 17, 50–58.

Khan, L. M. L., & Lewis, N. P. (2002). *Khan–Lewis. Phonological Analysis* (2nd Edition). Circle Pines, MN: American Guidance Service.

Kilminster, M. G. E., & Laird, E. M. (1978) Articulation development in children aged three to nine years. *Australian Journal of Human Communication Disorders*, 6(1), 23–30.

Kim, J., & Chin, S. B. (2008). Fortition and lenition patterns in the acquisition of obstruents by children with cochlear implants. *Clinical Linguistics & Phonetics*, 22, 233–251.

Kiparsky, P., & Menn, L. (1977). On the acquisition of phonology. In J. Macnamara (Ed). *Language Learning and Thought*. New York: Academic Press.

Kiran, S. (2007). Complexity in the treatment of naming deficits. *American Journal of Speech-Language Pathology*, 16(1), 18–29.

Kirkpatrick, J., Stohr, P., & Kimbrough, D. (1990a). *Moving Across Syllables*. Tucson, AZ: Communication Skill Builders.

Kirkpatrick, J., Stohr, P., & Kimbrough, D. (1990b). *Test of Syllable Sequencing Skills (TSSS)*. Tucson, AZ: Communication Skill Builders.

Kishon-Rabin, L., Taitelbaum-Swead, R., Ezrati-Vinacour, R., Kronnenberg, J., & Hildesheimer, M. (2004). Pre-first word vocalizations of infants with normal hearing and cochlear implants using the PRISE. *International Congress Series. Cochlear Implants. Proceedings of the VIII International Cochlear Implant Conference*, 1273, 360–363.

Klein, E. S. (1996a). Phonological/traditional approaches to articulation therapy: A retrospective group comparison. *Language, Speech, and Hearing Services in Schools*, 27, 314–323.

Klein, E. S. (1996b). *Clinical Phonology: Assessment and Treatment of Articulation Disorders in Children and Adults*. San Diego, CA: Singular Publishing Group, Inc.

Klein, H. B., Lederer, S. H., & Cortese, E. E. (1991). Children's knowledge of auditory / articulatory correspondences: Phonologic and metaphonologic. *Journal of Speech and Hearing Research*, *34*, 559–564.

Klein, N., & Gilkerson, L. (2000). Personnel preparation for early childhood intervention programmes. In J. P. Shonkoff and S. J. Meisels (Eds). *Handbook of Early Childhood Intervention* (2nd Edition). Cambridge: Cambridge University Press, pp. 454–483.

Knowles, M. S. (1970). *The Modern Practise of Adult Education: Andragogy Versus Pedagogy*. New York Association Press.

Koegel, L. K., Koegel, R. L., & Ingham, J. C. (1986). Programming rapid generalization of correct articulation through self-monitoring procedures. *Journal of Speech and Hearing Disorders*, *51*, 24–32.

Koegel, R. L. Koegel, L. K., Van Voy, K. V., & Ingham, J. C. (1988). Within-clinic versus outside-of-clinic self-monitoring of articulation to promote generalization. *Journal of Speech and Hearing Disorders*, *53*, 392–399.

Kollias, S., & Lester, R. (2004). *Nonspeech oral motor exercises in children's speech therapy: Clinicians' opinions and experiences*. Unpublished manuscript. University of Alberta, Edmonton, AB.

Kretzmann, J. P., & McKnight, J. L. (1993). *Building Communities from the Inside Out*. Chicago, IL: Acta Publications.

Kuehn, D. (1991). New therapy for treating hypernasal speech using continuous positive airway pressure (CPAP). *Plastic and Reconstructive Surgery*, *88*(6), 959–966.

Kuehn, D. (1997). The development of a new technique for treating hypernasality: CPAP. *American Journal of Speech-Language Pathology*, *6*(4), 5–8.

Kuerman, P., Bligh, S., & Goodban, M. (1980). Activating articulation skills through theraplay. *Journal of Speech and Hearing Disorders*, *45*, 540–545.

Kuhn, T. S. (1962). *The Structure of Scientific Revolutions*. Chicago, IL: The University of Chicago Press.

Kummer, A. W. (2001a). Perceptual assessment. In A. W. Kummer (Ed). *Cleft Palate and Craniofacial Anomalies: The Effects of Speech and Resonance*. San Diego, CA: Singular, pp. 265–292.

Kummer, A. W. (2001b). Speech therapy for effects of velopharyngeal dysfunction. In A. W. Kummer (Ed). *Cleft Palate and Craniofacial Anomalies: The Effects of Speech and Resonance*. San Diego, CA: Singular, pp. 459–482.

Kummer, A. W. (2008). *Cleft Palate and Craniofacial Anomalies: Effects on Speech and Resonance* (2nd Edition). Clifton Park, NY: Thomson Delmar Learning.

Kummer, A. W., Marty-Grames, L., Jones, D., Karnell, M., & Ruscello, D. M. (2006). Response to velopharyngeal dysfunction: Speech characteristics, variable etiologies, evaluation techniques, and differential treatments. *Language, Speech, and Hearing Services in Schools*, *37*, 236–238.

Kummer, A. W., Strife, J. L., Grau, W. H., Creaghead, N. A., & Lee, L. (1989). The effects of Le Fort I osteotomy with maxillary advancement on articulation, resonance, and velopharyngeal function. *Cleft Palate Journal*, *26*, 193–199.

Kwiatkowski, J., & Shriberg, L. D. (1992). Intelligibility assessment in developmental phonological disorders: Accuracy of caregiver gloss. *Journal of Speech and Hearing Research*, *35*, 1095–1104.

Kwiatkowski, J., & Shriberg, L. (1993). Speech normalization in developmental phonological disorders: A retrospective study of capability-focus theory. *Language, Speech, and Hearing Services in Schools*, *24*, 10–18.

Kwiatkowski, J., & Shriberg, L. D. (1998). The capability-focus treatment framework for child speech disorders. *American Journal of Speech-Language Pathology*, *7*, 27–38.

Labov, W. (1966). *The Social Stratification of English in New York City*. Washington DC: Center for Applied Linguistics.

Labov, W. (1994–2001). *Principles of Linguistic Change* (2 vols). Oxford: Blackwell.

Lacan, J. (2005). The mirror stage as formative of the function of the I as revealed in psychoanalytic experience. In B. McLaughlin and B. Coleman (Eds). *Everyday Theory: A Contemporary Reader*. New York: Pearson Education, pp. 547–553.

Lai, C. S. L., Fisher, S. E., Hurst, J. A., et al. (2000). The SPCH1 region on human 7q31: Genomic characterization of the critical interval and localization of translocations associated with speech and language disorder. *American Journal of Human Genetics*, 67, 357–368.

Lai, C. S. L., Fisher, S. E., Hurst, J. A., Vargha-Khadem, F., & Monaco, A. P. (2001). A forkhead-domain gene is mutated in a severe speech and language disorder. *Nature, 413*, 519–523.

Laing, S. P., & Espeland, W. (2005). Low intensity phonological awareness training in a preschool classroom for children with communication impairments. *Journal of Communication Disorders, 38*, 65–82.

Lalli, J. S., Casey, S., & Kates, K. (1995). Reducing escape behavior and increasing task completion with functional communication training, extinction, and response chaining. *Journal of Applied Behavior Analysis, 28*, 261–268.

Lancaster, G. (1991). *The effectiveness of parent administered input training for children with phonological disorders*. Unpublished Masters thesis, City University, London.

Lancaster, G. (2007). *Developing Speech and Language Skills*. London: David Fulton Publishers, Routledge.

Lancaster, G., Keusch, S., Levin, A., Pring, T., & Martin, S. (in press). Treating children with phonological problems: Does an eclectic approach to therapy work? *International Journal of Language & Communication Disorders*.

Lancaster, G., & Pope, L. (1989). *Working with Children's Phonology*. Oxon: Winslow Press.

Lane, H., & Perkell, J. S. (2005). Control of voice-onset time in the absence of hearing: a review. *Journal of Speech, Language, and Hearing Research, 48*(6), 1334–1343.

Lane, H., & Tranel, B. (1971). The Lombard sign and the role of hearing in speech. *The Journal of Speech and Hearing Sciences, 14*, 677–709.

LaRiviere, C., Winitz, H., Reeds, J., & Herriman, E. (1974). The conceptual reality of selected distinctive features. *Journal of Speech and Hearing Research, 17*, 122–133.

Larrivee, L. S., & Catts, H. W. (1999). Early reading achievement in children with expressive phonological disorders. *American Journal of Speech-Language Pathology, 8*, 118–128.

Larroudé, B. (2004). Multicultural-multilingual group sessions: Development of functional communication. *Topics in Language Disorders, 24*, 137–140.

Larson, V. L., & McKinley, N. L. (2003). *Communication Solutions for Older Students: Assessment and Intervention Strategies*. Eau Claire, WI: Thinking Publications.

Lass, N. J., & Pannbacker, M. (2008). The application of evidence-based practice to oral motor treatment. *Language, Speech, and Hearing Services in Schools, 39*(3), 408–421.

Law, J. (Ed). (1992). *The Early Identification of Language Impairment in Children*. London: Chapman and Hall.

Law, J., Boyle, J., Harris, F., Harkness, A., & Nye, C. (1998) Screening for speech and language delay: A systematic review of the literature. *Health Technology Assessment, 2*(9), 1–184.

Law, J., Garrett, Z., & Nye, C. (2003). Speech and language therapy interventions for children with primary speech and language delay or disorder. *Cochrane Database of Systematic Reviews, Issue 3*. Art. No.: CD004110. DOI: 10.1002/14651858.CD004110.

Law, J., Garrett, Z., & Nye, C. (2004). The efficacy of treatment for children with developmental speech and language delay/disorder: A meta-analysis. *Journal of Speech, Language, and Hearing Research, 47*, 924–943.

Lee, S., Potamianos, A., & Narayanan, S. (1999). Acoustics of children's speech: Developmental changes in temporal and spectral parameters. *Journal of the Acoustical Society of America*, *105*, 1455–1468.

Leitão, S., Hogben, J., & Fletcher, J. (1997). Phonological processing skills in speech and language impaired children. *European Journal of Disorders of Communication*, *32*(2), 91–113.

Leiter, V. (2004). Dilemmas in sharing care: maternal provision of professionally driven therapy for children with disabilities. *Social Science & Medicine*, *58*, 837–849.

Lejeune, B., & Demanez, L. (2006). Speech discrimination and intelligibility: outcome of deaf children fitted with hearing aids or cochlear implants. *B-ENT*, *2*(2), 63–68.

Lenneberg, E. (1967). *The Biological Foundations of Language*. New York: Wiley.

Leonard, L. B. (1973). The nature of disordered articulation. *Journal of Speech and Hearing Disorders*, *38*, 156–161.

Leonard, L. B. (1985). Unusual and subtle phonological behavior in the speech of phonologically disordered children. *Journal of Speech and Hearing Disorders*, *50*, 4–13.

Leonard, L. B., & Brown, B. L. (1984). Nature and boundaries of phonologic categories: A case study of an unusual phonologic pattern in a language-impaired child. *Journal of Speech and Hearing Disorders*, *49*, 419–428.

Leonard, L. B., Camarata, S., Schwartz, R. G., Chapman, K., & Messick, C. (1985). Homonymy and the voiced-voiceless distinction in the speech of children with specific language impairment. *Journal of Speech and Hearing Research*, *28*, 215–224.

Leonard, L. B., Schwartz, R. C., Allen, G., Swanson, L., & Loeb, D. (1989). Unusual phonological behavior and the avoidance of homonymy in children. *Journal of Speech and Hearing Research*, *32*, 583–590.

Leonard, L. B., Schwartz, R. G., Swanson, L., & Loeb, D. (1987). Some conditions that promote unusual phonological behavior in children. *Clinical Linguistics & Phonetics*, *1*, 23–34.

Leonard, L. B., & Webb, C. E. (1971). An automated therapy program for articulatory correction. *Journal of Speech and Hearing Research*, *14*, 338–344.

Leopold, W. F. (1947). *Speech Development of a Bilingual Child, Vol. 2. Sound Learning in the First Two Years*. Evanston, IL: Northwestern University Press.

Lewin, K. (1951). *Field Theory in Social Science: Selected Theoretical Papers*. New York, NY: Harper & Row.

Lewis, B. A. (1990). Familial phonological disorders: Four pedigrees. *Journal of Speech and Hearing Disorders*, *55*, 160–170.

Lewis, B. A., Ekelman, B. L., & Aram, D. M. (1989). A familial study of severe phonological disorders. *Journal of Speech and Hearing Research*, *32*, 713–724.

Lewis, B. A., & Freebairn, L. (1992). Residual effects of preschool phonology disorders in grade school, adolescence, and adulthood. *Journal of Speech and Hearing Research*, *35*, 819–831.

Lewis, B. A., Freebairn, L. A., Hansen, A. J., Miscimarra, L., Iyengar, S. K., & Taylor, H. G. (2007). Speech and language skills of parents of children with speech sound disorders. *American Journal of Speech-Language Pathology*, *16*(2), 108–118.

Lewis, B. A., Shriberg, L. D., Freebairn, L. A., et al. (2006). The genetic basis of speech sound disorders: Evidence from spoken and written language. *Journal of Speech, Language, and Hearing Research*, *49*, 1294–1312.

Lewis, B. A., Freebairn, L. A., & Taylor, H. G. (2000a). Academic outcomes in children with histories of speech sound disorders. *Journal of Communication Disorders*, *33*, 11–30.

Lewis, B. A., Freebairn, L., & Taylor, H. G. (2000b). Follow-up of children with early expressive phonology disorders, *Journal of Learning Disabilities*, *33*(5), 433–444.

Lewis, B. A., Freebairn, L. A., & Taylor, H. G. (2002). Correlates of spelling abilities in children with early speech sound disorders. *Reading and Writing: An Interdisciplinary Journal*, *15*, 389–407.

Lewis, J. R., Andeassen, M. L., Leeper, H. A., Macrae, D. L., & Thomas, J. (1993). Vocal characteristics of children with cleft lip/palate and associated velopharyngeal incompetence. *Journal of Otolaryngology, 22,* 113–117.

Liberman, A. M. (1996). *Speech: A Special Code.* Cambridge, MA: MIT Press.

Liberman, M., & Prince, A. (1977). On stress and linguistic rhythm. *Linguistic Inquiry, 8,* 249–336.

Lidz, C. S., & Pena, E. D. (1996). Dynamic assessment: The model, its relevance as a nonbiased approach, and its application to Latino American preschool children. *Language, Speech, and Hearing Services in Schools, 27,* 367–372.

Lim, S. Y., & Simser, J. (2005). Auditory-verbal therapy for children with hearing impairment. *Annals, Academy of Medicine, Singapore, 34*(4), 307–312.

Lindamood, C. H., & Lindamood, P. C. (1979). *Lindamood Auditory Conceptualization Test.* Austin, TX: Pro-Ed, Inc.

Linville, S. (1998). Acoustic correlates of perceived versus actual sexual orientation in men's speech. *Pholia Phoniatrica et Logopaedica, 50,* 35–48.

Lister, J. J., & Roberts, R. A. (2005). Effects of age and hearing loss on gap detection and the precedence effect: Narrow-band stimuli. *Journal of Speech, Language, and Hearing Research, 48*(2), 482–493.

Litchfield, R., & MacDougall, C. (2002). Professional issues for physiotherapists in family-centred and community-based settings. *Australian Journal of Physiotherapy, 48,* 105–112.

Lleo, C., & Printz, M. (1996). Consonant clusters in child phonology and the directionality of syllable structure assignment. *Journal of Child Language, 23,* 31–56.

Lloyd, S. (1998). *The Phonics Handbook* (3rd Edition). UK: Jolly Learning.

Locke, J. L. (1979). Homonymy and sound change in the child's acquisition of phonology. In N. Lass (Ed). *Speech and Language: Advances in Basic Research and Practice.* New York, NY: Academic, pp. 257–282.

Locke, J. L. (1980). The inference of speech perception in the phonologically disordered child. Part II: Some clinically novel procedures, their use, some findings. *Journal of Speech and Hearing Disorders, 45,* 445–468.

Locke, J. L. (1983). Clinical phonology: The explanation and treatment of speech sound disorders. *Journal of Speech and Hearing Disorders, 48,* 339–341.

Locke, J. L. (1983). *Phonological Acquisition and Change.* New York, NY: Academic.

Locke, J. L. (1993). *The Child's Path to Spoken Language.* Cambridge, MA: Harvard University.

Lof, G. L. (1996). Factors associated with speech-sound stimulability. *Journal of Communication Disorders, 29,* 255–278.

Lof, G. L. (2002). Special forum on phonology: Two comments on this assessment series. *American Journal of Speech-Language Pathology, 11,* 255–256.

Lof, G. L. (2003). Oral motor exercises and treatment outcomes. *Perspectives on Language Learning and Education, 10*(1), 7–12.

Lof, G. L. (2006). Logic, theory, and evidence against using nonspeech oralmotor exercises. *Paper presented at the American-Speech-Language-Hearing Association Convention, Miami Beach.*

Lof, G. L. (2007, November 15). Reasons why non-speech oral motor exercises should not be used for speech sound disorders. Paper presented at the *American Speech-Language-Hearing Association Convention*, Boston, MA. Retrieved December 19, 2007 from: http://convention.asha.org/handouts/1137_1597Lof_Gregory_057291_Nov08_2007_Time_105638AM.pdf.

Lof, G. L., & Synan, S. T. (1997). Is there a speech discrimination/perception link to disordered articulation and phonology? A review of 80 years of literature. *Contemporary Issues in Communications Sciences and Disorders, 24,* 63–77.

Lof, G. L., & Watson, M. M. (2004, November). Speech-language pathologist's use of nonspeech oral-motor drills: National survey results. Poster presented at the *American Speech-Language-Hearing Association Convention*, Philadelphia, PA.

Lof, G. L., & Watson, M. M. (2008). A nationwide survey of non-speech oral motor exercise use: Implications for evidence-based practice. *Language, Speech, and Hearing Services in Schools*, 39(3), 392–407.

Lohman, P. (2000). Results of summer 2000 apraxia-kids parental survey. Retrieved December 20, 2007 from: http://www.apraxia-kids.org/site/apps/nl/content3.asp?c=chKMI0PIIsE&b=788461&ct=464273.

Loncar-Belding, L. (1998). *Take Home™ Oral-Motor Exercises*. East Moline, IL: LinguiSystems.

Long, S. (2007). *Computerized Profiling*. Downloaded December 30, 2007 from: http://www.computerizedprofiling.org/downloads.html

Louko, L. J., Edwards, M. L., & Conture, E. G. (1990). Phonological characteristics of young stutterers and their normally fluent peers: Preliminary observations. *Journal of Fluency Disorders*, 15, 191–210.

Lous, J., Burton, M. J., Felding, J. U., Ovesen, T., Rovers, M. M., & Williamson, I. (2005). Grommets (ventilation tubes) for hearing loss associated with otitis media with effusion in children [see comment]. *Cochrane Database of Systematic Reviews*, 1, CD001801.

Louw, B. (2004) Culture. In I. Eloff and L. Ebersöhn (Eds). *Keys to Educational Psychology*. Cape Town: UCT Press, pp. 258–271.

Louw, B. (2006). Family focused early intervention for young children affected by Aids: A paradox? *42nd South African ENT Congress* in conjunction with SA Head and Neck Oncology Society, SASLHA and SAAA. 8–11 October 2006, Cape Town.

Louw, B., & Avenant, C. (2002). Culture as context for intervention: Developing a culturally congruent early intervention programme. *International Pediatrics*, 17(3), 145–150.

Louw, B., & Delport, R. (2006). Contextual challenges in South Africa: The role of a research ethics committee. *Journal of Academic Ethics*, 4, 39–60.

Louw, B., Shibambu, M., & Roemer, K. (2006). Facilitating cleft palate team participation of culturally diverse families in South Africa. *Cleft Palate-Craniofacial Journal*, 43(1), 47–54.

Love, R. J. (2000). *Childhood Motor Speech Disability* (2nd Edition). Toronto: Maxwell Macmillan Canada.

Lowe, R. J. (1993). *Speech-Language Pathology and Related Professions in the Schools*. Boston, MA: Allyn & Bacon.

Lowe, R. J. (1994). *Phonology: Assessment and Intervention Application in Speech Pathology*. Baltimore, MD: Williams & Wilkins.

Lowe, R. J. (2000) *ALPHA-R: Assessment Link between Phonology and Articulation – Revised*. Mifflinville, PA: ALPHA Speech & Language Resources.

Lowe, R. J. (2002). *Workbook for the Identification of Phonological Processes and Distinctive Features* (3rd Edition). Austin, TX: Pro-Ed.

Lowe, R. J., & Weitz, J. (1992a). *Activities for the Remediation of Phonological Disorders*. Dekalb, IL: Janelle Publications, Inc.

Lowe, R. J., & Weitz, J. (1992b). *Picture Resources for the Remediation of Articulation and Phonological Disorders*. Dekalb, IL: Janelle Publications, Inc.

Lubianca Neto, J. F., Hemb, L., & Brunelli, E. S. D. (2006). Systematic literature review of modifiable risk factors for recurrent acute otitis media in childhood. *Jornal de Pediatria*, 82(2), 87–96.

Lum, C. (2002). *Scientific Thinking in Speech and Language Therapy*. Mahwah, NJ: Lawrence Erlbaum Associates.

Lundberg, I., Frost, J., & Peterson, O.-P. (1988). Effects of an extensive program for stimulating phonological awareness In preschool children. *Reading Research Quarterly*, 23, 263–284.

Luterman, D. M. (2001). *Counseling Persons with Communication Disorders and their Families* (4th Edition). Austin, TX: Pro-Ed.

Lynch, E. W. (1998). Developing cross-cultural competence. In E. W. Lynch and M. J. Hanson (Eds). *A Guide for Working with Children and their Families: Developing Cross-Cultural Competence*. Baltimore, MD: Paul H. Brookes, pp. 47–86.

Maassen, B. (2002). Issues contrasting adult acquired versus developmental apraxia of speech. *Seminars in Speech and Language*, 23(4), 257–266.

MacKean, G., Thurston, W., & Scott, C. (2005). Bridging the divide between families and health professionals' perspectives on family-centred care. *Health Expectations*, 8, 74–85.

Macken, M. A. (1980). The child's lexical representations: the 'puzzle - puddle - pickle' evidence. *Journal of Linguistics*, 16, 1–17.

Macken, M. A., & Ferguson, C. A. (1983). Cognitive aspects of phonological development: Model, evidence and issues. In K. E. Nelson (Ed). *Children's Language, 4*. Hillsdale, NJ: Lawrence Erlbaum.

Madding, C. C. (2000). Maintaining focus on cultural competence in early intervention services to linguistically and culturally diverse families. *Infant-Toddler Intervention. The Transdisciplinary Journal*, 10(1), 9–18.

Major, E., & Bernhardt, B. (1998). Metaphonological skills of children with phonological disorders before and after phonological and metaphonological intervention. *International Journal of Language & Communication Disorders*, 33, 413–444.

Malone, T. W., & Lepper, M. R. (1987). Making learning fun: A taxonomy of intrinsic motivations for learning. In R. E. Snow and M. J. Farr (Eds). *Aptitude, Learning and Instruction: III. Conative and Affective Process Analysis*. Hillsdale, NJ: Erlbaum, pp. 223–253.

Mann, V. A., & Foy, J. G. (2007). Speech development patterns and phonological awareness in preschool children. *Annals of Dyslexia*, 57, 51–74.

Manning W. H., Keappock, N. E., & Stick, S. L. (1976). The use of auditory masking to estimate automatization of correct articulatory production. *Journal of Speech and Hearing Disorders*, 41, 143–149.

Markham, C., & Dean, T. (2006). Parents' and professionals' perceptions of quality of life in children with speech and language difficulty. *International Journal of Language & Communication Disorders*, 41(2), 189–212.

Marquardt, T. P., Sussman, H. M., Snow, T., & Jacks, A. (2002). The integrity of the syllable in developmental apraxia of speech. *Journal of Communication Disorders*, 35, 31–49.

Marshalla, P. (2001). *Oral Motor Techniques in Articulation and Phonological Therapy*. Kirkland, WA: Marshalla Speech and Language.

Marshalla, P. (2004). Oral-motor techniques in articulation and phonological therapy (Millennium Ed., rev. 2000). Kirkland, WA: Marshalla Speech and Language.

Massaro, D. W., & Light, J. (2004). Using visible speech to train perception and production of speech for individuals with hearing loss. *Journal of Speech, Language, and Hearing Research*, 47(2), 304–320.

Massie, R., & Dillon, H. (2006). The impact of sound-field amplification in mainstream cross-cultural classrooms: part 1 educational outcomes. *Australian Journal of Education*, 50, 62–77.

Masterson, J., & Bernhardt, B. (2001). *Computerized Articulation and Evaluation Phonology System (CAPES)*. San Antonio, TX: The Psychological Corporation.

Masterson, J. A., Bernhardt, B. H., & Hofheinz, M. K. (2005). A comparison of single words and conversational speech in phonological evaluation. *American Journal of Speech-Language Pathology*, 14, 229–241.

Maxwell, E. M. (1984). On determining underlying representations of children: a critique of the current theories. In M. Elbert, D. A. Dinnsen and G. Weismer (Eds). Phonological theory and the misarticulating child. *ASHA Monographs*, 22, Rockville, MD: ASHA.

McAllister, L., & Lincoln, M. (2004). *Clinical Education in Speech-Language Pathology*. London: Whurr.

McCabe, P., Rosenthal, J. B., & McLeod, S. (1998). Features of developmental dyspraxia in the general speech-impaired population? *Clinical Linguistics & Phonetics*, 12(2), 105–126.

McCarthy, J. (1988). Feature geometry and dependency: a review. *Phonetica*, 43, 84–108.

McCartney, E., Boyle, J., Bannatyne, S., Jessiman, E., Campbell, C., Kelsey, C., Smith, J., McArthur, J., & O'Hare, A. (2005). 'Thinking for two': A case study of speech and language therapists working through assistants. *International Journal of Language & Communication Disorders*, 40, 221–235.

McCauley, R. J. (2003). Review of Screening Test for Developmental Apraxia of Speech, 2nd Edition. In B. Plake, J. C. Impara, and R. A. Spies (Eds). *The Fifteenth Mental Measurements Yearbook*. Austin, TX: Pro-Ed, pp. 786–789.

McCauley, R. J., & Fey, M. (Eds) (2006). *Treatment of Language Disorders in Children*. Baltimore, MD: Paul Brookes.

McCauley, R. J., & Strand, E. A. (2008). A review of standardized tests of nonverbal oral and speech motor performance in children. *American Journal of Speech-Language Pathology*, 17(1), 1–11.

McCurry, W. H., & Irwin, O. C. (1953). A study of word approximations in the spontaneous speech of infants. *Journal of Speech and Hearing Disorders*, 18(2), 133–139.

McKinnon, D. H., McLeod, S., & Reilly, S. (2007). The prevalence of stuttering, voice, and speech-sound disorders in primary school students in Australia. *Language, Speech, and Hearing Services in Schools*, 38, 5–15.

McLeod, S. (2004). Speech pathologists' application of the ICF to children with speech impairment. *Advances in Speech-Language Pathology*, 6(1), 75–81.

McLeod, S. (2006). The holistic view of a child with unintelligible speech: Insights from the ICF and ICF-CY. *Advances in Speech-Language Pathology*, 8(3), 293–315.

McLeod, S. (Ed). (2007a). *The International Guide to Speech Acquisition*. Clifton Park, NY: Thomson Delmar Learning.

McLeod, S. (2007b). Speech acquisition and participation in society. In S. McLeod (Ed). *The International Guide to Speech Acquisition*. Clifton Park, NY: Thomson Delmar Learning.

McLeod, S. (2009). Speech sound acquisition. In J. E. Bernthal, N. W. Bankson, and P. Flipsen, Jr. (Eds). *Articulation and Phonological Disorders: Speech Sound Disorders in Children* (6th Edition). Boston, MA: Pearson Education, pp. 63–120.

McLeod, S., & Baker, E. (2004). Current clinical practice for children with speech impairment. In B. E. Murdoch, J. Goozee, B.-M. Whelan, and K. Docking (Eds). *26th World Congress of the International Association of Logopedics and Phoniatrics*. Brisbane: University of Queensland.

McLeod, S., & Bleile, K. M. (2004). The ICF: A framework for setting goals for children with speech impairment. *Child Language, Teaching and Therapy*, 20(3), 199–219.

McLeod, S., & Bleile, K. M. (2007). The ICF and ICF–CY as a framework for children's speech acquisition. In S. McLeod (Ed). *The International Guide to Speech Acquisition*. Clifton Park, NY: Thomson Delmar Learning.

McLeod, S., Hand, L., Rosenthal, J. B., & Hayes, B. (1994). The Effect of Sampling Condition on Children's Productions of Consonant Clusters. *Journal of Speech and Hearing Research*, 37, 868–882.

McLeod, S., & McCormack, J. (2007). Application of the ICF and ICF-CY to children with speech impairment. *Seminars in Speech and Language*, 28(4), 254–264.

McLeod, S., & Threats, T. T. (2008). The ICF-CY and children with communication disabilities. *International Journal of Speech-Language Pathology*, 10(1), 92–109.

McNeilly, L., Fotheringham, S., & Walsh, R. (2007). *Future directions in terminology*. Symposium: Terminology in communication sciences and disorders: a new approach. Copenhagen: 27th World Congress of the International Association of Logopedics and Phoniatrics.

McReynolds, L. V. (1972). Articulation generalization during articulation training. *Language and Speech*, *15*, 149–155.

McReynolds, L. V., & Bennett, S. (1972). Distinctive feature generalization in articulation training. *Journal of Speech and Hearing Disorders*, *37*, 462–470.

McReynolds, L. V., & Jetzke, E. (1986). Articulation generalization of voiced-voiceless sounds in hearing-impaired children. *Journal of Speech and Hearing Disorders*, *51*, 348–355.

McReynolds, L. V., & Kearns, K. P. (1983). *Single-Subject Experimental Designs in Communicative Disorders*. Baltimore, MD: University Park.

McReynolds, L. V., & Thompson, C. K. (1986). Flexibility of single-subject experimental designs. Part I: Review of the basics of single-subject designs. *Journal of Speech and Hearing Disorders*, *51*, 194–203.

McWilliams, B. J. (1954). Some factors in the intelligibility of cleft palate speech. *Journal of Speech and Hearing Disordorders*, *119*, 524–528.

McWilliams, B. J., Morris, H. L., & Shelton, R. L. (1984). *Cleft Palate Speech*. Philadelphia, PA: B. C. Decker, Inc.

Mendoza-Denton, N. (2007). *Homegirls: Symbolic Practices in the Making of Latina Youth Styles*. Malden, MA: Blackwell.

Menn, L. (1976). Evidence for an interactionist discovery theory of child phonology. *Papers and Reports on Language Development*, *12*, 169–177. Stanford, CA: Stanford University.

Meredith, A. (2002). Disordered Prosody and Articulation in Children with Childhood Apraxia of Speech: What's the Relationship? Retrieved Mar 20, 2008 from http://www.apraxia-kids.org/site/c.chKMI0PIIsE/b.980831/apps/s/content.asp?ct=464245.

Meyer, S. M. (2004). *Survival Guide for the Beginning Clinician* (2nd Edition). Austin, TX: Pro-Ed.

Miccio, A. W. (2002). Clinical problem solving: Assessment of phonological disorders. *American Journal of Speech-Language Pathology*, *11*, 221–229.

Miccio, A. W. (2005). A treatment program for enhancing stimulability. In A. G. Kamhi and K. E. Pollock (Eds). *Phonological Disorders in Children: Clinical Decision Making in Assessment and Intervention*. Baltimore, MD: Paul H. Brookes, pp. 163–173.

Miccio, A. W., & Elbert, M. (1996). Enhancing stimulability: a treatment program. *Journal of Communication Disorders*, *29*, 335–352.

Miccio, A. W., Elbert, M., & Forrest, K. (1999). The relationship between stimulability and phonological acquisition in children with normally developing and disordered phonologies. *American Journal of Speech-Language Pathology*, *8*, 347–363.

Michael, D. D., Siegel, G. M., & Pick, H. L., Jr. (1995). Effects of distance on vocal intensity. *Journal of Speech and Hearing Research*, *38*(5), 1176–1183.

Michie, S., & Abraham, C. (2004). Identifying techniques that promote health behaviour change: Evidence based or evidence inspired? *Psychology and Health*, *19*, 29–49.

Milisen, R. (1954). A rationale for articulation disorders. *Journal of Speech and Hearing Disorders* (Monograph supplement), *4*, 6–17.

Milroy, L. (1987). *Language and Social Networks* (2nd Edition). Oxford: Blackwell.

Minke, K., & Scott, M. (1995). Parent-professional relationships in early intervention: A qualitative investigation. *Topics in Early Childhood Special Education*, *15*(3), 335–352.

Mirabito, K., & Armstrong, E. (2005). Parent reactions to speech therapy involvement. Paper presented at the *Speech Pathology Australia National Conference*, Canberra.

Mirenda, P. (2003). Toward functional augmentative and alternative communication for students with autism: Manual signs, graphic symbols, and voice output communication aids. *Language, Speech, and Hearing Services in Schools*, *34*, 202–215.

Miyamoto, R. C., Cotton, R. T., Rope, A. F., et al. (2004). Association of anterior glottic webs with velocardiofacial syndrome (chromosome 22q11.2 deletion). *Otolaryngology–Head & Neck Surgery*, *130*:415–417.

Moats, L. C. (1994). The missing foundation in teacher education: knowledge of the structure of spoken and written language. *Annals of Dyslexia, 44*, 81–102.

Moeller, M. P., Hoover, B., Putman, C., et al. (2007). Vocalizations of infants with hearing loss compared with infants with normal hearing: Part I–phonetic development. *Ear & Hearing, 28*(5), 605–627.

Moller, K. T. (1994). Dental-occlusal and other oral conditions and speech. In J. E. Bernthal and N. W. Bankson (Eds). *Child Phonology: Characteristics, Assessment and Intervention with Special Populations*. New York, NY: Thieme Medical Publishers, pp. 3–28.

Monahan, D. (1984). *Remediation of Common Phonological Processes*. Tigard, OR: CC Publications.

Monahan, D. (1986). Remediation of common phonological processes. Four case studies. *Language, Speech, and Hearing Services in Schools, 17*, 187–198.

Montgomery, E. B., & Turkstra, L. S. (2003). Evidence-based practice: let's be reasonable. *Journal of Medical Speech-Language Pathology, 11*(2), ix–xii.

Morgan Barry, R. (1995a). The relationship between dysarthria and verbal dyspraxia in children: A comparative study using profiling and instrumental analyses. *Clinical Linguistics & Phonetics, 9*, 277–309.

Morgan Barry, R. (1995b). A comparative study of the relationship between dysarthria and verbal dyspraxia in adults and children. *Clinical Linguistics & Phonetics, 9*, 311–332.

Morrisette, M. L., Farris, A. W., & Gierut, J. (2006). Applications of learnability theory to clinical phonology. *Advances in Speech-Language Pathology, 8*(8), 207–219.

Morrisette, M. L., & Gierut, J. (2002). Lexical organisation and phonological change in treatment. *Journal of Speech, Language, and Hearing Research, 45*, 143–159.

Morrison, J. A., & Shriberg, L. D. (1992). Articulation testing versus conversational speech sampling. *Journal of Speech and Hearing Research, 35*, 259–273.

Moriarty, B. C., & Gillon, G. T. (2006). Phonological awareness intervention for children with childhood apraxia of speech. *International Journal of Language & Communication Disorders, 41*(6), 713–734.

Morley M. E., Court, D., Miller, H. (1954). Developmental dysarthia. *British Medical Journal, 2*(1), (4852), 8–10.

Morosan, D. E., & Jamieson, D. G. (1989). Evaluation of a technique for training new speech contrasts: Generalization across voices, but not word-position or task. *Journal of Speech and Hearing Research, 32*, 501–511.

Moskowitz, B. A. (1980). Idioms in phonology acquisition and phonological change. *Journal of Phonetics, 8*, 69–83.

Mowrer, D. E. (1985). The behavioral approach to treatment. In N. A. Creaghead, P. W. Newman, and W. A. Secord (Eds). *Assessment and Remediation of Articulatory and Phonological Disorders*. Columbus, OH: Merrill, pp. 159–192.

Mowrer, O. (1952). Speech development in the young child: The autism theory of speech development and some clinical applications. *Journal of Speech and Hearing Disorders, 17*, 263–268.

Mowrer, O. (1960). *Learning Theory and Symbolic Processes*. New York: John Wiley and Sons.

Müller, N. (Ed). (2006). *Multilayered Transcription*. San Diego, CA: Plural Publishing.

Müller, N., Ball, M. J., & Rutter, B. (2006). A profiling approach to intelligibility problems. *Advances in Speech-Language Pathology, 8*(3), 176–189.

Mullins, G., & Kiley, M. (2002). It's a PhD, not a Nobel Prize: how experienced examiners assess research theses. *Studies in Higher Education, 27*(4), 369–386.

Munro, J. (1999). *A study of the efficacy of speech and language therapy for particular speech sounds in children*. Unpublished Master's thesis, City University London.

Munson, B., & Babel, M. (2007). Loose lips and silver tongues, or, projecting sexual orientation through speech. *Language and Linguistics Compass, 1*, 416–449.

Munson, B., Baylis, A., Krause, M., & Yim, D.-S. (2006). Representation and access in phonological impairment. Paper presented at the *10th Conference on Laboratory Phonology*, Paris, France, June 30–July 2.

Munson, B., Bjorum, E., & Windsor, J. (2003). Acoustic and perceptual correlates of stress in nonwords produced by children with suspected developmental apraxia of speech and children with phonological disorder. *Journal of Speech, Language, and Hearing Research, 46*(1), 189–202.

Munson, B., Edwards, J., & Beckman, M. E. (2005). Relationships between nonword repetition accuracy and other measures of linguistic development in children with phonological disorders. *Journal of Speech, Language, and Hearing Research, 48*, 61–78.

Munson, B., McDonald, E. C., DeBoe, N. L., & White, A. R. (2006). The acoustic and perceptual bases of judgments of women and men's sexual orientation from read speech. *Journal of Phonetics, 34*, 202–240.

Munson, B., & Zimmerman, L. (2006). *Perceptual Bias and the Myth of the 'Gay Lisp'.* Poster presentation at the annual meeting of the American Speech-Language-Hearing Association, Miami, FL, November 16. Retrieved December 3, 2007 from http://convention.asha.org/2006/handouts/855_1165Munson_Benjamin_073148_111306114227.pdf.

Murai, J. (1963). The sounds of infants, their phonemicization and symbolization. *Studia Phonologica, 3*, 18–34.

Myklebust, H. (1952). Aphasia in childhood. *Journal of Exceptional Children, 19*, 9–14.

Nail-Chiwetalu, B., & Bernstein Ratner, N. (2007). An assessment of the information-seeking abilities and needs of practicing speech-language pathologists. *Journal of the Medical Library Association, 95*(2), 56–57.

Nathan, L., Stackhouse, J., Goulandris, N., & Snowling, M. J. (2004). The development of early literacy skills among children with speech difficulties: A test of the 'Critical Age Hypothesis'. *Journal of Speech, Language, and Hearing Research, 47*(2), 377–391.

Nation, K., & Norbury, C. F. (2005). Why reading comprehension fails. *Topics in Language Disorders, 25*, 21–32.

National Enquiry into the Teaching of Literacy (2005). *Teaching Reading.* Australian Government: Department of Education, Science and Training. Retrieved on December 10, 2007 from: http://www.dest.gov.au/nitl/documents/report_recommendations.pdf.

National Institute on Deafness and Other Communication Disorders. (1994). National strategic research plan for speech and speech disorders. Bethesda, MD: Department of Health and Human Services. Author.

National Institute of Child Health and Human Development. (2000). *Report of the National Reading Panel. Teaching children to read: an evidence-based assessment of the scientific research literature on reading and its implications for reading instruction.* Retrieved December 10, 2007, from http://www.nichd.nih.gov/publications/nrp/smallbook.cfm

National Research Council. (2001). *Educating Children with Autism.* Washington, DC: National Academy Press, Committee on Educational Interventions for Children with Autism, Division of Behavioral and Social Sciences and Education.

Neilson, R. (2003a). *Sutherland Phonological Awareness Test - Revised.* Wollongong: Author.

Neilson, R. (2003b). *Astronaut Invented Spelling Test (AIST).* Wollongong: Author.

Nemoy, E., & Davis, S. (1937). *The Correction of Defective Consonant Sounds.* Boston MA: Expression Company.

Niedzielski, N. (1999). The effect of social information on the perception of sociolinguistic variables. *Journal of Language and Social Psychology, 18*, 62–85.

Nijland, L., Maassen, B., & Meulen, S. (2003). Evidence of motor programming deficits in children diagnosed with DAS. *Journal of Speech, Language, and Hearing Research, 46*(2), 437–450.

Nippold, M. A. (2002). Stuttering and phonology: Is there an interaction? *American Journal of Speech-Language Pathology, 11*, 99–110.

Northern, J. L., & Downs, M. P. (2002). *Hearing in Children* (5th Edition). Philadelphia, PA: Lippincott, Williams, and Wilkins.

Nunes, A. (2002). *The Price of a Perfect System: Learnability and the Distribution of Errors in the Speech of Children Learning English as a First Language.* University of Durham: unpublished PhD dissertation.

Nunes, A. (2006). The space between. *Speech and Language Therapy in Practice.* Summer, 4–6.

O'Grady, W., Archibald, J., Aronoff, M., & Rees-Miller, J. (2005). *Contemporary Linguistics: An Introduction* (5th Edition). Boston, MA: Bedford/St. Martin's.

Odell, K. H., & Shriberg, L. D. (2001). Prosody-voice characteristics of children and adults with apraxia of speech. *Clinical Linguistics & Phonetics, 15,* 275–307.

Ohala, D. K. (1999). The influence of sonority on children's cluster reductions. *Journal of Communication Disorders, 32,* 397–422.

Ohala, J. J. (1990). 'There is no interface between phonetics and phonology: a personal view'. *Journal of Phonetics, 18,*153–171.

Ohde, R. N., & Sharf, D. J. (1988). Perceptual categorization and consistency of synthesized /r-w/ continua by adults, normal children and /r/-misarticulating children. *Journal of Speech and Hearing Research, 31,* 556–568.

Oller, D. K., Wieman, L. A., Doyle, W. J., & Ross, C. (1976). Infant babbling and speech. *Journal of Child Language, 3,* 1–11.

Olmstead, D. (1971). *Out of the Mouths of Babes.* The Hague: Mouton.

Olswang, L. B. (1998). Treatment efficacy research. In C. M. Frattali (Ed). *Measuring Outcomes in Speech-Language Pathology.* New York: Thieme, pp. 134–150.

Olswang, L. B. (1990a). Treatment efficacy: The breadth of research. In L. B. Olswang, C. K. Thompson, S. F. Warren, et al. (Eds). *Treatment Efficacy Research in Communication Disorders.* Rockville, MD: ASHA Foundation.

Olswang, L. B. (1990b, January). Treatment efficacy research: A path to quality assurance. ASHA, 45–47.

Olswang, L. B., & Bain, B. A. (1985). The natural occurrence of generalization during articulation treatment. *Journal of Communication Disorders, 18,* 109–129.

Olswang, L. B., & Bain, B. A. (1991). When to recommend intervention. *Language, Speech, and Hearing Services in Schools, 22,* 255–263.

Olswang, L. B., & Bain, B. A. (1996) Assessment information for predicting upcoming change in language production. *Journal of Speech and Hearing Research, 39,* 414–423.

Orr, C. (1998). *Mouth Madness: Oral Motor Activities for Children.* San Antonio, TX: Therapy Skill Builders.

Orton, S. T. (1937). *Reading, Writing and Speech Problems in Children: A Presentation of Certain Types of Disorders in the Development of the Language Faculty.* New York: W. W. Norton.

Osgood, C. (1957). *A Behavioristic Analysis of Perception and Language as Cognitive Phenomena, Contemporary approaches to Cognition.* Cambridge: Harvard University Press.

Overby, M., Carrell, T., & Bernthal, J. (2007). Teachers' perceptions of students with speech sound disorders: A quantitative and qualitative analysis. *Language, Speech, and Hearing Services in Schools, 38*(4), 327–341.

Overturf, G. D. (2000). American Academy of Pediatrics. Committee on Infectious Diseases. Technical report: prevention of pneumococcal infections, including the use of pneumococcal conjugate and polysaccharide vaccines and antibiotic prophylaxis. *Pediatrics, 106*(2 Pt 1), 367–376.

Ozanne, A. (1995). The search for developmental verbal dyspraxia. In B. Dodd (Ed). *Differential Diagnosis and Treatment of Children with Speech Disorder.* London: Whurr, pp. 91–109.

Ozanne, A. (2005). Childhood apraxia of speech. In B. Dodd (Ed). *Differential Diagnosis and Treatment of Children with Speech Disorder* (2nd Edition). London: Whurr, pp. 71–82.

PIRLS Report Progress in International Literacy Study 2005/2006. Available from: http://www. educationcounts.govt.nz/publications/series/2539/pirls_0506/16400.

Paatsch, L. E., Blamey, P. J., Sarant, J. Z., & Bow, C. P. (2006). The effects of speech production and vocabulary training on different components of spoken language performance. *Journal of Deaf Studies & Deaf Education, 11*(1), 39–55.

Paden, E. (2007). Foreword. *Evaluating and Enhancing Children's Phonological Systems: Research and Theory to Practice.* Greenville, SC: Thinking Publications/Super Duper, p. ix.

Paden, E. P., Matthies, M. L., & Novak, M. A. (1989). Recovery from OME-related phonologic delay following tube placement. *Journal of Speech and Hearing Disorders, 54,* 94–100.

Pamplona, M. C., Ysunza, A., & Espinoza, J. (1999). A comparative trial of two modalities of speech intervention for compensatory articulation in cleft palate children: Phonological approach versus articulatory approach. *International Journal of Pediatric Otorhinolaryngology, 49,* 21–26.

Pantelemidou, V., Herman, R., & Thomas, J. (2003). Efficacy of speech intervention using electropalatography with a cochlear implant user. *Clinical Linguistics & Phonetics, 17*(4–5), 383–392.

Paradise, J. L., Rockette, H. E., Colborn, D. K., et al. (1997). Otitis media in 2253 Pittsburgh-area infants: Prevalence and risk factors during the first two years of life. *Pediatrics, 99*(3), 318–333.

Parsloe, R. (1998). Use of the speech pattern audiometer and the electropalatograph to explore the speech production/perception relationship in a profoundly deaf child. *International Journal of Language & Communication Disorders, 33*(1), 109–121.

Pascoe, M. (2006). Review of the book *Phonological disorders in children: Clinical decision making in assessment and intervention,* A. G. Kamhi and K. E. Pollock (Eds). *Child Language Teaching and Therapy, 22*(2), 243–245.

Pascoe, M., Stackhouse, J., & Wells, B. (2005). Phonological therapy within a psycholinguistic framework: promoting change in a child with persisting speech difficulties. *International Journal of Language & Communication Disorders, 40*(2), 189–220.

Pascoe, M., Stackhouse, J., & Wells, B. (2006). *Children's Speech and Literacy Difficulties III: Persisting Speech Difficulties in Children.* Chichester: John Wiley and Sons.

Passy, J. (1990). *Cued Articulation.* Ponteland, Northumberland: STASS Publications.

Paterson, J. E., Carter, S., Wallace, J., Ahmad, Z., Garrett, N., & Silva, P. A. (2006). Pacific Islands families study: the prevalence of chronic middle ear disease in 2-year-old Pacific children living in New Zealand. *International Journal of Pediatric Otorhinolaryngology, 70*(10), 1771–1778.

Paterson, J. E., Carter, S., Wallace, J., Ahmad, Z., Garrett, N., & Silva, P. A. (2007). Pacific Islands Families Study: risk factors associated with otitis media with effusion among Pacific 2-year-old children. *International Journal of Pediatric Otorhinolaryngology, 71*(7), 1047–1054.

Paul, R. (2007). *Language Disorders from Infancy Through Adolescence: Assessment and Intervention* (3rd Edition). St. Louis, MO: Mosby, Inc.

Paul, R., & Shriberg, L. D. (1982). Associations between phonology and syntax in speech-delayed children. *Journal of Speech and Hearing Research, 25,* 536–547.

Pena-Brooks, A., & Hegde, M. (2000). *Assessment and Treatment of Articulation and Phonological Disorders in Children.* Austin, TX: ProEd.

Peng, S. C., Weiss, A. L., Cheung, H., & Lin, Y. S. (2004). Consonant production and language skills in Mandarin-speaking children with cochlear implants. *Archives of Otolaryngology – Head & Neck Surgery, 130*(5), 592–597.

Pennington, L., Goldbart, J., & Marshall, J. (2003). Speech and language therapy to improve the communication skills of children with cerebral palsy. *The Cochrane Database of Systematic Reviews,* Issue 3, Art. No. CD003466. DOI: 10.1002/14651858.CD003466. pub2.

Peppe, S., & McCann, J. (2003). Assessing intonation and prosody in children with atypical language development: the PEPS-C test and the revised version. *Clinical Linguistics & Phonetics, 17*(4-5), 345–354.

Peter, B., & Stoel-Gammon, C. (2005). Timing errors in two children with suspected childhood apraxia of speech (sCAS) during speech and music-related tasks. *Clinical Linguistics & Phonetics, 19*(2), 67–87.

Peterson-Falzone, S., Hardin-Jones, M., & Karnell, M. (2001). *Cleft Palate Speech* (3rd Edition). St. Louis, MO: Mosby.

Peterson-Falzone, S., Trost-Cardamone, J., Hardin-Jones, M., & Karnell, M. (2006). *The Clinician's Guide to Treating Cleft Palate Speech*. St. Louis, MO: Mosby.

Petinou, K., Schwartz, R. G., Mody, M., & Gravel, J. S. (1999). The impact of otitis media with effusion on early phonetic inventories: A longitudinal prospective investigation. *Clinical Linguistics & Phonetics, 13*(5), 351–367.

Pickstone, C. (2007). Triage in speech and language therapy. In S. Roulstone (Ed). *Prioritising Child Health*. London: Routledge.

Pickstone, C., Hannon, P., & Fox, L. (2002). Surveying and screening preschool language development in community-focused intervention programmes: a review of instruments. *Child: Care, Health and Development, 28*(3), 25–264.

Piggott, G. L., & Kessler Robb, M. (1999). Prosodic features of familial language impairment: Constraints on stress assignment. *Folia Phoniatrica et Logopaedica, 51*, 55–69.

Pittman, A. L., Stelmachowicz, P. G., Lewis, D. E., & Hoover, B. M. (2003). Spectral characteristics of speech at the ear: implications for amplification in children. *Journal of Speech, Language, and Hearing Research, 46*(3), 649–657.

Pollock, K. E. (2005). Early language growth in children adopted from China: Preliminary normative data. *Seminars in Speech and Language, 26*, 22–32.

Pollock, K. E. (2007). Speech acquisition in second first language learners (children who were adopted internationally). In S. McLeod (Ed). *The International Guide to Speech Acquisition*. Clifton Park, NY: Thomson Delmar Learning, pp.137–145.

Pollock, K. E., & Berni, M. C. (2001). Transcription of vowels. *Topics in Language Disorders, 21*, 22–40.

Pollock, K. E., & Berni, M. C. (2003). Incidence of non-rhotic vowel errors in children: Data from the Memphis Vowel Project. *Clinical Linguistics & Phonetics, 17*, 393–401.

Pollock, K. E., Chow, E., & Tamura, M. (2004). Phonology and prosody in preschoolers adopted from China as infants/toddlers. Poster presented the *American Speech-Language-Hearing Association Convention*, Philadelphia, PA, November.

Pollock, K. E., & Hall, P. K. (1991). An analysis of the vowel misarticulations of five children with developmental apraxia of speech. *Clinical Linguistics & Phonetics, 5*(3), 207–224.

Pollock, K. E., & Keiser, N. J. (1990). An examination of vowel errors in phonologically disordered children. *Clinical Linguistics & Phonetics, 4*, 161–178.

Pollock, M., Gaesser, G., Butcher, J., Despres, J, Dishman, R., Franklin, B., et al. (1998). The recommended quantity and quality of exercise for developing and maintaining cardiorespiratory and muscular fitness, and flexibility in healthy adults. *Medicine & Science in Sports & Exercise, 30*, 975–991.

Pollock, K. E., & Price, J. R. (2005). Phonological skills of children adopted from China: Implications for Assessment. *Seminars in Speech and Language, 26*, 54–63.

Pollock, K. E., Price, J. R., & Fulmer, K. (2003). Speech-language acquisition in children adopted from China: a longitudinal investigation of two children. *Journal of Multilingual Communication Disorders, 1*, 184–193.

Poole, I. (1934). Genetic development of articulation of consonant sounds in speech. *Elementary English Review, 11*, 159–161.

Popich, E., Louw, B., & Eloff, I. (2007). Caregiver education as a prevention strategy for communication disorders in South Africa. *Infants and Young Children, 20*(1), 64–81.

Powell, J., & McReynolds, L.V. (1969). A procedure for testing position generalization from articulation training. *Journal of Speech and Hearing Research, 12*, 629–645.

Powell, T. W. (1991). Planning for phonological generalization: An approach to treatment target selection. *American Journal of Speech-Language Pathology, 1*, 21–27.

Powell, T. W. (2003). Stimulability and treatment outcomes. *Perspectives on Language Learning and Education, 10*(1), 3–6.

Powell, T. W. (2007). A model for ethical practices in clinical phonetics and linguistics. *Clinical Linguistics & Phonetics, 21*, 851–857.

Powell, T. W. (2008a). The use of nonspeech oral motor treatments for developmental speech sound production disorders: Interventions and interactions. *Language, Speech, and Hearing Services in Schools, 39*(3), 374–379.

Powell, T. W. (2008b). An integrated evaluation of nonspeech oral-motor treatments. *Language, Speech, and Hearing Services in Schools, 39*(3), 422–427.

Powell, T. W., & Elbert, M. (1984). Generalization following the remediation of early-and later-developing consonant clusters. *Journal of Speech and Hearing Disorders, 49*, 211–218.

Powell, T. W., Elbert, M., & Dinnsen, D. A. (1991). Stimulability as a factor in the phonologic generalization of misarticulating preschool children. *Journal of Speech and Hearing Research, 34*, 1318–1328.

Powell, T. W., Elbert, M., Miccio, A. W., Strike-Roussos, C., & Brasseur, J. (1998). Facilitating [s] production in young children: an experimental evaluation of motoric and conceptual treatment approaches. *Clinical Linguistics & Phonetics, 12*, 127–146.

Powell, T. W., & Miccio, A. W. (1996). Stimulability: A useful clinical tool. *Journal of Communication Disorders, 29*, 237–253.

Powers, G., & Starr, C. D. (1974). The effects of muscle exercises on velopharyngeal gap and nasality. *Cleft Palate Journal, 11*, 28–35.

Powers, M. H. (1959). Functional disorders of articulation. In L. E. Travis (Ed). *Handbook of Speech Pathology and Audiology*. London: Peter Owen.

Prather, E. M., Hedrick, D. L., & Kern, C. A. (1975). Articulation development in children aged two to four years. *Journal of Speech and Hearing Disorders, 40*, 179–191.

Prezas, R., & Hodson, B. (2007). Diagnostic evaluation of children with speech sound disorders. In S. Rvachew (Ed). *Encyclopedia of Language and Literacy Development*. London, Ontario: Canadian Language and Literacy Research Network. Retrieved April 28, 2008 from: http://www.literacyencyclopedia.ca/.

Price, J. R., Pollock, K. E., & Oller, D. K. (2006). Speech and language development in six infants adopted from China. *Journal of Multilingual Communication Disorders, 4*, 108–127.

Pugh, K. C., Burke, H. W. K., & Brown, H. M. (2004). Tympanometry measures in native and non-native Hawaiian children. *International Journal of Pediatric Otorhinolaryngology, 68*(6), 753–758.

RCSLT (2006). *Communicating Quality 3: RCSLT's Guidance on Best Practice in Service Organisation and Provision*. London: Royal College of Speech and Language Therapists.

Raitano, N. A., Pennington, B. F., Tunick, B. F., Boada, R., & Shriberg, L. D. (2004). Pre-literacy skills of subgroups of children with speech sound disorders. *Journal of Child Psychology and Psychiatry, 45*, 821–835.

Ramakrishnan, K., Sparks, R. A., & Berryhill, W. E. (2007). Diagnosis and treatment of otitis media [summary for patients in *Am Fam Physician* 2007 Dec 1;76(11):1659–60; PMID: 18092707]. *American Family Physician, 76*(11), 1650–1658.

Ratner, N. B. (2006). Evidence-Based Practice: An Examination of Its Ramifications for the Practice of Speech-Language Pathology. *Language, Speech, and Hearing Services in Schools, 37*(4), 257–267.

Rauscher, F. B., Krauss, R. M., & Chen, Y. (1996). Gesture, speech and lexical access: The role of lexical movements in speech production. *Psychological Science, 7*, 226–231.

Ray, J. (2002). Treating phonological disorders in a multilingual child: A case study. *American Journal of Speech-Language Pathology, 11*(3), 305–315.

Raz, M. G. (1993). *How to Teach a Child to Say the "S" Sound in 15 Easy Lessons.* Scottsdale, AZ: Gersten Weitz Publishers.

Raz, M. G. (1996). *How to Teach a Child to Say the "R" Sound in 15 Easy Lessons.* Scottsdale, AZ: Gersten Weitz Publishers.

Raz, M. G. (1999). *How to Teach a Child to Say the "L" Sound in 15 Easy Lessons.* Scottsdale, AZ: Gersten Weitz Publishers.

Rees, R. (2001). What do tasks really tap? In J. Stackhouse and B. Wells (Eds). *Children's Speech and Literacy Difficulties: Book Two: Identification and Intervention.* London: Whurr.

Reid, J. (2003). The vowel house: a cognitive approach to vowels for literacy and speech. *Child Language Teaching and Therapy, 19*, 152–180.

Reilly, S. (2004). The move to evidence-based practice within speech pathology. In S. Reilly, J. Douglas, and J. Oates (Eds). *Evidence-Based Practice in Speech Pathology.* London: Whurr, pp. 3–17.

Reilly, S., Douglas, J., and Oates, J. (Eds). (2004). *Evidence-Based Practice in Speech Pathology.* London: Whurr Publishers.

Renfrew, C. E. (1997). *Action Picture Test* (4th Edition). Bicester, England: Winslow Press.

Rescher, N. (1998). *Complexity: A Philosophical Overview.* New Brunswick, NJ: Transaction.

Rescorla, L., & Bernstein Ratner, N. (1996). Phonetic profiles of typically developing and language-delayed toddlers. *Journal of Speech and Hearing Research, 39*, 153–165.

Reynolds, J. (1990). Abnormal vowel patterns in phonological disorder: Some data and a hypothesis. *British Journal of Disorders of Communication, 25*, 115–148.

Rhoades, E. A. (2006). Research outcomes of auditory-verbal intervention: Is the approach justified? *Deafness & Education International, 8*, 125–143.

Rivers, K. L. (2000). Working with caregivers of infants and toddlers with special needs from culturally and linguistically diverse backgrounds: Infant-toddler intervention. *The Transdisciplinary Journal, 10*(2), 61–71.

Robb, M. P., Bleile, K. M., & Yee, S. S. L. (1999). A phonetic analysis of vowel errors during the course of treatment. *Clinical Linguistics & Phonetics, 13*(4), 309–321.

Robbins, S. D., & Robbins, R. (1937). *Corrections of Speech Defects of Early Childhood.* Boston, MA : Expression Co.

Roberts, J. (2002) Child language variation. In Chambers, Trudgill, and Schilling-Estes (Eds). *The Handbook of Language Variation and Change.* Oxford: Blackwell, pp. 333–348.

Roberts, J., & Hunter, L. (2002, May) Otitis media and language learning sequelae: Current research and controversies. Symposium conducted in Arlington, Virginia.

Roberts, J., Pollock, K., Krakow, R., Price, J., Fulmer, K., & Wang, P. Language development in preschool-aged children adopted from China. *Journal of Speech, Language, and Hearing Research, 48*, 93–107.

Roberts, J. E., Rosenfeld, R. M., & Zeisel, S. A. (2004). Otitis media and speech and language: a meta-analysis of prospective studies [see comment]. *Pediatrics, 113*(3 Pt 1), e238–e248.

Robertson, M. (2007). Speech sound disorders: Comments on Prezas and Hodson, *Encyclopedia of Language and Literacy Development.* London, ON: Canadian Language and Literacy Research Network, pp. 1–7. Retrieved December 3, 2007 from: http://www.literacyencyclopedia.ca/pdfs/topic.php?topId=37.

Robey, R. R. (2004). A five-phase model for clinical-outcome research. *Journal of Communication Disorders, 37*, 401–411.

Robey, R. R., & Schultz, M. C. (1998). A model for conducting clinical-outcome research: An adaptation of the standard protocol for use in aphasiology. *Aphasiology, 12*, 787–810.

Roca, I., & Johnson, W. (1999). *A Course in Phonology.* Oxford: Blackwell Publishers.

Rockman, B. K., & Elbert, M. (1984). Untrained acquisition of /s/ in a phonologically disordered child. *Journal of Speech and Hearing Disorders, 49*, 246–253.

Roehrig, S., Suiter, D., & Pierce, T. (2004, November). An examination of the effectiveness of passive oral-motor exercises. Poster presented at the *American Speech-Language-Hearing Association Convention*, Philadelphia, PA.

Rose, J. (2006). *Independent Review of the Teaching of Early Reading*. Retrieved December 10, 2007 from http://www.standards.dfes.gov.uk/phonics/report.pdf

Rose, M., & Baldac, S. (2004). Translating evidence into practice. In S. Reilly, J. Douglas, and J. Oates (Eds). *Evidence-Based Practice in Speech Pathology*. London: Whurr Publishers, pp. 317–329.

Rosen, G. M., & Davidson, G. C. (2003). Psychology should list empirically supported principles of change (ESPs) and not credential trademarked therapies or other treatment packages. *Behavior Modification, 27*(3), 300–312.

Rosenbaum, P., King, S., Law, M., King, G., & Evans, J. (1998). Family-centred service: A conceptual framework and research review. *Physical & Occupational Therapy in Pediatrics, 18*, 1–20.

Rosenbeck, J. C., Lemme, M. L., Ahern, M. B., Harris, E. H., & Wertz, R. T. (1973). A treatment for apraxia of speech in adults. *Journal of Speech and Hearing Disorders, 38*, 462–472.

Rosenbek, J., & Wetz, R. T. (1972). A review of 50 cases of developmental apraxia of speech. *Language, Speech, and Hearing Services in Schools, 3*, 23–33.

Rosenfeld-Johnson, S. (1999). *Oral Motor Exercises for Speech Clarity*. Tucson, AZ: Ravenhawk.

Rosenfeld-Johnson, S. (2001). *Oral-Motor Exercises for Speech Clarity*. Tucson, AZ: Innovative Therapists International.

Rosenthal, J. B. (1994). Rate control therapy for developmental apraxia of speech. *Clinics in Communication Disorders, 4*(3), 190–200.

Roth, F. P., & Paul. R. (2002). Principles of intervention. In R. Paul (Ed). *Introduction to Clinical Methods in Communication Disorders*. Baltimore, MD: Paul H. Brookes, pp. 160–181.

Roth, F. P., Troia, G. A., Worthington, C. K., & Dow, K. A. (2002). Promoting awareness of sounds in speech: An initial report of an early intervention program for children with speech and language impairments. *Applied Psycholinguistics, 23*, 535–565.

Roth, F. P., & Worthington, C. K. (2005). *Treatment Resource Manual for Speech-Language Pathology*. San Diego, CA: Singular.

Rothman, A. J. (2004). 'Is there nothing more practical than a good theory?': Why innovations and advances in health behavior change will arise if interventions are used to test and refine theory. *International Journal of Behavioral Nutrition and Physical Activity, 1*(11), 1–7.

Ruder, K. F., & Bunce, B. H. (1981). Articulation therapy using distinctive feature analysis to structure the training program: Two case studies. *Journal of Speech and Hearing Disorders, 46*, 59–65.

Rudolph, M., Kummer, P., Eysholdt, U., & Rosanowski, F. (2005). Quality of life in mothers of speech impaired children. *Logopedics Phoniatrics Vocology, 30*, 3–8.

Ruscello, D. M. (1982). A selected review of palatal training procedures. *Cleft Palate Journal, 18*, 181–193.

Ruscello, D. M. (1993). A motor skill learning treatment program for sound system disorders. *Seminars in Speech and Language, 14*, 106–118.

Ruscello, D. M. (2004). Considerations for behavioral treatment of velopharyngeal closure for speech. In K. Bzoch (Ed). *Communicative Disorders Related to Cleft Lip and Palate* (5th Edition). Austin, TX: Pro-Ed, pp. 763–796.

Ruscello, D. M. (2007). Treatment of Velopharyngeal Closure for Speech: Discussion and Implications for Management. *Journal of Speech and Language Pathology and Applied Behavior Analysis, 1*, 62–82.

Ruscello, D. M. (2008a). *Treating Articulation and Phonological Disorders in Children*. St. Louis, MO: Elsevier.

Ruscello, D. M. (2008b). Oral motor treatment issues related to children with developmental speech sound disorders. *Language, Speech, and Hearing Services in Schools, 39(3)*, 380–391.

Ruscello, D. M., St. Louis, K. O., & Mason, N. (1991). School-aged children with phonologic disorders: Coexistence with other speech/language disorders. *Journal of Speech and Hearing Research, 34*, 236–242.

Ruscello, D. M., Tekieli, M. E., & Van Sickels, J. E. (1985). Speech production before and after orthognathic surgery: A review. *Oral Surgery, Oral Medicine, and Oral Pathology, 59*, 10–14.

Rutter, M., & The English and Romanian Adoptees Study Team (1998). Developmental catch-up and deficit following adoption after severe global early deprivation. *Journal of Child Psychology and Psychiatry, 39*, 465–476.

Rvachew, S. (1994). Speech perception training can facilitate sound production learning. *Journal of Speech and Hearing Research, 37*, 347–357.

Rvachew, S. (2005a). The importance of phonetic facotrs in phonological intervention. In A. G. Kamhi and K. E. Pollock (Eds). *Phonological Disorders in Children: Clinical Decision Making in Assessment and Intervention*. Baltimore, MD: Paul H. Brookes, pp. 175–187.

Rvachew, S. (2005b). Stimulability and treatment success. *Topics in Language Disorders, 25(3)*, 207–219.

Rvachew, S. (2006a). Longitudinal predictors of implicit phonological awareness skills. *American Journal of Speech-Language Pathology, 15*, 165–176.

Rvachew, S. (2006b). Effective interventions for the treatment of speech sound disorders. *Encyclopedia of Language and Literacy Development*. London, ON: Canadian Language and Literacy Research Network, pp. 1–9. Retrieved December 3, 2007 from: http://www.literacyencyclopedia.ca/pdfs/topic.php?topld=17.

Rvachew, S. (2007a). Perceptual foundations of speech acquisition. In S. McLeod (Ed). *International Guide to Speech Acquisition*. Clifton Park, NY: Thomson Delmar Learning, pp. 26–30.

Rvachew, S. (2007b). Phonological processing and reading in children with speech sound disorders. *American Journal of Speech-Language Pathology, 16*, 260–270.

Rvachew, S., Chiang, P.-Y., & Evans, N. (2007). Characteristics of speech errors produced by children with and without delayed phonological awareness skills. *Language, Speech, and Hearing Services in Schools, 38(1)*, 60–71.

Rvachew, S., Creighton, D., Feldman, N., & Sauve, R. (2005). Vocal development of infants with very low birth weight. *Clinical Linguistics & Phonetics, 19(4)*, 275–294.

Rvachew, S., & Grawburg, M. (2006). Correlates of phonological awareness in preschoolers with speech sound disorders. *Journal of Speech, Language, and Hearing Research, 49*, 74–87.

Rvachew, S., & Jamieson, D. G. (1989). Perception of voiceless fricatives by children with a functional articulation disorder. *Journal of Speech and Hearing Disorders, 54*, 193–208.

Rvachew, S., & Nowak, M. (2001). The effect of target selection strategy on phonological learning. *Journal of Speech, Language, and Hearing Research, 44*, 610–623.

Rvachew, S., & Nowak, M. (2003). Clinical outcomes as a function of target selection strategy: A response to Morrisette and Gierut. *Journal of Speech, Language, and Hearing Research, 46*, 386–389.

Rvachew, S., Nowak, M., & Cloutier, G. (2004). Effect of phonemic perception training on the speech production and phonological awareness skills of children with expressive phonological delay. *American Journal of Speech-Language Pathology, 13*, 250–263.

Rvachew, S., Ohberg, A., Grawburg, M., & Heyding, J. (2003). Phonological awareness and phonemic perception in 4-year-old children with delayed expressive phonology skills. *American Journal of Speech-Language Pathology, 12*, 463–471.

Rvachew, S., Rafaat, S., & Martin, M. (1999). Stimulability, speech perception and the treatment of phonological disorders. *American Journal of Speech-Language Pathology, 8*, 33–43.

Rvachew, S., Slawinski, E. B., Williams, M., & Green, C. L. (1999). The impact of early onset otitis media on babbling and early language development. *Journal of the Acoustical Society of America*, *105*(1), 467–475.

Saben, C. B., & Ingham, J. C. (1991). The effects of minimal pairs treatment on the speech-sound production of two children with phonologic disorders. *Journal of Speech and Hearing Research*, *34*, 1023–1040.

Sackett, D. L., Haynes, R. B., Guyatt, G. H., & Tugwell, P. (1991). *Clinical Epidemiology: A Basic Science for Clinical Medicine* (2nd Edition). Boston, MA: Little Brown and Company.

Salt, A., & Redshaw, M. (2006). Neurodevelopmental follow-up after preterm birth: follow up after two years. *Early Human Development*, *82*(3), 185–197.

Sander, E. (1972). When are speech sounds learned? *Journal of Speech and Hearing Disorders*, *37*, 55–63.

Scarborough, H. S., & Brady, S. A. (2002). Toward a common terminology for talking about speech and reading: A glossary of the 'phon' words and some related terms. *Journal of Literacy Research*, *34*, 299–334.

Schmidt, A. M., & Meyers, K. A. (1995). Traditional and phonological treatment for teaching English fricatives and affricates to Koreans. *Journal of Speech and Hearing Research*, *38*, 828–838.

Schmidt, R. A., & Lee, T. D. (2000). *Motor control and learning: A behavioral emphasis* (3rd Edition). Champaign, IL: Human Kinetics.

Schonweiler, R., Ptok, M., & Radu, H. J. (1998). A cross-sectional study of speech- and language-abilities of children with normal hearing, mild fluctuating conductive hearing loss, or moderate to profound sensoneurinal hearing loss. *International Journal of Pediatric Otorhinolaryngology*, *44*(3), 251–258.

Schuele, C. M., & Hadley, P. A. (1999). Potential advantages of introducing specific language impairment to families. *American Journal of Speech-Language Pathology*, *8*, 11–22.

Scott, K., Roberts, J., & Krakow, R. (2008). Oral and written language development of children adopted from China. *American Journal of Speech-Language Pathology*, *17*(2), 150–160

Sherman, D., & Geith, A. (1967). Speech sound discrimination and articulation skill. *Journal of Speech and Hearing Research*, *10*, 277–280.

Shott, S. R., Joseph, A., & Heithaus, D. (2001). Hearing loss in children with Down syndrome. *International Journal of Pediatric Otorhinolaryngology*, *61*(3), 199–205.

Shuster, L. I. (1998). The perception of correctly and incorrectly produced /r/. *Journal of Speech, Language, and Hearing Research*, *41*, 941–950.

Schwartz, R. G. (1992). Advances in phonological theory as a clinical framework. *Language, Speech, and Hearing Services in Schools*, *23*, 269–276.

Schwartz, R. G., & Leonard, L. (1982). Do children pick and choose? *Journal of Child Language*, *9*, 319–336.

Schwartz, R. G., Leonard, L., Folger, M., & Wilcox, M. (1980). Evidence for a synergistic view of language disorders: Early phonological behavior in normal and language disordered children. *Journal of Speech and Hearing Disorders*, *45*, 357–377.

Secord, W., Boyce, S. Donohue, J., Fox, R., & Shine R. (2007). *Eliciting Sounds: Techniques and Strategies for Clinicians* (2nd Edition). Clifton Park, NY: Thompson Delmar Learning.

Seddoh, S. A. K., Robin, D. A., Sim, H.-S., Hageman, C., Moon, J. B., & Folkins, J. W. (1996). Speech timing in apraxia of speech versus conduction aphasia. *Journal of Speech and Hearing Research*, *39*, 590–603.

Selkirk, E. O. (1984). *Phonology and Syntax*. Cambridge, MA: The MIT Press.

Shelton, R. L. (1993). Grand rounds for sound system disorder. Conclusion: What was learned? *Seminars in Speech and Language*, *14*, 166–177.

Shelton, R. L. (2005). Oral motor treatments [letter to the editor]. *ASHA Leader*, *10*(12), 36.

Shelton, R. L. Johnson, A. F., & Arndt, W. B. (1972). Monitoring and reinforcement by parents as a means of automating articulatory responses. *Perceptual and Motor Skills, 35,* 759–767.

Shelton, R. L., Johnson, A., Ruscello, D., & Arndt, W. (1978). Assessment of parent administered listening training for preschool children with articulation deficits. *Journal of Speech and Hearing Disorders, 43,* 242–254.

Shelton, R. L., Johnson, A. F., Willis, V., & Arndt, W. B. (1975). Monitoring and reinforcement by parents as a means of automating articulatory responses: II. Study of pre-school children. *Perceptual and Motor Skills, 40,* 599–610.

Shprintzen, R. J. (1999). *The Velo-Cardio-Facial Syndrome Educational Foundation Clinical Database Project.* Retrieved April 10, 2008 from http://www.vcfsef.org/pp/vcf_facts/index.htm.

Shprintzen, R. J., & Croft, C. B. (1981). Abnormalities of the Eustachian tube orifice in individuals with cleft palate. *International Journal of Pediatric Otorhinolaryngology, 3,* 15–23.

Shprintzen, R. J., & Golding-Kushner, K. J. (2008). *Velo-Cardio-Facial Syndrome: Volume 1.* San Diego, CA: Plural Publishing.

Shprintzen, R. J., Sher, A. E., & Croft, C. B. (1987). Hypernasal speech caused by hypertrophic tonsils. *International Journal of Pediatric Otorhinolaryngology, 14,* 45–56.

Shriberg, L. D. (1975). A response evocation program for http://jshd.asha.org/cgi/content/abstract/40/1/92. *Journal of Speech and Hearing Disorders, 40,* 92–105. Reprinted in *Contemporary Readings in Articulation Disorders.* C. Bennett, N. Bountress, and G. Bull. Dubuque, IA: Kendall-Hunt.

Shriberg, L. D. (1982). Diagnostic assessment of developmental phonological disorders. In M. Crary (Ed). *Phonological Intervention, Concepts and Procedures.* San Diego: College-Hill Inc.

Shriberg, L. D. (1993). Four new speech and prosody-voice measures for genetics research and other studies in developmental phonological disorders. *Journal of Speech and Hearing Research, 36,* 105–140.

Shriberg, L. D. (1994). Five subtypes of developmental phonological disorders. *Clinics in Communication Disorders, 4,* 38–53.

Shriberg, L. (1997). Developmental phonological disorders: One or many? In B. W. Hodson and M. L. Edwards (Eds.). *Perspectives in Applied Phonology.* Gaithersburg, MD: Aspen, pp. 105–132.

Shriberg, L. D. (2003). Diagnostic markers for child speech-sound disorders: Introductory comments. *Clinical Linguistics & Phonetics, 17,* 501–505.

Shriberg, L. D. (2004). Diagnostic classification of five sub-types of childhood speech sound disorders (SSD) of currently unknown origin. Paper presented at the *International Association of Logopedics and Phoniatrics Congress,* Brisbane, Australia.

Shriberg, L. D. (2006, June). Research in idiopathic and symptomatic childhood apraxia of speech. Paper presented at the *5th International Conference on Speech Motor Control* Nijmegen, the Netherlands.

Shriberg, L. D., Aram, D. M., & Kwiatkowski, J. (1997a). Developmental apraxia of speech: I. Descriptive perspectives. *Journal of Speech, Language, and Hearing Research, 40,* 273–285.

Shriberg, L. D., Aram, D. M., & Kwiatkowski, J. (1997b). Developmental apraxia of speech: II. Toward a diagnostic marker. *Journal of Speech, Language, and Hearing Research, 40,* 286–312.

Shriberg, L. D., Aram, D. M., & Kwiatkowski, J. (1997c). Developmental apraxia of speech: III. A subtype marked by inappropriate stress. *Journal of Speech, Language, and Hearing Research, 40,* 313–337.

Shriberg, L. D., Austin, D., Lewis, B. A., McSweeny, J. L., & Wilson, D. L. (1997). The percentage of consonants correct (PCC) metric: extensions and reliability data. *Journal of Speech, Language, and Hearing Research, 40,* 708–722.

Shriberg, L. D., & Campbell, T. F. (2002). *Proceedings of the 2002 Childhood Apraxia of Speech Research Symposium.* Carlsbad, AZ: The Hendrix Foundation.

Shriberg, L. D., Campbell, T. F., Karlsson, H. B., McSweeney, J. L., Nadler, C. J. (2003). A diagnostic marker for childhood apraxia of speech: The lexical stress ratio. *Clinical Linguistics & Phonetics*, *17*(7), 549–574.

Shriberg, L. D., Flipsen, P., Jr., Karlsson, H. B., & McSweeny, J. L. (2001). Acoustic phenotypes for speech-genetics studies: An acoustic marker for residual / 6 /distortions. *Clinical Linguistics & Phonetics*, *15*, 631–650.

Shriberg, L. D., Flipsen, P., Jr., Kwiatkowski, J., & McSweeny, J. L. (2003). A diagnostic marker for speech delay associated with otitis media with effusion: The intelligibility-speech gap. *Clinical Linguistics & Phonetics*, *17*, 507–528.

Shriberg, L. D., Flipsen, P., Jr., Thielke, H., et al. (2000). Risk for speech disorder associated with early recurrent otitis media with effusion: Two retrospective studies. *Journal of Speech, Language, and Hearing Research*, *43*, 79–99.

Shriberg, L. D., Green, J. R., Campbell, T. F., McSweeny, J. L., & Scheer, A. (2003). A diagnostic marker for childhood apraxia of speech: The coefficient of variation ratio. *Clinical Linguistics & Phonetics*, *17*, 575–595.

Shriberg, L. D., & Kent, R. D. (2003). *Clinical Phonetics* (3rd Edition). Boston, MA: Allyn & Bacon.

Shriberg, L. D., Kent, R. D., Karlsson, H. B., McSweeny, J. L., Nadler, C. J., & Brown, R. L. (2003). A diagnostic marker for speech delay associated with otitis media with effusion: Backing of obstruents. *Clinical Linguistics & Phonetics*, *17*(7), 529–547.

Shriberg, L. D., & Kwiatkowski, J. (1980). *Natural Process Analysis*. New York: Academic Press.

Shriberg, L. D., & Kwiatkowski, J. (1982a). Phonological disorders I: A diagnostic classification system. *Journal of Speech and Hearing Disorders*, *47*, 226–241.

Shriberg, L. D., & Kwiatkowski, J. (1982b). Phonological disorders II: A conceptual framework for management. *Journal of Speech and Hearing Disorders*, *47*, 242–256.

Shriberg, L. D., & Kwiatkowski, J. (1982c). Phonological disorders III: A procedure for assessing severity of involvement. *Journal of Speech and Hearing Disorders*, *47*, 256–270.

Shriberg, L. D., & Kwiatkowski, J. (1987). A retrospective study of spontaneous generalization in speech-delayed children. *Language, Speech, and Hearing Services in Schools*, *18*, 144–157.

Shriberg, L. D., & Kwiatkowski, J. (1988). A follow-up study of children with phonologic disorders of unknown origin. *Journal of Speech and Hearing Disorders*, *53*, 144–155.

Shriberg, L. D., & Kwaitkowski, J. (1990). Self-monitoring and generalization in preschool speech-delayed children. *Language, Speech, and Hearing Services in Schools*, *21*, 157–170.

Shriberg, L. D., & Kwiatkowski, J. (1994). Developmental phonological disorders I: A clinical profile. *Journal of Speech and Hearing Research*, *37*, 1100–1126.

Shriberg, L. D., Kwiatkowski, J., Best, S., Hengst, J., & Terselic-Weber, B. (1986). Characteristics of children with phonologic disorders of unknown origin. *Journal of Speech and Hearing Disorders*, *51*, 140–161.

Shriberg, L. D., Kwiatkowski, J., & Gruber, F. A. (1994). Developmental phonological disorders II: Short-term speech sound normalization. *Journal of Speech and Hearing Research*, *37*, 1127–1147.

Shriberg, L. D., Kwiatkowski, J., & Snyder, T. (1986). Articulation testing by microcomputer. *Journal of Speech and Hearing Disorders*, *51*, 309–324.

Shriberg, L. D., Kwiatkowski, J., & Snyder, T. (1989). Tabletop versus microcomputer-assisted speech management: Stabilization phase. *Journal of Speech and Hearing Disorders*, *54*, 233–248.

Shriberg, L. D., Kwiatkowski, J., & Snyder, T. (1990). Tabletop versus microcomputer-assisted speech management: Response evocation phase. *Journal of Speech and Hearing Disorders*, *55*, 635–655.

Shriberg, L. D., Lewis, B. A., Tomblin, J. B., McSweeny, J. L., Karlsson, H. B., & Scheer, A. R. (2005). Toward diagnostic and phenotype markers for genetically transmitted speech delay. *Journal of Speech, Language, and Hearing Research*, *48*, 834–852.

Shriberg, L. D., & Smith, A. J. (1983). Phonological correlates of middle-ear involvement in speech-delayed children: A methodological note. *Journal of Speech and Hearing Research*, *26*, 293–297.

Shriberg, L. D., Tomblin, J. B., & McSweeny, J. L. (1999). Prevalence of speech delay in 6-year-old children and comorbidity with language impairment. *Journal of Speech and Hearing Research*, *42*, 1461–1481.

Shuster, L. I., Ruscello, D. M., & Smith, K. D. (1992). Evoking [r] using visual feedback. *American Journal of Speech-Language Pathology*, *1*, 29–34.

Simpson, S. A., Thomas, C. L., van der Linden, M. K., Macmillan, H., van der Wouden, J. C., & Butler, C. (2007). Identification of children in the first four years of life for early treatment for otitis media with effusion [update of *Cochrane Database Syst Rev* 2003;(2):CD004163; PMID: 12804500]. *Cochrane Database of Systematic Reviews*, *1*, CD004163.

Skinder, A. (2000). *The Relationship of Prosodic and Articulatory Errors Produced by Children with Developmental Apraxia*. Unpublished Doctoral Dissertation, University of Washington, Seattle.

Skinder-Meredith, A. (2000, May). A Descriptive Analysis of Speech Characteristics in Children with Developmental Apraxia of Speech. Child Phonology Conference, Wichita, KS.

Skinder-Meredith, A., Carkowski, S., & Graff, N. (2004). Comparison of nasalance measures in children with childhood apraxia of speech and repaired cleft palate, to their typically developing peers. Retrieved March 21, 2008 from http://www.speechpathology.com/articles/index.asp.

Skinder-Meredith, A., Lommers, K., & Yoder, J. (2007). Trends in the case histories of 15 children with Childhood Apraxia of Speech. Poster presented at the *American Speech-Language-Hearing Association Convention*, Boston, MA.

Smit, A. B. (2004a). Speech sampling, articulation tests, and intelligibility in children with phonological errors. In R. D. Kent (Ed). *The MIT Encyclopedia of Communication Disorders*. Cambridge, MA: The MIT Press, pp. 213–215.

Smit, A. B. (2004b). Speech sampling, articulation tests, and intelligibility in children with residual errors. In R. D. Kent (Ed). *The MIT Encyclopedia of Communication Disorders*. Cambridge, MA: The MIT Press, pp. 215–218.

Smit, A. B., & Bernthal, J. E. (1983). Voicing contrasts and their phonological implications in the speech of articulation-disordered children. *Journal of Speech and Hearing Research*, *26*, 486–500.

Smit, A. B., Hand, L., Freilinger, J. J., Bernthal, J. E., & Bird, A. (1990). The Iowa Articulation Norms Project and its Nebraska replication. *Journal of Speech and Hearing Disorders*, *55*, 779–798.

Smith, B. L., & Stoel-Gammon, C. (1983). A longitudinal study of the development of stop consonant production in normal and Down' s syndrome children. *Journal of Speech and Hearing Disorders*, *48*, 114–118.

Smith, E. C., & Lewicki, M. S. (2006). Efficient auditory coding. *Nature*, *439*, 978–982.

Smith, N. V. (1973). *The Acquisition of Phonology: A Case Study*. Cambridge: Cambridge University Press.

Smith, N. V. (1978). Lexical representation and the acquisition of phonology. Paper given as a forum lecture, Linguistic Institute, *Linguistic Society of America*.

Smith, R. J. H., Bale, J. F., & White, K. R. (2005). Sensorineural hearing loss in children. *The Lancet*, *365*(9462), 879–890.

Snowling, M., Bishop, D. V. M., & Stothard, S. E. (2000). Is pre-school language impairment a risk factor for dyslexia in adolescence? *Journal of Child Psychology & Psychiatry*, *41*(5), 587–600.

Snowling, M., Goulandris, N., & Stackhouse, J. (1994). Phonological constraints on learning to read: Evidence from single case studies of reading difficulty. In C. Hulme and M. Snowling (Eds). *Reading Development and Dyslexia*. London: Whurr, pp. 86–104.

So, L. K. H., & Dodd, B. (1994). Phonologically disordered Cantonese speaking children. *Clinical Linguistics & Phonetics*, 8, 235–255.

Solomon, N., & Munson, B. (2004). The effect of jaw position on measures of tongue strength and endurance. *Journal of Speech, Language, and Hearing Research*, 47, 584–594.

Sommers, R. K. (1992). A review and critical analysis of treatment research related to articulation and phonological disorders. *Journal of Communication Disorders*, 25, 3–22.

Sommers, R. K., Leiss, R. H., Delp, M., et al. (1967). Factors related to the effectiveness of articulation therapy for kindergarten, first and second grade children. *Journal of Speech and Hearing Research*, 13, 428–437.

Stackhouse, J. (1985). Segmentation, speech and spelling difficulties. In M. Snowling (Ed). *Children's Written Language Difficulties*. Windsor, Berkshire: The NFER-Nelson Publishing Company, pp. 96–115.

Stackhouse, J. (1992). Developmental verbal dyspraxia I: A review and critique. *European Journal of Disorders of Communication*, 27, 19–34.

Stackhouse, J. (1996). Speech, reading and spelling: Who is at risk, and why? In M. Snowling and J. Stackhouse (Eds). *Dyslexia, Speech and Language: A Practitioner's Handbook*. London: Whurr Publishers, pp. 12–30.

Stackhouse, J. (1997). Phonological awareness: Connecting speech and literacy problems. In B. W. Hodson and M. L. Edwards (Eds). *Perspectives in Applied Phonology*. Gaithersburg, MD: Aspen, pp. 157–196.

Stackhouse, J., Pascoe, M., & Gardner, H. (2006). Intervention for a child with persisting speech and literacy difficulties: A psycholinguistic approach. *Advances in Speech-Language Pathology*, 8(3), 231–244.

Stackhouse, J., Vance, M., Pascoe, M., & Wells, B. (2007). *Children's Speech and Literacy Difficulties IV: Compendium of Auditory and Speech Tasks*. Chichester: John Wiley and Sons.

Stackhouse, J., & Wells, B. (1997). *Children's Speech and Literacy Difficulties I: A Psycholinguistic Framework*. London: Whurr Publishers.

Stackhouse, J., & Wells, B. (2001). *Children's Speech and Literacy Difficulties II: Identification and Intervention*. London: Whurr Publishers.

Stackhouse, J., Wells, B., Pascoe, M., & Rees, R. (2002). From phonological therapy to phonological awareness. *Seminars in Speech and Language*, 23(1), 27–42.

Stampe, D. (1969). The acquisition of phonetic representation. *Papers from the 5th Regional Meeting of the Chicago Linguistic Society*, 443–454.

Stampe, D. (1973). *A dissertation on natural phonology*. Unpublished doctoral dissertation, University of Chicago.

Stampe, D. (1979). *A Dissertation on Natural Phonology*. New York: Academic Press.

Starr, C. D. (1990). Treatment by therapeutic exercises. In J. Bardach and H. L. Morris (Eds). *Multidisciplinary Management of Cleft Lip and Palate*. Philadelphia, PA: W.B. Saunders Company, pp. 792–798.

Stemberger, J. P., & Bernhardt, B. H. (1997). Optimality Theory. In M. Ball and R. Kent (Eds.) *The New Phonologies*. San Diego, CA: Singular Publishing Group, pp. 211–245.

Stephens, H., & Elton, M. (1986). Description of Systematic Use of Articulograms. *College of Speech and Language Therapists Bulletin*: December.

Steriade, D. (1990). *Greek prosodies and the nature of syllabification* (Doctoral dissertation, Massachusetts Instituted of Technology, 1982). New York: Garland Press.

Sternberg, D. (1981). *How to Complete and Survive a Doctoral Dissertation*. New York, NY: St. Martin's Press.

Stinchfield, S., & Young, E. H. (1938). *Children with Delayed or Defective Speech: Motor-Kinesthetic Factors in their Training.* Stanford, CA: Stanford University Press.

Stinchfield-Hawk, S. (1950). *Speech Therapy for the Physically Handicapped.* Stanford, CA: Stanford University Press.

Stoel-Gammon, C. (1988). *Evaluation of Phonological Skills in Pre-School Children.* New York: Thieme Medical Publishers.

Stoel-Gammon, C. (1990). Issues in phonological development and disorders. In J. Miller (Ed). *Progress in Research on Child Language Disorders.* Austin, TX: Pro-Ed.

Stoel-Gammon, C. (2007). Variability in speech acquisition. In S. McLeod (Ed). *International Guide to Speech Acquisition.* Clifton Park, NY: Thomson Delmar Learning, pp. 55–60.

Stoel-Gammon, C., & Cooper, J. A. (1984). Patterns of early lexical and phonological development. *Journal of Child Language, 11,* 247–271.

Stoel-Gammon, C., & Dunn, C. (1985). *Normal and Disordered Phonology in Children.* Baltimore, MD: University Park Press.

Stoel-Gammon, C., & Pollock, K. E. (2008). Vowel development and disorders. In M. Ball, M. Perkins, N. Muller, et al. (Eds). *Handbook of Clinical Linguistics.* Oxford: Blackwell Publishers.

Stoel-Gammon, C., Stone-Goldman, J., & Glaspey, A. (2002). Pattern-based approaches to phonological therapy. *Seminars in Speech and Language, 23,* 3–13.

Stone, J. R. (1992) Resolving relationship problems in communication disorders treatment: A systems approach. *Language, Speech, and Hearing Services in Schools, 23,* 300–307.

Stone, J. R., & Olswang (1989). The hidden challenge in counseling. *ASHA, 27*–31.

Stone, J. R., & Stoel-Gammon, C. (1995). Phonological disorders and development in children. In F. Minifie (Ed). *Introduction to Communication Sciences and Disorders.* Singular Press.

Storkel, H. L., Armbruster, J., & Hogan, T. P. (2006). Differentiating phonotactic probability and neighborhood density in adult word learning. *Journal of Speech, Language, and Hearing Research, 49,* 1175–1192.

Storkel, H. L., & Morrisette, M. L. (2002). The lexicon and phonology: Interactions in language acquisition. *Language, Speech, and Hearing Services in Schools, 33,* 22–35.

Stothard, S. E., Snowling, M. J., Bishop, D. V. M., Chipchase, B. B., and Kaplan, C. A. (1998). Language impaired preschoolers: A follow-up into adolescence. *Journal of Speech, Language, and Hearing Research, 41,* 407–418.

Strand, E. A., & Debertine, P. (2000). The efficacy of integral stimulation with developmental apraxia of speech. *Journal of Medical Speech-Language Pathology, 8*(4), 295–300.

Strand, E., & Johnson, K. (1996). Gradient and visual speaker normalization in the perception of fricatives. In D. Gibbon (Ed). *Natural Language Processing and Speech Technology: Results of the 3rd KONVENS Conference, Bielfelt, October 1996.* Berlin: Mouton de Gruyter, pp. 14–26.

Strand, E., & McCauley, R. J. (1999). Assessment procedures for treatment planning in children with phonologic and motor speech disorders. In A. Caruso and E. Strand (Eds). *Clinical Management of Motor Speech Disorders in Children.* New York, NY: Thieme-Stratton, pp. 73–107.

Strand, E., McCauley, R., & Stoeckel, R. (2006). Dynamic assessment of acquired and developmental apraxia of speech in children. Presented to the 2006 *Conference on Motor Speech*: San Antonio, TX, March 23–26, 2006.

Strand, E., & Skinder, A. (1999). Treatment of developmental apraxia of speech: Integral Stimulation Methods. In A. Caruso and E. Strand (Eds). *Clinical Management of Motor Speech Disorders in Children.* New York, NY: Thieme-Stratton, pp. 109–148.

Strand, E., Stoeckel., R., & Baas, B. (2006). Treatment of severe childhood apraxia of speech: A treatment efficacy study. *Journal of Medical Speech Pathology, 14,* 297–307.

Strode, R., & Chamberlain, C. (1997). *Easy does it*™ *for Articulation: An Oral-Motor Approach*. E. Moline, IL: LinguiSystems.

Stromswold, K. (1998). Genetics of spoken language disorders. *Human Biology*, 70, 297–324.

Sudbery, A., Wilson, E, Broaddus, T., & Potter, N. (2006, November). Tongue strength in preschool children: Measures, implications, and revelations. Poster to the *American Speech-Language-Hearing Association Convention*, Miami Beach, FL.

Sutherland, D., & Gillon, G. T. (2005). Assessment of phonological representations in children with speech impairment. *Language, Speech, and Hearing Services in Schools*, 36, 294–307.

Sutherland, D., & Gillon, G. T. (2007). The development of phonological representations and phonological awareness in children with speech impairment. *International Journal of Language & Communication Disorders*, 14(2), 229–250.

Sweet, H. M. A. (1908). *The Sounds of English: An Introduction to Phonetics*. Oxford: Clarendon Press.

Swift, W. B. (1918). *Speech Defects in School Children and How to Treat Them*. Boston, MA: Houghton Mifflin.

Taylor-Goh, S. (Ed). (2005). *Royal College of Speech and Language Therapists: Clinical Guidelines*. Brackley: Speechmark.

Templin, M. C. (1957). Certain language skills in children. *Monograph Series No. 26*. Minneapolis, MN: The Institute of Child Welfare, University of Minnesota.

Tharpe, A. M. (1998). Treatment fads versus evidence-based practice. In F. H. Bess (Ed). *Children with Hearing Impairment: Contemporary Trends*. Nashville, TN: Vanderbilt Bill Wilkerson Press, pp. 179–188.

Thelwall, J. (1812). *Selections for the Illustration of a Course of Instructions on the Rhythms and Utterances of the English Language: with an introductory essay on the application of rhythmical science to the treatment of impediments and the improvement of our national oratory; and an elementary analysis of the science and practice of elocution.*

Thinking Publications (2004). Barbara Hodson: Phonological intervention guru. *Thinking Big News*, Issue 22, December.

Thomas, E. (2007). Phonological and phonetic characteristics of African-American English. *Language and Linguistics Compass*, 1, 450–475.

Thomlison, B. (2002). *Family Assessment Handbook. An introductory Practice Guide to Family Assessment and Intervention*. Canada: Brooks/Cole.

Thompson, C. K. (2007). Complexity in language learning and treatment. *American Journal of Speech-Language Pathology*, 16(1), 3–5.

Thompson, C. K., & Shapiro, L. P. (2007). Complexity in treatment of syntactic deficits. *American Journal of Speech-Language Pathology*, 16(1), 30–42.

Thompson, K. (1998). Early intervention services in daily family life: mothers' perceptions of 'ideal' versus 'actual' service provision. *Occupational Therapy International*, 5(3), 206–221.

Tomes, L. A., Kuehn, D. P., & Peterson-Falzone, S. J. (2004). Research considerations for behavioral treatments of velopharyngeal impairment. In K. Bzoch (Ed). *Communicative Disorders Related to Cleft Lip and Palate* (5th Edition). Austin, TX: Pro-Ed, pp. 797–846.

Torgesen, J. K., & Bryant, B. (1994). *Test of Phonological Awareness*. Austin, TX: Pro-Ed.

Travis, L. E. (1931). *Speech Pathology: A Dynamic Neurological Treatment of Normal Speech and Speech Deviations*. New York: D. Appleton Co.

Trost-Cardamone, J. E., & Bernthal, J. E. (1993). Articulation assessment procedures and treatment decisions. In K. T. Moller and C. D. Starr (Eds). *Cleft Palate: Interdisciplinary Issues and Treatment*. Austin, TX: Pro-Ed, pp. 307–336.

Trudgill, P. (2004). *New-Dialect Formation: The Inevitability of Colonial Englishes*. Edinburgh: Edinburgh University Press.

Tunmer, W., Chapman, J., & Prochnow, J. (2006). Literate cultural capital at school entry predicts later reading achievement: A seven year longitudinal study. *New Zealand Journal of Educational Studies*

Turnbull, A. P., Turbiville, V., & Turnbull, H. R. (2000). Evolution of family-professional partnerships. Collective empowerment as the model for the early twenty first century. In J. P. Shonkoff and S. J. Meisels (Eds). *Handbook of Early Childhood Intervention* (2nd Edition). Cambridge: Cambridge University Press, pp. 638–646.

Twitmeyer, E. B., & Nathanson, Y. S. (1932). *Correction of Defective Speech*. Philadelphia, PA: P. Blakiston's Son and Co.

Tyler, A. A. (2002). Language-based intervention for phonological disorders. *Seminars in Speech and Language*, 23, 69–82.

Tyler, A. A. (2005). Planning and monitoring intervention programs. In A. G. Kamhi and K. E. Pollock (Eds). *Phonological Disorders in Children: Clinical Decision Making in Assessment and Intervention*. Baltimore, MD: Paul H. Brookes, pp. 123–137.

Tyler, A. A., Edwards, M. L., & Saxman, J. H. (1987). Clinical application of two phonologically based treatment procedures. *Journal of Speech and Hearing Disorders*, 52, 393–409.

Tyler, A. A., Edwards, M. L., & Saxman, J. H. (1990). Acoustic validation of phonological knowledge and its relationship to treatment. *Journal of Speech and Hearing Disorders*, 55, 251–261.

Tyler, A. A., & Figurski, G. R. (1994). Phonetic inventory changes after treating distinctions along an implicational hierarchy. *Clinical Linguistics & Phonetics*, 8, 91–107.

Tyler, A. A., Figurski, G. R., & Langsdale, T. C. (1993). Relationships between acoustically determined productive knowledge and phonological treatment progress. *Journal of Speech and Hearing Research*, 36, 746–759.

Tyler, A. A., & Lewis, K. E. (2005). Relationships among consistency/variability and other phonological measures over time. *Topics in Language Disorder: Clinical Perspectives on Speech Sound Disorders*, 25(3), 243–253.

Tyler, A. A., Lewis, K. E., Haskill, A., & Tolbert, L. C. (2002). Efficacy and cross-domain effects of a morphosyntax and phonology intervention. *Language, Speech, and Hearing Services in Schools*, 33, 52–66.

Tyler, A. A., Lewis, K. E., & Welch, C. M. (2003). Predictors of phonological change following intervention. *American Journal of Speech-Language Pathology*, 12(3), 289–298.

Tyler, A. A., & Tolbert, L. C. (2002). Speech-language assessment in the clinical setting. *American Journal of Speech-Language Pathology*, 11, 215–220.

Tyler, A., & Watterson, K. (1991). Effects of phonological versus language intervention in preschoolers with both phonological and language impairment. *Child Language Teaching and Therapy*, 7, 141–160.

UK National Screening Committee (n.d.). *What is screening?* Retrieved December 11, 2007 from: http://www.nsc.nhs.uk/whatscreening/whatscreen_ind.htm.

UN Millennium Project (2005). *Investing in Development: A Practical Plan to Achieve the Millennium Development Goals*. Washington: Communication Developments, Inc. (Also available from http://www.unmillenniumproject.org/reports/fullreport.htm.)

Uffen, E. (2006). Alex Johnson, ASHA President. *The ASHA Leader*, 11(1), 6–7.

Ullrich, A. (2007). *Nichtlineare phonologische Diagnostik, NILPOD*. Unpublished manuscript. [Nonlinear phonological assessment].

Ullrich, A., & Bernhardt, B. (2005). Neue Perspektiven der phonologischen Analyse - Implikationen für die Untersuchung phonologischer Entwicklungsstörungen. *Die Sprachheilarbeit*, 5, 221–233. [New perspectives in phonological analysis – Implications for the investigation of developmental phonological impairments.]

Vallino-Napoli, L. D., and Reilly, S. (2004). Evidence-based health care: A survey of speech pathology practice. *Advances in Speech-Language Pathology*, 6(2), 107–112.

Van Borsel, J., Van Rentergem, S., & Verhaeghe, L. (2007). The prevalence of lisping in young adults. *Journal of Communication Disorders, 40*(6), 493–502.

Van Demark, D. R., & Hardin, M. A. (1990). Speech therapy for the child with cleft lip and palate. In J. Bardach and H. L. Morris (Eds). *Multidisciplinary Management of Cleft Lip and Palate*. Philadelphia, PA: W.B. Saunders Company, pp. 799–806.

Van Riper, C. (1939). *Speech Correction: Principles and Methods*. Englewood Cliffs, NJ: Prentice-Hall.

Van Riper, C. (1963). *Speech Correction: Principles and Methods*. Englewood Cliffs, NJ: Prentice-Hall.

Van Riper, C. (1978). *Speech Correction: Principles and Methods* (6th Edition). Englewood Cliffs, NJ: Prentice-Hall.

Van Riper, R., & Emerick, L. (1984). *Speech Correction: An Introduction to Speech Pathology and Audiology*. Englewood Cliffs, NJ: Prentice-Hall.

Van Riper, C., & Irwin, J. V. (1958). *Voice and Articulation*. Englewood Cliffs, NJ: Prentice Hall.

Van Weel, C., & Knottnerus, J. A. (1999). Evidence-based interventions and comprehensive treatment. *Lancet, 353,* 916–918.

Vargha-Khadem, F., Watkins, K., Alcock, K.,. Fletcher, P., & Passingham, R. (1995). Praxic and nonverbal cognitive deficits in a large family with a genetically transmitted speech and language disorder. *Proceedings of the National Academy of Science USA, 92,* 930–933.

Velleman, S. L. (1998). *Making Phonology Functional: What Do I Do first?* Boston, MA: Butterworth-Heinemann.

Velleman, S. (2002). Phonotactic therapy. *Seminars in Speech and Language, 23,* 43–57.

Velleman, S. L. (2003). *Resource Guide for Childhood Apraxia of Speech*. Clifton Park, NY: Thomson Delmar Learning.

Velleman, S. (2005). Perspectives on assessment. In A. Kamhi and K. Pollock (Eds). *Phonological Disorders in Children*. Baltimore, MD: Brookes, pp. 23–34.

Velleman, S. L., & Shriberg, L. D. (1999). Metrical analysis of the speech of children with suspected developmental apraxia of speech. *Journal of Speech, Language, and Hearing Research, 42,* 1444–1460.

Velleman, S. L., & Strand, K. (1994). Developmental verbal dyspraxia. In J. E. Bernthal and N. W. Bankson (Eds). *Child Phonology: Characteristics, Assessment, and Intervention with Special Populations*. New York, NY: Thieme Medical Publishing, pp. 110–139.

Velleman, S. L., & Vihman, M. M. (2002). Whole-word phonology and templates: Trap, bootstrap, or some of each? *Language, Speech, and Hearing Services in Schools, 33,* 9–23.

Velten, H. (1943). The growth of phonemic and lexical patterns in infant language. *Language, 19,* 281–292.

Von Bremen, V. (1990). *A nonlinear phonological approach to intervention with severely phonologically disordered twins*. Unpublished Master's thesis, University of British Columbia.

Vygotsky, L. S. (1978). Mind in society. In M. Cole, V. John-Steiner, S. Scribner, et al. (Eds). *The Development of Higher Psychological Processes*. London: Harvard University Press.

Walton, J. H., & Pollock, K. E. (1993). Acoustic validation of vowel error patterns in developmental apraxia of speech. *Clinical Linguistics & Phonetics, 7,* 95–111.

Warren, S., Fey, M., & Yoder, P. (2007). Differential treatment intensity research: A missing link to creating optimally effective communication interventions. *Mental Retardation and Developmental Disabilities Research Reviews, 13*(1), 70–77.

Warrick, N., Rubin, H., & Rowe-Walsh, S. (1993). Phoneme awareness in language-delayed children: comparative studies and intervention. *Annals of Dyslexia, 43,* 153–173.

Waterson, N. (1971). Child phonology: A prosodic view. *Journal of Linguistics, 7,* 170–221.

Waterson, N. (1981). A tentative development model of phonological representation. In T. Myers, J. Laver, and J. Anderson (Eds). *The Cognitive Representation of Speech*. Amsterdam: North Holland.

Watts, N. (2004). Assessment of vowels summary. *ACQuiring Knowledge in Speech, Language and Hearing*, Speech Pathology Australia, 6(1), 22–25.

Watts Pappas, N., & Bowen, C. (2007). Speech Acquisition and the Family. In S. McLeod (Ed). *The International Guide to Speech Acquisition*. Clifton Park, NY: Thomson Delmar Learning.

Watts Pappas, N., & McLeod, S. (2008). Working with families of children with speech impairments. In N. Watts Pappas and S. McLeod (Eds). *Working with Families in Speech-Language Pathology*. San Diego, CA: Plural Publishing.

Watts Pappas, N., McLeod, S., McAllister, L., & Daniel, G. (2006). Parental involvement in phonological intervention. Paper presented to *International Clinical Linguistics & Phonetics Association Conference*, Dubrovnik, Croatia.

Watts Pappas, N., McLeod, S., McAllister, L., & McKinnon, D. H. (2008). Parental involvement in speech intervention: A national survey. *Clinical Linguistics and Phonetics*, 22(4), 335–344.

Watts Pappas, N., McLeod, S., McAllister, L., & Simpson, T. (2005). Partnerships with parents in speech intervention: A review. *Speech Pathology Australia National Conference*. Melbourne: Speech Pathology Australia.

Weatherby, A., & Prizant, B. (2002). *Communication and Symbolic Behavior Scales – Developmental Profile*. Baltimore, MD: Brookes.

Weiner, F. (1979). *Phonological Process Analysis*. Baltimore, MD: University Park Press.

Weiner, F. (1981a). Treatment of phonological disability using the method of meaningful contrast: Two case studies. *Journal of Speech and Hearing Disorders*, 46, 97–103.

Weiner, F. (1981b). Systematic sound preference as a characteristic of phonological disability. *Journal of Speech and Hearing Disorders*, 46, 281–286.

Weismer, G. (1984). Acoustic analysis strategies for the refinement of phonological analysis. In M. Elbert, D. A. Dinnsen, and G. Weismer (Eds). *Phonological Theory and the Misarticulating Child* (ASHA Monographs No. 22). Rockville, MD: ASHA, pp. 30–52.

Weismer, G. (1997). *Assessment of oromotor, nonspeech gestures in speech-language pathology: A critical review* (Videotape recording Telerounds 35). Tucson, AZ: National Center for Neurologic Communication Disorders.

Weismer, G. (2006). Philosophy of research in motor speech disorders. *Clinical Linguistics & Phonetics*, 20, 315–349.

Weismer, G., Dinnsen, D., & Elbert, M. (1981). A study of the voicing distinction associated with omitted, word-final stops. *Journal of Speech and Hearing Disorders*, 46, 320–328.

Weiss, A. L. (2004). The child as agent for change in therapy for phonological disorders. *Child Language Teaching and Therapy*, 20(3), 221–244.

Weiss, C. E., Gordon, M. E., & Lillywhite, H. S. (1987). *Clinical Management of Articulatory and Phonological Disorders, Treatment of Special Populations*. Baltimore, MD: Williams and Wilkins, pp. 259–260.

Wellman, B. L., Case, I. M., Mengert, I. G., & Bradbury, D. E. (1931). Speech sounds of young children. *University of Iowa Studies in Child Welfare*, 5(2). Iowa City: The Iowa Child Welfare Research Station: University of Iowa.

Wells, J. C. (1982a). *Accents of English 1: An Introduction*. Cambridge: Cambridge University Press.

Wells, J. C. (1982b). *Accents of English 2: The British Isles*. Cambridge: Cambridge University Press.

Wells, J. C. (1982c). *Accents of English 3: Beyond the British Isles*. Cambridge: Cambridge University Press.

Wenke, R., Goozee, J., Murdoch, B., & LaPointe, L. (2006). Dynamic assessment of articulation during lingual fatigue in myasthenia gravis. *Journal of Medical Speech-Language Pathology*, 14, 13–32.

Werner, E. E. (2000). Protective factors and individual resilience. In J. P. Shonkoff and S. J. Meisels (Eds). *Handbook of Early Childhood Intervention* (2nd Edition). Cambridge: Cambridge University Press, pp. 115–132.

West, R., Kennedy, L., & Carr, A. (1937). *The Rehabilitation of Speech*. New York: Harper and Bros.

Weston, A., & Irvin, J. (1971). Use of paired stimuli in modification of articulation. *Perceptual Motor Skills*, *32*, 947–957.

Williams, A. L. (1991). Generalization patterns associated with training least phonological knowledge. *Journal of Speech and Hearing Research*, *34*, 722–733.

Williams, A. L. (2000a). Multiple oppositions: Theoretical foundations for an alternative contrastive intervention approach. *American Journal of Speech-Language Pathology*, *9*, 282–288.

Williams, A. L. (2000b). Multiple oppositions: Case studies of variables in phonological intervention. *American Journal of Speech-Language Pathology*, *9*, 289–299.

Williams, A. L. (2001). Phonological assessment of child speech. In D. M. Ruscello (Ed). *Tests and Measurements in Speech-Language Pathology*. Woburn, MA: Butterworth-Heinemann, pp. 31–76.

Williams, A. L. (2002a). Prologue: Perspectives in the phonological assessment of child speech. *American Journal of Speech-Language Pathology*, *11*, 211–212.

Williams, A. L. (2002b). Epilogue: Perspectives in the phonological assessment of child speech. *American Journal of Speech-Language Pathology*, *11*, 259–263.

Williams, A. L. (2003a). Target selection and treatment outcomes. *Perspectives on Language Learning and Education*, *10*(1), 12–16.

Williams, A. L. (2003b). *Speech Disorders: Resource Guide for Preschool Children*. Clifton Park, NY: Thomson Delmar Learning.

Williams, A. L. (2005). From developmental norms to distance metrics: Past, present, and future directions for target selection practices. In A. G. Kamhi and K. E. Pollock (Eds). *Phonological Disorders in Children: Clinical Decision Making in Assessment and Intervention*. Baltimore, MD: Paul. H. Brookes Publishing, pp. 101–108.

Williams, A. L. (2006a). *Sound Contrasts in Phonology (SCIP)*. Eau Claire, WI: Thinking Publications.

Williams, A. L. (2006b). A systemic perspective for assessment and intervention: A case study. *Advances in Speech-Language Pathology*, *8*(3), 245–256.

Williams, G. C., & McReynolds, L. V. (1975). The relationship between discrimination and articulation training in children with misarticulations. *Journal of Speech and Hearing Research*, *18*, 401–412.

Williams, K. T. (1997). *Expressive Vocabulary Test*. Circle Pines, MN: American Guidance Service, Inc.

Williams, P., & Corrin, J. (2004), Developmental verbal dyspraxia: A review of the literature. In P. Williams and H. Stephens (Eds). *Nuffield Centre Dyspraxia Programme*. Windsor, UK: The Miracle Factory.

Williams, P., & Stackhouse, J. (1998). Diadochokinetic skills: Normal and atypical performance in children aged 3–5 Years. *International Journal of Language & Communication Disorders*, *33* (Supp), 481–486.

Williams, P., & Stephens, H. (Eds). (2004). *Nuffield Centre Dyspraxia Programme*. Windsor, UK: The Miracle Factory.

Williams, P., Stephens, H., & Connery, V. (2006). What's the evidence for oral motor therapy? A response to Bowen 2005. *ACQuiring Knowledge in Speech, Language and Hearing*, Speech Pathology Australia, June, *8*(2), 89–90.

Williams, R., Ingham, R., & Rosenthal, J. (1981). A further analysis for developmental apraxia of speech in children with defective articulation. *Journal of Speech and Hearing Research*, *24*, 496–505.

Williams, R., Packman, A., Ingham, R., & Rosenthal, J. (1980). Clinical agreement on behaviours that identify developmental articulatory dyspraxia. *Australian Journal of Human Communication Disorders, 8*, 16–26.

Wilson, L., Lincoln, M., & Onslow, M. (2002). Availability, access, and quality of care: Inequities in rural speech pathology services for children and a model for redress. *Advances in Speech-Language Pathology, 4*(1), 9–22.

Windsor, J., Glaze, L., Koga, S., & the Bucharest Early Intervention Project Core Group. (2007). Language acquisition with limited input: Romanian institution and foster care. *Journal of Speech, Language, and Hearing Research, 50*, 1365–1381.

Winitz, H. (1969). *Articulatory Acquisition and Behavior*. New York: Appleton-Century-Crofts.

Winitz, H. (1975). *From Syllable to Conversation*. Baltimore, MD: University Park.

Winitz, H. (1984). *Treating Articulation Disorders: For Clinicians by Clinicians*. Baltimore, MD: University Park.

Winner, M., & Elbert, M. (1988). Evaluating the treatment effect of repeated probes. *Journal of Speech and Hearing Disorders, 53*, 211–218.

Wolk, L., Edwards, M. L., & Conture, E. G. (1993). Coexistence of stuttering and disordered phonology in young children. *Journal of Speech and Hearing Research, 36*, 906–917.

Wolk, L., & Meisler, A. W. (1998). Phonological assessment: a systematic comparison of conversation and picture naming. *Journal of Communication Disorders, 31*, 291–313.

Wood, K. S. (1971). Terminology and nomenclature. In L. E. Travis (Ed). *Handbook of Speech Pathology and Audiology*. Englewood Cliffs, NJ: Prentice-Hall.

World Health Organization. (1980). *ICIDH: International Classification of Impairment, Disabilities and Handicaps*. Geneva: World Health Organization.

World Health Organization. (2001). *ICF: International Classification of Functioning, Disability and Health*. Geneva: World Health Organization.

World Health Organization. (2005). *Bridging the 'know-do' gap meeting on knowledge translation in global health*. Retrieved on August 28, 2007 from: http://www.who.int/kms/WHO_EIP_KMS_2006_2.pdf.

World Health Organization (WHO Workgroup for development of version of ICF for Children & Youth). (2007). *International Classification of Functioning, Disability and Health - Version for Children and Youth: ICF-CY*. Geneva: World Health Organization.

Wren, Y., & Roulstone, S. (2006). *Phoneme Factory Sound Sorter*. Manchester: Granada Learning.

Wren, Y., Hughes, T., & Roulstone, S. (2006). *Phoneme Factory Phonology Screener*. London: NFER Nelson Publishing Company.

Wyllie-Smith, L., McLeod, S., & Ball, M. J. (2006). Typically developing and speech-impaired children's adherence to the sonority hypothesis. *Clinical Linguistics & Phonetics, 20*(4), 271–291.

Yaruss, J. S., & Logan, K. (2002). Evaluating rate, accuracy, and fluency of young children's diadochokinetic productions: A preliminary investigation. *Journal of Fluency Disorders, 27*, 65–86.

Yavas, M. (2006). Sonority and the acquisition of #sC clusters. *Journal of Multilingual Communication Disorders, 4*(3), 159–168.

Yavas, M. (2007). Multilingual speech acquisition. In S. McLeod (Ed). *The International Guide to Speech Acquisition*. Clifton Park, NY: Thomson Delmar Learning, 2007, pp. 96–110.

Yavas, M., & Core, C. W. (2006). Acquisition of #sC clusters in English speaking children. *Journal of Multilingual Communication Disorders, 4*(3), 169–181.

Yoshinaga-Itano, C., Johnson, C. D., Carpenter, K., & Brown, A. S. (2008). Outcomes of children with mild bilateral hearing loss and unilateral hearing loss. *Seminars in Hearing, 29*(2), 196–211.

Yoss, K., & Darley, F. (1974). Developmental apraxia of speech in children with defective articulation. *Journal of Speech and Hearing Research, 17,* 399–416.

Young, E. C. (1991). An analysis of young children's ability to produce multisyllabic words. *Clinical Linguistics & Phonetics, 5,* 297–316.

Young, E. C. (1995). An analysis of a treatment approach for phonological errors in polysyllabic words. *Clinical Linguistics and Phonetics, 9,* 59–77.

Zimmerman, I. L., Steiner, V. G., Pond, R. E. (1991). *Preschool Language Scale-3.* San Antonio, TX: The Psychological Corporation.

Index

Note: Italicized page numbers to boxes, figures and tables